Executive Editor and Publisher: Stephen D. Dragin
Editorial Assistant: Anne Whittaker
Marketing Manager: Jared Brueckner
Production Editor: Gregory Erb
Editorial Production Service: Omegatype Typography, Inc.
Composition Buyer: Linda Cox
Manufacturing Buyer: Megan Cochran
Electronic Composition: Omegatype Typography, Inc.
Cover Designer: Linda Knowles

For related titles and support materials, visit our online catalog at www.pearsonhighered.com

Library of Congress Cataloging-in-Publication Data

Haynes, William O.
   Understanding research and evidence-based practice in communication disorders: a primer for students and practitioners / William O. Haynes, Carole E. Johnson.
        p.   ;   cm.
   Includes bibliographical references and index.
   ISBN-13: 978-0-205-45363-4 (hardcover)
   ISBN-10: 0-205-45363-5 (hardcover)
  1. Communicative disorders—Research—Methodology.   2. Speech therapy—Research—Methodology.   3. Audiology—Research—Methodology.   4. Evidence-based medicine.   I. Johnson, Carole E.   II. Title.
   [DNLM: 1. Communication Disorders.   2. Evidence-Based Medicine.   3. Research Design.   4. Statistics as Topic—methods.   WL 340.2. H424u 2009]
   RC428.H39 2009
   616.85'50072—dc22   2008028649

Printed in the United States of America

10   9   8   7   6   5   4   3   2   1   HAM   12   11   10   09   08

Allyn & Bacon
is an imprint of

www.pearsonhighered.com   ISBN-13:   978-0-205-45363-4
                                 ISBN-10:   0-205-45363-5

Understanding Research and Evidence-Based Practice in Communication Disorders

A Primer for Students and Practitioners

William O. Haynes
Auburn University

Carole E. Johnson
Auburn University

Boston   New York   San Francisco
Mexico City   Montreal   Toronto   London   Madrid   Munich   Paris
Hong Kong   Singapore   Tokyo   Cape Town   Sydney

Dr. William O. Haynes earned his bachelor's and master's degrees in speech-language pathology from Northern Michigan University and his Ph.D. from Bowling Green State University in Ohio. He has written six textbooks in communication disorders, published over forty research articles in peer-reviewed national and international journals, and has presented numerous research papers at professional meetings. Dr. Haynes has been an editorial consultant for many professional journals in communication disorders. He has also directed over thirty master's theses in speech-language pathology. Dr. Haynes has been on the faculty in the department of communication disorders at Auburn University, Alabama, for over thirty years and currently holds the rank of professor emeritus at that institution. His teaching specialties have been child and adolescent language development and disorders and research methodology.

Dr. Carole E. Johnson is a professor in the Department of Communication Disorders at Auburn University and runs its Auditory Rehabilitation Laboratory. She received her bachelor's degrees in psychology and speech and hearing sciences from the University of California, Santa Barbara. She received her Ph.D. from the University of Tennessee at Knoxville in 1989 and her Au.D. from the Pennsylvania College of Optometry, School of Audiology (now Salus University) in 2006. Her area of expertise is auditory rehabilitation. She has published forty-five research articles, made over 100 presentations at professional meetings, and has coauthored two books, *Guidebook for Support Programs in Aural Rehabilitation* and *Handbook of Outcomes Measurement in Audiology*. In the past, her research has been funded by the American Speech-Language-Hearing Foundation and the National Institute of Deafness and Other Communicative Disorders of the National Institutes of Health. In addition, she was recipient of the Larry Mauldin Award for Excellence in Education in 2007.

CONTENTS

SECTION II: The Nature of Scientific Inquiry and Essentials
of Experimental Control   41

2 Scientific Principles and Methods Used by Researchers   41

3 Crafting Scientific and Answerable Questions   73

4 Controlling Threats and Confounding Variables through Experimental Design   99

SECTION III: Design and Analysis of Research on Groups and Single Cases   143

5 Levels of Measurement and Distribution of Scores   143

6 An Introduction to Hypothesis Testing with Inferential Statistics 165

7 Common Statistical Analyses for Finding Differences among Two or More Groups or Conditions on One Independent Variable 189

8 Studies That Analyze Differences in Groups Using Factorial Designs with More Than One Independent Variable—Between, Within, and Mixed   221

9 Studies That Measure Relationships among Variables or Attempt Prediction   243

A knowledge and appreciation of research methods has never been more important at any time in the history of communication sciences and disorders. First, the scientific information base has exploded in our field and in other related disciplines. There are more journals, research articles, scientific papers, and technological advances than ever before. Moreover, most of this new information is available via the Internet with a click of a mouse. Students and practitioners must somehow process all of this information and be able to discriminate good from poor quality research and strong from weak evidence.

Second, our national professional associations have demonstrated a commitment to evidence-based practice in the fields of audiology and speech-language pathology. This means that our practitioners, university professors, clinical supervisors, and students must be able to talk not only about disorders of speech, hearing, and language but also *scientifically supported* methods of assessing and treating these problems. Evidence-based practice implies an understanding of hierarchies of scientific rigor and a firm grasp of valid and reliable scientific methods. This means that a course in research methods and a required textbook should not be a mere addendum to an interesting clinical curriculum but rather one of its *central* features. Hopefully, in this new era of training, the instructors of research courses and their required textbooks will be the springboard from which information in *all* clinical courses is interpreted. The relevance of information presented in disorders courses should be determined to a large extent by critical analysis of basic and applied clinical research.

Third, information is transmitted so quickly and is accessible to millions of people on the Internet. Research, just as many other commodities, has become as ubiquitous as fast food. If you want to know "the truth" about something, just Google it and you are guaranteed to find a plethora of information. Unfortunately, the pseudoscience gets lumped right in with the science, and the uninitiated often have difficulty discriminating the wheat from the chaff. The search engines have not yet reached a point where they interpret information for you or tell you good from poor research. That is why there is still no substitute for a solid knowledge base in research methods and why our students must learn it.

As mentioned above, there are many potent reasons for learning about research methods. However, learning about experimental design and developing a conceptual understanding of statistical methods has never been easy. Roger Brown, the famous authority in child language, used to say that those people who appreciated linguistics must have some "kinky gene" that accounted for such an interest. If our experience as teachers is a valid barometer, it must take an even kinkier gene to learn to love research methods. After years of teaching research methods courses, we are aware that just because of the nature of the material it is easily viewed by students as boring, not clinically relevant, and sometimes threatening. The present text is written for graduate students, first professional degree students, and clinicians. Therefore, it may be their initial foray into research methods, and we believe that it is important to make the trip as interesting and as gentle as possible. Some topics are best eased into. After all, the first impressions students form about research methods could influence their relationship with science for the rest of their careers, not to mention their use of evidence-based practice. We would like it to be a positive experience. For so long students and practitioners have viewed research as the province of university professors and those working in laboratories. Now our professional associations want these same students and practitioners to become critical scientific consumers, use evidence-based practice, embrace the research process, and make important contributions to science. One major step to making professionals in communication disorders appreciate the research process and embrace it is to first make it *accessible, relevant, and understandable.* That is what we have tried to do in this book.

The first course in research methods may play a significant role in stimulating a research interest in beginning students and practitioners. Based on such a course, students may elect to do a master's thesis or other research project and go on as practitioners to continue in research endeavors. So in this text we have tried to strike the same kind of tone that we might use if a student came to us during office hours agonizing over a three-way analysis of variance. The tone of the book is collegial and interactive and immediately seeks to establish relationships with students and instructors. We want to assist instructors in helping students understand and *apply* this material in their classes and clinical work, not just memorize it for tests. We want students to develop confidence in their own research acumen. To that end, we have tried to talk to students about very complex phenomena in relatively simple ways without distorting the basic concepts. We have not hesitated to use humor, copious examples, and straight talk. We have also developed many visual representations (figures) that will hopefully be conceptual maps for students to use in navigating through, understanding, and remembering this material. By the end of the text, we hope that readers have taken ownership of the material by seeing its relevance to daily clinical practice and by hopefully participating in the research process.

We want students not only to understand the information, but to be excited about it. As a result, some who read this work might think it a bit informal compared to other texts on the subject. That is probably true. But it is important to consider that there are many ways to teach difficult material, and such information does not always have to be communicated in a dry and humorless way. However, let there be no mistake. We do not approach either the writing of this text or the research process frivolously. A perusal of the table of contents will reveal that this book covers research methodology in as much or more breadth and depth than most existing textbooks in our field. We wanted the material to meet and exceed expectations of professors who teach courses on research methods in communication disorders. In an introductory text, however, it is a challenge to determine what is *necessary* for students to learn in order to interpret professional literature and what is *overkill.* In walking this fine line, we made some judgments based on many years of being active research-ers and teaching courses in research methodology. When we made decisions, they were based on how often certain experimental designs and statistical methods are encountered in our scientific literature. When discussing information on research methods, we hope that we have provided enough necessary information for students to interpret the literature without overwhelming them with detail more in the realm of statisticians. This is not meant to be a statistics text that shows students how to compute analyses. The tone of the present text is more conceptual than statistical. The emphasis is on how a researcher selects an appropriate statistic based on the ex-perimental design and what critical elements of the statistical analysis are important for consumers of research to interpret in an investigation. When we discuss statistical methods, we make some general statements and do not try to cover *all* the possible nuances or controversies. Again it was a judgment call, but we have always tried to remain faithful to the basic material, even though we could not discuss all the issues associated with a particular procedure.

We have attempted to use clinical examples to illustrate all types of research dis-cussed in this text. More importantly, we have included five chapters on evidence-based practice into which have been folded the traditional types of research conducted in communication disorders. The goal of these chapters is to provide students with basic skills and methodologies to apply evidence-based practice in the clinical setting. For example, the earlier chapters of the book provide the foundation for evaluating re-search, and the later chapters on evidence-based practice provide a context for ap-plication of those skills in the clinical milieu. In other words, students not only will understand the basic nuances of research design, but understand why the results from one study may have more credibility than another based on its level of evidence. Furthermore, students will be provided with the basic skills for evidence-based prac-tice, from asking answerable questions, to searching for relevant studies, to commu-nicating evidence to patients for clinical decision making.

We hope that this text will serve to promote research collaboration between pro-fessionals from a variety of work settings and educational backgrounds and foster research collaboration between professionals from different disciplines (e.g., psy-chology, medicine, education, communication disorders). If clinicians can begin to see themselves as clinician-researchers, then they can reach out to others and join in a research collaboration. If university professors begin to see clinicians working in schools and clinics as potential research collaborators, then they can reach out to practitioners and form partnerships. The possibilities such research collaboration can address are endless. The questions these collaborators pose and answer may well be the salvation of both our profession and the clients with communication disor-ders whom we serve with such dedication. Get ready to touch the future.

> If I were to wish for anything, I should not wish for wealth and power, but for the passionate sense of potential—for the eye which, ever young and ardent, sees the possible. Pleasure disappoints; possibility never.
>
> Soren Kierkegaard, Danish philosopher, 1813–1855

Acknowledgments

We would like to thank several groups of people who contributed to our ability to write this textbook. The first group is our students, who have given us both formal and informal feedback over many years of teaching them about research concepts. These students trusted us when we told them that they could learn about research methods and that if they persevered, they could actually grow to like it. They allowed us to watch the light bulbs go on in their heads as they initially grasped scientific principles, and they let us eavesdrop on their discussion groups as they deftly used those concepts to critically review research. Those students, research sharks all, have been changed forever by learning about science, and we have in turn been changed by each succeeding class. We are proud of the way our students have turned into effective consumers and producers of research.

A second group we would like to acknowledge includes all of the participants who have been involved in our scores of research projects over the years. These people have taught us about the research process from the ground up. We made our empirical mistakes with them, completed satisfying research with them, and learned from both types of experiences. All of those data sets we analyzed over the years were first behaviors performed by real people who decided to help us out when they did not have to participate at all. They might not have cared about our research questions, but they helped anyway. Without all those studies of real children and adults, we could not have become researchers and would be relegated to talking about science as an abstraction.

The third group includes all of our many research collaborators over the years who have helped us to learn and gain critical insights into the research process. These colleagues, students, and practitioners have allowed us the opportunity to work together and share exciting research ideas. We met together in offices, classrooms, hospitals, and schools to plan projects that would eventually be completed and published. We drew experimental designs on bar napkins, chatted on airplanes, met at conventions, and talked long into the night to fuel our collective excitement. We shared the exhilaration that comes with every step of the research process from brainstorming and planning to gathering information, analyzing it, and writing it up for publication. We hope that many of the people who read this book will be lucky enough to have such satisfying relationships with their research colleagues. Finally, we would like to thank our executive editor, Steve Dragin, and the staff at Allyn and Bacon for their support during the creative process. Thanks also to Anne Bothe, University of Georgia; Michael W. Casby, Michigan State University; Miriam A. Henoch, University of North Texas; James Mahshie, Gallaudet University; Carmen McGee, University of Houston; Lois Weiss, University of Hawaii; and Carole Zangari, Nova Southeastern University, who gave us encouragement and feedback on various portions of the project.

W. O. H.
C. E. J.

CHAPTER 1

The Importance of Research in Communication Sciences and Disorders

As an adolescent I aspired to lasting fame, I craved factual certainty, and I thirsted for a meaningful vision of human life—So I became a scientist. This is like becoming an archbishop so you can meet girls.

—M. Cartmill

I drifted into medical science . . . initially I was doing it just to mark time . . . I suddenly discovered what I wanted to do in life.

—Dr. Priscilla Kincaid-Smith, former president of the Royal Australian College of Physicians

As illustrated in the quotations, people often have preconceived notions about phenomena only to find that these ideas do not match their experience. Cartmill thought that the life of a scientist would bring fame, certainty, and meaning to life, only to learn that this belief was unfounded. On the other hand, Kincaid-Smith approached science courses as a way to "mark time" until she found her *real* passion and was pleasantly surprised. Some of the people reading this textbook right now have the notion that research is boring, intimidating, and unrelated to clinical work. We hope to show you that such initial negative beliefs are just as unfounded as the concept of science as a route to fame. Other readers may have a genuine interest in science and approach the course in a positive manner. For you, we are truly grateful. Some of you really do not know how to think about a research course in communication disorders. For this undecided group we will show you that research can be not only challenging, but also rewarding, intriguing, and fun. The truth, as they say, lies somewhere in the middle.

LEARNING OBJECTIVES

This chapter will enable readers to:

- Understand how research supports the credibility of professions and professionals.
- Become familiar with the main types of professional literature in communication sciences and disorders.
- Understand parallels between the research process and clinical work.
- Understand the concept of clinician-researcher.

Preconceived Notions

One of the difficulties for any author is imagining the audience who will read a text, especially for authors writing for very large audiences. People who write works of fiction, for example, try to appeal to a mass audience. One advantage of writing a textbook on research methodology in communication disorders is that the present authors are very familiar with the intended audience, primarily because those in our audience had to choose speech-language pathology or audiology as a major. They are upper-level undergraduates, professional degree students, or graduate students. These facts alone increase the homogeneity of our audience in terms of intelligence, educational level, professional interests and to some degree, socioeconomic level. We have also had many years of experience in teaching courses in research methods, with many opportunities to learn from students their attitudes toward research, their abilities to learn the material, and the things that frustrate them to no end. Let us tell you a little bit about yourselves. First off, most of you are female. An interesting aspect of the field of communication disorders is that males are actually a minority of practitioners. Anyway, we will not dwell on this unpleasant topic lest we depress the largely female part of the audience.

Another general feature of our audience is that, for the most part, you are post-baccalaureate students. Most of you have firsthand experience that graduate school is quite different from undergraduate training. You are already rolling your eyes when the undergraduates (which you yourself were only a couple of semesters ago) whine about having to read a textbook or do a measly project. You, on the other hand, are in "the big time" and have to read research articles, do hours of preparation for clinical practicum, complete major term papers and projects and perform at a significantly higher level than you did only a few short semesters ago. We recently heard an undergraduate complain to a new graduate student that "We have a test on four chapters from the textbook on Wednesday," to which the graduate student replied in her best California accent, "Whatever!"

The present authors also know that most students equate taking a course in research methods with getting in line for a complimentary root canal. Most students feel that the course in unnecessary, too technical, and has nothing to do with why they got into the field, the desire to do clinical work. We don't delude ourselves into thinking that students are doing handsprings over learning about science, research, evidence-based practice, and quantitative methods. In fact, we *know* that you are not looking forward to the experience of learning about research in communication disorders, and we *know* that you will probably be resistant, at least at first, to allow yourselves to like it even a little bit. Do you know how we have figured this out? Well, first of all, it is important for you to remember that we were once students ourselves. Yes, we sat in those same classes you are taking, although it was years ago, and one thing for sure is that research methods have not changed drastically over the past quarter of a century. We initially thought it boring and intimidating just as you might right now. Why are courses dealing with research often perceived negatively by students? In some cases, research courses continue to be menacing and unsettling to students just because of inertia. It is interesting how a person ends up teaching at a university. We are here to tell you that, in most cases, nobody really "teaches you how to teach" a college course. In fact, many professors simply pattern their courses after those that *they* took during their degree program (that is the inertia). Some professors (a minority) even think that certain courses, and research courses in particular, are part of the "rite of passage" to get a degree. In other words, they feel that just because they had to take a boring and uninteresting research course, all the future cohorts of students must pass through the same initiation. Or some feel that just due to the nature of the material, research courses have to be dry, uninteresting, intimidating, and irrelevant to clinical work. And so it goes, paraphrasing the Bible, "pouring the new wines of possibility into the old bottles of tradition." Even when professors make their lectures interesting and relevant and the students become excited about research methods, they must still contend with textbooks written for research courses that are often not very exciting or student-friendly. This is one of the factors leading us to write the present textbook. Another source of knowledge about student's attitudes is by observing them over many years of teaching research courses. Students come in on the first day of class and suspiciously examine the syllabus, like it was a piece of spoiled food, wrinkling up their noses when they see statistical terms and scientific language. They simply are not ready to see the relevance, wonder, challenge, humor and clinical utility of this material. Most come into a research course with a negative mind-set. Thus, after many years of teaching, we have learned that part of our job as professors and scientists is to spend some time at the beginning of a research course showing students that there is another way to look at this material. To do so makes the material more relevant to students while also making the course more fun and the difficult material easier to digest. It is important for students to realize that we are not just attempting to drum up some bogus enthusiasm here; this material is very important to being a competent professional and you will use this information for the rest of your career. You might think that showing students that research is important to them and is actually fun and interesting would be a hard sell. Let us assure you that this is not the case. The arguments for the applicability of the material are irrefutable because they make so much sense. We have routinely observed students go through the metamorphosis from being skeptical about research methodology to actually becoming what we like to call "research sharks."

What is a research shark? You have no doubt seen movies in which sharks are swimming compatibly with scuba divers. They are enjoying each other's company and coexisting well. On the other hand, you have seen movies in which sharks go into a feeding frenzy where they smell blood in the water and rip some poor fish or human to shreds. A research shark swims around scientific studies and if the research is good the shark will know it and treat the study with admiration and respect. Conversely, if a study is uncontrolled and poorly done, the research shark will also know it, and like sharks smelling blood in the water, the study will progressively be nibbled at and ultimately ripped apart. One important insight about research is realizing the large differences in quality of studies that are published and presented to consumers. We should *always* be skeptical of someone who says that he or she has research that "shows" something to be true. That's where research sharks come in. By the end of this semester, you will be a research shark able to appreciate good research or pick apart weak research by asking pertinent questions. But before beginning your research shark training, it is important for you to really appreciate the critical necessity for you to either become intimately familiar with the research process or be left behind and relegated to a career of mediocrity. That's right, a knowledge of research can be the major difference between being a run-of-the-mill professional and one who is continually growing and reinventing his or her competence. The following sections illustrate why an appreciation of good research is essential to practitioners in speech-language pathology and audiology.

The Role of Research in Making a Profession Credible

Let us focus away from the individual student and concentrate for a bit on the profession as a whole. Let us consider the concept that research plays a significant role in establishing the credibility of a profession. Although a profession is made up of individual practitioners, a profession also has an identity and reputation of its own, regardless how much respect an individual practitioner develops from clients and society as a whole. For example, it is not unusual for certain professions to be degraded in the popular media. A person whose profession is used car salesperson carries a certain amount of baggage attached to that classification. Many people view used vehicle salespeople as seedy, untrustworthy sorts who will attempt to foist an unreliable automobile on some unsuspecting purchaser. As the late Rodney Dangerfield used to say, "They get no respect." We all know, however, that many salespeople who purvey "pre-owned vehicles" have great integrity, honesty and consideration for their customers. But this is the point. No matter how good the reputation of a particular car salesperson, the perception of the overall profession may overshadow the performance of this individual. As a result, the person is starting out at a disadvantage with customers and must continually reestablish his or her credibility and reliability during each sale to overcome the negative perceptions of the overall profession. So why is it that used car salespeople do not receive the respect from the public that many of them deserve? How does this apply to the clinical professions devoted to helping people with disabilities? How do the helping professions gain credibility and a good reputation?

Any profession with a clinical orientation has certain constituents that contribute to establishing credibility. Figure 1.1 shows the major common areas that the public

FIGURE 1.1

Seven of Eight Determinants of Professional Credibility Involve Research Either Directly or Indirectly

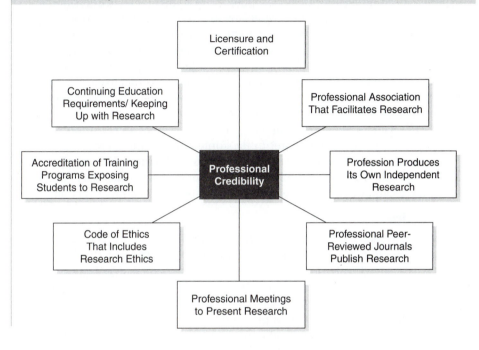

and other disciplines look for in defining a credible profession. Note that seven out of the eight areas involve research either directly or indirectly. We will briefly touch on each of these important components.

Credentialing

A major contributor to professional credibility is a credentialing mechanism that issues a "permit" to provide the services a person is trained to perform. This is the *one area* where research is not directly or indirectly involved. We do not want just anyone hanging out a shingle saying they are a physician, speech-language pathologist, audiologist, or physical therapist. In speech-language pathology and audiology, the American Speech-Language-Hearing Association (ASHA) offers the Certificate of Clinical Competence (CCC) to students completing an accredited training program and passing a national examination. Such certification shows the public and professionals from other disciplines that a practitioner has undergone adequate training and experience. Another credentialing mechanism used by most states is licensure. In most states, professionals in helping professions must have a license to practice their profession, and licensure requirements are typically identical to certification requirements.

Accreditation of Training Programs

Any profession that desires public acceptance has to somehow define standards of training and practice. For instance, clinicians in training must undergo some sort of common educational and practicum experience in order to "become" a professional in a given field. In communication disorders, we have very specific academic and practicum requirements in both audiology and speech-language pathology that must be completed prior to graduation and eventual certification. In order to ensure that training programs meet some level of consistency in training clinicians, professional organizations such as ASHA have developed criteria that university programs must meet in order to be sanctioned or "accredited" by the professional organization. So where does research come into the picture? In the context of a training program, students are *initially exposed to the research base* on communication disorders and the normal aspects of speech, hearing, and language. Exposure to this research base provides a basis for the techniques we use clinically and the rationale for employing them.

Code of Ethics

An important aspect of any profession is the presumption that its practitioners will be ethical. Clearly, ethics is an individual trait and people vary considerably in their view of what is or is not ethical in a particular situation. Professional organizations have an important role in setting ethical standards for people who practice under their auspices. In the field of communication disorders, ASHA has a code of ethics that outlines the parameters of ethical conduct for practitioners. The code of ethics also covers the conduct of research and even ethical issues in publishing research. The ethical prescriptions set by ASHA of commitment to continuing education, providing competent services, not misrepresenting any research you do, and crediting others with their contribution in publications and presentations all indirectly involve research. The fact that a profession has a well-defined code of ethics which, if violated, can result in loss of certification and licensure is of some comfort to those in the public who receive our services. It gives them some recourse if they are not treated ethically by a clinician.

Continuing Education

Most of the clinical professions have requirements that practitioners remain abreast of current literature and practices in the field to maintain their certification or licensure. This involves keeping up with current research by reading it or attending conferences where new research is presented. This is why almost all of the helping professions require a prescribed number of continuing education credits each year to maintain certification or licensure.

A National Association

One major step toward credibility is to establish a national association to represent the profession and set guidelines for practice. We have already said that such organizations develop accreditation criteria for training programs, certification mechanisms, and ethical codes of conduct for practitioners. National organizations also help to define research agendas for a profession and even develop grant support for specific lines of research.

Professional Journals

National organizations also produce professional literature in the form of peer-reviewed journals (*American Journal of Audiology; American Journal of Speech-Language Pathology*) and monographs. These publications provide practitioners with access to new research and are often included in the cost of membership in a national association.

Professional Conferences

National and state organizations hold annual meetings where professionals gather to present research, develop position papers on current issues by reviewing research, and take advantage of continuing education opportunities.

Discipline-Specific Research and Research from Other Fields

Now we come to the impact of research production on the credibility of a profession. We touched indirectly on research in the previous paragraphs mentioning professional journals and professional meetings where state-of-the-art research is presented to members. A professional organization such as ASHA or the American Academy of Audiology (AAA) has as a major goal to facilitate and encourage research in communication disorders, which is why these groups hold conventions, publish journals, and offer research grants to students and practitioners. But let's go a bit deeper. It has been said that a profession that does not produce its own research base is rudderless, buffeted about by the waves of change in other fields as research trends change. What if we had no research base in communication disorders and had to exclusively rely on psychology, education, and medicine to tell us about the nature of communication disorders and how to do clinical work? We would constantly be on the sidelines waiting for other professions to let us know about current trends in our own field. What if audiology exclusively relied on research conducted by the hearing instrument companies to tell them the types of hearing aids to dispense and how to fit them? Without our own body of research, that could easily be the case. Some often-quoted sentiments by experts in communication disorders appear below.

> A profession that provides its own research base is much more in charge of its own destiny than a profession that doesn't.
>
> R. Kent

> If we must rely on others both to achieve the scientific and technological advances and then to apply those advances within our field, we cannot pretend to be a mature and autonomous profession.
>
> R. Flower

> Unless a discipline quickly begins to produce its own experimental database, it will continue to borrow theories and methods that may or may not be appropriate for studying its subject matter.
>
> M. Hegde

Despite the truth of these quotes, it is important to note that *no* profession can be truly autonomous and produce *all* relevant research for its practitioners. Most fields are far too complex and research from many disciplines is relevant; however, any profession increases its credibility if it contributes to the research base and does not totally rely on other fields to produce the scientific support for its practice.

Three Examples of Professional Credibility

The history of chiropractic shows that it was initially perceived by many as quackery. Even today, there are people who will not go to a chiropractor if they have a bad back or other type of pain or movement disorder. Ask yourself who is the primary "go to" profession if you have strained your back? The answer is not unambiguous. There are people who would immediately think about going to their general practitioner. Others would pick an orthopedic clinic that specializes in sports injuries. Yet others may elect to go to a chiropractor. By no means is the chiropractor the unanimous professional of choice in this scenario. Then ask the various professionals if they feel competent to deal with the back strain. Probably all of the professionals mentioned would claim competence in treating such patients, bolstered partly from the credibility accorded to the various professions. Despite the persistence of early attitudes, currently the field of chiropractic is significantly more accepted by the medical community than in the past. We even see chiropractors on the staffs of certain medical centers with traditional physicians, which was not the case a few decades ago. How did the field of chiropractic begin to turn around the negative perceptions of the public and other professions? Interestingly, over the past quarter century, schools of chiropractic have developed accreditation guidelines for training programs, certification boards, and state licensure requirements. Most relevant to the present text, however, as little as twenty years ago, the chiropractic field was lamenting *the lack of well-controlled studies in their own field* (www.worldchiropracticalliance.org, 1987). At that time, professionals in chiropractic urged the development of research agendas *within the discipline* as a major priority in the field. As a result, many recent studies have shown the effectiveness of chiropractic for specific disabilities used in concert with traditional medical practice. This type of evidence-based practice is indispensable to a profession to prove its efficacy and potential contributions to treatment. It is especially important for a field to generate its own research base and not have to rely solely on other professions to define the scope and effectiveness of practice in that field. If you look at other clinical professions that command respect such as veterinary medicine, pharmacy, and optometry, *the one thing they have in common is that they have maintained a strong research base*. If someone wants to know about the effects of drug interactions, it would be a good bet that the pharmacy literature contains some important research. If we had questions about how to do a hip replacement on a Great Dane, we would be going to the research produced by veterinary medicine.

Now let us look at communication disorders. Are we credible as professions? Since speech-language pathology has been around the longest, we will start there. One question we might ask is "Who might a person seek out for help for a speech or language problem?" Most people would say a speech-language pathologist (SLP). Even other professionals such as psychologists, educators, or physicians would not represent themselves as being able to teach a nonverbal child to talk or remediate the language in a stroke patient. The fact that the SLP is the "go to" profession in these situations speaks directly to the credibility of the field. Even though people in neurosciences are interested in brain-injured adults, you rarely see them providing therapy for aphasia, apraxia, and motor speech disorders. Specialists in learning disabilities are interested in language, yet they do not often take on the primary responsibility for assessment and treatment of language disorders. Some occupational and physical therapists provide therapy for dysphagia or swallowing disorders, but it is still mostly SLPs who perform these treatments. Ironically, it may be research on evidence-based practice that ultimately will play the pivotal role in determining which profession ends up as the "go to" group for treating dysphagia. It seems to be clear that SLPs have commanded a significant level of credibility with the public and other professionals for dealing with speech and language disorders. In examining some of the other areas in Figure 1.1, speech-language pathology has clearly done many of the right things. For example, ASHA's Council of Academic Accreditation (CAA) is an accrediting agency for training programs and issues certification for speech-language pathologists. Most states have licensure laws for the practice of speech-language pathology. ASHA is a major professional organization of almost 100,000 people and it holds professional meetings to share information and offers continuing education resources for practitioners. Does speech-language pathology produce its own "inhouse" basic and clinical research? First of all, ASHA has a long history of encouraging research in speech, language, and hearing by providing grant support for students and practitioners and making many venues available for the presentation of research information at professional meetings and in ASHA journals. The professional journals produced by ASHA have been in existence since the 1930s and still constitute the "benchmark" publications for anything having to do with communication disorders. While we incorporate research from other fields into our knowledge base, we do most of the specific research on communication disorders ourselves. Any ASHA determination of a need for more research activity in a particular area is articulated in position papers by the association and in an increase in grant support for specific types of projects. For instance, ASHA has determined that we are sorely lacking in research in evidence-based practice (American Speech-Language-Hearing Association, 2004). Now, evidence-based practice is a major emphasis in our field and new research is emerging every month on this important topic. Rather than waiting for other fields to provide data on what we do, we have a research base of our own that is both wide and deep. In summary, the educational requirements, certification, research production, public/professional perceptions, and a strong national organization all establish strong credibility for speech-language pathology.

Is the audiology profession the clear leader in dealing with the diagnosis and treatment of hearing impairments? The answer to this question, on the surface at least, is not as clear as in speech-language pathology. For example, across the country, there are three distinct professions that do audiometric work: audiologists, hearing aid dealers, and hearing aid–dispensing otolaryngologists. Given these three sources of audiometric practice, how do we determine which profession is the "best" for dealing with diagnosis and treatment of hearing impairment? The answer lies in the criteria illustrated in Figure 1.1. An interesting study on this very question was done by Turner (1998), who wanted to compare the three professions mentioned in terms of several criterion variables to see which had the most credibility. The specific variables studied by Turner involved education (degree, length of training, type of training), research (research production, emphasis on research in training), knowledge transfer (communicating research findings to practitioners at national meetings), and quality/quantity of clinical service as measured by data gathered from clinics and clients. Let us briefly summarize the results for each of the professional groups. You might initially think that dispensing otolaryngologists would be difficult to compete with since they are physicians. Clearly, otolaryngologists have extensive formal medical education; however, they have precious little training dealing with hearing instruments and the nuances of diagnosing hearing ability. When you look at the contribution made by otolaryngologists to the literature specifically dealing with research on hearing instruments and patient assessment for these devices, their role is minor at best. At national meetings of otolaryngologists, only a small portion of the papers presented deal with information on hearing instruments and audiometry. Finally, only a small proportion of people who use hearing instruments received these devices directly from an otolaryngologist. Many times otolaryngologists hire audiologists to handle testing and prescription of hearing instruments and do not do the testing themselves. Thus, although otolaryngologists have a clear edge in dealing with diseases of the ear, surgical intervention, and medical treatment, they are not typically trained to deal with the diagnosis and remediation of hearing impairment and their research base is medical as opposed to audiometric.

Hearing aid dealers are in every city, typically in high-profile locations, and they advertise heavily to the public their claims of effectiveness in dealing with the effects of hearing impairment. They often offer free assessments and say that they can provide the most current technological solutions to hearing impairment. But are they the most credible profession to deal with audiometric issues? First of all, hearing aid dealers have no formal educational requirements. One can become a hearing aid dealer by graduating from high school and attending a short training course conducted by a hearing instrument manufacturer. Second, hearing aid dealers make virtually no contribution to the research literature, leaving it to the hearing instrument companies. Third, Turner found in examining the programs from national meetings that there was very little significant research information presented on hearing aids. Although hearing aid dealers still provide significant hearing aid services to many people, their contributions to dispensing hearing instruments have decreased in the last fifteen years. Thus, in the areas of educational preparation and production of research the hearing aid dealers are not doing the things necessary to develop credibility among the public and other professionals.

Finally, we consider the audiologist. Regarding educational preparation, the profession of audiology has mandated a professional doctorate as the entry level degree for clinical practice. All training programs can earn accreditation by the American Speech-Language-Hearing association if they train students to demonstrate very specific areas of knowledge and skill. ASHA also provides certification for audiologists who graduate from accredited programs. Contrary to the other two professions mentioned previously, audiologists are the only dispensing group whose formal educational requirements deal specifically with audiometric diagnosis, treatment, and hearing instruments. Audiologists have made outstanding contributions to the hearing research literature in the ASHA journals and other publications by the American Academy of Audiology (AAA). Their national meetings host more research presentations on hearing instruments and the diagnosis and treatment of hearing loss than those of other professions. Examining trends in hearing aid dispensing over the past fifteen years, audiologists have steadily increased in the numbers of instruments dispensed, while hearing aid dealers have gradually decreased. In studies of patient satisfaction, audiologists have better ratings than hearing aid dealers. Finally, the available data suggest that audiologists do not charge more for hearing instruments compared to hearing aid dealers, so when patients go to an audiologist they are getting services from a significantly more highly trained professional for a similar cost (Turner, 1998).

What should we conclude from the brief synopses of the three professions discussed above? First, it is easy to see that many of the elements in Figure 1.1 are critical in making decisions about the credibility of a profession. Audiologists are the clear choice over the other two professions based on accreditation, educational requirements, licensure/certification, professional associations, and independent research production. The reader should not lose sight of the importance of producing and presenting research as a major variable that helps to separate audiologists from the other practitioners. As we stated earlier in this chapter, this is true for any field that is seeking respect from other professions.

Our Professional Literature and the Information Base

Quality of Data in the Information Base

In the past, when our field was simpler and had far less of an information base, it was possible to remain current with very little effort. In that era, some people would even get "dual certification" in both speech-language pathology and audiology. Nowadays there is so much information in each field that it is very rare for a person to seek dual certification. It has been said that over 80 percent of the world's knowledge has been developed in the past century, and today, scientific information *doubles* every five years (Drucker, 1998). But is all information created equal? Is all research well controlled and of high quality? You may be surprised to hear this, but the answer is *definitely not*. Yes, you heard us correctly; there is a load of research, textbooks, presentations, courses, and Internet sites that present misinformation, incomplete information, or outright fabricated information. It is unfortunate but true. Much of our information base is composed of good research, but as long as there is poorly done research out there, it makes it difficult for consumers of research (students and practitioners) to believe everything they read. One important goal of a course on research methodology revolves around making research consumers more educated so that they can discriminate studies that are well done from those that are shoddy and come to conclusions not based on their data. Remember the research shark? That fish can smell a rotten study a mile away and start asking questions that will expose it for what it is. Research sharks can also appreciate studies that are well done and not rip them to shreds. So one solution to the problem of varying quality in our information base is to educate students and practitioners to become critical consumers of research. That doesn't mean not to trust people who do our scientific work; it just means that we do not take every study as being well done just because it is in print. Like Ronald Reagan said, "Trust, but verify." So how does one stay in tune with the information base in communication disorders? Students and practitioners are exposed to the information base in many ways as illustrated in Figure 1.2. We will deal with each of these in the following sections as we look at the information base. No matter which section of the information base we examine, research is (or should be) the underlying common thread that unites them all (see Figure 1.3).

Textbooks

Some of you might be thinking that if we must be suspect of our research base, then why not just get all our information from textbooks? After all, we use them in college

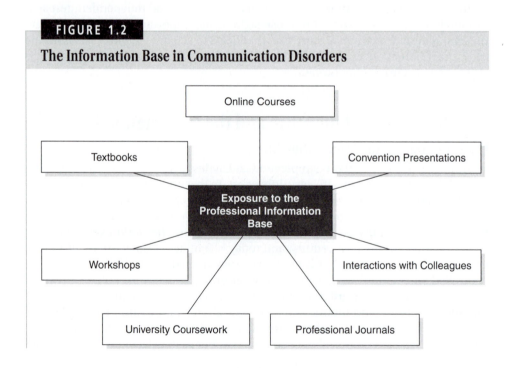

FIGURE 1.2

The Information Base in Communication Disorders

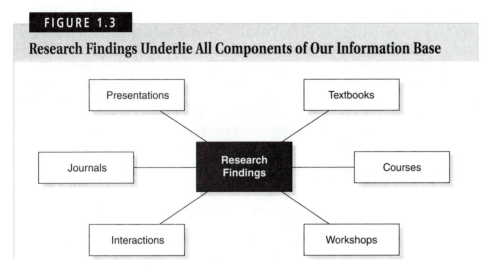

FIGURE 1.3

Research Findings Underlie All Components of Our Information Base

and spend all that money to build our professional library. It is important to realize that textbooks are really a "secondary" source. The "primary" sources of information are actually the research studies that the textbook author has reviewed and referenced in the book. Would you really like to read a book that provided information that had no empirical support? Without scientific research to support the points of view in a text, the writing just amount to nothing more than the author's opinion. A competent author in writing a book has reviewed piles of research information and distilled the findings into a reasonable synthesis of the work that was done. We see the research as filtered through the nervous system of the author. Readers of textbooks must be concerned about several important issues. First, we have to be satisfied that the author is actually qualified to write about the topic of interest. Do we want to read a book on psychology that was written by a talk show host? Second, we must be concerned about the depth and breadth of the literature review conducted by the author. Were all of the references from decades ago? Were all major points of view represented in the literature review? Were there controversies within the information base that were never dealt with? Third, it is possible that an author may have reviewed most of the pertinent research in an area but then interpreted it in an unconventional manner. The author may have misinterpreted studies and as a result made errors in reporting information in the textbook. Also, textbooks are typically not subjected to stringent peer review as are articles in professional journals. Although some publishing houses take great care to obtain reviews of manuscripts during their development and prior to publication, many other firms are not as careful to secure such feedback. Books also are reviewed in professional journals and on professional association websites, and these reviews can be helpful to prospective textbook purchasers in deciding on the quality of the work. If a book is of very low quality, the review will be negative, the text will not be widely adopted by professors, and it will go out of print in a relatively short time. A high-quality textbook is a good general source of information if the author has done a good job of reviewing existing literature and given a faithful interpretation of the studies reviewed, identifying observable and real trends in the existing data. In this way, textbooks can help us synthesize many individual studies into an interpretable framework so that we can make sense of the information in a particular area. Textbooks, however, are no substitute for the individual scientific studies that they review. A textbook can never provide enough detail about the individual research studies it is based on and diligent consumers must consult the original investigations to make a principled judgment about the worth of a particular study.

Presentations at Professional Meetings

As indicated in Figure 1.2, another source of information is found in presentations offered at professional meetings such as local, state, regional, and national conventions. Again, a presentation at a professional meeting is typically based on research. If it were not, we would again be dealing with someone standing up in front of a group merely expressing an opinion or selling their favorite treatment program. Although most convention presentations are subjected to peer review, this process is not as rigorous as in submitting a paper for a journal article. This is because most convention submissions require an extremely abbreviated summary of the research to be presented, typically under 1500 words. Thus, it is not possible to really evaluate the work in terms of its empirical quality since there is not enough detailed information provided. In fact, many researchers try to convert their convention presentations into journal articles, only to have their work rejected for empirical reasons after it is subjected to the glaring light of more rigorous peer review. At conventions, there are different types of presentations available. First, there are **short courses** and **mini-seminars** that constitute the longest presentations offered at conventions, often lasting from several hours to even a full day. Typically focusing on a particular area such as "Assessment of Children with Autism" or "Working with Children Who Have Cochlear Implants," these presentations often mention research without elaborating in detail. Rather, these presentations serve to summarize research in a given area and provide a continuing education opportunity for practitioners who want to catch up on a specific topic. A second type of presentation at conventions, the **traditional platform** session, is run by a moderator and typically focuses on a specific topic area. Individual researchers present results of their studies in fifteen- to twenty-minute lectures. An example of a topical focus might be "Use of Masking in the Treatment of Stuttering" and individual researchers will present the results of their studies related to this topic. There is typically little time left for questions and often no attempt is made to synthesize the research results by the moderator. A third type of presentation at conventions is the **poster session**. A large room is reserved and scores of forty-by-eight-foot bulletin boards are set up by topic areas. For instance, there may be forty poster boards on the topic of phonology, thirty boards on adult aphasia, and twenty boards on voice disorders, similar to a high school science fair where students display the results of a project that they have completed. Poster sessions are typically set up for ninety minutes during which people come by each poster and chat with the person who conducted the research. This provides a great opportunity for questioning and often the presenters learn as much from the interactions as the people who attend the poster sessions. A fourth type of convention presentation is the technical/computer session, providing opportunities to demonstrate new technology and software programs to practitioners and giving them "hands on" experience. It can be seen that conventions offer many opportunities for continuing education, but it is important for consumers of research to remember that such presentations are often not rigorously screened or reviewed. Another significant point to make is that all conventions are not of the same quality as far as the scientific rigor to which convention paper submissions are subjected. For example, it is much easier to have your presentation accepted at a local convention than it is at a state convention, and in turn state conventions are typically less rigorous in selecting research papers for presentation than regional or national conventions. Thus, if a person's research has been presented it is important to note whether this was local, state, regional, or national before making a judgment about the quality of the work. Even at national or international meetings we must remember that the quality of the research presented has typically not been evaluated in depth, even though such venues are more impressive than local, state, or regional levels. This makes it crucial that consumers of research critically evaluate the information being presented and ask questions of presenters about the nature of their scientific work rather than taking it at face value.

Scientific Journals

Ah yes, the professional literature! Doesn't the thought of it just make you want to curl up in front of the fireplace on a winter evening with a nice juicy copy of the *Journal of Speech-Language-Hearing Research* or the *Journal of the American Academy of Audiology* and sip on a steaming cup of hot chocolate? We didn't think so. Although journal articles are not always exciting, they will become a major source of your continuing education after you graduate. And again, as in Figure 1.2, most journal articles are based on reporting research findings or, in the case of tutorial articles, synthesizing research findings. It usually takes about a year for recent graduates to be able to approach journals again after their graduate school experience. Many of you are probably vowing to never crack a professional periodical again after you get out of graduate school, but the reality is that you probably will. When you get your first job you will no doubt run into some cases that are not as cut and dried as you were led to believe in graduate school. You may even have cases that represent totally new syndromes or types of disorder, which should help get you interested in any article you can find that will clarify things for you. We always smile when we get the inevitable telephone calls or e-mails from recent graduates asking us for the latest references that might help them with a clinical dilemma. Now you won't sit down with a journal and read it from cover to cover, reading articles on disorders that you are not even dealing with in your job, but you *will* focus on those pieces of research that are relevant to your practice. That is the way it is *supposed* to be. If you do not find yourself trying to remain abreast of the current research in your profession, you should begin to wonder about your ability to remain competent. Every professional worthy of respect should have a desire to keep up with current information, and this is no easy task. No one sets out to become a mindless gerbil on a treadmill who keeps thinking and doing the same things year after year even if they are outdated. One of our former professors said that there is big difference between having twenty-five years of experience and having the first year of experience repeated twenty-five times. Unfortunately, there are people in our profession, in every work setting from clinics all the way to university training programs, that are not in tune with current developments in our field. You will recognize them when you see them, especially if you make a concerted effort to not be left behind professionally. Don't let it happen to you. Let it be said by others throughout your career that you are a consummate clinician who is up to date with the current literature.

What are professional journals and how do articles end up in them? A very important part of the information base in any field is the contribution from peer-reviewed professional journals. Before discussing this important component of our professional literature, we will briefly talk about how a professional journal is organized and some steps in the editorial process. Figure 1.4 shows a typical organizational structure of a professional journal in speech-language pathology.

The basic organization is the same in audiology and other professions. The editor in charge of the journal manages the flow of manuscripts from authors and sees to it that the work is reviewed by professionals who are highly qualified to judge research in the particular topic area. Many journals use electronic submission of articles, but some still require authors to submit several "hard copies" for review. So

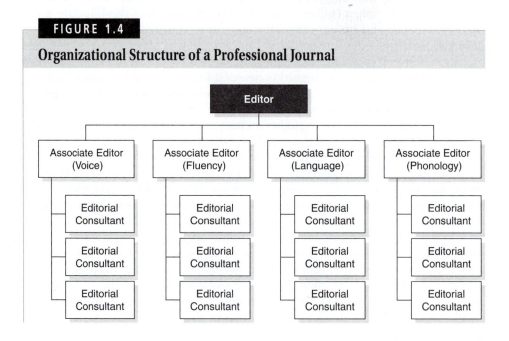

FIGURE 1.4

Organizational Structure of a Professional Journal

if an editor receives a research paper in the area of voice disorders, the manuscript will be forwarded to an associate editor who specializes in this topic. After receiving the manuscript, the associate editor must then decide who among the available editorial consultants (reviewers) would be most qualified to review the paper. For example, if the research is concerned with spasmodic dysphonia, there may be certain editorial consultants who have also done studies in this area and have a national reputation for expertise in this disorder. Typically, a manuscript is reviewed by three editorial consultants. When the associate editor decides which editorial consultants will review the manuscript, it is sent to these reviewers and they are typically given about two months to complete their analyses of the paper. Editorial consultants are usually asked to make specific decisions on the manuscripts that they review, typically representing three levels: (1) Accept the manuscript as submitted; (2) Accept the manuscript but with suggested revisions that the author must complete prior to publication; or (3) Reject the manuscript in its present form. It is quite rare for a manuscript to be accepted without revision; in fact, it is almost unheard of. Perhaps the most common decisions made by editorial consultants are numbers 2 and 3 listed above. Let's talk a bit about these two scenarios. In the case of a decision to accept the manuscript with revisions, there may be stylistic errors in grammar or spelling, there may be organizational problems, some critical information may be missing, the review of the literature may be incomplete, or the author may have made certain claims in the discussion section of the article that went beyond the scope of the study. In any of these cases it is possible for the author to remediate the problem by revising the manuscript. These are not "fatal" errors that would be irreparable, and the basic study is scientifically sound and potentially meaningful to the readership of the journal. When the manuscript is revised in accordance with the suggestions of the editorial consultant, it is returned to the same reviewers who made the revision suggestions to determine if the author has responded appropriately to the suggestions. Sometimes this process takes many months from the initial submission of the manuscript to the editor, through the review and revision process, and finally to the actual publication of the article. The time spent in the editorial process is often referred to as **publication lag**. If you look at the end of the next article that you read, you will find two dates listed. One date is the original date of submission, and the second date is the date of acceptance. This is the part of publication lag that accounts for the time spent in reviewing and revising the manuscript. After acceptance, the actual journal article may not appear in print for up to a year because the layout and content of a journal must be planned well in advance of its actual appearance in libraries and the mailboxes of subscribers. The upshot of this is that there may be a publication lag of two years between the completion of a study and its appearance in journals. What we may think is new information that is "hot off the press" may actually be fairly old by today's standards of exploding information. Several years ago one of the present authors read a new journal article and contacted the person who had done the study to ask some questions. The author of the study replied that she had trouble remembering the work since it was done three years earlier, and in fact, she no longer was even pursuing that line of research.

In the case of a decision to reject the manuscript the study suffers from a fatal flaw. It is possible that there was not sufficient justification for doing the study in the first place, or perhaps the issue has been studied enough. Another reason for rejection is that the study was not well controlled scientifically and the results cannot be interpreted unambiguously because of errors in the experimental design. Perhaps the author used the wrong statistical methods to analyze the data. Whatever the reason, if a study is rejected, the editorial consultants feel that the work cannot be salvaged or can only be saved by a major reworking, gathering more data, redesigning the study, or approaching the question from an entirely different direction. The perceptive reader may wonder if there is usually agreement among editorial consultants regarding a particular study. In most cases, there does tend to be agreement; however, the system has a method of dealing with cases where the reviewers may differ in their appraisal of an article. If the reviewers are split in the decision to accept a manuscript (say two-thirds want to accept the study) then the associate editor and editor must review the manuscript and render their judgment along with the editorial consultants. In this case, there may be as many as five experts that have reviewed a study (three editorial consultants, associate editor, and editor). If a decision still cannot be reached, it is also possible to send the paper out to more editorial consultants for review. When an author feels that the editorial process has unfairly reviewed a work, most journals have a provision for authors to write a rejoinder to the criticisms made by reviewers and have these arguments reviewed along with those of the editorial consultants.

It is important for students to know that professional journals have differing levels of "prestige" in any given field, and this reputation is highly correlated with the quality of the editorial staff and the rigor with which manuscripts are subjected to review. It is infinitely more difficult to succeed in getting an article published in the *Journal of Speech-Language-Hearing Research* than it is to have an article accepted in a state or regional journal. The criteria and expectations for the quality of the research question and conduct of the study are more rigorous in the more prestigious journals. Many journals publish their acceptance/rejection rates and there is quite a bit of variation among publications. Thus, it is not unusual for an author to initially submit an article to a high-level journal and receive a rejection only to resubmit the work to a less prestigious periodical on the national, regional, or state level where it is accepted. The lesson for consumers of research is that we must increase our "sharky" vigilance when reading studies in state and regional journals. National journals also vary in quality, so we must be careful to critically examine studies that we read rather than assume that "if it's in print, it must be good." Even in some high-level journals, it is wise to bear in mind that although editorial consultants are scientists who are encouraged to examine manuscripts critically, they are also people with families, troubles, job stresses, and time constraints. These consultants are not reviewing manuscripts as their sole occupation but have taken on these editorial responsibilities in addition to their full-time jobs at universities and clinics. Thus, there may be limited time to read manuscripts and think critically about every aspect of the study reported by the author. Human error can creep into the editorial system very easily and as a result, we find errors in articles published in even the most prestigious journals. This is why it is important to be a research shark. *Always* read a piece of research with a critical eye, knowing that studies vary considerably in quality, and it is always possible for a poorly controlled investigation to slip in under the empirical radar.

University Coursework and Online Courses

There is no escape from research findings in coursework, whether live or online. Any course in communication disorders worth its salt is firmly rooted in science. We want to learn about the treatment techniques that have been shown to be effective by empirical study. We are not interested in having to endure lectures from some insufferable gasbag that only talks about theories, personal experiences, and 150 ways to use *Mr. Potato Head* in language therapy. There *is* a literature out there that can tell us which techniques have the highest probability of being effective for our clients. Courses are actually an ideal format for discussing specific studies and synthesizing the research into an effective clinical perspective.

Workshops

A workshop is usually nothing more than a convention presentation or part of a course lecture that has not been subject to peer review. Most workshop presenters, in order to establish their own credibility, spend considerable time reviewing the research that supports whatever perspective they are presenting. How would you feel after sitting in a workshop all day if the following series of events transpired? The person presenting the workshop tells you how to do therapy for a particular type of disorder. You ask the presenter if there have ever been any studies done that show this therapy to be effective. The presenter replies that he does not know. You probably would have felt better if the presenter had laid a strong research foundation for the techniques being discussed. So again we must ask questions and be critical of things people tell us in workshops, just as we do with journal articles, convention presentations, and textbooks.

Interactions with Colleagues

A final way to learn professional information is to have discussions with colleagues. Other professionals can be a great source of information when they tell us about new procedures, clinical materials, journal references, and textbooks. But again, if the information your colleague gives you as "truth" is not based on adequate research, it only amounts to opinion. There are a couple of ways you can look at these professional interactions, either informally by exchanging your opinions and best guesses about certain issues over a cup of coffee or a beer or more formally by a colleague giving you instruction in how to do a procedure or in the case of supervisors, telling you how to approach a particular clinical problem. The informal sharing of information is fun and stimulates you to think about things from different perspectives. It may even encourage you to get into the literature to see if your brainstorming with another colleague has been studied scientifically. The more formal sharing of information whereby you are attempting to learn about something from your colleague (whether they are a peer or supervisor) is a bit more problematic. When a supervisor tells you to do something a particular way, you assume that this technique is widely used in this manner and there is some support for it in the extant literature. Unfortunately, this is not always the case. So again it is healthy for students and practitioners who learn from colleagues to ask about the research support for techniques so they can examine the efficacy of performing them.

The purpose of this section was to illustrate that research findings underlie all aspects of our information base in communication disorders. If you ignore research and believe that it is not important to communication disorders, you are closing your eyes to reality and severely limiting your own competence. To read about research findings and be able to discriminate good from poor research is the ethical responsibility of all clinicians in communication disorders. Research is what makes us credible as a profession and what determines the quality of the information we learn through a variety of professional venues. Without research, we might as well use Tarot cards, horoscopes, or a dartboard to make our clinical decisions. Research is what makes us effective as a profession and as individual professionals. Learn about it, embrace, it and develop into a hotshot research shark. You will *never* be sorry.

The Scientific Method and Clinical Work: The Notion of Clinician-Researcher

As far as we know, it was Silverman (1998) who coined the term "clinician-investigator" in the earliest editions of his book on research in communication disorders. He states that a clinician-investigator is "a speech-language pathologist or audiologist who functions both as a clinician and a clinical investigator, or researcher. A hyphen was inserted between 'clinician' and 'investigator' to indicate that the two roles are not independent but interdependent" (p. 12). We have used the term **clinician-researcher** because we feel it is a bit clearer to readers that clinicians can choose to be actively involved in the research process as consumers as well as producers of research. Interestingly, it is quite common for clinicians to resist their role in the research process. Many view "research" and "clinical work" as opposite ends of a continuum or incompatible notions. When they see terms like "clinician-researcher" they feel it is an oxymoron like "jumbo shrimp." Remember in the first part of this chapter we spent some time discussing the idea that students come into a research course with a preconceived notion that the material will not be relevant to their training because they entered the communication disorders major to become clinicians. This is similar to the thinking referred to above that clinical work and research are basically incompatible. Unfortunately, this line of thought is based on faulty logic and some degree of misinformation. Silverman (1998) and Schiavetti and Metz (2002) discuss a number of misconceptions or myths that help to perpetuate this type of thinking. We feel that these misconceptions are important to bring to a conscious level and we will discuss them here.

Research versus Clinic: The Dichotomy Myth

When we listen to people talk about research and clinical work they make certain stereotypical statements that illustrate dichotomous (either/or) thinking. Some people say, "There are research people and clinical people" or "I'm not a researcher, I'm a clinician." Obviously these statements suggest that a person must represent one category or another but cannot or should not be both. There are several problems with this line of thought. First, if you examine convention programs and professional journals it is fairly clear that at least 50 percent of the research presented involves people who are in clinical positions (e.g., public schools, hospitals, clinics) and do not consider themselves primarily researchers. Peruse the last convention program and note how many presenters list their affiliation in a school system, hospital, rehabilitation center, or private practice. Also note how many presentations were done exclusively by people with master's degrees. Then look at how many presentations were coauthored by a doctoral-level person and one or more master's-level clinicians. Look at how many presentations involved both a university and a school system or medical setting. If you add them all up, you will see that a large proportion of the research presented at conventions and published in our journals involves people who have master's degrees and work in clinical environments. Research is typically not produced by the stereotypical "scientist" in a white coat who works in a laboratory setting. In fact, surveys of ASHA members suggest that less than 3 percent of professionals in speech-language pathology and audiology classify themselves as "full-time researchers." Even university professors are usually not full-time researchers. Although you might think of people who work at universities as primarily engaged in research, the vast majority of university professors spend only a small part of their time in the research process. Most of them have several classes to teach each semester and administrative duties within the department, and many have limited clinical assignments in terms of supervision of practicum students. Thus, it is just not true to think of all people working in a university setting as being researchers to the exclusion of their role as teachers and clinicians. If you look at the multitude of research publications and presentations produced each year, it is just not possible for the 3 percent of the ASHA membership who consider themselves to be researchers to generate all the studies completed annually. Most of the research is done by people who primarily view themselves as academics or clinicians, and even the academic types either do clinical supervision as part of their job or they often collaborate with clinicians in schools and medical settings on research projects. So if you look at it from a "people" perspective, there is no way around the fact that in most cases "research people" *are* "clinical people." It is not an either/or issue.

A misconception related to the dichotomy between clinicians and researchers is seen when people characterize information and its usefulness. For instance, a common statement might be "Research is esoteric and has little practical clinical application." This is just another way of saying that something is either "research" or "clinical" and they really represent opposite ends of a continuum of usefulness or practicality. The stereotypes are many and varied. Automatically, one who does research is seen as interested in some arcane issue hovering up in the clouds that surround the ivory tower, an issue that would never be of interest to a working clinician. Conversely, a clinician only does practical things and is not interested in finding new ways of approaching clinical issues, or discovering which methods work best, or finding out the causes of certain clinical phenomena. Both of these perspectives are a disservice to researchers and clinicians alike. Actually, most clinical techniques began with a research project of some type. The research may have appeared to be esoteric at first (e.g., delayed auditory feedback, otoacoustic emissions, impedence audiometry, phonological process analysis), but then it is applied to clinical work and becomes a standard part of practice. We use delayed auditory feedback in stuttering treatment. Audiologists now commonly use otoacoustic emissions and impedence audiometry in clinical work as a standard part of assessment. Speech-language pathologists now routinely examine patterns of phonological errors based on the early research on phonological processes. Thus, what might appear initially to be "esoteric" research may develop into a clinical technique that has widespread applicability. Also, think about it from the point of view of a "researcher." Who would want to study a phenomenon that would have no applicability? The answer is no one. Researchers always hope that their work will be practical, if not now, in the future. Another argument for rejecting the dichotomy between esoteric research and practical clinical techniques is that most of our current research directly deals with assessment and treatment. While there is still "basic" research going on, the majority of studies in our journals and at conventions have to do with assessment and/or treatment. We challenge you to examine your next issue of a convention program or professional journal. Look at the titles of the studies represented and you will find that the overwhelming majority of the investigations have to do with assessment and/or treatment of communication disorders. So the bottom line is that our research is *not* esoteric and anathema to clinical work; rather, it is focused directly on clinical issues. The few studies that seem to be "esoteric" to you now may actually be investigating technology or techniques that could be the routine clinical practices of tomorrow. Don't bet against it.

Research Qualifications: The Mensa Myth

You can join a group called Mensa if you have an intelligence quotient in the top 2 percent of the general population. Most people think of scientists as being superintelligent, educated to the doctoral level, associated with a university, and experts in statistics. When clinicians say why they are not interested in research they often intone such remarks as "I'm not smart enough to do research," "You have to know all about statistics to do research," "You have to have a Ph.D. to do research," or "You have to work at a university to do research." None of these statements are totally true. They are part of the Mensa myth. Let's take intelligence first. Most research is done by people of normal intelligence who have learned a set of research skills. Look at any university faculty. These are mostly folks that are not extraordinary, just focused. Most have knowledge that is an inch wide and a mile deep. And of course, perhaps in greater proportion than in other occupations, we have our share of eccentrics on university faculties. But the fact is that university faculty are required to do research for tenure and promotion and they manage to crank out the research projects despite not being members of Mensa. The majority of faculty members got to where they are by taking one step at a time through bachelor's, master's and doctoral degrees, which are all achievable goals for any person of average intelligence. Interestingly, ASHA is predicting a critical drought in the availability of doctoral-level faculty as the "baby boomers" begin to retire from the university. Who will replace us? It is in many ways easier to get into a doctoral program today than it is to gain admission to a master's program. There are more financial incentives in the form of assistantships for doctoral students and yet our programs are very sparsely populated (ASHA, 2004). Doctoral programs are out recruiting master's students with more zeal than ever before. So it's a good bet that if you are a master's student and would like to join that august group of Ph.D.-level faculty, you will no doubt be welcomed into the fold—average intelligence, eccentricities, and all.

The second part of this myth is that one has to have a doctorate to do research. As we stated earlier, much of our research is done by people on the master's degree level either independently, or in collaboration with doctoral-level colleagues. At any rate, people without doctorates are routinely involved in research. Many people publish their master's theses. Master's-level clinicians across many work settings contribute to research presentations at national conventions and in national journals. So it is just not true to say that one needs a doctoral degree for the conduct of research, although it is certainly helpful to have a Ph.D. on your research team.

A third part of the Mensa myth is that one has to be associated with a university or laboratory to do research. Wrong. Much research comes from hospitals, school systems, private clinics and rehabilitation centers. A large proportion of research involves people from universities collaborating with other professionals in nonuniversity settings. In this way, a person in a school system or hospital can do research and rely on expertise from a person in a university. The person from the university has the opportunity to collaborate in a real-life clinical setting and gain access to cases that ordinarily may not be accessible in the university setting. In such a collaboration, each professional makes a unique contribution that makes the project richer because everyone brings different perspectives and resources to the table.

The final part of this myth is that researchers need to know all the details of statistical analysis and the computer programs that accomplish them. Again, this is not necessarily true. When a problem arose in our household like a broken pipe or malfunctioning air conditioner, my mother used to say "Aren't there people for that?" and proceed to look in the yellow pages for the appropriate "person." So it is with statistics. Even among university faculty who all had to sit through a series of courses in statistics and research design, there is considerable variability in expertise in these areas. Take it from us that this type of information is not like a fine wine. It does not get better with age. The point here is that even on the university faculty a professor may have to seek the help of a statistical consultant to plan a study or analyze and interpret data. You can hire a consultant or work with someone at a university who will be more than willing to help with the statistics and design issues. Also, you should know that statistics and experimental design are not rocket science. You could learn them by taking a couple of courses or learn them when you are actually doing research. The authors have had master's-level research assistants and thesis students who easily mastered the mechanics of statistical analysis peculiar to a specific project. It is not necessary for you to know everything there is to know about statistics. To participate in research it is just important that you know the statistic that will analyze your data and get some help in selecting which one to use in the first place. We will deal with statistics to a greater extent in later chapters.

When and Where: The Time and Place Myth

One stumbling block people often use as an excuse for not participating in research is that they don't have the time. Well, when you think about it, not having adequate time can be an excuse for just about anything. But let's focus on research. First of all, some types of research (e.g., retrospective) involve the use of clinical records that are already available. A clinician in the public schools or in a clinic may already have significant amounts of assessment or treatment data on a specific type of case. It is especially important, however, that such data were gathered systematically with the researcher ensuring quality control. Such data may just require organization and evaluation by a clinician. Although there are some caveats about the types of retrospective data that are appropriate for research, the point here is that such research may not take an inordinate amount of time to do because data may be already available. Now obviously, if a person working in the public schools embarks on a research program involving a study of brain activity in patients who have suffered strokes, this is clearly over and above the call of duty for a public school SLP. This type of research will have to be done after hours at a local hospital or university and will detract from family or recreation time. Despite the attraction for some people, such extracurricular research *does* take time and a person would need a fervent interest in doing it. A second point is that many research projects involve single case experimental designs, which means that you can do a study on a single client by being systematic in how you do therapy. Even the most prestigious journals routinely publish single case designs because they provide very important information. So if you are doing therapy with a particular client anyway, why not systematically study how it works. Obviously, this may not take a significant amount of time because you are simply organizing the way you approach your existing clinical work. As explained in a later chapter, a clinician will have to follow good single case procedure and adhere to ethical guidelines for conducting such research. Third, a useful first step in conducting research is to report a case study. If you have a client who represents an unusual syndrome or clinical profile, you can write up a detailed history, summary of assessment data, and the response to treatment. Most journals publish case studies because clinicians all over the country would be interested in such reports, especially if they have similar clients. A fourth point is that you do not have to do research alone. Collaboration with colleagues in your work setting or another work setting divides up the work involved. If you collaborate, you may only have to score tests or give tests or review literature, and the rest of the steps can be done by others. Fifth, you may use research to address issues that you are interested in as part of your job. Let's say your boss wants you to be able to show the effectiveness of your clinical program. How do you do it? How about a person working in the schools who wants to develop a screening test, an assessment program, or treatment materials and activities. In such cases you have to determine if the procedures are reliable and valid, develop cutoff scores for screening instruments, and decide which types of treatment work best. All of this is accomplished by research. What if you wanted to determine whether certain types of clients can make the same amount of progress with fewer treatment sessions? What if you wanted to compare the effectiveness of a home therapy program to treatment without a home program? There are literally hundreds of relevant questions that you might address with research that really are part of your job and not some additional, unrelated enterprise. ASHA currently has a major emphasis on evidence-based practice and applied clinical research. This is the kind of research usually done by practitioners out in the field as part of their daily job routines, often in collaboration with others. The bottom line is that research can fit into a person's daily routine without taking a lot of extra time.

This second part of the time and place myth concerns the issue of place. Where should relevant research be conducted and by whom? One view is to believe that all the clinically relevant research will be done by scientists in laboratories. These scientists know what we need to study, and they are familiar with all the best methods for carrying out research. The truth of the matter is that the people who will probably solve clinical problems and make important applied research contributions are clinicians that are able to participate in collaborative research on meaningful issues related to assessment at treatment. It will probably not be some scientist in a laboratory. So the "where" of much of our future research is right where you will be working as a communication disorders specialist, and the "who" is you.

There is a warning that goes along with becoming a clinician-researcher. Research is serious business and there are definite skills associated with conducting it. We are not advocating that clinicians participate in research without the appropriate skills or involvement of a collaborator who has those skills. Science is far too important for people to "dabble" in a research project. If you are going to do research, you must learn the skills and/or collaborate or consult with a researcher who has had experience. If you don't do it right, you'll be shark bait.

Clinical and Research Skills: Two Sides of the Same Coin

Research and clinical skills overlap to some degree in many significant areas. Let's talk first about the general attributes of a good clinician and a good researcher and some of the common activities of both. First of all, to be a good clinician or a good researcher fundamentally requires the ability to ask pertinent questions and solve problems. Clinicians ask relevant questions when they assess a patient. They use clinical techniques to solve a patient's communication problem. Researchers ask scientific questions and try to solve problems empirically. Figure 1.5 shows six areas that relate to both clinical and research skills. We will discuss each of them individually.

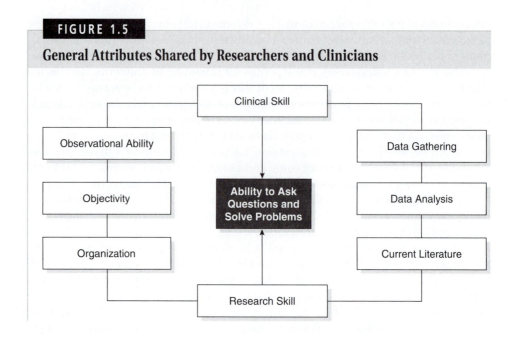

FIGURE 1.5

General Attributes Shared by Researchers and Clinicians

Observational Ability

A good clinician uses trained observational ability to absorb relevant details and detect nuances in a patient's communicative performance. We attend to many subtle aspects of communication when we evaluate children by examining their play, their gestures, their phonology, and other behaviors. We must be organized in observing a patient in clinic by selecting specific performance tasks so that we can watch particular aspects of patient communication. The researcher must also attend to specific phenomena and observe these in a systematic manner. Researchers are always counting events and phenomena and creating operational definitions of more complex behaviors just as clinicians do in assessment and treatment. Observational ability is a prerequisite for both clinicians and researchers; also, the more time you spend in either the research or clinical arena the more you will develop your ability to critically observe events in general.

Objectivity

Everyone has hunches about what might be causing a particular event. It is human nature to have a pet theory or hypothesis about why things happen. Clinicians are not immune from this tendency. For example, you might see an adult who is referred after having a stroke. You might expect the person to have a language problem and you set up your evaluation to assess adult language ability. But a good clinician also recognizes the possibility that the person's language may be fine, so the clinician is also prepared to examine other areas such as motor speech disorders or apraxia.

A clinician, despite hunches about a given client, tries to remain objective and open to other possibilities. So it is with researchers. The researcher may have a pet hypothesis such as "I'll bet that people who stutter process language with the right hemisphere of their brain." When they do the study in a controlled manner, however, they may find that only certain types of stuttering are associated with right hemispheric processing. Scientists have to be objective and open to whatever their results turn out to be. No matter the theory, if the data do not support it, you probably have to adjust your thinking on the matter. You can see how this applies to the clinic as well as research. You may feel that a particular treatment approach will be successful with a certain client, but if the person is not making measurable progress, you need to rethink your approach. Research and clinical skills both require objectivity, and the more time you spend doing either clinical work or research, the more objective you will become.

Organization

Any competent clinician will tell you that being organized is important to good clinical work. You have to organize case history information on your client and even organize how you ask questions in a diagnostic interview. You have to keep test data organized and fill out all the important identifying information. You have to be systematic in how you conduct the evaluation or structure treatment in order to accomplish goals in a logical manner. Clinical work requires you to be highly organized on many levels from planning assessment and treatment to producing reports and case staffings. One of the hallmarks of scientists also is their organization. Any research study must follow stringent guidelines and every aspect must be planned and controlled to reduce scientific errors. Thus, the more research you do, the more organized you will become. Clinicians, trained to be organized, will take to research like a duck takes to water.

Data Gathering

We usually think of data gathering as the province of the researcher, but just think of all the types of data we gather in clinical practice during assessments and treatment sessions. We count disfluencies in people who stutter, measure length of utterance in language cases, take vocal measurements with instruments for voice clients and tally gestural communications in preverbal children. These are only a few of the types of data gathered by clinicians. Similarly, researchers gather exactly the same types of data when they do a study. A researcher examining the occurrence of disfluency under certain specific conditions would be counting behaviors in the same way as a clinician approaches the task in assessment. The skill of being able to objectively gather data on any behavior is built through practice. Thus, the more we gather data, whether part of a research project or a clinical interaction, the better our skills will be for research or clinical work. You can no doubt see that many of the attributes common to clinicians and researchers also overlap. For example, gathering reliable data either clinically or for research requires good observational ability and an objective definition of what you are counting, as well as being systematic in counting and cataloging the data acquired.

Data Analysis

Earlier we discussed statistics as a tool typically used by researchers. When you think of data analysis, we will wager you are conjuring images of statistical formulas in your head. But before they actually perform a statistical procedure, scientists have to do a lot of basic analysis, a process often called **data reduction**. A researcher studying the development of pointing behavior in babies would have to view videotapes of communication samples, count pointing behaviors, place the pointing behaviors in specific categories of interest (distal point, proximal point, arm point, finger point, etc.), and summarize the pointing results for each child. Then these data are statistically analyzed. After I do a statistical procedure I need to further analyze the data in terms of what it means. So when we refer to "analysis" here, we are also meaning "interpretation" of the data. A researcher must examine the data analysis and determine how these results fit into the context of existing research and what implications flow from the results. Similarly, a clinician who gathers assessment data on a client is faced with a myriad of scores, behavioral data, interview information, and reports from other professionals. To get these numbers and behavioral tallies the clinician must score tests, count behaviors, elicit historical information, and study reports from other professionals related to the client. The "analysis" of the totality of existing assessment data also requires that the clinician put each individual bit of information into the context of other evidence gathered during the diagnostic session before making a clinical judgment about the person. Clinicians analyze data just as researchers do, "crunching" numbers, consolidating information, and arriving at an interpretation of what the data really mean. The more practice one has in thinking analytically about data, the better clinician or researcher one will become.

Keeping Up with the Current Literature

It is axiomatic that research should be on the "cutting edge" of knowledge in a particular area. No one wants to read old news. Therefore, a researcher is obligated to keep up with the current literature because he or she must be aware of what other researchers have studied and the methods used to investigate a particular subject. Every empirical study begins with a detailed review of the existing literature that serves to (1) show that the researcher is familiar with the knowledge base in the area of study and (2) provide a rationale for the researcher's present study. Perhaps no one has looked at the research topic from this perspective, or prior studies have methodological problems that make their results uninterpretable. There is no substitute for an acquaintance with past and current research findings. In the clinical realm, no one wants treatment from a person using outdated therapy methods. Our patients assume that clinicians providing services will be familiar with current methods of assessment and treatment. Good clinicians strive to keep up with the current literature by updating their knowledge through reading journals, attending professional conferences, and going to workshops. The drive to remain abreast of past and current trends is a shared characteristic of the good researcher and the good clinician. Keeping up with contemporary literature improves the ability to do both research and clinical work.

We have attempted to show that the general attributes discussed above are critical to both research and clinical work. They are indispensable because these characteristics give us the ability to ask pertinent questions and solve problems, whether in the context of a research study or a case you are seeing in the clinic. Good observation, objectivity, organization, gathering data, analyzing data, and keeping up with current literature are all critical attributes for clinical and empirical problem solving. Cultivate these characteristics during your training and in your later career because they are essential for effective research and clinical practice.

Parallels in Clinical and Research Processes

Let us now focus for a moment on the "processes" involved in research and clinical work. We go through a series of steps in order to do a research project, and we also proceed through a sequence of events as we engage in clinical diagnosis and treatment programs. Figure 1.6 illustrates the steps involved in research, diagnosis, and treatment. You can see how the processes of all three enterprises are somewhat analogous. Obviously, clinical work is *not* research and research is *not* clinical work. There are, however, certain parallels between the two that can be seen without too much stretching.

Diagnosis as a Research Activity

A clinician engaging in assessment is dealing with the unknown. We do not know what kind of communication disorder is being presented when a person comes to the clinic for an evaluation. Granted, we sometimes know some general information from the case history forms or the complaint a client articulates when setting up an appointment, but we certainly do not know all the details. So if a mother says that her child does not seem to hear her when she tells him things, we might suspect that the youngster has a hearing loss. But this is a long way from knowing the details or even if hearing impairment is the culprit in this situation. It could be that the child has attention deficit disorder or some other condition that might make him not pay attention. If the child does have a hearing loss, we do not know its extent or if it is conductive, sensorineural, or mixed. Thus, in our assessments we are constantly dealing with the unknown. Scientists as well are charting unknown territories when they study a phenomenon of interest. The way a researcher initially approaches the unknown is quite similar to the diagnostician (Haynes & Pindzola, 2008).

As Figure 1.6 demonstrates, a researcher must do a thorough review of the existing literature prior to designing and implementing a scientific investigation. We have said before that this review provides a solid rationale for doing the research. A clinician engaged in a diagnostic evaluation must spend considerable time reviewing historical information on a client. Many clients have had prior evaluations or have been referred by another professional for the assessment. We routinely have clients fill out case history information prior to the evaluation so that we can focus on areas of interest that we suspect may be related to their problem. In addition to the paper and pencil kind of historical information we always conduct an in-depth interview

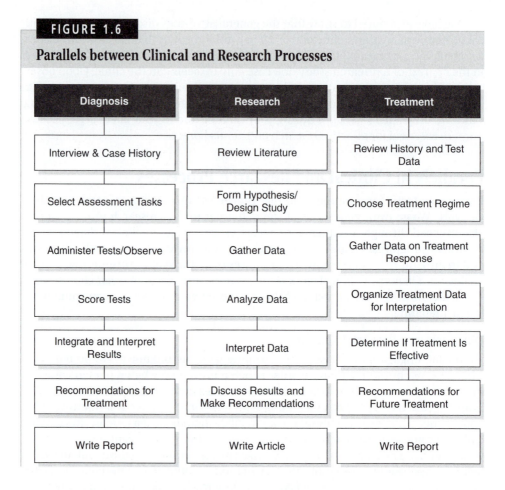

FIGURE 1.6

Parallels between Clinical and Research Processes

Diagnosis	Research	Treatment
Interview & Case History	Review Literature	Review History and Test Data
Select Assessment Tasks	Form Hypothesis/ Design Study	Choose Treatment Regime
Administer Tests/Observe	Gather Data	Gather Data on Treatment Response
Score Tests	Analyze Data	Organize Treatment Data for Interpretation
Integrate and Interpret Results	Interpret Data	Determine If Treatment Is Effective
Recommendations for Treatment	Discuss Results and Make Recommendations	Recommendations for Future Treatment
Write Report	Write Article	Write Report

with the client or the parents to obtain even more background data that might help in our evaluation. One can easily see that this step in either research or diagnosis is highly similar in both types of activity.

Once a researcher has reviewed the literature, an answerable scientific question is formulated and an empirical investigation is designed to answer it. You might think that this is the point where researchers and clinicians part company, but that is not so. Every evaluation is different, or at least it should be. We do not simply run all of our clients through the same set of tests and observations as part of a package; instead, we typically select assessment tasks based on questions we might have about the client. Diagnosticians must develop some questions about the client and design an assessment plan to address these queries. We wonder if a client who has had a stroke has visual difficulties, paralysis, paresis, swallowing difficulties, aphasia, apraxia, dysarthria, cognitive problems, hearing impairment, or reading or writing difficulties. Our examination must be designed to differentially diagnose one problem from another, and we must plan to administer enough tests and tasks so that all of our questions can be answered at the end of our evaluation. This is invariably different for each client and no standardized diagnostic protocol can possibly account for the potential individual difficulties presented by every patient. In this way, diagnosis is built from the ground up by the clinician selecting a number of tasks to do based on the client's historical information and complaints. Clinicians have particular questions that need to be answered about a client before a treatment plan can be formulated. It is very similar to a researcher asking unique questions and designing a specific study to answer them.

One of the clearest parallels between research and diagnosis is gathering data. In diagnosis, clinicians administer tests and obtain many nonstandardized measures of communicative behavior. Scientists often give tests as part of a research project and many of their measurements are of clinically relevant behaviors. Thus, we should not have to do much convincing to prove that both clinicians and researchers gather data.

We have made the point in an earlier section that data, once gathered, must be analyzed. The analysis includes such steps as organizing scores and behavioral information, scoring tests, and tallying instances of behaviors that are of interest. Both researchers and diagnosticians must organize data before making judgments about the interpretation of the data.

Without interpretation, any data that we gather in research or diagnosis represents just a lot of unrelated numbers. The data become meaningful to the researcher or diagnostician when patterns can be discerned among the numbers and these patterns relate to relevant clinical or empirical constructs. Thus, a particular pattern of clinical performance across a variety of tests and tasks may suggest a "diagnosis" of a specific type of disorder. In research, a particular type of statistical result may suggest a strong relationship between several variables and allow us to predict future behavior with more accuracy. Whether for diagnosis or research, the clinician or researcher must interpret the data in order to make it meaningful and useful. The process is highly similar in both enterprises.

Researchers will tell you that the results of a scientific study will often raise more questions than it answers. A researcher who finds that the incidence of a particular communication is more prevalent in a particular population now wonders about other populations not studied or the reason for the higher occurrence in one group over another. At the end of most journal articles you will find a paragraph that talks about suggestions for further research in which the researcher outlines possible lines of investigation for the future. Similarly, a diagnostic evaluation raises more questions than it answers and results in further testing or referral. Most of the time, diagnostic evaluations are confined to a particular slot of time, depending on the work setting. Some settings like universities allot a two-hour time frame for an evaluation. Other sites such as hospitals may only allow thirty minutes to complete a diagnostic evaluation. Even in the university setting where we have two hours, we rarely are able to complete all of the diagnostic tasks that we would ideally like to administer.

As a result, we have to indicate in our diagnostic report that further testing should be administered in the beginning phases of treatment. We may also determine that the client needs to be referred to another professional (e.g., audiologist, psychologist) for further evaluation. We may even have a section in our report that suggests further evaluation tasks that we did not have the opportunity to administer. That sounds very much like the researcher who suggests a course of future research to more completely answer a research question.

Both in research and diagnosis there is some written summary of the process. For researchers, the summary of the investigation may be in the form of a journal article or a written handout designed to accompany a convention presentation. For diagnosticians, an assessment report is generated that summarizes what was done in the evaluation and made a permanent part of the client's record. Summarizing research or diagnostic evaluations generally pulls together all of the steps discussed in this section. A good diagnostic report or journal article summarizes the background of the study or client, the design of the study or evaluation, the types of data gathered, the analysis of the data, the interpretation of the data into a meaningful form, and suggestions for future research or assessment. It is easy to see the similarities.

Treatment as a Research Activity

As illustrated above, the process of doing a diagnostic evaluation has parallels with the scientific method. We will now examine the steps illustrated in Figure 1.6 having to do with the relationship between treatment and the research process.

We can easily dispense with the first step in the process. Earlier sections have shown the importance of reviewing the literature prior to designing a research study. In clinical treatment of communication disorders, it would be foolhardy to prescribe a particular kind of treatment for a client without thoroughly examining diagnostic reports and recommendations. In both research and treatment processes, review of pertinent background information is critical.

The second step in the research process is to form a hypothesis and design a study. For example, a researcher reviews the literature on fluency disorders in adults and finds that stuttering is reduced in the presence of masking noise. The researcher wants to determine if the same is true in children with fluency disorders. Now this researcher might guess or hypothesize that a reduction of stuttering in children would occur based on the studies done on adults in the past but cannot with certainty predict how a study will turn out. Despite the reasonable belief that a particular outcome is probable, until the study is done the result will not be known. What a weird position in which to find yourself. You believe an event will turn out a certain way, but you really do not know if it will, in fact, materialize. Welcome to the clinic! Let's talk about how we do therapy for stuttering. There are probably twenty different treatments for stuttering. All of them have been shown to work on at least *some* people who stutter, but none of them have been agreed by experts to work on *all* people with fluency disorders. No matter what the disorder area, we always have a variety of approaches to take in treatment. How do we select a particular treatment? Are there treatments for any communication disorder that work 100 percent of the time? Probably not. So your choice of a treatment regimen for a client is influenced by many factors such as what you learned in school, efficacy studies in the current literature, your past experience in having success with a technique, the availability of materials for a particular method, time constraints, specific symptoms of the client, certain client behavioral or psychological characteristics, and many other variables. Most often, selection of a treatment mode is arbitrary. The same client seen at a different clinic by a different clinician may receive a totally different approach in treatment. And now we have to ask, "Will the treatment that we have selected work for the client?" Actually, this is a fairly easy question to answer. We simply do not know if the treatment that we initially select will be effective. It could, or it could not. That is the nature of clinical intervention. If we had techniques that would work 100 percent of the time there would be no question. But clinicians vary in their skill in therapy and judgment about the true nature of the client's problem. Perhaps there is incomplete diagnostic information and the client has issues that are unknown to the clinician. Also, clients vary in motivation, severity, intelligence, and commitment. Treatment can fail for many reasons, including clinician variables, client variables, or a combination of both. So we are in the same position as the researcher. Will the study come out as anticipated, with all the strong reasons to think it should? Will the treatment be successful, even though the clinician knows it has worked in the past for other similar clients? It has been said that all therapy is really a single case experiment. That is, we do not know what will truly work, but we will select a probable approach, take data on client performance, and make any necessary changes in the program to result in progress. Think about that idea, because it is quite profound. Therapy is like a single case experiment. We start out a particular way and then we tweak the program if the client's progress stalls. The choice of a treatment regimen is only an educated guess, just like a researcher's hypothesis. Will it be correct? Only an analysis of the data will tell.

As we said in the prior section, we will not know if treatment is successful until we gather data on the client's performance. If it is fluency we are interested in we count moments of disfluency and hope they diminish as treatment progresses. Without data, clinicians are not able to tell if their treatment is working. Similarly, researchers must gather data to see if children are more fluent when they are listening to masking noise. Gathering data is critical to both treatment and research.

Once we gather data in either clinical treatment sessions or in a research project, it must be organized so that we can make some judgments about its meaning. In treatment, data usually are arranged by therapy session so that we can see if certain behaviors increase or decrease over time. In a research project, data must be organized for statistical analysis and interpretation.

After data are gathered and organized, we can make some determinations about what the findings mean. In treatment, our most important determination is whether therapy has been successful or if we need to modify our approach. If the clinical behaviors we are attempting to train have increased over time, we generally believe that our decision about the type of therapy to use is substantiated. However, we said before that a treatment plan is only a guess. The data will let us know if it is successful or not. Similarly, in a research project, the scientist might find that children's fluency is significantly better when they listen to masking noise as compared to performance without masking noise. Again, an analysis of the data show that a particular hypothesis is supported, very similar to the way our clinical treatment data support our therapy plan.

Often in the research process the data analysis and interpretation show that the researcher's study was not optimally designed or that there were errors in how the study was conducted. This results in the researcher making suggestions for modifying future research projects designed to answer a particular question. Science is always evolving because there are better ways to answer questions and new information to consider. In treatment, we are faced with the same issue. Let's say that the treatment data do not show client improvement over the course of therapy. Knowing that the initial therapy plan was only an educated guess about what is likely to work for the client, we should not be surprised or disappointed if we have to modify our attack on the problem. Even a good clinician is not always able to initially select a successful treatment approach at the outset of therapy. If such a thing were knowable, everyone would do it and we would all be master clinicians. Since we have no certainty in knowing what approach will work for a given client, this is an unrealistic goal. The mark of a good clinician is more related to how one deals with adversity and failure of an initial treatment approach. It involves being able to systematically modify the treatment plan when it is not working for the client by knowing as many variables as possible to manipulate in the face of failure. To paraphrase Charles Van Riper, "The more therapeutic arrows you have in your quiver, the better clinician you will be." And don't think that only one modification will always be enough. Gathering and analyzing more treatment data after you change the program may suggest that you need to make further modifications to your approach. This is not failure; it is just being a good clinician.

The Benefits of Becoming a Clinician-Researcher

In an earlier section we introduced the concept of clinician-researcher, someone who although employed in primarily a clinical capacity also contributes to the research base in communication disorders. We tried to make the point that there is a critical need for applied clinical research in communication disorders and this type of investigation is most appropriately done by clinicians, either independently or in collaboration with professionals in university settings. Why, you might ask, should I consider becoming a clinician-researcher? What benefits might I gain? Will I get a membership card and a secret code ring? Believe it or not, there are actually some reasons why people might want to become a clinician-investigator (see Figure 1.7).

Some of you have already decided that you would be open to participating in research at some point in your career. And we know that there are others who, even if we did give them a membership card and secret code ring, would still not do it. That's OK. This section is for those people who are on the fence.

1. *Make a contribution.* A major benefit of becoming a clinician-researcher is that you will be able to contribute important applied clinical research to the field of

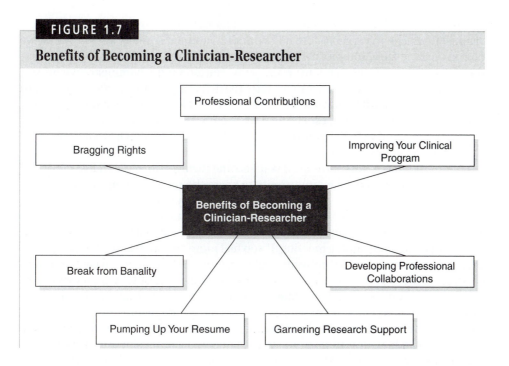

FIGURE 1.7

Benefits of Becoming a Clinician-Researcher

communication disorders. Our field is in dire need of applied research into evaluation and treatment issues. You will be in a good position to provide such data from a real-world caseload rather than in the rarefied atmosphere of a university or laboratory. This type of contribution should not be underestimated, and it is a good way for you to give something back to our field.

2. *A refreshing break from banality.* As faculty members, we are perennially refreshed by the optimism, drive, and excitement of our students. We set them adrift on the job market with hopes and dreams and the thought that they will change the world by helping people, as Van Riper said, "who talk with words that have broken wings." This enthusiasm in our students is infectious and helps to keep us older and jaded faculty members going for yet another semester. It is interesting, however, to see our students after they are five or ten years past graduation. After years of presenting the same pure tones and telling children how to make speech sounds, they are sometimes less than enthusiastic. Some, as in any profession, are suffering from "burnout" and have changed job settings a couple of times. Others are bored with therapy and assessment and are looking for something to get them "fired up" again. One of the present authors once asked a local pediatrician to collaborate on a research project on language development in children. The doctor's eyes lit up as he excitedly agreed, recounting his frustration that over 90 percent of the cases he sees are children with upper respiratory infections. He said it was tiresome to do the same type of examination time after time and prescribe the same medications over

and over again. Where were all those interesting cases he learned about in medical school? The same thing can happen in communication disorders. Much of what we do can become fairly routine after a number of years. And we are only talking about the assessment and therapy; don't even get us started on the administrative hassles and paperwork requirements. At any rate, participating in a research project with your colleagues or with someone in another setting like a university will open up a whole new world of interest, especially if it is a clinically oriented study. It could very well be that becoming a clinician-researcher will be a key element in saving your sanity as your career progresses.

3. *Pumping up your resume.* If you become involved in research as a clinician-researcher, you will have the opportunity to share the results of your work with colleagues on many levels. Let's say you work in a school system and you develop a new screening instrument in collaboration with a faculty member at a local university. You can share the development and use of this new clinical tool with your colleagues during an in-service training meeting. If you feel more ambitious, you can submit the project to a state or national convention and present the research to a wider range of colleagues. If you receive favorable feedback, you might want to write up an article summarizing your research for a state, regional or national journal. Every step of this process can be documented in your resume as an accomplishment. Most resumes have a section for presentations and another section for publications. As you engage in more research, your resume grows to reflect your accomplishments. How do employers distinguish among students or professionals that they will hire for a vacant position? First of all, everyone has a master's degree, so that is not a significant discriminator. Second, if you have a master's degree, most programs demand that you have maintained above a 3.0 grade point average (GPA) for graduation, so most students have a "B" average or above. That is not much of a discriminator. A third discriminator might be the type of program from which you graduated. In order to be certified, one must graduate from an ASHA-accredited program, and nowadays almost all master's programs are accredited. Certainly, there are differences among programs in terms of their national ranking and the prestige of the faculty, but overall accredited programs must ensure that a graduate meets specific knowledge and skill requirements for clinical practice. A fourth discriminator might be job experience; however, for this example let us assume that two job applicants both have three years of clinical practice. Again, the candidates are roughly similar. If an employer is deciding between two resumes that both show candidates having master's degrees earned with similar GPAs, from similar accredited programs and having similar postgraduate experience, there is precious little to differentiate one from the other. If, on the other hand, one candidate has a resume that reflects state and local convention presentations, some publications, and some grant money received for research, this represents a real discriminator that an employer could use. The candidate with a research background has done everything the other candidate has done but also has a whole other dimension of expertise and involvement. Thus, being a clinician-researcher can be an important way to show that you are professionally active and a "cut above" the average graduate in communication disorders.

4. *Improving your clinical program.* We have suggested that if a person becomes a clinician-researcher, a logical focus of scientific studies would be his or her own caseload or work setting. By concentrating research efforts on current activities, a clinician is not required to set aside research time on a totally unrelated topic and will not be doing the study on evenings and weekends. A clinician focusing on his or her own caseload will find all sorts of interesting issues to address. By doing research, you can demonstrate the effectiveness of your own clinical program (Wambaugh & Bain, 2002). You can gather normative data for the local population you are dealing with in clinical work. For example, we have very few local norms for language and phonology for different cultural groups and most normative data available are based on white, middle class children. Gathering local norms will benefit your own clinical program and be of interest to others who work with similar populations. As mentioned previously, you can develop assessment and screening protocols and generate norms for these procedures to use in daily clinical practice. You may also have ideas for unique treatment protocols or materials that require some study to determine if they are more or less effective than existing approaches. All of these projects can be addressed by the clinician-researcher in the context of the work setting and add to the effectiveness of the clinical program.

5. *Developing professional collaborations.* Research is one of the most effective ways to foster collaboration among professionals, both within and between work settings. All across the country there are university faculty who need to produce research to be eligible for promotion and tenure. Likewise, schools, hospitals, rehabilitation centers, physicians' offices, and other settings are replete with clinicians who have access to caseloads but little research experience. These professionals would like to answer clinical questions, validate their treatment regimens with outcome data, and develop more efficient methods of service delivery. If university faculty and professionals in work settings could collaborate on applied clinical research, everyone would benefit, including our clients (Williams & Fagelson, 2003). We challenge you to develop collaborative relationships with university faculty when you get into the workforce. If you visited a university faculty member, described your caseload, and indicated a desire to participate in research, it is very probable that the faculty member will be elated and grateful for the opportunity to work with you. Remember, university faculty have research expertise but typically lack a population to study. You have a caseload, some knowledge of research, and may only need some advice about how to proceed in a scientific investigation. One impediment to such collaboration is that clinicians and researchers are often not encouraged to work together, or one assumes that the other may not be interested in collaboration. One of the basic principles of the current text is to provide encouragement and many examples of collaboration in action. Collaboration between clinician-researchers and other professionals that have greater research expertise should be encouraged. A clinician-researcher with a good basic knowledge of the scientific method, essentials of research design, and a conceptual knowledge of statistical procedures would be an ideal collaborator with a university faculty member. Knowledge of these essentials is available in the present text and will promote collaboration with more experienced researchers, allowing

the mutual development of more sophisticated research designs and statistical treatments. One barrier to collaboration has been that practitioners are often unfamiliar with the basic aspects of research design, experimental control, and statistical treatment. This may lead to a feeling that they are unequal participants in collaboration or a feeling that the more experienced researcher is "directing" the practitioner as a student. If the practitioner can approach the collaboration with a good working knowledge of basic experimental design and the scientific method as presented in the present textbook, these perceptions should be minimized. However, although these concepts are basic to the process, they may not include the subtleties required for a successful design or analysis, which is why we encourage clinicians to collaborate with other professionals in universities and clinical settings who have more experience and specific expertise. But they must come to the table with some basic knowledge of the research process such as asking answerable questions, choosing valid and reliable measurements, controlling for contaminating variables, and some conceptual appreciation of how statistical procedures can be used to answer questions. Those are exactly the issues that we deal with in this book. It is our belief that a person who develops an appreciation for the scientific method and a basic expertise in experimental design will develop confidence in the ability to critically evaluate research, produce simple research projects, and effectively participate as a collaborator with other professionals having more experience. These collaborations can be some of the most satisfying professional relationships you will ever experience.

　　6. *Research begets research support.* An interesting phenomenon is how one research project leads to another. We mentioned earlier that the results of a particular study usually raise additional questions for the scientist. If a public school clinician gathered normative data on utterance length from three-year-old African American children in the local area, then a logical follow-up might be to examine four and five year olds. Having the results from the study of three year olds, a clinician-researcher might approach the local school district for support on purchasing audiotapes or a digital recorder to use in a study of four to five year olds in the system. If the results from the study of three year olds has proven to be clinically useful for the speech-language pathologists in the school system, chances are that the school district would at least consider supporting future studies that also promise a benefit. Also, the clinician-researcher shown to be capable and dependable in terms of designing and completing a research project will find greater access to the grant support available through many private foundations and government agencies. One has a much better chance of obtaining grant support with a track record of successful research. A clinician-researcher can obtain all sorts of tests, materials, equipment, and even research assistants to help with an investigation by applying for the millions of dollars that are available. You have nothing to lose and everything to gain by applying for grant support. The more research you do, the easier it is to succeed in obtaining grant monies.

　　7. *Bragging rights.* By becoming a clinician-researcher, you can bring prestige to yourself and your facility. We have already indicated that research is one important way to add to one's professional resume. By doing so, you can show the world that

you are a multidimensional professional. But this only serves to showcase your own capabilities. Let us assure you that bragging is not only a phenomenon seen on an individual level, but it is also an integral part of organizations. For instance, in a school system the special education coordinator may be asked to provide an annual report to the school superintendent about accomplishments in the special education area. If in addition to the regular provision of special education services, some members of the department have done research and presented it at state or national meetings and published in a journal, you can be assured that the special education coordinator will be very interested in making this part of the annual report. Why? Because it allows the special education department to "toot its own horn." The same thing is true in hospital settings. If a clinician-researcher develops a new bedside screening procedure for stroke patients this is presented and published, the head of the speech pathology section will no doubt want to include this in a report to the hospital administration. And it doesn't stop there. When the school superintendent gets word that the special education department is doing research, you can be sure that this will be presented as part of the school system accomplishments to the city council. When the hospital administrator learns of the research on the bedside screening test developed in the hospital, you can be certain that the administrator will let the board of directors know about it. When a clinician-researcher publishes an article or does a presentation on a research project, the authors and *their affiliations* are always included right under the title of the article or presentation. So the world can see "Susan Smith, Montgomery County School System, PA" or "Susan Smith, East Rutherford General Hospital, IL" and it amounts to free advertising for you and your facility. At any rate, do not underestimate the importance and impact of public relations and bragging rights. Most facilities absolutely love it when they can talk about research produced, papers presented, articles published, and grant support received. You can almost see the pay raises marching over the horizon.

Summary

Communication sciences and disorders is a profession that has achieved significant credibility and respect over the years from other disciplines as well as the public at large. One major component of professional credibility is the emphasis that our field places on the importance of research. We facilitate it, produce it, publish it, present it, teach it to students in training, and keep up with it through continuing education requirements. Clinical work and research have many parallels in diagnosis and treatment. The attributes of a good researcher are similar to those possessed by a good clinician. It is not productive for us to view the clinical and research enterprises as incompatible. Since we are an applied clinical field, there are many opportunities for collaboration among clinicians and those interested in research to provide important data related to the nature, assessment, and treatment of communication disorders. Especially in this era of evidence-based practice, it is important to foster collaboration between professionals in a variety of work settings to produce clinically relevant research.

LEARNING ACTIVITIES

1. Borrow a copy of a recent professional journal and look at the authors' affiliations (where they work) for every article in that issue of the periodical. Pay attention to the different types of work settings and the degrees held by the researchers.
2. For that same issue of the journal, tally how many articles focus on assessment, treatment, and general topics of research. Are most of them laboratory studies or applied clinical research?
3. Interview two SLPs or audiologists in your local area who have engaged in research but are not working in the university setting. Summarize the types of research they did and their feelings about the research process.
4. Locate three different journals and see if you can find their acceptance rate for submitted articles.
5. Locate the "call for papers" for a national and state convention and outline the criteria for paper submission and peer review.
6. Interview a faculty member at your university regarding the process and perceived pitfalls in submitting research for publication.
7. Locate sources of student research support on your campus.

CHAPTER 2

Scientific Principles and Methods Used by Researchers

> Science is best defined as a careful, disciplined, logical search for knowledge about any and all aspects of the universe, obtained by examination of the best available evidence and always subject to correction and improvement upon discovery of better evidence. What's left is magic. And it doesn't work.
>
> —James Randi, aka The Amazing Randi, magician and author

In order to understand science, one must learn to appreciate the philosophical framework from which scientists operate. The methods used by researchers to understand the world are unique to scientists and separate them from other groups such as philosophers, artists, theologians, and historians. Scientists must also have strong ethical principles, which have evolved over the past century for the conduct of their work. Finally, there are many published works that claim to be scientific in nature but in actuality are pseudoscientific, junk science, or quackery. This chapter attempts to outline scientific principles and methods used by researchers so that you will be able to distinguish scientific from nonscientific work in the extant literature.

LEARNING OBJECTIVES

This chapter will enable readers to:

- Understand the various ways in which we learn about the world.
- Become familiar with the characteristics of science and how it differs from other ways of knowing.
- Understand ethical issues in research involving scientific misconduct and treatment of human and animal participants.
- Differentiate among legitimate science, pseudoscience, junk science, and quackery.

Sinister Stereotypes

Many people have a stereotypical view of scientists and researchers, perceiving them as objective, cold, calculating, eccentric, uncaring, obsessive, and often quite mad. A quick computer search generated the following list of defining characteristics of a "mad scientist," which unfortunately, is how some people seem to view researchers in general (http://en.wikipedia.org):

- Pursuit of science without regard to its ethical implications
- Self-experimentation
- Playing God, tinkering with nature
- Lack of normal relationships
- Perpetually unkempt appearance or physical deformity
- Speaking with a German or Eastern European accent
- In villains, maniacal laughter, especially pronounced when their experiments reach their climax

Not all that flattering, is it? But we are sure you can recall characters in films or books that pretty much embodied those characteristics. Early prototypes in literature included Mary Shelley's *Frankenstein* written in 1818 and Robert Louis Stevenson's *Dr. Jekyll and Mr. Hyde* penned in 1886. Later these same characters were portrayed in films before 1945. Scores of more recent films show scientists exhibiting many of the characteristics mentioned above (*Dr. Strangelove,* 1964; Dr. Loveless in *Wild, Wild West,* 1999; and Dr. Totenkopf in *Sky Captain and the World of Tomorrow,* 2004). Why have scientists been depicted this way in literature and in films? Do all researchers have the same personality characteristics? Is there any truth to these stereotypes? In general, it is a good practice to avoid thinking in stereotypes, because they almost always distort characteristics of the group in question. On the other hand, you have no doubt heard that there is probably a kernel of truth in most stereotypes, because the group is at least recognizable from the generalization. A major source of the "mad scientist" stereotype probably flows from the beliefs held by scientists and the scientific methods themselves that are used by researchers. One connection binding all scientists together is that there is a *method* to our madness. The "process" of research, known as the scientific method, will make researchers appear similar because the approach they take to answering questions embodies many of the same steps, no matter what they are studying. Also, the beliefs that most scientists have regarding the most valid ways of learning about the world also contribute to their similarity. This chapter will discuss some of the principles that underlie scientific inquiry and the procedures that have historically been the process of science. But first, we will discuss nonscientific ways of learning about the world.

Ways of Knowing about the World

Classical introductions to science usually include the seminal philosophical and metaphysical work of Charles Sanders Peirce, who discussed four ways of knowing or fixing belief (*The Fixation of Belief,* 1877, in Houser and Kloesel, 1992). Peirce has been credited with pioneering a school of thought known as *pragmatism* which partially flowed out of a series of discussions at Harvard University with Oliver Wendell Holmes and William James and other members of "the Metaphysical Club." Some of the ways we learn about the world are more susceptible to distortion and error than others, but even our most reliable methods cannot escape a certain degree of error.

Although most authorities feel that science has certain advantages over other ways of knowing, even science has imperfections that must be dealt with. We will discuss the classical ways of fixing belief below. Figure 2.1 illustrates the ways of knowing we will discuss in this chapter.

The first of Peirce's ways of knowing is called the **method of tenacity** in which people persist in believing a particular view just because that is what they have always done. Tenacity implies that a person holds on to a perspective, sometimes even when faced with new information that suggests the old belief may be in error. In *The Fixation of Belief,* Peirce says:

> This method of fixing belief . . . will be unable to hold its ground in practice. The social impulse is against it. The man who adopts it will find that other men think differently from him, and it will be apt to occur to him, in some saner moment, that their opinions are quite as good as his own, and this will shake his confidence in his belief. . . . Unless we make ourselves hermits, we shall necessarily influence each other's opinions; so that the problem becomes how to fix belief, not in the individual merely, but in the community. (1877, pp. 116–117)

Obviously, if the method of tenacity were our only means of "knowing," an individual or society as a whole would not progress very far. When we believe something because "that is the way it has always been" we are eliminating the opportunity to see things from a new and different perspective. For example, some people continue to keep all of their money in a standard passbook savings account earning less than one half of one percent interest per year because that is what they have always done. They tenaciously hold on to this view of saving money even though they might earn significantly higher interest with little risk if they put the money in certificates of deposit or bonds. Similarly, when mothers tell their kids they will get a cold if they go outside with wet hair, they will ruin their eyes if they sit too close to the television screen, or they must wait one hour after eating before they swim, they are passing on beliefs that have little scientific support. They are just passing on beliefs tenaciously held by their families and it's easier to go with the inertia than really investigate the truth of the matter. One can readily see that the method of tenacity is probably not

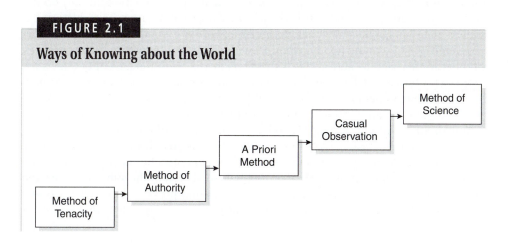

FIGURE 2.1

Ways of Knowing about the World

the most effective way of learning about the world or advancing our level of technology and thinking.

The second way of knowing is the **method of authority** and it, to some degree, builds on the method of tenacity. If we extend the method of tenacity to a social group, such as a government or a church, we essentially "institutionalize" belief and these institutions tell people what is true and false in the world. This will result in a kind of coherency in the beliefs and actions of a community, and everyone will be happy. But Peirce finds some problems with this method of fixing belief:

> There will be men who possess a wider sort of social feeling; they see that men in other countries and in other ages have held to very different doctrines from those which they themselves have been brought up to believe; and they cannot help seeing that it is the mere accident of their having been taught as they have, and of their having been surrounded with the manners and associations they have, that has caused them to believe as they do and not far differently. Nor can their candour resist the reflection that there is no reason to rate their own views at a higher value than those of other nations and other centuries; thus giving rise to doubts in their minds. (1877, p. 119)

In our contemporary society, we have several ways that "authorities" on particular topics can communicate "the truth" to the rest of the world. Written materials in the form of books, periodicals, newspapers, and information on the Internet are outlets for many authorities to pontificate on a variety of topics. Certainly, the credibility of an "authority" is enhanced by degrees and credentials that suggest the person has expertise in a specific area. Large institutions such as governments and religious organizations are not shy about telling people what to believe and how to behave. Whatever these institutions say is truth carries a large degree of gravitas simply because they are authoritative and have credibility. So if a spokesperson for the government says that a particular model of automobile is unsafe or safe, many people will tend to believe this information. When an authority from the church says that you should vote for a particular political party because it will support family values, you will tend to believe this information. Unfortunately, an authority can make such statements as simply a personal opinion or with an incomplete review of the existing data on the topic. Authorities are often champions of a particular point of view and they do not care about information that conflicts with their bias. On a darker level, history has shown that demagogues have passed on beliefs of hate, genocide, and racism that were embraced by many people who listened unquestioningly to these authorities. Another forum used by authorities is the mass media. With the advent of television, radio, the Internet, satellite radio, and movies, authorities have even more resources to reach masses of people around the world. With every news event, the networks assemble a group of "authorities" to tell people how to interpret current events. Another venue for authorities to dispense knowledge about the world is through "live" verbal communication in classes, speeches, and lectures. As you sit in classes listening to professors talk about "the truth" in their discipline, you must be constantly aware that they may be presenting either a biased or a balanced view of the subject matter. You are relying on authority when you believe information presented in your textbooks and classes. Now obviously, the method of authority as a way of knowing about the world is not all bad. Learning about the world from authorities is an essential means of gaining knowledge in today's world (Kerlinger, 1973). Clearly, relying on authorities can save us significant time that we would otherwise have to spend individually investigating a particular issue. But the obvious caveat is that we must be very careful about which authorities we give credence to before we internalize what they want us to believe. Be wary of who you regard as an authority. Ask authorities where they got their information to make their judgments about "the truth" of the matter. The Internet is a veritable hotbed of information on any topic you wish to explore. With the software available to create impressive websites, many of these web pages are very slick and may seem credible. Yet try inputting "alien abduction" into your favorite search engine and you will find hundreds of websites that deal in abductions, crop formations, alien implant removal, deprogramming, and many other topics that have not been generally accepted as "truth." To its credit, the Internet has sites solely devoted to debunking myths, misinformation, and half truths presented to the public on the World Wide Web by "authorities" from a variety of areas (www.snopes.com). So while we do rely on authority as a means of knowing the world, we must be vigilant about where these authorities got their information and how completely they have investigated the area in question.

The third way of knowing about the world is what Peirce called the **a priori method** and it builds on the other two methods discussed previously. Others have called this the *method of intuition* or the *method of pure rationalism* (Schiavetti & Metz, 2002), because this method involves the use of discussion and reasoning to acquire knowledge. According to Peirce:

> A different new method of settling opinions must be adopted, that shall not only produce an impulse to believe, but shall also decide what proposition it is which is to be believed. Let the action of natural preferences be unimpeded, then, and under their influence let men, conversing together and regarding matters in different lights, gradually develop beliefs in harmony with natural causes. . . . Systems of this sort have not usually rested upon observed facts, at least not in any great degree. They have been chiefly adopted because their fundamental propositions seemed "agreeable to reason." (1877, p. 119)

Rationalists are most associated with using deductive reasoning in which general principles are used to make conclusions about specific cases. Logic or reason to divine the "truth" about a particular topic can be useful, but it can also lead to error and distortion. Logic is only as good as the assumptions underlying logical thought. For instance, if one believed, as they did in ancient Greece, that "humors" circulated in the bloodstream, then perhaps the practice of bleeding or bloodletting might be a logical medical procedure to use in treating physical ailments. Again, Peirce finds flaws in the a priori method as in the others mentioned above:

> This method is far more intellectual and respectable from the point of view of reason than either of the others which we have noticed. But its failure has been the most manifest. It makes of inquiry something similar to the development of taste; but taste, unfortunately, is always more or less a matter of fashion, and accordingly metaphysicians have never come to any fixed agreement, but the pendulum has swung backward and forward between a more material and a more spiritual philosophy, from the earliest times to the latest. (1877, p. 119)

Thus, discussion among individuals, intuition, logic, and rationalism are capricious and subject to change over time and evidently are not the royal road to discovering truth.

Before we discuss the scientific method, we would like to discuss a process that underlies all forms of fixing belief. Although we certainly defer to Peirce when it comes to knowing about knowing, we would like to spend some time focusing on the act of observing "reality." We are talking here about casual, **uncontrolled observation,** which is certainly alive and well in the world. In science, observation is highly controlled in terms of who is doing the observing, how it is measured, and how it is interpreted. Thus, there is a big difference between scientific observation and casual, uncontrolled observation. So what can be wrong with casual observation as a method of knowing about the world? There are several problems. First, it has long been held that no person can observe *everything* about an event. So many things are happening simultaneously and sometimes very quickly. Think of a car accident taking place on a busy street corner downtown. Could you really observe everything that occurred in that split second, everything that led up to the crash, and everything that ensued after the accident? It would not be possible. So even when observing a fairly simple event, a person may not be able to see it from all possible angles and perspectives. As you know, two people observing from different directions may report the events of an accident quite differently. Just the process of observation is incomplete unless you have multiple sources of video recording an event. A second problem with observation is that people and events are always different. The generalization you might make from watching one event (a car accident) may not even apply to crashes involving other types of cars, differing speeds, different drivers, or other road conditions. So any "truth" you extrapolate from a casual, uncontrolled observation may be incomplete. The Greek philosopher Heraclitus (c. 535–475 BC) suggested that people and events are constantly changing when he said "you never step into the same river twice." The river has changed, and time has changed you as well. So if you observed that car accident several years later after many other experiences, you may have attended to different aspects of the event with quite different interpretations about what you have seen. So far, we have just talked about the act of observing; it really gets dicey when we come to *interpreting* what we have observed. What does it mean? We know that people who have observed a robbery may come up with all sorts of different stories and interpretations about the acts, feelings, and judgments made by the perpetrator and the victims. Interpreting observations is a very slippery slope. And finally, when we turn our observations and interpretations into *language* to communicate what we have seen, we are one more step removed from reality. Although language can be specific, most language users may not actually describe events in the most accurate way when they are faced with cobbling together the semantics and syntax used in their explanation. Casual observation, then, is infested with error when it comes to learning about the world.

Now we turn to Peirce's **method of science.** He states:

> To satisfy our doubts therefore, it is necessary that a method should be found by which our beliefs may be caused by nothing human, but by some external permanency—by something upon which our thinking has no effect. . . . It must be something which affects, or might affect,

every man. And, though these affects are necessarily as various as are individual conditions, yet the method must be such that the ultimate conclusion of every man shall be the same, or would be the same if inquiry were sufficiently persisted in. Such is the method of science. . . . I may start with known and observed facts to proceed to the unknown; and yet the rules which I follow in doing so may not be such as investigation would approve. The test of whether I am truly following the method is not an immediate appeal to my feelings and purposes, but, on the contrary, itself involves the application of the method. Hence it is that bad reasoning as well as good reasoning is possible; and this fact is the foundation of the practical side of logic. (Peirce, 1877, p. 119)

In a later publication called *How to Make Ideas Clear* (1878) Peirce describes the elegance of a scientific approach to gaining knowledge:

This activity of thought by which we are carried, not where we wish, but to a fore-ordained goal, is like the operation of destiny. No modification of the point of view taken, no selection of other facts for study, no natural bent of mind even, can enable a man to escape the predestinate opinion. This great law is embodied in the conception of truth and reality. The opinion which is fated to be ultimately agreed to by all who investigate, is what we mean by the truth, and the object represented in this opinion is the real. That is the way I would explain reality. (Houser and Kloesel, 1992, pp. 138–139)

Peirce is saying that it is important for a person to develop beliefs and knowledge about the world through a process that is removed from personal biases, influences, and prejudices. Only science, as a methodology, can allow a person to examine phenomena apart from self. A certain amount of "objectivity" is built into the scientific method that reduces human bias, measurement error, and emotional and moral judgments. We will discuss these aspects of the scientific method in a later section.

Characteristics of Science

As we indicated in our discussion of Peirce's method of science, the scientific approach to gaining knowledge has traditionally been characterized by some very specific attributes. Kerlinger and Lee (2000) lament the difficulty in developing a universally agreed on definition of *science* or for that matter *scientific research*. Fortunately for us, they took the risk and provide the following definition of scientific research:

Scientific research is systematic, controlled, empirical, amoral, public and critical investigation of natural phenomena. (p. 14)

This definition is very tightly constructed and contains many critical points. Below, we will attempt to expand a bit on these issues and a few others not directly stated but implied in the definition. We view these issues as critical characteristics of scientific research.

The Systematic Nature of Science

Earlier in this chapter we referred to the "scientific method" as a procedure common to most scientists. This classical method discussed long ago by Pearson (1937) and further developed by others can be generally described as encompassing the following steps: 1) formulating a "problem," 2) reviewing background information, 3) developing a hypothesis, 4) designing an investigation or experiment, 5) gathering data, 6) analyzing data to confirm or disconfirm the hypothesis, and 7) revising the problem or hypothesis in light of the results of the experiment. It is not uncommon for some introductory textbooks about science to list the steps of the scientific method. Even though the present section is calculated to illustrate that researchers are "systematic," it is certainly not meant to imply that scientists use a cookie cutter approach to their work. It is also not meant to communicate that science is just a bunch of rigid procedures that stifle creativity and innovation in practitioners. Although it is true that the general procedures mentioned above are commonly used in a wide variety of research projects, epitomizing the notion that science is systematic, the actual practice of research will reveal that scientists using the "method" often do it in many different ways. In fact, many authorities in science indicate that when you examine the actual behavior of researchers performing their studies, there does not appear to be evidence of any single method that is generally applied (Carey, 1994; Gibbs & Lawson, 1992; Chalmers, 1990; Gjertsen, 1989). Carrier further illustrates the variety in the methods of science:

> [T]he methods that work well will vary according to what is being studied, and so "the scientific method" ends up a multifarious hodge-podge of "methods," some shared across fields, some specific to certain subjects of study, and these methods are themselves always subject to scrutiny and change over time, as their efficacy, or lack thereof, is discovered, and as new effective methods are found out. The exact same problem can even be explored using several different methods, and in fact scientists often seek to use several, as there is even greater certainty in the results if these same results are arrived at by completely different means. (2001, p. 4)

Interestingly, Medawar (1963) points out that one factor in perpetuating the perception that all scientists approach their work in the same manner is the conventions that we use to write up a research project after it is finished. Scientific journals and the papers they contain must be organized and reported in a specific way, and it gives the impression that all researchers approached their problem using the same steps in the same order. This, of course, is not the case in practice.

The systematic character of science then is not that researchers all use exactly the same methods but that they are meticulous in applying the methods they do use. Scientists are systematic in crafting answerable questions and designing their studies to minimize sources of error. Researchers are systematic in their methods of gathering data and analyzing their observations. Researchers, out of necessity, must be highly organized in their work, even though the stereotype of scientists is that they are absentminded. One cannot carry out a valid scientific investigation without significant attention to detail in every aspect of the research project. It is important to remember that these are not necessarily "personal" characteristics. They are part of the method of doing science. Although a scientist can have a messy garage at home, you will generally find that he or she is highly organized in the business of research. You cannot keep everything straight any other way and still have something relevant to analyze at the end of the study. Things must be done in a certain order for the experiment to work. Finally, a scientist must be able to report to other researchers exactly how a study was conducted so that the work can be evaluated and replicated by others.

Experimental Control

We have a major section on **experimental control** coming up in a later chapter, but we will briefly mention it here because it is a critical characteristic of research. When we say "control" we are referring to the researcher taking charge of certain extraneous sources of error that could affect the outcome of a particular study. Let's say that a researcher wants to see if three-year-old girls have a longer mean length of utterance (MLU) compared to three-year-old boys. On the surface, this seems to be a fairly simple study in which we could assemble 100 three year olds comprised of fifty boys and fifty girls. We decide to take a language sample from all of the children and calculate the MLU for each child. We then can compare the average MLU for the boys with the MLU for the girls. After analyzing our data, we find that the girls have an MLU of 5.00 and the boys have an MLU of 3.00. Now we can conclude that girls have a higher MLU than boys. Well, not so fast. Other researchers will ask what you "controlled for" in this study. You hope, of course, that the only explanation for the girls' MLU being higher than the boys' is the gender of the groups. But could someone come up with a competing explanation for the results? Let's try:

- Did you control for hearing ability? Could the boy group have had more kids with hearing loss and poorer language ability?
- Did you control for socioeconomic class? Could the boy group have had more children of lower socioeconomic status (SES), who have been shown in some studies to have shorter utterance lengths compared to middle SES children?
- Did you control for cultural variables? Did the boy group have more African American, Hispanic, or Asian children in it who speak dialects of English that reduce bound morphemes that are counted in MLU calculations?
- Did you have the same person take the samples from the boy and girl groups? If not, maybe the girl group had a more experienced language sampler and thus got longer samples.

These are among many possible extraneous variables we could ask the researcher about controlling for in this study. If the researcher "controlled" for them, the study is sound. If the researcher did not control for extraneous variables, then the finding that girls have a longer MLU than boys at age three and that it is due mainly to gender is susceptible to attack. Critics could say to the researcher, "The MLU difference could have been due to SES, hearing ability, ethnicity, or the sample elicitation method, so what are you going on about gender for? Any of these other explanations for the MLU difference is just as good as your gender explanation." The researcher who can answer these attacks by explaining the controls in the study is in good shape. For instance, a good researcher could control for hearing by screening all participants and control for SES by creating gender groups with equal numbers of middle and lower socioeconomic class children. Further, culture could be controlled for by balancing the groups by cultural group or just studying all white children (of course, then you could not generalize the results to boys and girls from other cultures). Finally, the language samples could be gathered by people with comparable levels of experience and training. The researcher interested in the effects of gender has to rule out all other variables that could affect the MLU that are *not* gender. Science is all about controlling sources of error that could contaminate the results of a study.

The notion of control also refers to gathering data under controlled conditions. For example, a scientist wanting to gather data on how people listen should do it under controlled conditions, such as placing participants in a sound-treated booth and presenting information through earphones that give consistent sound levels of the stimulus. By controlling the stimuli, task, and environment, all participants will experience comparable listening conditions. Thus, control is a critical characteristic of science and we will be discussing it frequently throughout this text.

The Public Nature of Science

It is extremely important that the scientific pursuit of knowledge is shared with other researchers and is open to public scrutiny. When an investigator reports a new finding, it is usually published in a scientific journal. In order to be published, as discussed in Chapter 1, the study must be written, submitted to a journal, and subjected to a rigorous peer review process. The reviewers must be provided with the exact methods, stimuli, tasks, data analysis procedures, and statistical treatment of the data in order to render a judgment on the quality of the research. In fact, when a topic of research is important enough, it is not unusual for scientists to visit the laboratory of a researcher and ask to see the data and how it was analyzed just to confirm that the study was done in accordance with scientific methods. If a researcher does not share this information with the scientific community, the study will not be accepted. In fact, scientists who do their experiments independently and refuse to share the details of their methods with other researchers are viewed as unethical by their peers. In the research community, one cannot make "scientific" statements without subjecting their work to the scrutiny of other scientists. Sometimes a person will say that they have done research supporting a particular result, but instead of detailing this in scientific journals they go straight to the popular media such as newspapers, magazines, television, or the Internet. On these media outlets they can easily say that they have done research and not be pressed to go into the details. Such behavior is often one of the first symptoms of "junk science" or "pseudoscience." For instance, it is not uncommon for a person who is trying to promote a particular product or point of view to claim "scientific support" to further their cause. Many people, whether they are scientists or not, can "talk the talk," but the proof of real scientific evidence is in "walking the walk." It is not unusual at all to hear proponents of the most wacky ideas say that they have research support in their corner, which is why we have a section in this chapter about junk science, pseudoscience, and quackery. In these cases, the practitioners may not have really used methods based on scientific principles, or they may have taken shortcuts in the scientific method. Unfortunately, anyone can say that they have done research on a particular topic, but will that study hold up to scientific scrutiny? Science is a process that a researcher must go through in order to answer questions. There are no shortcuts and just because someone claims to have "studied" something, it is not scientific unless certain procedures, methods, and safeguards have been performed and are *publicly* verifiable. As Carrier states:

> Science sets the highest bar, requiring the highest standards of verification, employing the most experienced and well-trained judges, and that is what makes it scientific (and superior to all other endeavors that claim to produce knowledge). Moreover, science does not conceal its evidence or rest its case on mysteries or private revelations, but makes everything public, so that all experts, and even the layman, can examine and weigh the claims and arguments of scientists to an extent not possible in any other field, creating the most effective check against individual bias that humans can devise. (2001, p. 3)

Replication in Science

An interesting and predictable characteristic of many neophyte researchers, whether students or faculty, is that they may think that their study will be the definitive investigation about their topic of inquiry. The world is waiting, with bated breath, for their results to finally "know the truth" about this important issue. Unfortunately, it rarely works this way. When we do a study, we are typically just adding another "data point" to a chain of studies that have examined the problem. We may have done it in a different way or added another variable to the equation, but we still are just putting our results out there for others to see and evaluate. Hegde points out the importance of **replication:**

> Replication, which is the repetition of a study with or without variations, is the method of establishing generality of research findings. A single study, no matter how well done, cannot establish generality. . . . A study must be repeated to find out if the evidence holds under different circumstances. (2003, p. 375)

One can readily see how replication can add significant strength to a particular hypothesis when the same results are found by a different investigator using different participants and gathering data under slightly different conditions. This is an obvious manifestation of how science takes a research issue away from any personal preferences or biases and through a series of related studies that show a clear trend in the data. Long ago, Peirce described the process by which the work of different scientists working within the constraints of science coalesces to reveal the "truth":

> (Scientists) may at first obtain different results, but as each perfects his method and his processes, the results are found to move steadily together toward a destined center. . . . Different minds may set out with the most antagonistic views, but the progress of investigation carries them by a force outside of themselves to one and the same conclusion. (1878, p. 138)

The progress of science thus can be seen as a series of individual data points (studies) that begin to form a "trend" that clearly and discernably points in a given direction, allowing scientists to make generalizations about the "truth" of a particular matter. Unfortunately, we do not see many replications in the literature on communication disorders. This could be due to researchers wanting to probe new areas or scientific journals emphasizing original research at the expense of publishing replication studies. Lately, more journals are reserving a section for "research notes" and replication studies, which is a positive development in our literature. We will discuss replication in more depth in a later section.

Empirical Testing

Empirical testing means that information is derived from experimentation, observation, and evidence rather than just theory. Kerlinger and Lee state that

> scientific investigation is empirical. If the scientist believes something is so, that belief must somehow or other be put to an outside independent test. (2000, p. 14)

It is important to go a bit beyond a rigid definition of empiricism as exclusively observation and evidence when we are discussing science. Part of empiricism involves the "interpretation" of evidence from observing test results, and this moves us into the realm of subjectivity. Interestingly, scientists study many directly unobservable phenomena such as magnetic fields and psychological states that must be operationally defined and taken with a certain degree of faith as being reality. It would be far simpler if science only dealt with readily measurable and agreed-on notions like height, weight, and chemical composition, but alas, it does not. For some, this creates a conundrum for a scientist that pits empirical measurement against subjective interpretation. Carrier says:

> Science builds up faith in its concepts, principles and conclusions through repeated practice or testing, and when its faith is challenged it returns again to examine the facts and see if its faith is justified by them. This is what makes science an *empirical* enterprise, the fact that it ultimately grounds and justifies its faith by appeal to observable evidence. The idea of an empirically-based faith is hard for many people to grasp, especially if they have been raised or indoctrinated into believing that "faith" is only a reason for believing something when you *don't* have evidence. (2001, p. 3)

Thus, even though science may not be able to observe everything it studies, researchers do their best to operationally define the phenomena of study, test their hypotheses, and make these operations available for public view so others can see that assumptions were tested and exactly how they were tested. This sets science apart from other enterprises of gaining knowledge.

Probabilistic Knowledge

Many students are surprised when we tell them that scientists do not believe in absolute certainty but in **probabilistic knowledge.** In their experiments, scientists are content to live with probabilities instead of certainties. Kerlinger and Lee state:

> Let us flatly assert that nothing can be "proved" scientifically. All one can do is to bring evidence to bear that such-and-such a proposition is true. (2000, p. 218)

On the one hand, most people would find it frustrating to accept that one cannot absolutely "know the truth" about a particular issue. Certainly, belief systems other than science such as religion have no trouble suggesting that they have the answer to specific questions and even faith in an afterlife. If you talk to religious people, many will say they have no doubt about certain issues. Religion, of course, has different requirements for belief as compared to science. In religious systems, all you have to do is have faith in a concept and choose to believe it. In science, as we discussed previously, there must be empirical evidence to support a particular point of view.

There are several reasons that researchers do not take a leap of faith and say that they have found the absolute truth about a matter. First, scientists know that every experiment will contain a certain degree of error. Error is ubiquitous and there is no way to avoid it. We can control our studies, but the most we can do is reduce error, not eliminate it. This is why researchers use statistical methods to tell them the "probability" that their results could be due to chance. The lower the probability that the results of an experiment are due to chance, the more confidence researchers can have in the results. For instance, if the statistics told the researcher that an experiment would turn out the same way ninety-nine times out of a hundred he or she would have quite a bit of confidence in the results. This is a very good probability to "believe in." However, the scientist who is happy to accept that findings are not just luck or chance is always mindful of that one time in a hundred that the results might turn out differently. So most scientists talk about their results in terms of probability and always know that their study has not revealed an immutable truth because all research involves a certain degree of error.

A second reason why scientists talk about their results probabilistically is that their study has not evaluated all of the possible variables that could have affected the results. Researchers know that most phenomena they study are affected by multiple influences and their experiment can only control for so many. Thus, while their study may have shown a relation between two variables, there may well be other variables that influence this relationship as well. So the researcher tends to be very specific about reporting the results of an experiment and usually indicates that the findings reveal only a part of the potential puzzle being investigated.

A third cause of the tentativeness of scientific conclusions is that most researchers know that science is an *ongoing process* and that it is unusual to find absolute scientific truth. Think of how our conceptions of the universe, medicine, and psychology have changed over time. All of these areas have changed their "truth" in light of new research findings, because new research data lead to modifications of theories, principles, and how we view the world. Scientists know this process and cannot let themselves become too excited and complacent with a finding that they know is at best probabilistic and tentative. You might wonder how scientists can live with the absence of absolute truth and the fact that all scientific knowledge is tentative. In fact, you may wonder if lack of true knowledge is tantamount to no knowledge at all. In research, however, we have seen over the course of history that tentative knowledge with a high probability of being correct has slowly moved us toward higher levels of science and technology. We certainly do not require a "sure thing" to win a bet at a casino—just a good probability of winning. When you really think about it, satisfaction with the "truth" of the status quo would make our society stagnant and unchanging, rather like Peirce's method of tenacity. It is exactly the tentative and probabilistic nature of science that moves us away from incomplete knowledge and toward a more complete understanding of phenomena. The transient nature of truth coupled with the skepticism, questioning, and doubt of scientists is the engine that moves us away from the inertia and complacency of "knowing the truth."

Objectivity

We always imbue a scientific approach with some degree of objectivity. One persistent myth about scientists is that they, as people, possess more objectivity than other people on the planet. Just like the stereotype of the mad scientist at the beginning of this chapter, scientists are viewed as cold, calculating, and objective. Most often laypeople confuse the scientist as a practitioner with the scientist as a person. Although it is hoped that scientists will evaluate their results with a metric outside their own biases, researchers are only human. Even if scientists will not admit it, they probably have a "pet" hypothesis and a result that they hope will be supported in a given experiment. Sometimes the researcher is not even aware of bias because it is totally on an unconscious level. So if scientists as people are not any more objective than anyone else, how can we say that science has the characteristic of objectivity? The answer is that the process of "doing science" is designed to foster objectivity and reduce bias. Most of the parts of this self-correcting process have been talked about previously, but we will discuss them here as they relate to the concept of objectivity.

Figure 2.2 shows a fox watching a chicken, which any farmer will tell you is not a great idea. The fox has a vested interest in the chicken because it represents a good candidate for an afternoon snack. Thus, we would not want to trust the fox to watch the chicken. In this metaphor the scientist is the fox and the experiment is represented by the chicken. As we said earlier, most scientists (foxes in this metaphor) have

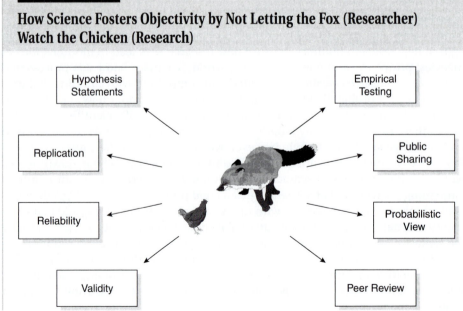

FIGURE 2.2

How Science Fosters Objectivity by Not Letting the Fox (Researcher) Watch the Chicken (Research)

Hypothesis Statements

Empirical Testing

Replication

Public Sharing

Reliability

Probabilistic View

Validity

Peer Review

some sort of human bias, whether conscious or unconscious, about the outcomes of their studies (the chickens). We cannot depend on scientists as humans to resist these biases, but we can construct scientific principles that serve to reduce bias as much as possible. Figure 2.2 illustrates eight arrows moving away from the fox/chicken scenario that represent how the scientific method serves to increase objectivity in scientists and reduce their bias. Many of these overlap in reality; however, we will discuss each one individually.

Empirical testing is a scientific requirement that forces a researcher to test hypotheses outside of himself or herself. The hypothesis must be testable and the outcome of the empirical test will either support or not support the hypothesis. If it were not for the requirement of empirical testing, scientists could just "say" that something was found without providing evidence, and not just any evidence will do. It must be a well-designed experiment that will stand up under the scrutiny of other scientists. If the study was not designed appropriately, or if the scientist built bias into the investigation, it will be noted by others and not given credence as reliable scientific information. This fosters objectivity because it makes the scientist evaluate the issue under study outside of himself or herself.

We have stated earlier that public sharing of scientific information is one of the hallmarks of valid research. As stated above, it is the public sharing of an empirical study with the scientific community and society as a whole that reduces the chance of coming to a biased conclusion. The movement of the experiment into the public domain takes it out of the personal control of the researcher.

Another characteristic of science is that all findings are to some degree probabilistic. One way that scientists evaluate the probability that their results are "real" or may have occurred by chance and sampling error is through the use of quantitative methods or statistics. If your statistical analysis indicates that your results not "real" and are likely to have occurred due to chance, it's "game over." Scientists cannot make nonsignificant findings significant, and if they try, other scientists will point out the error of their ways. Thus, your data analysis will tell you the "truth" about your data, not your opinion or desire for a particular result.

The notion of peer review for scientific work overlaps with the public sharing of information. We wanted to mention it separately, however, because "the public" is not necessarily well trained in scientific matters. Peer review implies that the work of scientists is critically examined by other researchers who are equally educated and experienced in the scientific method. No matter how badly you wanted your experiment to turn out a certain way, it is not possible to get the result you wanted if the data do not support it. Peers will look at your study and if you are interpreting it in an inappropriate way, they will let you know. Of course, a scientist can fabricate a study or change data to come out as wanted, but this violates ethical codes and in the long run will be exposed as either a fraud or some anomaly in the chain of data points on the topic that is not supported by the research of others. Peer reviews take the science out of the individual researcher and put it in the hands of others, which increases objectivity. Even the thought of other people having to review one's work makes the individual researcher more diligent and careful with interpretations.

Hypothesis statements, according to Kerlinger and Lee (2000, p. 26) constitute "a conjectural statement of the relation between two or more variables." Kerlinger (1973) differentiates between a substantive hypothesis and a statistical hypothesis. An example of a substantive hypothesis might be, "Children with articulation disorders will produce more misarticulations in syntactically complex sentences than they do in syntactically simple sentences of the same length."

In this substantive hypothesis we are conjecturing that syntactic complexity relates to misarticulation in such a way that as syntactic complexity increases, there will be a concomitant increase in articulation errors. In a statistical hypothesis we try to predict the possible results of a quantitative (statistical) analysis of the substantive hypothesis. According to Kerlinger:

> Statistical hypotheses must be tested against something. . . . The alternative usually selected is the null hypothesis, . . . which states essentially, that there is no relation between the variables (of the problem). (1973, p. 201)

Essentially, in a classical statement of statistical hypotheses, the researcher knows that the **null hypothesis** is always a possibility right along with the other hypotheses that could be proved true. In the articulation example, the statistical hypotheses might be:

H_1: Significantly more misarticulations will occur in sentences of high syntactic complexity as compared to sentences of low syntactic complexity.

H_2: Significantly more misarticulations will occur in sentences of lower syntactic complexity as compared to sentences of high syntactic complexity.

H_0: There will be no significant difference in misarticulations between sentences of high and low syntactic complexity (the null hypothesis).

Although scientists typically do not write down all the alternative possibilities for hypotheses including the null hypothesis, researchers know that any of the possibilities could occur in any given study. That is, scientists are forced to at least consider on some level that a study could turn out a number of possible ways, just because this is the way statistical methods are set up. Researchers intuitively know that their "pet" hypothesis may be substantiated by the statistics, but they also know that there may not be a significant difference and their preferred outcome may not occur. Hypothesis statements, whether implicit or explicit, keep researchers honest, unbiased, and objective. They at least have to acknowledge the possibility that a study can turn out any number of different ways regardless of their preferences.

Earlier we stated that the generality of research findings was primarily achieved through replication. If a study is repeated and comparable results are obtained, we are a little closer to the "truth." We have begun to see a chain of data points that suggest a direction in the research. In replication, we see a clear means of taking a study out of the control of an individual and inoculating a research finding against subjective bias. When we physically turn over the conduct of a study to another person in another laboratory, we are relinquishing the opportunity to affect the results with our personal bias. Replication, as a valued characteristic of science, fosters objectivity by encouraging many different researchers to examine an issue and report whatever results they obtain. Let the empirical chips fall where they may.

We will have a section in a forthcoming chapter on the issue of reliability in research, but it is appropriate to mention it briefly now in our discussion of objectivity. One type of reliability that clearly relates to objectivity is interjudge reliability. An important part of any research report is some indication of reliability of measurements. For example, a researcher doing research on vocal qualities in people undergoing therapy for vocal nodules may want to rate the hoarseness and breathiness in the participants being studied. Perhaps the researcher is interested in determining if vocal quality improves with treatment by dividing a group of patients into a treatment group and a control group of people who do not desire therapy. If the vocal quality of the treatment group improves more than the control group, then the treatment is thought to have "worked" better than a no-treatment condition. Of course, the researcher could rate the vocal qualities of the participants, but would this be a case of the fox watching the chicken house? Yes, it probably would. Who knows what conscious or unconscious agenda the researcher may have or vested interest in the ratings turning out a particular way? Maybe the researcher wants to show that treatment works. So in almost every worthwhile investigation there is some mention of reliability. In the case of interjudge reliability, the investigator might ask some other trained professional to rate the vocal qualities of the participants, preferably in a random order so the new rater would not know who was in the therapy or nontherapy groups nor which samples were taken at the beginning or the end of the study. If there is a high level of agreement between the researcher and the reliability judge then there is high reliability. You can see how forcing a researcher to report reliability information moves the study away from experimenter biases and increases objectivity. Having another person or group of judges recheck your results is another way that the scientific method reduces bias and individual control by the experimenter. During the peer review process, a researcher submitting a study for publication without any mention of reliability is almost certain to be rejected or asked to provide such information before the work is processed further. We will discuss reliability again in a later chapter.

Validity has to do with whether the measurement you have taken in an investigation is really tapping the construct of interest. For example, a researcher interested in anxiety as a construct must measure it in a way that is considered valid by the scientific community. Let's say that a researcher decided that he or she could tell anxiety level by looking at a person's facial expressions. This researcher wants to determine if people who stutter are more anxious than people who are fluent. So the researcher makes video recordings of the faces of research participants and rates their anxiety based on facial expressions. It may even be possible that the scientist could train a graduate assistant to recognize particular aspects of facial expressions supposedly related to anxiety and the two researchers could come to fairly acceptable interjudge reliability. When the researcher submits this work for peer review, however, it is unanimously rejected because editorial consultants opine that the use of facial expression is not a well-accepted or *valid* means of measuring the construct of anxiety. Perhaps the use of a standardized anxiety scale, a physiological measurement such as galvanic skin response, or some other indicator that has been established and agreed on as a valid indicator of anxiety would have been more appropriate. Thus, whatever an individual might think is a valid measurement is not important. If you do a study with a measurement that lacks validity, your study is doomed from the beginning. Validity is established by consensus of the scientific community for each area of study. This is just another way that the scientific method takes the research away from an individual and allows others to make judgments about the worth of a particular investigation.

Scientific Neutrality and Limitations

Another way that people tend to stereotype science is to assume that it has some sort of moral agenda to help the world or improve life in some way. Of course, many scientists, *as people,* do engage in their work with the initial goal of improving conditions on the planet. On the other hand, many studies are designed to simply understand natural phenomena without any "good or bad" connotation. At any rate, the value judgments of good and bad are not the business of science. Scientists would probably say that *science is neutral.* First of all, the value judgments of bad and good are not universal for all phenomena and even if they were, changes can occur over time. Take for example the development of the atomic bomb. Scientists worked on the Manhattan Project intensively for years and developed one of the most powerful devices known to mankind. Was this good or bad? Some of the Japanese people would probably say it was bad. Some Americans would say it was good because it allegedly shortened the war in the Pacific and ultimately saved American and Japanese lives. One can easily see both sides of this moral judgment. But with the development of this technology, we unleashed nuclear proliferation and as other countries built nuclear arsenals we felt less safe. On the other hand, nuclear medicine has been helpful in the treatment of cancer and other diseases. Good or bad? Did "science" have the intention to be good or bad? Every new scientific development can be used for good or evil and has its upside and downside. Development of new pharmaceuticals has increased our life span, but now we have overpopulation and an overloaded health care system. Even if scientists as people may have motives that relate to the betterment of mankind, science as an approach to gaining knowledge is a rather impartial process. Scientific results, of course, can be viewed from philosophical or moral standpoints, but this is not part of science itself, merely perceptions by nonscientists. Lest the reader think we are marginalizing moral values and those who study them, let us assure you that we are not. Science is just not equipped to deal in such issues, just as it cannot deal with aesthetic issues, but other disciplines such as music, art, philosophy, and religion certainly can. Philosophy, the arts, and religion are not constrained by the scientific method and practitioners can develop knowledge and belief with nonempirical means. These disciplines have accepted processes of accumulating relevant knowledge and belief that have been developed over thousands of years. But science by its very characteristics is limited in the types of questions it can attempt to answer, the kinds of evidence it can gather, and the interpretations of data it can put forth. Thus, science can never answer a question about good or bad, right or wrong, best or worst, or beautiful or ugly because these are aesthetic or moral beliefs that do not lend themselves to empirical study. In a similar vein, science is not designed for **engineering questions** such as: "How do we build a bridge?" or "How do we teach children to read?" Science can certainly answer questions about which materials for a bridge have a greater tensile strength as compared to other materials. Science can tell us which types of reading materials result in lower reading comprehension scores for groups of children. But processes such as building or teaching have so many components that must come together that they are difficult to study empirically. Also, complicating engineering with **value questions** becomes especially difficult for science. So a question like "How can we build the best bridge in the world?" would be scientifically unanswerable. The term "best" could refer to strength, aesthetic beauty, ability to process the most traffic in the least amount of time, or the greatest span or height. Researchers leave the moral, aesthetic, and engineering questions to other disciplines and focus on the questions that are answerable with scientific principles.

Ethics in Science

After spending some time in the previous section making the argument that science is neutral and amoral, we are now about to present the case that science is most definitely concerned with ethical standards. On the surface it sounds like we are contradicting our prior statements by saying that science is, after all, concerned with right and wrong. However, the ethical issues that we discuss below have to do with *the way studies are conducted* and with *the protection of those who participate* in scientific investigations. We still maintain, as we said above, that *the questions scientists ask* are not about "right and wrong." The first area we discuss has to do with **scientific misconduct.**

Scientific Misconduct

Case 1

In the fall of 1912 Charles Dawson discovered an old hominid skull in Piltdown quarry located in England and rocked the world of paleontologists of the time. The skull was reputed to be a "missing link" between man and ape since it had a cranium that appeared to be human and a jaw that was more apelike. Dawson named his discovery *Eoanthropus dawsoni* and the artifact became known as the Piltdown man. It was not until almost 1950 that other scientists discovered the Piltdown man to be a fabrication after fluorine absorption tests, a detailed microscopic examination revealing suspicious file marks on the teeth, and further dating of the gravel beds at Piltdown quarry. The Piltdown man was finally exposed as a hoax in 1953, some forty years after Dawson's announcement.

Case 2

Dr. John Darsee was thought to be a brilliant researcher who worked at such universities as Emory, Notre Dame, Indiana, and Harvard in the 1970s studying the effects of heart drugs on dogs. By 1981 Darsee had published over one hundred articles and abstracts in cardiovascular research. In the spring of 1981 several of Darsee's colleagues began to suspect that he had fabricated and falsified data. When these colleagues reported their suspicions to the director of the laboratory, Darsee was asked to produce his raw data and notes on a recent investigation. Remarkably, Darsee went into the lab and began to take data on a single dog and record that these readings had been taken in several experiments over many different times and dates. Unbeknownst to Darsee, as he was in the process of falsifying his data he was being watched by other research fellows and a lab technician. Ultimately, Darsee admitted falsifying the data but did not admit any other wrongdoing. He lost his research fellowship and a job offer for a faculty position at Harvard. With further investigation, it was later found that Darsee had engaged in scientific misconduct at other universities dating back to his undergraduate program at Notre Dame and many of his papers and abstracts had to be retracted (Lock, Wells, & Farthing, 2001).

Case 3

Between 1979 and 1983 about one-third of the existing research dealing with psychopharmacology in the treatment of people with mental retardation was contributed by Dr. Stephen Breuning. He had received a lot of grant money from the National Institute of Mental Health (NIMH) and his work on the use of Ritilin affected public policy on the use of psychotropic drugs in dealing with mental retardation (Holden, 1987). When Dr. Robert Sprague from the University of Illinois raised questions about the conduct of Breuning's research, investigations revealed that some of the studies were in fact never done and some data were fabricated. Unfortunately, while Sprague initially sent his concerns to NIMH in 1983, it was not until 1989 that the case was finally resolved. Sprague believes that the process was probably moved along faster because the popular media (e.g., CBS' *60 Minutes*) became involved. Ultimately, Breuning was the first researcher convicted in federal court for fraudulent research practices. He was sentenced to a short prison term and had to pay financial restitution to the University of Pittsburgh.

The researchers profiled in these capsules are often singled out in textbooks and university courses on research as representing some of the most egregious examples of scientific misconduct. Most definitions of scientific misconduct include data that are fabricated or falsified, which means that the researcher never did the study and made up the data, most likely skewed to reflect a particular bias. While this represents "faking" data, another level of scientific misconduct is "fudging, manipulating, or massaging" data that are actually gathered so that a certain result is obtained. If a researcher ignores the data obtained in a study that do not support a pet hypothesis and only retains scores that go along with a bias, it is scientific misconduct. Why would a researcher engage in misconduct? Goodstein states:

> Among the incidents of scientific fraud that I have looked at, three motives, or risk factors, have been present. In all cases, the perpetrators (1) were under career pressure, (2) knew, or thought they knew, what the result would be if they went to all the trouble of doing the work properly, and (3) were in a field in which individual experiments are not expected to be precisely reproducible. Simple monetary gain is seldom, if ever, a factor in scientific fraud. (2002, p. 5)

How widespread is scientific misconduct? Actually, the figures on this matter are difficult to find. In the year 2000, Dooley and Kerch reported that as many as 170 researchers were suspected of scientific misconduct by agencies such as the National Institutes of Health and the National Science Foundation and twenty individuals were found guilty of such acts. A survey of over a thousand researchers commissioned by the American Association for the Advancement of Science reported that almost a quarter of those surveyed had witnessed some instance of scientific misconduct in the past decade (Marsa, 1992). In a discussion of scientific responsibility a panel composed of members of the National Academy of Sciences, the National Academy of Engineering and the Institute of Medicine concluded that

> the number of confirmed cases of misconduct in sciences is low compared to the level of research activity in the United States. However, as with all forms of misconduct, underreporting may be significant; federal agencies have only recently imposed procedural and reporting requirements that may yield larger numbers of reported cases. Any misconduct comes at a price to scientists, their research institutions, and society. Thus every case of misconduct in science is serious and requires attention. (NAS, NAE, IOM, 1996, p. 9)

It has been said that science is "self-correcting" and that the process is robust enough to withstand a certain degree of scientific misconduct. If a person falsifies or fudges data, the results will be subjected to peer review before publication. Because science thrives on knowledge derived from multiple sources, fabricated data points will eventually be exposed as not representing "the truth" as the trend of legitimate data points forms the "real" trend and outliers are left behind because their findings are not substantiated. Maybe the researcher who falsified data will not be caught, but any findings will be disregarded if the research of others does not support them. Thus, the process of science can stand a bit of abuse and ultimately land on its feet, but scientific misconduct is unethical and unfortunate. It is a shame when other scientists who *are* ethical have to spend their time investigating a spurious finding only to find out it was a blind alley built on the foundation of scientific misconduct. Robert Sprague, the researcher who "blew the whistle" on Stephen Breuning, laments:

> There is a myth that science is beautifully self-correcting. The few students of scientific misconduct who have written about the topic point out that the correction is slow and often painful and that peer review seldom catches the misconduct. Usually an insider with information generally not available to others blows the whistle on the scientist who is cheating. Quite often the whistleblower pays dearly for the action. (1989, p. 2)

So what can we do about scientific misconduct? First, most large governmental agencies such as the National Science Foundation, the National Institutes of Health, the Public Health Services, the Office of Scientific Integrity, and the National Academy of Sciences have developed policies relating to identifying and dealing with acts of scientific misconduct. Most professional associations such as the American Psychological Association, the American Speech-Language-Hearing Association, and the American Academy of Audiology have put standards and procedures in place to deal with scientific misconduct. Additionally, almost all universities have mechanisms in place to deal with scientific misconduct. These are good initial steps by organizations, but it will obviously take more than large organizations overseeing scientific research to reduce the incidence of scientific misconduct. Bolton (2002) suggests that fostering scientific integrity must be an effort of the scientific community as a whole to inculcate ethical scientific values in students from the beginning of their training and then for researchers to police themselves for the occurrence of scientific misconduct. She outlines a number of useful measures that could reduce scientific misconduct:

- Students going into science professions should receive strong training in research methodology.
- New researchers should be exposed to mentors who are ethical role models.
- Collegial interactions with other researchers should be developed and reinforced.
- There should be some oversight and management of research projects by institutions.
- A workplace culture of research integrity should be emphasized and cultivated.
- If detected, a person committing scientific misconduct should receive appropriate and swift sanctions.
- Students should be socialized from the beginning into ethical conduct by emphasizing these issues in coursework and other venues of academia.

Although the prevalence of scientific misconduct is widely regarded to be small, its very existence is a threat to research. Even though science has the self-correcting mechanisms previously noted, this is tantamount to closing the barn door after the horse has escaped. The strong positions taken by governmental agencies and professional associations will go a long way to deter those tempted to engage in scientific misconduct. The suggestions by Bolton are even more proactive because they will help to create self-monitoring within the community of scientists, and even better, may actually prevent a young scientist from engaging in misconduct in the first place because of a strong research ethic instilled during training. This is precisely why we have this section in the present text.

Protection of Research Participants

Case 1

The Nuremberg Military Tribunal convened in December 1946. Part of these criminal proceedings involved twenty-three prominent German physicians who were accused of war crimes and crimes against humanity. Medical experiments were routinely conducted on prisoners without their consent that involved freezing and hypothermia, infectious diseases, torture, killing, high altitude exposure, pharmacology, sterilization, and traumatic injuries. The majority of these studies resulted in the death of the prisoners, most often in cruel and painful ways. Many of these "experiments" were really not valuable scientific work but simply arbitrary decisions made by the physicians who were curious about an issue. Some of the "experiments" were not really research at all but nothing more than different variations on ways to kill a human being. Ultimately, the tribunal judges found sixteen doctors guilty in August 1947, and seven of the doctors were executed the following year. The result of this trial was "The Nuremberg Code" which put forth directives for any future human experimentation and is the template for most current policies on protection of human participants in research.

Case 2

Between 1932 and 1972 the United States Public Health Service studied 399 African American men in the late stages of syphilis in what has become known as the Tuskegee syphilis experiment. During the course of this "experiment" the men, who were largely sharecroppers from Alabama with limited formal education, were told that they suffered from "bad blood" and the true seriousness of their condition was kept from them. As the investigation progressed, these men were predictably ravaged by heart disease, neurological disorders, blindness, mental illness, and ultimately death. In many cases, because of the secrecy, the disease was passed on to spouses and some children were born with congenital syphilis. The saddest part of all is that the United States Public Health Service actively saw to it that these patients never received treatment for their condition even when antibiotic treatment was routinely available. On May 16, 1997, President Bill Clinton issued an apology on behalf of the United States Government to the eight remaining survivors of the Tuskegee Syphilis Experiment.

The two examples portrayed above represent outlandish examples of people suffering abuse in the name of science. Incredibly, even with the Nuremberg Code which was published in 1949, the Tuskegee Experiment still continued for another twenty years until media attention finally exposed this horrific mistreatment of human beings by an agency of the United States government. The Tuskegee case coupled with other reports detailing abuse of research participants led to major legislative initiatives in the mid-1970s. For instance, the National Research Act of 1974 and the National Commission for the Protection of Human Subjects of Biomedical and Behavioral Research made specific recommendations that were later approved by the Department of Health and Human Services (DHHS) in Title 45, Code of Federal Regulations (CFR), Part 46, Protection of Human Subjects (45 CFR 46) which later became the official policy governing all research receiving federal support. There are also similar guidelines in place for research involving animals. The Animal Welfare Act of 1985 governs the use and care of research animals. Every institution using animals in research must have an **Animal Care and Use Committee (ACUC)** to review research protocols using animals as participants. Similar guidelines are used by national and international boards (e.g., American Association for the Accreditation of Laboratory Animal Care) well as ethical codes put forth by various professional organizations (e.g., American Psychological Association).

Following the guidelines mentioned previously, all major institutions in which research is conducted have developed systematic review and approval processes for the safe conduct of research. For example, every university, hospital, and school system must have in place an **institutional review board (IRB)** that evaluates and approves any research that is conducted within those settings. Ideally, the IRB should comprise a panel that possesses expertise in a variety of areas. Of course, most of the board members should understand appropriate research design, but it is equally important that the members represent a variety of disciplines (e.g., behavioral sciences, biological sciences) so that a given protocol can be fairly evaluated. For a psychological study, it is important that someone on the board is familiar with psychological research, appropriate controls, and possible risks for participants in this type of research. Some IRB members may also represent professions in the community such as attorneys, members of the clergy, or local physicians. It may come in handy to have the input of a lawyer or doctor on certain issues involved in educational research. Thus, a researcher working in a university, public school, or hospital setting cannot simply decide to do a study and then commence gathering data. There is a very specific procedure that must be followed. First, the researcher must develop a detailed protocol for the study, which is submitted to the IRB for evaluation; the research cannot be initiated until final approval by the board is obtained. Sometimes the IRB will have questions, comments, or changes that they want the investigator to make prior to beginning the project. In some cases, the IRB will disapprove the project or demand significant changes in the investigation because they feel that it represents potential risks to human participants that will outweigh the scientific benefits gained by completing the study. One might think that a study that uses existing information, about participants (e.g., clinical records, computer databases) would be immune from the IRB process. However, with the passage of the Health Insurance Portability and Accountability Act (HIPAA) and the Family Educational Rights and Privacy Act (FERPA), most identifiable personal information, whether stored on paper or electronic media, is protected by law (Horner and Wheeler, 2005). We cannot just go rooting around in client folders to complete a research project without a participant's permission. A research protocol submitted to the IRB is likely to include the following:

- A description of the experimental research design that is detailed enough for the IRB to determine if the study is scientifically sound and will not impose unnecessary risks on participants.
- A statement of the potential benefits that will accrue from the study and some evidence that the risk to human participants is worth the scientific advances that will be made.
- A detailed description of how participants will be selected, where they will be solicited from, and why some groups of participants, if any, will be excluded from the investigation. For instance, a researcher who wants to include or exclude a certain cultural group will have to provide justification for its necessity.
- Especially when studying "vulnerable populations" (e.g., pregnant women, children, persons with mental illness), the researcher must detail how coercion of these participants and any additional risks will be avoided.
- The researcher must provide an "informed consent" (discussed in more detail below) outlining the study that must be signed by the participant or an authorized representative.
- The researcher must describe all potential risks to participants and how these will be minimized during the study.

- All procedures used in the study to protect participant confidentiality and privacy should be outlined in the protocol.

Of all the protections included in the research protocol submitted to the IRB for consideration, the **informed consent** is one of the most important. The informed consent serves to explain the study in detail using language that potential participants can understand (e.g., no technical jargon). All pertinent information about the research is explained in writing so there are no surprises and the participant will know exactly what participation will entail. The informed consent also constitutes a written legal record which has to be signed and dated by the researcher, the participant, and a witness. According to federal regulations the following guidelines must be considered:

- The informed consent must be obtained from all participants or their authorized representative before the study begins.
- Potential participants should be given ample time to read and understand the informed consent and to ask questions about the study before they decide whether or not to participate.
- There should be no coercion to participate, either directly or indirectly.
- The language of the informed consent should be understandable and appropriate for potential participants.
- No legal rights of the participant should be waived in the informed consent.
- The informed consent must not release the investigator or the institution from liability for negligence.

It is generally understood, based on federal legislation, that the informed consent should have a number of required components:

- A statement that the study involves research, the purpose of the research, the expected duration of the study, a description of the procedures, and a specific identification of any procedures that are experimental in nature
- A statement describing any foreseeable risks to the participants
- A statement describing any general societal benefits potentially arising from the study (e.g., determining a more efficient method of early diagnosis of hearing loss) and any specific benefits that the participant will receive (e.g., monetary compensation, specific training, an evaluation)
- Some statement of alternatives to participating in the study, especially in cases where more than one treatment or intervention is possible (for example, if the researcher was studying a new method of training vocabulary, participants should be apprised of other existing alternatives that they could take advantage of instead of participating in the study)
- A statement of how the **confidentiality** of participant information will be maintained during the study and if any of their information will be shared with another agency or if someone not involved with the study will have access to their records
- For studies involving more than minimal risk, an explanation of any compensation or treatments available if injury occurs and where these can be obtained

- A statement that the participation in the study is strictly voluntary and that if a person opts not to participate there will be no prejudice or penalty directed toward that person nor will there be any penalty or loss of benefits to which the participant is entitled, if a person who initially volunteered to participate in the research decides to terminate involvement in the study and that on leaving a study any information gathered by the investigators can be taken by the person

There are some additional and more specific elements of informed consent that should be included under special circumstances (e.g., experimentation with embryos or fetuses) that we will not go into here. It is enough to say that the typical informed consent must include the critical elements mentioned above or the IRB will not approve the research project. Both of the present authors have had the experience of serving as members of a university IRB.

One of the present authors (WH) was selected to serve on an IRB early in his career and quite frankly thought it would be a waste of time. Just another worthless committee assignment. After all, the days of abusing human participants simply had to be a thing of the past! What kinds of things could we do nowadays to mistreat research participants? The first protocol was a rude awakening. We were asked to review a proposal from a department studying the effects of large leather belts worn by weightlifters to determine if these belts had an effect on lifting. One of the measurements the researchers were interested in was intra-abdominal pressure. In order to measure the pressure within the abdominal cavity, the researchers intended to place a balloon up the participant's rectum and inflate it. The amount of displacement of the balloon inside the abdominal cavity during weight lifting was measured through sensors and thus intra-abdominal pressure was recorded. As I gazed aghast at the protocol trying to place myself in the position of the potential participants, all sorts of questions occurred to me. Where were the participants coming from? Were they majors in this department who could be subtly coerced to take part in the study? Who would be inserting the balloons? Exactly how much "inflation" of the balloon would occur? Was there any privacy? What if the participants experienced extreme discomfort? What if there were ill effects after the study? For how long a time would the balloon be inserted? What would be done with the balloons after the experiment? Would medical personnel be present during the study? I had a host of other questions that were not dealt with on the protocol, and I assure you I had no trouble whatsoever fulfilling my responsibilities as a new member of the institutional review board. If you are planning to do a master's thesis, you will become intimately familiar with IRB procedures as they are explained in the guidelines published by your university. Submission of protocols to the IRB for approval is required by federal regulations and is a necessary process to protect research participants, but it is often not on the researcher's top ten list of favorite things to do. No matter how careful we are in developing a research protocol, the IRB will invariably find deficiencies that we overlooked and must change. Because of such time-consuming and often frustrating constraints, some researchers view the IRB as an impediment to their research. They would prefer to just get on with their research without getting "permission" from people not involved or acquainted with their field of expertise. In our experience, however, it is *good* to have other people examine our proposal with the welfare of human participants in mind. Any short delay, if it adds to the protection of participants, is well worth the time. We bring this up only to let potential student researchers know that the approval of your protocol by the IRB is not a slam dunk. You will no doubt have to go through one or two versions of your protocol before it is finally approved. But don't lose heart, because ultimately you will probably receive approval. Resist the urge to view the process as an administrative hassle or just a series of meaningless time-consuming steps we have to go through. It is very serious business that is the legacy of all those tortured and abused souls from places like Auschwitz, Dachau, and Tuskegee.

Junk Science, Pseudoscience, and Quackery

According to Snow (1998), prior to the 1950s there were two cultures involved with science and its interpretation. One culture comprised scientists who did research but did not communicate with society at large. The other culture was composed of the intellectuals who interpreted scientific findings based on theoretical and philosophical information but most often produced writings mostly for each other and sometimes for the public. Today, communication between scientists and lay people has changed.

In *The Third Culture*, Brockman (1995) describes how our society has gradually evolved with regard to science and its interpretation:

> Scientists are communicating directly with the general public. Traditional intellectual media played a vertical game; journalists wrote up and professors wrote down. Today, third-culture thinkers tend to avoid the middleman and endeavor to express their deepest thoughts in a manner accessible to the intelligent reading public. . . . Scientific topics receiving prominent play in newspapers and magazines over the past several years include molecular biology, artificial intelligence, artificial life, chaos theory, massive parallelism, neural nets, the inflationary universe, fractals, complex adaptive systems, superstrings, biodiversity, nanotechnology, the human genome. . . . Unlike previous intellectual pursuits, the achievements of the third culture are not the marginal disputes of a quarrelsome mandarin class; they will affect the lives of everybody on the planet. (1995, p. 18)

With scientists communicating directly with the public instead of just with each other and society no longer needing "intellectuals" to interpret science for them, the third culture has moved science to some extent into the public domain. Interestingly, whereas in politics, the economy, entertainment, and fashions, the same news often repeats over and over again, science produces newsworthy information that has the potential of actually revolutionizing our world. Those interested in cutting-edge topics often gravitate toward scientific subject matter. We thus see reporters from television and newspapers "interpreting science" as they read popular books written by scientists themselves. The public is therefore more comfortable with science because they read and hear about it in the media, and as a result, they think they "know" about science, even though they have not been trained as scientists. Many organizations invoke science in their advertising of products. People make decisions about their health based on "scientific evidence" cited on supplements, foods, exercise equipment, and medications. However, an unfortunate byproduct of this popularization of science is some distortion and misinterpretation of research by reporters and the public in general as they read popular books written by authors who represent the third culture. As the third culture has developed, we have also seen a rise in junk science, pseudoscience, and quackery, all of which are based on exaggerations, misinterpretations, and sometimes intentional distortion of scientific research.

Junk science can be characterized as "shoddy," "worthless," and "superficial" investigations and analysis that misinterpret scientific data. For example, someone may be trying to promote an ideology or realize financial gain by selectively interpreting scientific data to further their own ends. Junk science may actually involve legitimate research investigations, but these studies are not presented in the context of all the research done on a given topic. For example, a person trying to sell a vitamin supplement phones the offices of ten local doctors and asks whoever answers (e.g., nurse, physician's assistant, doctor, nurse's aide, secretary) whether they recommend the use of supplements. The advertisement for the product then says, "Nine out of ten medical professionals recommend the use of our vitamin supplement." It is easy to see that this "study" was not scientific at all but was used because citing "science" in an advertisement lends some credibility to an organization or product. Another example of junk science involves a person trying to promote a procedure for helping to increase word retrieval in patients with aphasia. The person finds a published study that shows the procedure was effective in a group of participants. Unfortunately, a more thorough review of literature in this area reveals that there are ten studies on this topic and eight of the ten studies do not show any significant benefit from using the procedure. Yet this person tells clients that research has shown that the procedure is effective and tells student interns that this is a "clinically proven" way to approach treatment for word retrieval. Many statements seen in popular advertising may reflect junk science, but as the old saying goes, "*Caveat emptor*" ("Let the buyer beware"):

- Scientifically proven to help . . . (Who was studied? How many? How were they diagnosed? What is meant by "help"? Where were results published? Any studies not showing positive results?)
- Studies have shown . . . (Where were studies published? Were there any studies not showing these results?)
- Doctors recommend . . . (Who were they? What were their specialties? How many? Where is the study published?)
- Laboratory studies prove . . . (Whose laboratory? What were the studies? Any studies not agreeing with results?)
- Our (product) lasts three times longer . . . (Where is the research? Who did it? Any disagreement?)

It is easy to invoke science and give a scientific spin to any product or procedure, so we must always be wary of the possibility of junk science in the popular media and advertising.

It is sometimes difficult to distinguish between junk science and pseudoscience. For our purposes we will characterize **pseudoscience** as any practice that "simulates science" or claims to have a scientific basis, but in reality does not incorporate the philosophy and methods of science. For example, astronomy is a science, but astrology is not. Yet it is common to find terms such as "astrological research" and "astrological science" on the Internet and in popular periodicals. Sometimes the term **quackery** is used in reference to pseudoscience related to the medical profession. The *American Heritage Dictionary* (1985) defines *quack* as "a person who pretends to have medical knowledge. . . . a charlatan." Some people practicing quackery do it to intentionally bilk the public, while other practitioners believe sincerely that their methods are sound. In both cases, however, there is no real scientific basis for the efficacy of their practices.

How can we tell if someone is promoting junk science, pseudoscience, or quackery? Such authors as Carl Sagan, Robert Park, Michael Shermer, and others have provided guidelines for detecting pseudoscience. There are many websites such as www.quackwatch.org, http://skepdic.com, and http://junkscience.com that are devoted to exposing pseudoscience. Some of the most common indicators of these practices are the following:

1. *Lack of support by controlled, repeated experiments.* Any theory worth believing in should receive consistent support from the scientific community by researchers representing a variety of laboratories and backgrounds.

2. *Results are presented in a nonscientific arena of proof.* Any scientific enterprise will be introduced in professional, peer-reviewed journals. If it is introduced first to the mass media, bypassing the scientific community, we should be suspicious.

3. *Use of nonscientific evidence.* Typically proponents of junk science or pseudoscience only use anecdotal evidence such as success stories or testimonials from individuals. If there are no controlled scientific studies we should suspect pseudoscience.

4. *Use of questionable sources.* If the person making a scientific claim has been associated with questionable science in the past, is it logical to believe that the latest project is not also pseudoscience?

5. *Expressions of paranoia.* One of the hallmarks of pseudoscience is that its proponents have been discriminated against by the scientific community. They will tell the public that the government or scientific establishment is suppressing their work because they are not part of the elite research community. If anything, the scientific community is not into suppression but discovery. Anyone who provides a strong scientific basis for what they are studying will be accepted by the research community. If the basis for what you are espousing is bogus, with no scientific support, of course it will not be accepted.

6. *Lack of public sharing.* Any person or group of people who claim scientific proof should be willing to share their procedures in detail and desire independent replication of their results. We should be especially wary of people who say they will not share their data or methods with others for fear of someone stealing their

discovery. Remember, one of the characteristics of science is that it is public. A research result only gets stronger when it is replicated.

7. *Citing of ancient truths.* Remember that science advances slowly through changes based on empirical studies. We *expect* science to change over time. Whenever someone is pushing a "scientific" point of view that has remained static for decades or centuries, something is probably wrong with the picture. If we thought that we had medical science nailed down in 1900 and never continued research in multiple areas, think of the advances we would have missed. The "wisdom of the ancients" is often overrated.

8. *Finding small effects.* Generally if very controlled conditions and complicated statistical gymnastics result in a miniscule effect, then the "discovery" may be trivial or due to chance or systematic error. Some experiments on mind reading and telekinesis have shown such results.

9. *Making extraordinary claims which require extraordinary evidence (Carl Sagan).* A researcher claims to have found a way to reverse the aging process. The scientific community will not let this person get away with merely producing anecdotal reports, testimonials, and possibly "doctored" digital photographs to prove this claim. There will have to be many controlled and replicated studies to confirm the claim before it is accepted by other scientists.

10. *Complaining about observation effects.* Sometimes a person will say that a phenomenon cannot be measured because any attempt to do so will destroy the effect. This same notion is present when the "spirit world" will not communicate with us because "they sense that you disbelieve" in their existence. Something is either scientifically measurable or it is not.

11. *Inappropriate credentials of the proponents.* Science is far too complicated for a person to be an expert in several detailed fields. Sometimes a person who is well trained in one field such as physics may claim some sort of major "discovery" in the area of nutrition. The physicist, who may well know a lot about science in general and physics in particular, may not have adequate training to engage in research on nutrition. If the person making the claim has not been trained in the proper field of study, we should always be suspicious.

12. *Use of rhetoric, emotions, and propaganda.* Legitimate science relies on presenting data derived from controlled studies and replicated by others in the scientific community. There is little need to "sell" a result to other scientists. You will rarely hear scientists use terms such as "revolutionary" or "breakthrough" in scientific journals, although sometimes in popular media reports of the work reporters will use those descriptors. A person who has to use rhetoric and engender an appeal to emotion is most likely using pseudoscience.

13. *A mysterious lexicon.* In an effort to appear scientific, pseudoscientists often invent a whole new culture and vocabulary that is shared only by practitioners of the craft. To the outsider, it appears that there is whole new mysterious "world" inside the pseudoscience and one's initial feeling is that there must be something to this idea if it has its own terminology. Sometimes the pseudoscientists will simply rename phenomena that traditional science has already named, just to add to the mystery.

All of us who rely on the integrity of scientific research should constantly be on the alert for instances of pseudoscience or junk science. We must be very critical of research in our field and studies that relate to our field so that we base our clinical decisions only on the best information available. There is never a shortage of people who try to pass off their work as having scientific merit. Sometimes it is difficult to tell the real science from the pseudoscience and the real researchers from the charlatans. For example, Robert Park reports on a case (*Daubert v. Merrell Dow Pharmaceuticals, Inc.*) brought before the Supreme Court having to do with a woman who filed suit claiming that a medication she took caused birth defects:

> The case involved Bendectin, the only morning sickness medication ever approved by the Food and Drug Administration. It had been used by millions of women, and more than 30 published studies had found no evidence that it caused birth defects. Yet eight so-called experts were willing to testify, in exchange for a fee from the Daubert family, that Bendectin might indeed cause birth defects. In ruling that such testimony was not credible because of lack of supporting evidence, the court instructed federal judges to serve as "gatekeepers," screening juries from testimony based on scientific nonsense. Recognizing that judges are not scientists, the court invited judges to experiment with ways to fulfill their gatekeeper responsibility. Justice Stephen G. Breyer encouraged trial judges to appoint independent experts to help them. (2003, p. 1)

This case brings up an important point. Junk science and pseudoscience can work its way into the court system and is not just produced in the mass media. You can easily imagine a member of a jury inundated with technical jargon from both sides of a case, each of which seems impressive and plausible. With no background in science, jurors are at the mercy of the "expert" witnesses. As mentioned in the previous example, judges as well as attorneys must be ultimately responsible for the quality of information presented in their courtrooms.

As a student in communication disorders, it is your responsibility to critically read the scientific literature as a basis for your clinical work. But be aware that research varies in quality and that the pseudoscientific community is alive and well and communicating with your clients. They will always be asking you about some new fad in therapy that may or may not have sufficient empirical support. Just as the Supreme Court has directed federal judges to be gatekeepers for the quality of evidence presented in their courtrooms, you will also be the gatekeeper for evidence-based practice with your clients. You should be standing up for scientific integrity with your clients and colleagues every day of your professional life.

Summary

The scientific method is an important way of knowing about the world. It exists as a "process" carried out by individuals who are interested in answering questions. The method of science has specific characteristics that separates it from other ways of knowing and it involves experimental control, gathering empirical data, sharing data and procedures with others, and admitting that any single study reveals only probabilistic and possibly incomplete knowledge of what has been investigated. Scientists must adhere to a very strict ethical code in their conduct of research and the treatment of participants in their studies. Many who engage in pseudoscience and quackery try to imbue their work with a scientific mantle; however, failure to follow the scientific method always sets their findings apart from true science.

LEARNING ACTIVITIES

1. Find five outlandish claims on the Internet of "scientific support" for a product. Evaluate the evidence to see if it actually meets scientific criteria or not.

2. Go to the IRB web page at your university and read the guidelines for developing and submitting a research protocol.

3. Check your university website for material on scientific misconduct and how this is handled on your campus.

4. Go to one of the pseudoscience websites mentioned in this chapter and write a summary of five different examples of pseudoscience. Indicate why these are not viewed as legitimate science.

5. Search the ASHA website to find an article on pseudoscience in communication disorders and summarize the issues raised in the article.

CHAPTER 3

Crafting Scientific and Answerable Questions

Judge a man by his questions rather than by his answers.

—Voltaire (1694–1778)

In the movie *A Few Good Men* (1992) Tom Cruise plays an attorney named Lt. Kaffee and Jack Nicholson plays Colonel Jessup of the Marine Corps. In the courtroom the following interchange takes place:

Colonel Jessup: "You want answers?"
Lt. Kaffee: "I think I'm entitled."
Colonel Jessup: "YOU WANT ANSWERS?"
Lt. Kaffee: "I WANT THE TRUTH!"
Colonel Jessup: "YOU CAN'T HANDLE THE TRUTH!"

As illustrated in the exchange between Tom Cruise and Jack Nicholson, most people are typically very interested in answers. Unfortunately, it is most unusual for people to spend substantial time considering the questions for which they want answers. As the title of this chapter suggests, even when it is relatively easy to get answers, if the answer you obtain is not to a well-constructed, relevant question, your research project can be a rather unsatisfying experience. It is the feeling that a scientist has after spending a lot of time on a research project only to answer a question that other researchers feel is obvious, unimportant, or somehow ambiguous. There is a certain amount of regret when a researcher completes a study and wishes he or she would have designed the project differently or simply asked a different or more refined research question. In this textbook we will devote an entire chapter to the important issue of developing research questions. We will take our time, provide copious examples, and walk you through the process of crafting quality scientific questions.

Learning Objectives

This chapter will enable readers to:

- Understand the difference between theories, problems, hypotheses, and questions.
- Be able to explain the difference between inductive and deductive reasoning.

- Understand the nature of independent and dependent variables in research.
- Be able to determine if a research question is answerable or not.
- Understand the criteria for selecting an effective dependent variable in research.

In the old parlor game called *20 Questions* you have a limited number of queries (20) to determine the identity of some object that another person has in mind. Theoretically, by asking questions that can eliminate many possibilities (e.g., "Is the object alive?") you can gradually zero in on the identity of the object. If you cannot identify the object in twenty questions, you lose. If you ask a lousy question in the game (e.g., "Does the object exist?") you will get what you deserve—an answer that probably will not be very meaningful or helpful. Now let us think about research. It is much harder than the parlor game because you do not have twenty questions. You may only have one or two that can be answered by designing a scientific study. What this means to a good researcher is that a lot of time and effort must be spent crafting an answerable question so that when the answer is obtained the result will be meaningful. If you only have a limited number of questions to ask, they had better be good. In the movie quote, Tom Cruise does not really ask any good questions; rather, he is obsessed with getting answers so that he will know "the truth." Ideally, we hope that the answers we obtain will lead us to knowing more about a particular issue, but remember in the last chapter we said that scientists view these things probabilistically, and they may never really go as far as saying they have discovered "the truth" about anything. Answers to scientific questions, however, can increase our ability to accurately predict relations among variables but only if the questions are very carefully constructed.

Problems, Theories, Hypotheses, and Research Questions

Before we address exactly how to design an answerable research question we would like to get several definitions out of the way. Some of these terms overlap, and in fact, some authorities use them interchangeably. In some ways, you can view the terms **problem, theory, hypothesis,** and **research question** as being on a continuum from general to more specific (See Figure 3.1). We briefly discuss these terms because most books on experimental methods use them, and questions sometimes flow from theories and problems.

Problems

An undefined problem has an infinite number of solutions.

Robert A. Humphrey

The greatest challenge to any thinker is stating the problem in a way that will allow a solution.

Bertrand Russell (1872–1970)

A problem well stated is a problem half solved.

Charles F. Kettering (1876–1958)

The "research problem" is sometimes a difficult concept to define. Kerlinger and Lee state:

It is not always possible for a researcher to formulate the problem simply, clearly, and completely. The researcher may often have only a rather general, diffuse, even confused notion of the problem. . . . Nevertheless, adequate statement of the research problem is one of the most important parts of research. . . . If one wants to solve a problem, one must generally know what the problem is. (2000, p. 24)

FIGURE 3.1

Increasing Specificity in Approaching Research Questions

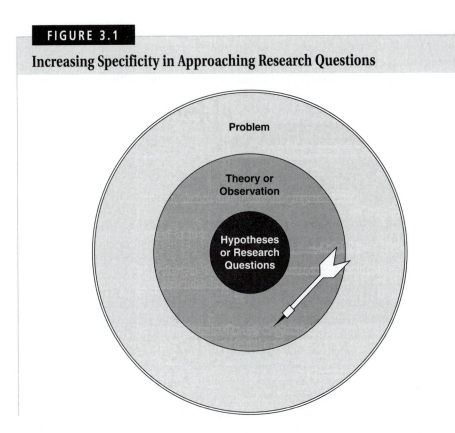

Given this perspective, it is easy to see that formulation of a research problem is one of the early stages in approaching a topic of research. It is necessarily a bit nebulous at first, and then as the scientist thinks about it, conceptualizing the problem at hand, he or she can form specific hypotheses and questions that can be answered empirically. According to Kerlinger and Lee (2000) a good problem statement should meet three criteria: (1) a relation between two or more variables should be expressed, (2) the problem should be clearly stated in unambiguous terms, and (3) the problem statement should be amenable to empirical evaluation. Kerlinger and Lee (2000) indicate that a problem can be articulated in either a statement or in question form, and they express their preference for the latter. Other researchers, however, express a more elaborate view of problem statements. For example, Cline and Clark (2000) state:

> The problem statement, in its entirety, is an internally consistent logical argument having structure, sequence and rationale. Although I have said that a problem statement is *not* a question, a problem statement necessarily leads into *at least one central research question* or objective from which numerous research questions and/or hypotheses could be generated.

Cline and Clark were referring to scientific writing of research proposals in which an entire section of the proposal is devoted to a "statement of the problem" which sets the stage for other sections of the research plan such as literature review, hypotheses, and methodology. Our point here is that whether a research problem is articulated in a statement, a question, or five pages of text in a research proposal, it is critically important in leading the researcher to more specific, measurable hypotheses and answerable questions.

Theories

> The scientific theory I like best is that the rings of Saturn are composed entirely of lost airline luggage.
>
> Mark Russell

> A theory must be tempered with reality.
>
> Jawaharlal Nehru (1889–1964)

According to Kerlinger and Lee, "A theory is a set of interrelated constructs (concepts), definitions, and propositions that present a systematic view of phenomena by specifying relations among variables, with the purpose of explaining and predicting the phenomena" (2000, p. 11). As we will discuss later in more detail, some research questions arise in an effort to verify or confirm a particular theory. In some respects, theories have taken a lot of heat from laymen and scientists. How often have you heard someone say, "It's only a theory"? Some college professors are criticized because all they do is talk about theories while neglecting practical matters. But it is important to remember that not all theories are equally validated. For example the theory of gravity (Newton), the theory of relativity (Einstein), and the theory that planets revolve around the sun (Copernicus) are all still regarded as "theories," because, as stated in Chapter 2, nothing can really be conclusively "proven." Yet we have used the implications of these theories to travel through space and account for many previously unexplainable phenomena in physics. On the other hand, there are theories that most people find absurd. Of course, what differentiates theories that have earned respectability from those on the fringes of science is their ability to explain and predict phenomena. The theory of gravity pretty much can account for most falling bodies, and although we cannot conclusively prove it impossible for you to step off the Empire State Building tomorrow and hover in the air, we wouldn't want to bet the ranch on it. Theories, of course, are subject to change as ongoing research provides new information. One can easily see that doing an experiment to validate a theory is a reasonable approach to scientific inquiry. In fact, Kerlinger and Lee state that the "basic aim of science is theory" (2000, p. 11). Theories are important because they are one way that we can perceive some coherence in the world or explain and predict the systematic occurrence of phenomena in the world. Theories thrive because of scientific validation, but they shrivel up and eventually disappear if the research fails to show results that support them. This is why, as the Nehru quote indicates, we must temper theories with reality. Bordens and Abbott (1999) discuss five factors that help to determine the longevity of a theory. First, a theory must be able to somehow account for the existing data on a particular topic. Second, a theory must have some explanatory value in accounting for phenomena. Third, the theory must be testable in that it can either pass or fail an empirical examination. A theory that is not amenable to empirical testing is probably not scientific in the first place and may be more in the realm of religion, philosophy, or art. Fourth, the theory must have some predictive value. If a theory predicts relations between or the occurrence of certain variables, it earns a degree of validation. Finally, a theory should be able to account for phenomena using the fewest unsupported assumptions, a notion referred to as **Occam's Razor** or the **Law of Parsimony.** Note that we are not saying that the "simplest" explanation or theory is the most acceptable. For instance, there might be a theory that accounts for the development of the Grand Canyon by positing that a large alien spaceship crashed on that site and created a large hole. On the other hand, there is the theory that the Grand Canyon is a gigantic gorge carved by the Colorado River. It is obviously simpler to assume the crash of an alien starship instead of assuming millions of years of erosion. However, the latter explanation is more acceptable because it accounts for the data, has greater explanatory power, is predictable from what we know about forces of erosion, and does not require us to believe outlandish assumptions that have little empirical support. We will talk a bit more about theories in a later section concerning how scientists approach the development of research ideas.

Hypotheses and Research Questions

It is a good morning exercise for a research scientist to discard a pet hypothesis every day before breakfast. It keeps him young.

Konrad Lorenz (1903–1989)

The great tragedy of Science—the slaying of a beautiful hypothesis by an ugly fact.

Thomas H. Huxley (1825–1895)

Kerlinger and Lee indicate that a "a hypothesis is a conjectural statement of the relation between two or more variables" (2000, p. 26). In this sense, it is very similar to the criteria for a good problem statement mentioned previously because the hypothesis describes a relation between variables and implies some possibility of testing that relationship. Perhaps the biggest difference between problem statements and hypothesis statements is their specificity.

Problem Statement
What is the relationship between intelligence and misarticulation in children with mental retardation?

Hypothesis Statement
As scores on the Stanford Binet Intelligence Scales increase, total errors on the Goldman-Fristoe Test of Articulation will decrease.

Note that in the problem statement, no prediction is made about the relationship between intelligence and misarticulation, only that there is some question about the relationship between the two variables. Note also, that the terms *misarticulation* and *intelligence*, although general, have some implication for testing if the scientist can find examinations that provide valid measurements of these constructs. Implicit in stating hypotheses, as mentioned in Chapter 2, is the notion that an experiment can produce a variety of possible results. So even though it may not be formally stated, the researcher interested in the previous hypothesis must also admit that the following possibilities could occur:

> As scores on the Stanford Binet Intelligence Scales increase, total errors on the Goldman-Fristoe Test of Articulation will increase.

Or:

> There will be no relationship between scores on the Stanford Binet Intelligence Scales and total errors on the Goldman-Fristoe Test of Articulation.

Recall that in Chapter 2 we included the fact that scientists either implicitly or explicitly state hypotheses in order to maintain some degree of objectivity in research. A researcher may have a "pet hypothesis" but still knows that it may not be supported by empirical testing. By stating what is being looked for in a study, the researcher is being very specific about why the study was done and what problem is being addressed. Some may view this as a certain type of bias on the part of the experimenter (Hegde, 2003), but others view considering hypotheses as productive (Kerlinger & Lee, 2000).

Other authorities (Hegde, 2003; Bachrach, 1969; Sidman, 1960; Skinner, 1972) do not place as much importance on stating hypotheses but instead emphasize asking questions. If the previous examples were addressed as questions, they would look like this:

> What is the relationship between scores on the Stanford Binet Intelligence Scales and total errors on the Goldman-Fristoe Test of Articulation?

Hegde states:

> Skinner (1972) said that one can ask a question and immediately proceed to answer it through an experiment. He saw the intermediate step of hypothesis formulation as an unnecessary exercise. Whether predicted or not, a well-designed experiment may produce results that throw light on the relation between the variables investigated. Because the experimental results are the final test of a relation between variables, the need to predict those results beforehand is not clear. (2003, p. 65)

There are other disadvantages of hypothesis statements often mentioned by researchers. Stating a hypothesis can reinforce bias in the investigator, even though the researcher is ideally supposed to consider *all* possible outcomes of a study. A focus on a favorite outcome might influence some scientists. Also, hypotheses not be necessary for certain types of research (e.g., ethnographic studies that simply try to describe phenomena of interest). Moreover, hypotheses may not account for unexpected or serendipitous results in research. Many of our most significant discoveries have been the results of accidental outcomes of research that could never have been hypothesized prior to the investigation (Roberts, 1989). However, despite these caveats, we can see the utility of both hypothesis statements and questions in terms of narrowing the focus of research from the general problem statement. Note that whether one uses hypotheses or questions, the statement of the problem is articulated in a more specific and testable manner. In questions, you are still asking about the relationship between two variables in a testable way. In hypotheses, you are suggesting what the relationship might be in a testable way.

Deductive and Inductive Approaches to Generating Questions

Most textbooks on research methods discuss deductive and inductive approaches to designing a scientific investigation. The deductive approach involves approaching the problem from a general idea, usually a theory, and moving toward specific controlled observations that ultimately will confirm or disconfirm the theory. The inductive approach starts with individual observations that lead to a question/hypothesis and finally result in development of an overall theory. Thus, **deductive reasoning** goes from general to specific and **inductive reasoning** proceeds from specific to general. We will give two examples of approaching research from both deductive and inductive perspectives. First, we have a speech-language pathologist who has meticulously combed through the extant literature in the local university library and found many articles concerning the occurrence of behavior problems in children with specific language impairment (SLI), some theorizing that a major reason for behavior problems in these children stems from their difficulty communicating. As the theory goes, children with language impairment "act out" because it is an efficient means of making their needs known to others in the environment. This theory got the SLP thinking about a research project. She wondered if the severity of the language impairment was somehow related to the severity of the behavior problems in SLI children. None of the studies she found had addressed this relationship, so she decided to design a study of her own. Her problem statement was: *What is the relationship between severity of SLI and severity of behavior problems in preschool children?* She then hypothesized the following theory: *As the severity of language disorder increases on the Smith Test of Language, the severity of behavior problems will increase on the Jones Behavior Disturbance Inventory.* Like any good scientist, however, the SLP kept all possible hypothetical outcomes, including the null hypothesis, in the back of her mind. After the study was completed, she was delighted to see that her initial hypothesis was confirmed and that as the severity of SLI increased, there was a concomitant increase in behavior problems. The theory that stimulated the research problem had now been strengthened by the results of the SLP's study. Note that in her research she began with a general theory and moved toward gathering data on specific children to determine if the theory was supported.

Meanwhile, on the other side of town, there was a clinical audiologist who owned a private practice. In the course of his practice, he sometimes offered four sessions of group aural rehabilitation therapy as an added incentive to purchase a hearing instrument from his clinic. Like clockwork, the audiologist would offer his "aural rehab special" three times a year. After five years of practice, he began to notice a pattern in client satisfaction. He had the subjective feeling that the clients who purchased their hearing instruments during his "aural rehab special" seemed more satisfied than those who purchased aids without any opportunity for aural rehabilitation. Many of the specific clients reported to him that the aural rehabilitation sessions helped them to use their hearing instruments in real situations. After seeing all of these specific cases over a period of years, the audiologist noticed a possible pattern and began to wonder about the effects of aural rehabilitation. The research problem that he formulated was: *What is the difference in hearing aid satisfaction between clients with similar types of hearing loss who experience post-fitting aural rehabilitation and those who do not?* This research problem could then be turned into a specific hypothesis or research question, which the audiologist formulated as the following: *Is there a significant difference in client satisfaction ratings on the Smith Hearing Aid Satisfaction Questionnaire between clients who experienced post-fitting aural rehabilitation and those who did not?* He had five years of clinical records, including hearing aid satisfaction questionnaires that had been routinely administered to every client who purchased a hearing instrument. He also had records of who purchased hearing aids during the "aural rehab special" periods. As it turned out, a statistical analysis of the two groups of clients showed that those receiving post-fitting aural rehabilitation were significantly more satisfied than those who did not receive the extra training. Note that the audiologist began his research quest by talking to many individual clients and then hypothesizing a possible pattern that he noticed over a five-year period. A systematic analysis revealed that at least for his clients, those who had undergone the aural rehabilitation reported higher degrees of hearing aid satisfaction. This result made him wonder if overall, there is more than just a knowledge of technology to being a successful practitioner. Maybe the lesson to be learned is that you not only have to know about the latest in hearing aid technology to treat clients successfully, but you also need to show people how to use it effectively for communication to achieve optimal client results. "Hmmmm, sounds like a pretty good theory to me," said the audiologist. In the process, he had moved from looking at specific cases to formulating a question to gathering data and finally to developing an overarching theory that would guide his future practice.

> If Edison had a needle to find in a haystack, he would proceed at once with the diligence of the bee to examine straw after straw until he found the object of his search. . . . I was a sorry witness of such doings, knowing that a little theory and calculation would have saved him ninety per cent of his labor.
>
> Nikola Tesla (1857–1943)

The steps involved in the deductive approach are summarized in Figure 3.2. You can see that the process starts with a theory, then moves to a hypothesis, then to a scientific observation and finally to a confirmation or disconfirmation of the original theory. As a result of this process theories undergo change with the implications

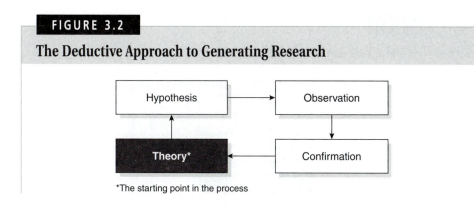

FIGURE 3.2

The Deductive Approach to Generating Research

*The starting point in the process

of new scientific data. The inductive approach is depicted in Figure 3.3. Note that the process begins with observation of specific instances of behavior which results in the researcher noticing a pattern in the performance. Knowledge of this pattern of behavior helps the researcher to generate a research question or hypothesis and conduct a scientific investigation. The results of the study may then direct the researcher to develop an overall theory to account for the phenomena that have been observed.

It is clear that valid research questions and procedures can arise from both deductive and inductive thinking. Figure 3.4 shows how the two types of reasoning could be viewed as different arms of a model with theory at its center. Recall the earlier quote by Kerlinger and Lee (2000) that "the basic aim of science is theory." As long as research can somehow be linked to theoretical formulations, it does not matter how we arrive there. As Kerlinger and Lee state:

> The ultimately most usable and satisfying relations, however, are those that are the most generalized, those that are tied to other relations in a theory. (2000, p. 13)

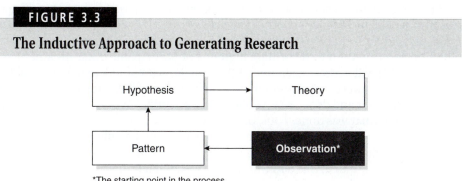

FIGURE 3.3

The Inductive Approach to Generating Research

*The starting point in the process

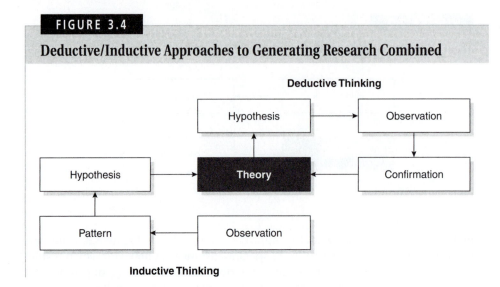

FIGURE 3.4

Deductive/Inductive Approaches to Generating Research Combined

Deductive Thinking

Inductive Thinking

Independent and Dependent Variables: Critical Elements

In our discussion of problems and hypotheses we stated that a major part of scientific inquiry is to determine relations between two or more variables. The terms **independent variable (IV)** and **dependent variable (DV)** come to us from the field of mathematics, which is why uttering them probably creates some measure of angst among our students. These terms, however, form the basis for comprehending *any* scientific investigation and we will take our time and give many examples to make sure that you understand them well. Figure 3.5 depicts four common examples of the relation between independent and dependent variables and illustrates the basic concept that *independent variables do exert some level of influence over or covariation with dependent variables.* It is sometimes a difficult task to determine the identity of the independent and dependent variable in a study. Figure 3.5 demonstrates that one reason independent variables may be especially elusive is because they can represent different conditions that are manipulated, show cause-effect relations, form prediction models, or be used to determine if groups of participants differ on a particular variable. We will address each one of these major uses of independent variables below. For now, however, it is important for you understand that knowing the identity of the independent and dependent variables in a scientific investigation is critical to understanding what was done. Thus, one of the first questions you should ask yourself in reading a study is "What are the independent and dependent variables?" We know it's difficult for you to even imagine yourself uttering those words, but take it from us that by the end of this book, they will be second nature to you.

As mentioned above, determining which variable is the IV and which variable is the DV is not always an easy task. The terms are described differently depending on

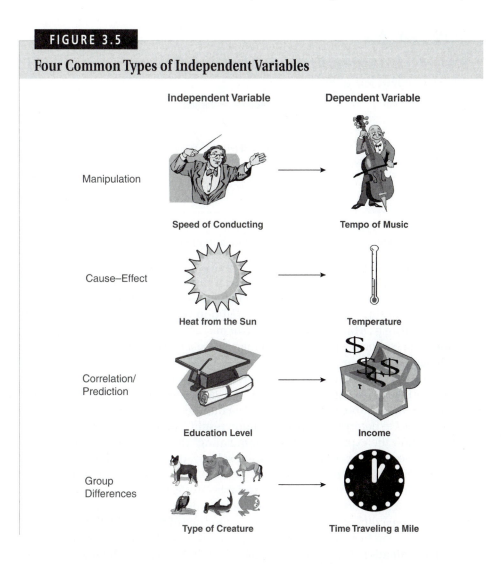

FIGURE 3.5

Four Common Types of Independent Variables

Independent Variable	Dependent Variable

Manipulation — Speed of Conducting → Tempo of Music

Cause–Effect — Heat from the Sun → Temperature

Correlation/ Prediction — Education Level → Income

Group Differences — Type of Creature → Time Traveling a Mile

which textbook you read and often in a study multiple measurements are reported by the researcher. Table 3.1 contains some common words and phrases associated with distinguishing between independent and dependent variables. Some of these terms are clearly related to the pictures in Figure 3.5.

Independent Variables That Manipulate

The notion of "manipulation" conjures up images of a scientist overtly directing parts of an experiment, rather like the conductor directing the cellist in Figure 3.5. In some cases, studies involving experimental manipulation may be focused on "cause-effect" relationships, and in some cases such relations may not be of primary

TABLE 3.1

Selected Terms Commonly Associated with Independent and Dependent Variables

Independent Variable	Dependent Variable
Cause	Effect
Antecedent	Consequent
Influences Dependent Variable	Influenced by Independent Variable
Manipulated Variable	Measured Variable
Predictor Variable	Predicted Variable
Causes Variation	Varies

interest. Let's look at some examples that represent clear manipulation on the part of the researcher:

• A researcher wants to find out the effects of three different tasks on the occurrence of phonological errors in preschool children. In the study, the researcher has children perform three tasks. In the first condition (single-word task), the child is shown a picture (e.g., a bicycle) and asked to name it. In the second condition (phrase task), the child is shown a picture (e.g., a man riding a bicycle), given the first part of the sentence (e.g., "The man is . . .), and the child is expected to produce the rest of the sentence (e.g., "riding the bicycle"). In the third condition, the child is expected to tell a story incorporating several pictures (e.g., a bicycle, a man, a park). Each child participates under all three conditions and the number and type of their articulation errors are tallied to determine which condition resulted in the most misarticulations. Can you see how the experimenter is "manipulating" the child by placing him or her into these three different conditions? In this example, the three conditions represent the independent variable. If the conditions are the IV, what is this IV supposed to have an effect on? In this case, the dependent variable (DV) is the number of misarticulations under each condition. The researcher wants to determine if the type of sampling mode (conditions) differentially affects the occurrence of misarticulations.

• Another researcher wants to determine the effects of masking noise level on speech discrimination. Can you already identify the IV and DV? The researcher develops four conditions that participants will experience. In the first condition, the participants will be given a speech discrimination task of telling if pairs of words presented at 50 dB are the same or different with no masking noise present. The second condition asks participants to do the discrimination task with 15 dB of masking noise presented through speakers. The third condition does the same thing with 25 dB of masking noise, and the fourth condition uses 35 dB of masking noise. In this study the IV is the level of masking noise presented across the four conditions. The DV is the score on the speech discrimination task. You can almost see the experimenter, hand on the attenuator, manipulating the level of masking noise.

These scenarios are very simple examples of independent variables that manipulate participants; we will consider more complex examples in later chapters concerning experimental design. Note that in all these studies, the researchers were not trying to determine the "cause" of anything. They were merely "describing" what happened to the dependent variable under various conditions.

Cause and Effect Independent Variables

Of all the scientific articles you will ever read as a student or a professional, very few of them will actually address the issue of cause and effect. In Figure 3.5 our example of cause and effect involves the sun (independent variable) having an effect on the temperature (dependent variable). There is clearly an effect on temperature when the sun is shining as opposed to when it is not. Temperatures should be higher in the presence of sunshine compared to when it is cloudy or dark. Cause and effect are dealt with most handily in the physical and biological sciences where variables can be tightly controlled, as in the study of chemistry or physics, and we do not have to worry as much about human participants. If we want to determine if a substance will explode when ignited with a spark, all we have to do is obtain a sample of the chemical and apply some ignition. If it explodes on a regular basis, we than know that we can "cause" an explosion by igniting this chemical. Even in biology, we can see the effects of administering various medications to human participants under controlled conditions. Thus, if we administer insulin to a person with diabetes we can reliably reduce the concentration of glucose in the blood. Inject the person and the glucose level goes down; do not inject them and the glucose level stays high—cause and effect. In behavioral sciences, however, investigation of cause and effect is much more problematic. Determining "cause," especially in the behavioral sciences, is difficult because cause is a very complicated issue. Many phenomena have multiple causes that act together to change a given variable. For example, we have not found the "cause" of stuttering. Over the years authorities have theorized that this disorder may arise from neurological, biological, psychological, behavioral, or other causal areas. It is also possible that two or more of these areas may interact together to "cause" stuttering. Adding to the complexity, it is also feasible that stuttering is comprised of various subtypes that each may be caused by a different combination of variables. Let us illustrate some limited examples of studies that may suggest cause and effect in communication disorders.

• A researcher is interested in determining if exposure to loud noise causes hearing loss in chinchillas. Remember the IRB from the previous chapter? It is possible that the "animal" IRB may not approve a study that is attempting to cause hearing loss in chinchillas, but let's say it is approved for this example. Four groups of animals are selected randomly and exposed systematically to varying levels of noise (independent variable) at 40 dB, 60 dB, 90 dB and 120 dB. Hearing function (dependent variable) was measured using auditory evoked potentials. If the hearing function for the groups exposed to the highest noise levels is lowest, then we may be able to say that excessive levels of noise exposure "caused" the hearing loss. This, of course, assumes that the groups of chinchillas were similar in their genetic makeup, age, and other relevant variables, which should have been accounted for in the random assignment (we will talk more about randomization in a later chapter.)

- The notion of "cause" does not always refer to accounting for the occurrence of a particular disorder as in the chinchilla example. In another sense, experimenters "manipulate" an independent variable to determine the effects of this control on a dependent variable. Thus, as Hegde indicates:

> There is no experiment unless the researcher has clearly identified at least one causal factor whose influence on a dependent variable is assessed while other potential causes are controlled for . . . an independent variable is manipulated whenever a treatment technique is introduced, withdrawn, reversed, or varied in some systematic manner. (2003, p. 63)

In our second example of "cause-effect" the researcher wants to determine the effect on disfluency when a person who stutters speaks in time to a metronome versus speaking without the timing device. In this experiment, five people who stutter are sampled as they talk spontaneously without a metronome and their disfluencies are counted (dependent variable.) Then each person is asked to speak in time to a metronome as disfluencies are counted again. These two techniques (independent variable) are alternated systematically four times for each of five participants. The results demonstrated that for all five participants, disfluency levels reduced to zero when speaking in time to the metronome, and disfluency increased significantly when speaking without the timing device. In this study we are not trying to say anything about the "cause" of stuttering, only that when we manipulate the IV (metronome/no metronome) fluency is systematically altered. We can "cause" a person to be more fluent by introducing a timing device and we can "cause" them to be more disfluent when we take the metronome away.

As this example shows, much of our research on the effects of treatment for various communication disorders assumes that the therapy or clinical manipulation has some sort of cause-effect relationship to client success. This is a very important concept known as *efficacy of treatment,* which basically boils down to knowing that the treatment is responsible for progress as opposed to other internal and external factors. You can imagine the challenges of attempting to control the manifold variables internal to the client (e.g., IQ, socioeconomic status, motivation, type of disorder, other complicating impairments, etc.) and external influences (e.g., parental involvement, language models, treatment provided by other sources, etc.) in showing that a particular treatment method is solely responsible for progress. We will discuss treatment research in detail later in the text. Attempting to determine any type of causation is a very difficult endeavor and as we said above, you will find very few studies in communication disorders that really address this issue well. We will be discussing in later chapters how people often believe that a particular study supports a cause-effect relationship when it in fact does not.

Correlation/Prediction Independent Variables

Much of the business of science involves *prediction* and *correlation.* Later portions of the present text will consider these types of research in more detail, but for now we would just like to introduce the material as it relates to independent and dependent variables. Recall that the basic notion of an independent variable is that it has an "effect" on a dependent variable. These "effects" were illustrated in our examples of independent variables that *manipulate* a dependent variable and those that *cause* a dependent variable to systematically vary. Independent variables that correlate or predict are a bit more subtle and differ from the first two types in a couple of ways. First, an IV that manipulates or causes a change in a DV clearly makes some sort of causal connection between manipulations of an experimenter and changes in the dependent variable. The conductor makes the cellist play faster and the sun causes the temperature to rise. In the case of correlational independent variables we are no longer talking about causal relationships in which an experimenter manipulates an IV for an effect on a DV. Correlational independent variables certainly are not thought to "cause" anything. Any "effect" you see of "manipulating" the IV is really seen in the two variables (IV and DV) moving together or *covarying*. For instance, our example in Figure 3.5 shows educational level as an independent variable and income as a dependent variable. The researcher may want to "manipulate" educational level (IV) by examining different levels of education among participants to determine any "effects" on annual income. It is easy to see that education does not "cause" changes in income level. There are many people with little formal education who have developed businesses or invented products that provide very high annual incomes. On the other hand, there are many people with college degrees in the ranks of the homeless. Yet there are many studies that show a general trend that the higher one's educational level, generally the greater the annual income. There is a high correlation between the two. In fact, it is possible to make a fairly accurate prediction of annual income range for groups of people if you know their educational level. You cannot predict accurately for an individual, but you can get in the ballpark for a group. Does this mean that educational level "causes" annual income? Certainly not. What it does mean is that statistically, for groups of people, educational level and income tend to *move together in the same direction,* up and down. Sure, there are many exceptions, but by and large, there is a strong relationship between the two variables for most people. You have no doubt heard the old phrase "correlation does not imply causation." We will remind you of that phrase many times in this book.

The second way correlational independent variables differ from the first two in Figure 3.5 is that researchers can use them for prediction of specific types of scores. Let's say we want to find out which students will be successful in graduate school. We have several variables at our disposal which include undergraduate GPA and the score on the Graduate Record Examination (GRE). If we wanted to predict a student's GPA at the end of graduate school, we might develop a formula that included undergraduate GPA and GRE to see if we can accurately predict the graduate GPA. In this case, the independent (or predictor) variables would be the undergraduate GPA and GRE and the dependent (predicted) variable would be the graduate GPA. We want to see the "effect" of the IVs on the DV. In this case the "effect" is really the ability of the

IVs to correlate or predict the DV and not any type of "manipulation" in a cause-effect sense. We just want to see in what directions these things move and use them to predict graduate performance. Here are some examples of correlational/predictive independent variables:

• A researcher wants to determine the relationship between age and hearing impairment. In this study the researcher gathers data on client age (IV) and hearing thresholds on an audiometric test (DV). The results of the study show that as age increases, hearing thresholds also increase. The study shows that as people get older, their hearing ability becomes worse. Does this mean that age "causes" hearing loss? Not really. Age is a "macrovariable" that includes many things such as physical deterioration, effects of medications taken over long periods of time, exposure to noise, and so forth. Also, there are many exceptions involving a young person with hearing loss and an older person whose hearing is still good. But there is certainly a significant relationship for groups of people. If you get a group of people who are in their 70s and compare them to a group of people in their 20s you will probably find more hearing loss in the older group. It has probably occurred to you that the selection of an IV in correlational studies is a bit arbitrary. You are absolutely correct! It depends a lot on the researcher's interest and framing of the research question. The hearing loss researcher may have a primary interest in hearing threshold and use this as the independent variable. In this case, the dependent variable would be age. Really, the main thing that changes is the wording of the question. In the first case you are asking, "What is the relationship between age and hearing threshold?" In the second example, you are asking "What is the relationship between hearing threshold and age?" Basically, the same issue is addressed either way, but there is a difference in which variable is independent and which is dependent.

• Another researcher wants to determine the most efficient predictor of vocabulary size in children who are eighteen months of age. Data are gathered on frequency of weekly parental book reading, interaction time with parents per week, and parent educational level (IVs). Children's vocabulary is measured using the MacArthur Communicative Development Inventory. There are statistical techniques that can tell us how effectively each of the three IVs predict vocabulary size both individually and in combination (we will talk about these methods later in the present text). The statistical analysis might show that if we use the parent book reading variable and the parent interaction variable we have a pretty good ability to predict a child's vocabulary score at eighteen months. That is, the more parents read to their children and interact with them, the higher the vocabulary score will become. In this study, we are not just interested in determining relationships among variables but are interested in being able to predict vocabulary (DV) based on knowledge of certain parental behaviors (IVs). The identity of "predictor" and "predicted" variables depends to a large degree on the way the researcher asks the question. It is possible that the researcher may want to use the child's vocabulary score (IV) to predict the frequency of parental book reading interactions (DV). Again, as in the correlation example above, prediction does not imply causation.

Independent Variables That Involve Group Differences

The final type of independent variable is one in which the experimenter wants to determine if groups differ on some relevant variable. In this type of study, the experimenter systematically "manipulates" the composition of groups of participants and then takes a measurement of some variable that is hypothesized to occur differentially among the groups. In Figure 3.5, our example involves six groups of various creatures (IV) and we want to measure their speed traveling the distance of one mile (DV). In this study, the researcher must be sure to select animals for membership in each group based on rigid criteria. For example, the researcher would not want to populate the dog group with a bunch of greyhounds and leave out chihuahuas. This would certainly affect the average speed of the group. Likewise, the bird group would perform differently if falcons were selected and no hummingbirds included. On the other hand, the researcher *may* want to operationally define the dog group as being composed of exclusively greyhounds and label it the "greyhound group." We will discuss the important role of operational definitions in the next section. The point here is that group membership in a study where the IV is "group" must be very carefully defined and controlled so we know what we are truly studying. We will talk much more about participant selection in studies evaluating group differences, but for now we just want to emphasize that the grouping of participants itself can constitute an independent variable. Now we will consider a couple of examples related to communication disorders.

• A researcher wants to determine if people who stutter differ from fluent speakers in terms of their anxiety level. One group of participants was selected based on their enrollment in speech clinics for treatment of stuttering. A conversational sample was taken to verify the existence of stuttering. A second group of age-matched fluent speakers was identified from a university population and a conversational sample verified that no stuttering occurred in this group. Thus, two groups (IV) were identified and compared on a valid and reliable psychological scale (DV) on which participants rated their level of anxiety for different situations. In this study, the two groups were found to differ significantly, with the stuttering group showing higher levels of anxiety than the nonstuttering group. How would the researcher interpret these results? Could he or she say that stuttering is caused by increased anxiety? Just like in the previous correlational example, there is absolutely no proof of any cause-effect relation between anxiety and stuttering. In fact, one could make the case that people who stutter are more anxious *because* they stutter rather than increased anxiety causing their fluency failure. Again we make the point that cause-effect relationships are *very* difficult to find in most empirical investigations.

• In another study using groups as an independent variable an audiologist was interested in determining if people with different types of hearing loss differed in their speech discrimination ability. The researcher found three groups of participants with comparable degrees of hearing loss that represented sensorineural, conductive, and mixed hearing loss. The measurement of interest in this study was percentage correct on a word discrimination test presented under controlled conditions. Can you guess the IV and DV in this study? If you said the IV is the type of hearing loss and the DV is the discrimination score, you are absolutely right!

A Final Word on Independent Variables

We have discussed independent variables in some detail because they are very important in understanding how a study was designed. Remember the progression from a general statement of the problem moving toward a specific hypothesis or research question. Usually the independent and dependent variables are clearly specified in the hypothesis or research question. They will not necessarily be called "independent variable" and "dependent variable" in the article you are reading, but the researcher will somehow juxtapose these two types of variables in some type of language. Take this example: "The present study was designed to determine the effects of different masking levels on the occurrence of disfluency in people who stutter." Even though the researcher did not specifically label them as such, you should be able to see that the IV is the different masking levels and the DV is disfluency. See how you do on the following:

• This study examined the use of distal pointing in children at six-month intervals between the ages of six to twenty-four months. (IV = age; DV = distal pointing)
• The present investigation was designed to determine if a group of participants who regularly take aspirin differs from a group of participants who do not take aspirin in hearing threshold. (IV = aspirin/nonaspirin; DV = hearing threshold)
• This study compared the use of time-out procedures versus response cost on the occurrence of behavior problems in children with language disorder. (IV = timeout/ response cost; DV = occurrence of behavior problems)
• This study compared two different types of aural rehabilitation treatment regimens to determine their effects on client satisfaction. (IV = type of treatment; DV = client satisfaction)
• Self-esteem was measured in children with language disorders (LD), children with phonological disorders, and those with normal communication skills. (IV = normal group, LD group, phonological group; DV = self-esteem)
• The present study was designed to determine the value of dynamic versus static assessment in predicting response to treatment in children with language impairment. (IV = dynamic/static assessment data; DV = response to treatment)

You can see that it is not always easy to determine the IV and DV in studies just because of the way things are worded in the article, and there are at least two major factors adding to the confusion when trying to determine the identity of the independent and dependent variables, as discussed in the following paragraphs.

Testing of Participants to Form Groups or to Qualify for the Study

We can use the example presented on self-esteem in three groups of children to illustrate this point. We have already said that the IV in this study is the three groups of children (language impaired, phonologically impaired, normal) and that the DV is a measurement of their self-esteem. The researcher reporting this project, however, provides a lot of test data on language production, language comprehension, and phonological ability. These are all measurements, and did we not say in an earlier section that the DV is usually the "measurement" that the researcher takes on the participants? What are all these language and phonological scores? Aren't we really interested in self-esteem? The answer is that the measurements of language and phonology were taken simply to place participants in appropriate groups so the IV of "group" could be validated. Certainly, if a child was placed in the language impaired group, we would want some evidence of language disorder. Therefore, when reading a study remember not to confuse measurements taken for purposes of grouping participants with measurements representing the dependent variable. A good way of thinking about this is to try and hook up the IV of the study with the measurement in which the researcher is *most* interested. Are we most interested in language ability or self-esteem? Another tipoff is to think specifically about whether the IV involves grouping of participants. If it does, then you should expect that measurements will be used to populate those groups even before the DV is actually measured.

Measurements That Could Be Either a DV or an IV

A second confusing issue in discriminating independent and dependent variables in a study involves an investigation where many of the variables studied *could be either* a DV or IV depending on the wording of the experimental question. For example: *The present investigation was designed to determine if a group of participants who regularly take aspirin differs from a group of participants who do not take aspirin in hearing threshold.* The wording in this example suggests that the participants were grouped by their use of aspirin, presumably by identifying people who were on consistent aspirin regimens and others who did not take aspirin at all. Because the researcher grouped the participants by aspirin/nonaspirin regimen and then measured hearing threshold, it is fairly clear that the medication status of the participants was the independent variable. The hearing threshold was the variable that was thought to be "influenced" by taking or not taking the medication. The experimenter, however, could have reversed the variables in the study. For instance, the researcher could have found participants who represented differing levels of hearing thresholds and then conducting in-depth interviews to determine the frequency and dosage of taking aspirin in all of the hearing threshold groups. In this case the independent variable would be hearing threshold group and the dependent variable would be the ingestion of aspirin. You can see why it is confusing when the variables in a study could be used in either way. It is very important to consider the way research questions or problems are worded to try and discern which is the independent and dependent variable. As we progress through the text, you will have many chances to practice identifying these important variables.

Answerability

Earlier in this text we indicated that science can only answer certain types of questions. As mentioned previously, the types of questions that science *cannot* answer are *engineering questions* and *value questions*. So as we construct our research questions, it is a "no-brainer" to steer clear of questions that deal with the "how to" of an issue or moral/aesthetic judgments about phenomena. Part of making a question answerable is to make sure it deals with measurable constructs and that there is some agreement in the scientific community as to how the measurement should be taken. Let's look at some questions that would make a competent scientist cringe:

> How can we cure stuttering?
> How can we teach children with language disorders to spell?
> Is it ethical to do therapy over the Internet?
> Should we recommend the most expensive hearing aids to our clients before
>   the less expensive options?

The first two questions have to do with engineering or "how to" issues. We are sure you could raise all sorts of issues about the first question. For instance, the notion of "cure" is problematic because we don't really know what this means. Does it mean total remission or just functional improvement in fluency? Think about the impossibility of designing a study to answer the "how" part of the question. How to do something requires that a procedure be developed with some sort of sequence of events. We could develop a treatment program for stuttering, but that would not be research. It would be developing a program. It is not an answerable question scientifically. Now if we had developed a program and wanted to determine whether it reduced stuttering, that is a different matter. It is certainly possible to compare two therapies, or compare a therapy condition against a control group who received no treatment. But these do not really answer the original question about a cure or address the "how" issue. The best we could do is to indicate whether stuttering is reduced under certain conditions, or maybe even to say that one stuttering treatment resulted in more fluency gains than another. The second question also involves engineering, this time about how to teach a child to spell. Again, when we come up against the "how" of an issue, we need to develop a procedure to teach spelling, but this is not research. We can evaluate a program once it is developed by comparing it to other programs or even determining if certain components of a treatment regime make significant contributions to client progress, but the original development of the program is not really a research question. The third question has to do with a moral judgment about ethics. Whenever we get into such judgments there are always differing perspectives and extenuating circumstances that could change the judgment. Such questions are best dealt with by professional ethics boards that will not be doing research on the issue; they will consult moral and ethical codes and make a judgment based on those. Similarly, the fourth question deals with ethics and the order in which you present treatment options to clients. Again, research cannot answer this question, because it deals with standards of practice and ethical prescriptions. It would be possible to study whether or not more expensive hearing instruments are purchased by clients if they are presented first in a list of options as compared to last. If the study found that more expensive instruments were, in fact, purchased when presented as a first option rather than last, this still does not answer the question of "should we do it that way?" As we zero in on crafting a competent research question, we should make sure to avoid asking questions that are scientifically unanswerable.

Selecting Dependent Variables

One of our wise old statistics teachers once said, "Your study is only as good as your dependent variable." The dependent variable is the measurement that you are taking in your study. It is the skill or behavior you are interested in measuring to see if it changes as the result of experimental manipulation, membership in a group, or can be predicted in some lawful way by knowing about the independent variable. A good way to recall this notion is to remember that the dependent variable *depends* on the independent variable. A scientist should do a lot of thinking and researching before choosing a dependent variable, because once it is selected, it must remain for the duration of the study and on through the publication phase of the investigation. Nothing is more regrettable than choosing a DV only to find out later that it is a lousy measurement that has little credibility or respect from the scientific community. Think of a researcher who has tested hundreds of participants, on a weak measurement that means nothing, wasting everyone's time. Researchers can avoid this scenario if they would only think of the three important factors discussed next.

Validity

In this chapter we will discuss validity only in terms of selecting dependent variables. Later in the text we will consider both validity and reliability as they relate to other aspects of research design. Validity refers to the notion that you are actually measuring what you intend to measure. On the surface, this seems to be an obvious statement. After all, why would any researcher choose a measurement that does not really tap the construct in which he or she is interested? Unfortunately, researchers do this all the time. One of the biggest prey that research sharks can attack when reading a study is the validity of the dependent variable. As stated in an earlier section, research in physical and biological sciences is much more straightforward than the behavioral sciences. This is true for validity as well. If a scientist is interested in the weight of particular metals, it is easy to find an instrument that everyone would agree measures the heaviness of objects down to fractions of a gram. Thus, finding a scale to make a valid measurement of weights of metals would be relatively uncontroversial. In behavioral sciences, however, it is a much different scenario. Think about this carefully as you read the following example.

> A researcher is interested in determining if patients with vocal nodules have improved after participating in a voice therapy program. Voice samples of the patients reading a paragraph were recorded prior to therapy and after a six-week treatment period. The researcher developed the following scale to evaluate hoarseness: 1 = normal voice, 2 = mild hoarseness, 3 = moderate hoarseness, 4 = severe hoarseness. The pretherapy and posttherapy samples were played in a random order to a class of undergraduate students in communication disorders, and the students were asked to rate each patient's voice quality on the hoarseness scale. At the end of the study it was found that the average rating for pretherapy samples was 3.7 and the average rating for posttherapy samples was 2.2. Statistical analysis showed that these scores were significantly different beyond chance. The researcher concludes that the treatment program was successful.

The first thing you should do is to determine the identity of the independent and dependent variables in this example. In this study the IV was pre/post samples and the DV was student ratings on the hoarseness scale. After completing the study, this researcher writes it up in article form and sends it to a journal. Much to the researcher's dismay, the article is promptly rejected. Some of the reasons that the article was rejected centered around the choice of the dependent variable. The reviewers of the manuscript had some of the following concerns:

- Where did this rating scale come from? Did the researcher just make it up? How do we know it can be used reliably to discriminate between different gradations of hoarseness?
- Why is the measure just of hoarseness? We know that "breathiness" is also present in people who have vocal nodules, and it was never evaluated.
- Why would you use undergraduate students in communication disorders as judges? Shouldn't you have used people with more experience in rating vocal quality?
- Why did you not use any instrumental measures of vocal performance (e.g., jitter, shimmer) that are readily available in most speech science laboratories to supplement the listener quality ratings?

Well, you can see where this is going. The researcher is already regretting the choice of the dependent variable, and justifiably so. It is easy to just "pick" a measurement, but if it is not viewed as a valid measure of the construct of interest, the researcher has wasted his or her time and effort. Like we said earlier: A study is only as good as the dependent variable. Validity is a big part of this issue.

How does a researcher avoid validity problems with choosing a dependent variable? Perhaps the best advice is to start with a meticulous review of the existing research literature on the topic of interest. You should make certain that you especially review the work of respected researchers in the area of interest and inspect studies published in the most prestigious journals. After a while you will see that respected researchers tend to measure your construct of interest in particular ways and that there is some consensus about the most valid dependent variables. It is almost always preferable to use a known measurement for your dependent variable. If you do, it is easy to justify your selection by citing other published investigations also using that measure. Any reviewer who objects to your dependent variable would have to reject not only your study but also a host of other investigations already published in scientific journals that used the same measurement. It is very difficult for a researcher to develop a brand new measurement and be assured that it will be received positively by others in the scientific community. In cases where a measurement is not currently available for a particular construct, the researcher must put in the time to systematically develop a new measurement and show its validity and reliability. This is a study in itself and should be shared with other researchers in a journal article. The work required to develop a new valid and reliable dependent measure that has credibility among other scientists attests to the central importance of dependent variables in the research process.

Reliability

As in our discussion of validity, we will consider reliability only in terms of selection of dependent variables present. In later chapters we will discuss reliability again in relation to conducting research. Any dependent measurement must have at least two types of reliability. The first type is called **interjudge reliability,** which has to do with agreement between two or more judges about the occurrence of an observable event. If a researcher is in the process of selecting a dependent variable, it had better be one that two people can observe and agree on the score for that measurement. Again, you might be thinking that this is a no-brainer, but it is more complicated than most people think. As in our example of finding a valid method of determining the weight of various metals, reliability is often easier to obtain in physical and biological sciences. We have decided to use a very sensitive scale as a valid measure of the weight of metals. If the scale has a digital readout two judges can look at the display and write down the weight of each metal. Probably, the judges would be in close agreement about the numbers they saw on the digital display. Their interjudge reliability would probably be quite high. But behavioral sciences are, again, a different story. Take for example a dependent measure like "symbolic/pretend play." A researcher wants to determine if children with language impairment exhibit more or less symbolic play than their normal language peers. In this study the IV is the group (language impaired/normal language) and the DV is occurrence of symbolic play. On the surface, one might think that everyone could agree about whether symbolic play occurs; however, you may be surprised that judges may differ in their perceptions. Here are some child behaviors:

- The child pushes a toy car. Is he pretending that the car is real?
- The child puts an empty cup to his mouth. Is he pretending to drink or *trying* to drink.
- The child makes an engine noise while pushing a car. Is he pretending to be a motor?
- The child watches an adult make a toy cow "walk." Then the child makes a horse walk. Is he pretending or imitating?
- The child feeds a doll with a toy bottle. Is he pretending or really trying to feed the doll?

It is easy to see how judges might have some lively discussions about whether some of these behaviors do or do not represent symbolic play. You can also understand how two judges could look at a video of a child's behavior and score it differently. Any dependent variable worth using will have an established record of interjudge reliability. If two people cannot agree on whether a behavior occurred or not, the dependent measure is not much good.

The second type of reliability is **test-retest reliability,** which is an index of the stability of a particular measurement. No one would think a dependent measure has value if it changes drastically every time you use it. What would you think if you put a piece of the aluminum on that scale we talked about earlier and it registered a different weight each time you used it? Which is the "real" weight of the aluminum? Whatever the dependent variable is, it must have some degree of stability over time or your study will not find an answer to the research question. Thus, if a researcher is going to measure a construct, the measurement should have stability. If a child is language impaired on Monday, we should have some confidence that he or she will be language impaired on Wednesday. If a person has poor motor skills on Tuesday, you should be able to find similar motor skill scores on Thursday. If you cannot, and the measurements fluctuate wildly from day to day, what is the point of using them?

Perhaps the best way to ensure that your dependent variable will have interjudge reliability and be a stable measurement is to again look at what other researchers have used. Typically, measurements that have a history of use among well-respected researchers and published in prestigious journals are high in both validity, interjudge reliability, and stability. If a researcher is developing a new measurement, however, it is incumbent on that scientist to demonstrate validity, reliability, and stability in that new measure. Again, establishing reliability, and stability data for a new measure is a laudable effort and should be shared with the scientific community through a published article, again showing that proper dependent variables are crucial in research.

Operational Definitions

Sometimes there is a fair amount of agreement about acceptable ways to measure a particular construct. Often, the researcher just has to make a choice among several acceptable options. In some cases, however, the construct that the researcher wants to measure may be difficult to define or there may be considerable disagreement about how to measure it. In such instances, researchers may characterize the construct in terms of an **operational definition.**

Complicated constructs such as social skills, racism, client satisfaction, academic achievement, or attraction must be operationally defined in some measurable way, realizing that by reducing the construct down to a measurable form you almost always distort it. Consider the construct of "client satisfaction." A researcher might operationalize this construct as a score on some sort of client satisfaction questionnaire that has been used in many investigations. Certainly, a score on a questionnaire addresses some aspects of client satisfaction, but clearly this is a limited evaluation of such a broad construct. By making the construct observable and measurable the researcher has made some compromises in terms of fully evaluating this elusive variable. Many researchers have studied "social skills" in children with various communication disorders, and this construct has been defined in many different ways using operational definitions. In some studies they have used the number of close friends reported by students. In other investigations they have used teacher ratings of social skills. Other studies have used pupil ratings of friendship. Yet other projects have operationally defined social skill by measuring length of social interactions on the playground. It is like the old metaphor of all the blind men feeling different portions of an elephant and coming to disparate conclusions about what type of beast they were touching. Scientists know that some constructs are just too complicated to define and measure ideally, but because they are scientists they will be specific about what they are measuring. When scientists develop operational definitions about what they are studying, they know that not everyone will agree with their measurement, but at least everyone knows how they measured it. So when a researcher claims to measure "language ability," it may have been operationally defined as the score on a particular language test. If the severity of stuttering is the measurement, the operational definition may be a score on a particular stuttering severity scale or instrument. Every study somehow operationalizes the dependent variable, whether the researcher calls it an operational definition or not. Readers of research should always remember that even though the title of an article may use an overarching term for a construct (e.g., "social skills") the study has most likely distilled that construct down into a measurable entity by operationalizing it.

Evaluating Research by Asking Questions about Questions

It should be clear to you by now that whether you are a consumer or a producer of research, issues such as defining independent and dependent variables and framing answerable research questions are critically important. In a later chapter we devote some time to talking about how to develop research ideas and form researchable questions. As you evaluate a study or design one yourself, you should ask yourself some of the questions listed below.

The Research Problem
- Where does the research problem come from? Does it come from a theory (deductive) or from examination of specific observable events (inductive)?
- Is there enough empirical justification from the literature to show that this problem is significant enough to warrant research?
- Has the literature been reviewed adequately to include older as well as more recent studies? Have a wide variety of scientific journals been included in the review?

The Research Question or Hypothesis
- Is the question unanswerable because it deals with engineering or values?
- Can you easily determine the identity of independent and dependent variables by reading the question or hypothesis?
- Does the question include measurable phenomena that are operationally defined?

The Dependent Variable
- Does the dependent variable validly represent the construct of interest (validity)?
- Is there some evidence that the dependent variable has interjudge reliability?
- Is the dependent variable known to be stable over time?

The researcher who can answer these questions adequately is well on the way to designing a worthwhile study. A good research shark will be able to munch and crunch on a lot of studies just because they have errors in their questions or variables. But there is *much* more to developing good research than just specifying independent and dependent variables and writing answerable questions. Although these are critical to a successful project, we will see in the following chapter that the issue of experimental design and control will make or break a study. In fact, the sharks are already circling.

Summary

A scientific investigation begins with theories, problems, hypotheses, and questions. These different levels of thought about a study move from more general to very specific. The researcher arrives at questions by deductive reasoning, inductive reasoning, or a combination of both. The research question must be answerable through use of the scientific method. Two critical decisions in any study are the identity of the independent and dependent variables under investigation. In order to understand any study from the perspective of the researcher or consumer, the independent and dependent variables must be identified clearly and given considerable thought prior to selection.

LEARNING ACTIVITIES

1. Find five different research articles and try to determine the independent and dependent variables.

2. Make up three research problems of your choice and try to develop specific research questions from these general problem statements. Ensure that your research questions are empirically measurable.

3. List five questions that are not answerable by science and explain why they are unanswerable.

4. Explain the thought process involved in using deductive reasoning to develop a research question. Provide an example of a study as an illustration.

5. Explain the thought process involved in using inductive reasoning to develop a research question. Provide an example of a study as an illustration.

CHAPTER 4

Controlling Threats and Confounding Variables through Experimental Design

Where no plan is laid, where the disposal of time is surrendered merely to the chance of incidence, chaos will soon reign.

—Victor Hugo (1802–1885)

A goal without a plan is just a wish.

—Antoine de Saint-Exupery (1900–1944)

Planning is bringing the future into the present so that you can do something about it now.
—Alan Lakein, Author of *How to Get Control of Your Time and Your Life*

Everybody's got plans…until they get hit.

—Mike Tyson, former heavyweight boxing champion

In the previous chapter we spent considerable time discussing the importance of crafting answerable research questions. You now know that a good question with measurable variables that are reliable and valid is necessary for the scientist to address the research issue of interest. But there is much more to a competent scientific investigation than just the question posed. Even when the researcher can develop an outstanding research question, the actual empirical investigation can fail to answer it if the study is poorly designed. The experimental design of a study can result in a tightly controlled investigation that is widely respected by the scientific community, or the study can be so infested with errors that the data are uninterpretable. In the case of a poor experimental design, the investigator cannot undo how the data were gathered. The result is a waste of time and effort while the empirical question remains unanswered. In the case of a strong experimental design, the results are readily interpretable and show a clear answer to the research question or demonstrate support for an experimental hypothesis. In fact, one of the main differences between a strong and a weak study is the experimental design. But what is it that makes one design strong and another weak? If you already have an answerable question, why must you worry about the experimental design? Why is design so important? The answer to these questions has a lot to do with variables that threaten the integrity of your investigation. Many sources of error threaten scientific investigations. One of the first lines of defense is to know the types of error that are your enemies. The other side of the equation is to learn techniques of experimental control and be confident in your ability to use them in combating error.

LEARNING OBJECTIVES

This chapter will enable readers to:

- Understand our experimental design notation.
- Be able to list and understand the threats to internal validity from maturation, history, testing effects, statistical regression, experimenter bias, participant bias, instrumentation, participant selection, and mortality.
- Be able to list and understand the threats to external validity from

participant selection bias, experimental arrangements, reactive testing, and multiple treatment interactions.
- Be able to explain the linkage between internal and external validity in research.
- Be aware of compromise in the conduct of research.

Threats and Experimental Design

> If you know the enemy and know yourself, you will not fear the result of a hundred battles. If you know yourself but not the enemy, for every victory gained, you will also suffer a defeat. If you know neither the enemy nor yourself, you will succumb in every battle.
>
> Sun Tzu, 544–496 BC, *The Art of War*

Figure 4.1 presents some common terms that have become associated with threats to scientific investigations. We refer to these terms as the "axis of error" because they all represent problems that can ruin a research project. The terms generally refer to the same basic concept: *Unless you can be relatively certain that your independent variable has accounted for most of the changes in your dependent variable, your study is fundamentally flawed.* We will talk about this at more length and give some examples, because this concept is important and is the reason that we need experimental design. The real axis of error is anything that can compete with your independent variable as an explanation for changes in the dependent variable. So the four terms in Figure 4.1 are just different ways of referring to some variable that might explain changes in your dependent variable as well as your independent variable. If someone has a competing explanation that sounds as plausible as your IV, then you might as well have not conducted your study. Experimental design is the way that a researcher controls confounding variables, competing explanations, extraneous variables and alternative interpretations that interfere with a clear, unambiguous interpretation of the effects of the IV on the DV (Diamond, 1981; Kirk, 1995; Montgomery, 1991). The better the experimental design, the more threats are eliminated. It is easy to see why a competent researcher would very carefully consider any and all variables that could compete with the independent variable. When designing a study, some researchers try to shoot some holes in their own design just to see if it is strong enough. If they find a possible confounding variable, they alter the design to compensate for it. An

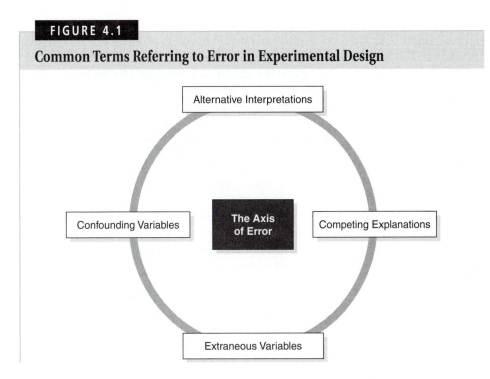

FIGURE 4.1

Common Terms Referring to Error in Experimental Design

experimental design that is relatively impervious to threats is a beautiful thing to behold. A design that allows many alternative explanations for the results of the study can just break your heart. Since experimental design is done *before* the actual study, there is really no excuse for a researcher to not at least consider all reasonable threats to the integrity of the study.

Research design is proactive in that the scientist tries to reduce sources of error in a study before it is conducted so that fatal, irreversible flaws can be avoided. Kerlinger and Lee (2000, p. 450) state: "Research design has two basic purposes: (1) to provide answers to research questions and (2) to control variance." According to Kerlinger and Lee, we want to *maximize systematic variation associated with our independent variable.* That is, we want any variability associated with the IV to be visible in our study and not obscured by other sources of variance. To do this we must *control systematic variance associated with* other *variables that could compete with the IV* in having an effect on the dependent variable. This is why we would control for variables such as intelligence, language ability, hearing level, and so on in most studies in communication disorders. By making our groups similar on these related variables, we reduce or control the variance associated with them. Finally, *we should strive to reduce error variance* in our study. Error variance will be present in *any* investigation and stems from sampling differences, procedural inconsistencies in how we do our study, and just plain mistakes made when gathering, summarizing, and analyzing data. We can reduce error variance by tightening up on our procedures and being meticulous in how we conduct the study. So you can see that controlling variance is no small issue in research, and it is a major goal of experimental design.

Some of you may be thinking that the term *threat* somehow implies attack. There is actually some truth to this notion. Since science is a public enterprise, researchers must expose their work to the scrutiny of others. Especially in cases where studies are submitted to a journal for publication, the investigation will be thoroughly critiqued by other researchers who will determine if the experimental design has controlled for any threats to the integrity of the study. If they can find even one competing explanation for changes in the DV other than the IV, then the study may be rejected. In many cases, if such alternative interpretations are found, the study may not be salvageable by the researcher. Most of the time such threats revolve around how the data were gathered, how the tests were administered, the composition of the groups of participants, or some other variable that cannot be changed after the study is completed. Even in cases where research is not submitted for publication, most professional meetings review papers submitted for presentation and will not accept studies that have obvious errors in experimental design. In cases where a study with flaws is accepted for presentation at a professional meeting, the researcher still has to deal with peers who will ask pertinent questions about the study and how it is being interpreted. If there are errors in the design, it is not difficult for other professionals to find them by asking questions about how the study was designed and conducted. This is precisely why we are training you to be research sharks. Remember we said that research sharks appreciate a study that is well done but will start nipping away at those with poor experimental designs. A study with a weak experimental design is tantamount to throwing a big, bloody eye-of-the-round roast into the ocean so the sharks can have a feeding frenzy. Good research sharks are an important part of the scientific community. They are good producers and consumers of scientific research. Whenever you listen to a research presentation or read an article, you should *always* ask yourself these questions:

1. Are their any reasonable competing explanations for the results of this study other than the independent variable?
2. Could the dependent variable have been influenced by anything in the methodology such as the way the data were gathered or analyzed?

Interestingly, you should ask yourself the same questions when you are designing your own research projects. Pretend that you are a disinterested research shark with no vested interest in the study and ask those questions. In many cases, you will find "holes" in your study that can be filled by tightening up the experimental design. Later in this chapter we will discuss specific threats to look for when you are evaluating research. Any researcher worth his or her salt will appreciate any questions or comments about how their study was designed and conducted. In many cases, constructive criticism may even help them when they write up their work for submission to a journal. It is important to remember, however, that when research sharks take a bite out of a study, they do it politely and usually in the form of a question.

Introduction to Our Design Notation: Between and Within Subjects Experimental Designs

This is a very important section. Do not go on to another section unless you *really* understand what we are talking about. One goal of this text is to take a conceptual approach to discussing experimental design and statistics. To that end, we will employ a certain type of notation to describe various experimental designs that involve separate groups of participants who are sampled only once or groups where there are repeated measurements on the same participants. We would like to take our time to introduce this notation to you, because it will be expanded on in later chapters to illustrate more complex experimental designs. For now, we will use only simple designs and introduce you to a very basic concept in research— the difference in **between subjects** and **within subjects** experimental designs. It is a testament to the proliferation of political correctness in the past few decades that there has been a change in the term used to refer to those people studied in experiments. Historically, we called these people "research subjects." A scientist would say, "I have to run some subjects this afternoon," meaning that they would be testing or examining people in an experiment. Nowadays, it is required in scientific writing to refer to people studied in experiments as "participants" rather than subjects. Perhaps participant implies that the people consented to participate whereas subject may suggest they were studied just because a scientist wanted to examine them. To many, this is not an insignificant distinction. Most statistics books, however, still use terms like "between subjects" and "within subjects" to refer to experimental designs and quantitative methods and we will continue such usage in the present text. Although we have not seen a statistics book published recently that refers to "between participants" and "within participants" designs, it is probably only a matter of time.

When evaluating threats to a scientific investigation, it is important to consider whether the study examined different groups of participants (between subjects) or if it sampled the same participants multiple times (within subjects). This distinction will be dealt with again as we talk about specific experimental designs and statistical methods in later chapters, but for now we just want you to know that threats to a study are different based on how many times participants are sampled. First, we would like to orient you to the notation we will use to discuss these designs.

One way to characterize an experimental design is to draw a series of boxes representing "cells" that contain numbers of participants in the study. In Figure 4.2 we depict four studies illustrating use of this notation. Between subjects designs are those in which separate groups of participants are evaluated. Every independent variable has a number of different "levels" that correspond to the number of different groups studied in a between subjects design. This is an important concept to remember because we will be using it from now on in this text. Take a look at Figure 4.2 to familiarize yourself with the idea that a single IV can have differing numbers of "levels" associated with it. Remember, in between subjects designs the number of levels is equal to the number of groups being studied. Each group is made up of participants

---

FIGURE 4.2

Design Notation Depicting Four Single IV Between Subjects Studies with Differing Numbers of Levels

IV = Gender

Male	Female
10	10

$N = 20$ (Total participants in study)
$n = 10$ (Total participants in each group)

IV = Socioeconomic Status

Low SES	Middle SES	Upper SES
10	10	10

$N = 30$
$n = 10$

IV = Branch of Military

Army	Navy	Air Force	Marines
10	10	10	10

$N = 40$
$n = 10$

IV = Type of Vocal Pathology

Contact Ulcers	Vocal Nodules	Papilloma	Granuloma	Vocal Polyps
10	10	10	10	10

$N = 50$
$n = 10$

---

who are measured only once for a particular variable of interest. In the figure, we do not want to confuse you by listing dependent variables, but just for purposes of these examples pretend that we are measuring anxiety in all of them as the DV. In the first study, we are comparing the anxiety levels of 10 males and 10 females to see if there is a gender difference between these two groups. When we talk about the participants in a study we can characterize them in terms of the total number in the study (the "big N") or the number of participants in each group or cell of the design (the "little n"). This first study has a total number of participants of 20, and each group has 10 members. Note also that the study has one IV—gender—that has two levels. In the second study we are interested in measuring anxiety in people from different socioeconomic levels. We have three groups of 10 participants for a total N of 30. This study has only one IV with three different levels. In the third study, we are looking at anxiety in members of different branches of the military. There are four groups of

10 participants for an N of 40. This represents one IV with four levels. In the fourth study, we are examining anxiety in five groups of people with different vocal pathologies, representing one IV with five levels. After studying Figure 4.2 you should be able to see that each study had only one IV and that each IV had different numbers of levels associated with it. In experimental design parlance, we would say that the participant in a *between subjects design* experiences *only one level* of the independent variable. Again, think of levels in a between subjects design as the number of groups participating in the study. In the studies shown in Figure 4.2, the males do not experience being female, those of lower SES do not experience being of middle SES, the Army soldiers do not experience being Navy sailors, and the patients with contact ulcers do not experience having the other vocal pathologies. We provide several other examples of between subjects designs as follows:

• The researcher studies three groups of participants representing Asian, African American, and Hispanic cultures (one IV with three levels) to determine their use of metaphors (DV) as they speak their dialect of English. This is clearly a study between subjects because you cannot be both Asian and Hispanic or experience all three levels of culture. Also, each participant was only sampled one time to evaluate the use of metaphors in a language sample.

• Another researcher is studying patients with two types of hearing loss, sensorineural and conductive (one IV with two levels), to see if there is a difference between the groups in their history of using of ototoxic drugs (DV). In this study, participants were selected because of their type of hearing impairment, either sensorineural or conductive. Thus the sensorineural group, by definition, would not experience having a conductive loss nor would the conductive group experience having a sensorineural loss. Each participant was only sampled one time using a history form listing a large number of ototoxic drugs. Thus, the study was between subjects because each participant was sampled once and group members could only experience one level of the IV (sensorineural or conductive).

Within subjects designs involve participants who experience *every* level of the independent variable. They are sampled repeatedly over a time period. Some authors call this type of design **repeated measures** because it involves repeated measurement of the same participants. Figure 4.3 shows four studies using the design notation we introduced in the between subjects section above. Note that again we have cells, but this time each cell represents a different "condition" or "treatment" of the participants. These are *not* different groups of participants but rather the same ten people experiencing all levels of the IV. Note the thick black arrow indicating that the same ten participants in the first cell are actually exposed to all the other conditions in the remaining cells. In these four studies, just to make it simple, the dependent variable is number of words recalled in a memory task. In the first study, the researcher wanted to see if there was a difference in the number of words recalled if the participants were told they would receive a mild electrical shock for every word they could not recall as compared to a no shock condition. You can see that there is only

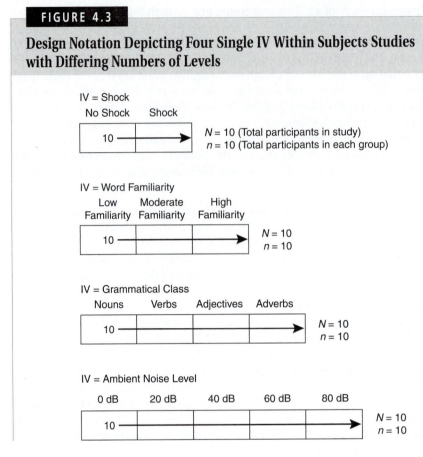

FIGURE 4.3

Design Notation Depicting Four Single IV Within Subjects Studies with Differing Numbers of Levels

IV = Shock

No Shock   Shock

10 ──────────→ $N = 10$ (Total participants in study)
                  $n = 10$ (Total participants in each group)

IV = Word Familiarity

Low   Moderate   High
Familiarity Familiarity   Familiarity

10 ──────────────────→ $N = 10$
                          $n = 10$

IV = Grammatical Class

Nouns   Verbs   Adjectives   Adverbs

10 ──────────────────────────→ $N = 10$
                                  $n = 10$

IV = Ambient Noise Level

0 dB   20 dB   40 dB   60 dB   80 dB

10 ──────────────────────────────────→ $N = 10$
                                           $n = 10$

one IV—"shock"—with two levels (presence of shock/absence of shock). What makes this study different than the previous between subjects example with males and females is that the ten participants experience *both* levels of the IV, shock and no shock. So in this experiment, participants first experience the condition of being shocked for every word not remembered and then another condition of remembering words without the threat of shock. In the second study, the researcher wanted to find if familiarity with the words to be remembered made any difference in the performance of the participants. Note that the same participants ($n = 10$) experience *all* levels of the IV and have the opportunity to try and remember words of three different levels of familiarity. In the fourth study, the researcher is trying to determine if the grammatical class of words affects the ability of participants to remember them. Each of the ten participants goes through four conditions or levels of the IV (grammatical class). Finally, in the last study, the researcher is attempting to see the effects of different levels of masking noise on the participant's ability to remember words. There are ten participants who experience *all* levels of the IV and try to remember words presented in each of the five masking conditions. Some other examples follow:

• A researcher wants to determine the difference among three different modes of language sampling (conversation, picture description, play with toys) on mean length of utterance (MLU). You probably have already noted that the IV in this study is the mode of language sampling, which has three levels, and the DV is MLU. For purposes of this example, let's say that the researcher has decided to do the study using a within subjects design. You should already be mentally picturing three boxes representing the three levels of the IV. If it is within subjects, then the same group of participants should experience all levels of the IV or all three sampling conditions. If the researcher used twenty participants, there will be a 20 in the first cell with that thick black arrow spanning all three cells of the design.

• In another study, the researcher is attempting to determine if analog or digital hearing instruments result in different discrimination scores for clients with hearing loss. The same clients are tested for speech discrimination in the two levels of the IV (analog and digital). Again, if there were twenty clients in the study ($N = 20$), each one of them would experience both levels of the IV. If you drew this design using our notation, you would have two cells with a 20 in the left hand cell and an arrow spanning the two conditions.

We have introduced you to our design notation, which will be used throughout the rest of the text. We have also illustrated the difference between experimental designs that examine differences between groups and those that sample participants multiple times. In the next section, we will discuss how the threats to a study differ in between and within subjects designs.

Threats to Internal Validity

Decades ago, Campbell (1957) and Campbell and Stanley (1963) revolutionized our way of thinking and talking about experimental design. Not only did they develop the elegant concepts of internal and **external validity,** but they specifically dealt with factors that threaten each of them and gave some suggestions on how to control those threats. In talking about internal and external validity, Kerlinger and Lee (2000, p. 475) indicate that these "notions constitute one of the most significant, important and enlightening contributions to research methodology in the past three or four decades." Rather than give a formal definition of internal validity we present Table 4.1, which illustrates some common differences between studies that have high and low **internal validity.**

Just looking at the differences between studies with high and low internal validity shown in Table 4.1 it is easy to see that internal validity is intimately connected to the level of control and care that a researcher uses in designing and conducting a study. Kerlinger and Lee (2000) suggest that any effective research design must (1) answer the research question, (2) control extraneous independent variables, and (3) allow for generalizability to other similar participants and conditions. Studies high in internal validity are in a much better position to fulfill these three criteria than investigations

TABLE 4.1

Attributes of Studies with Low and High Degrees of Internal Validity

Low Internal Validity	High Internal Validity
Weak research design that does not fully control for extraneous variables	Strong research design that controls extraneous variables as much as possible
Vague definitions of variables studied	Strong operational definitions of variables studied
Results of study are accounted for by alternative explanations other than the IV	Results of study are explained by effects of the IV on the DV with alternative explanations eliminated by the design
Conduct of the study was sloppy and not systematic	Study was conducted systematically with attention to detail

with low internal validity. Ideally, researchers design their investigations to have high degrees of internal validity, which maximizes the probability that the independent variable is the only factor responsible for changes in the dependent variable. Strong internal validity eliminates confounding variables, alternative explanations for results, or rival hypotheses from accounting for results of a study. As we said earlier, effective experimental design is how researchers compensate for the axis of error in their investigations.

Figure 4.4 shows the typical relationship between an independent and dependent variable in a study. Ideally, changes in the DV will be the result of influence from the IV, which is why the arrow representing the independent variable is pointing at the dependent variable. Note, however, that lurking just beneath the surface are multiple factors that can affect the dependent variable at the same time as the independent variable. The sharks shown "threatening" the dependent variable illustrate how research sharks can give possible alternative explanations for changes in the DV *in addition to* the IV. We said earlier that *even one* reasonable competing explanation for changes in the DV confounds your study. An effective experimental design with high internal validity will put your dependent variable in a shark-proof cage so you will not have to worry about rival explanations for your results. An ineffective experimental design with low internal validity is just an invitation to a feeding frenzy. As mentioned earlier and illustrated in Figure 4.4, Campbell and Stanley (1963) provide us with names for those threatening sharks. We would like to introduce the sharks to you one by one and give some examples of exactly *why* they have the potential to represent confounding variables in any study. It will also become very clear to you that the variables differ in their level of threat depending on whether your experimental design is within or between subjects.

The Maturation Threat

The threat of maturation is typically related to changes that take place *within the participants* over the passage of time. In both of the following examples researchers are

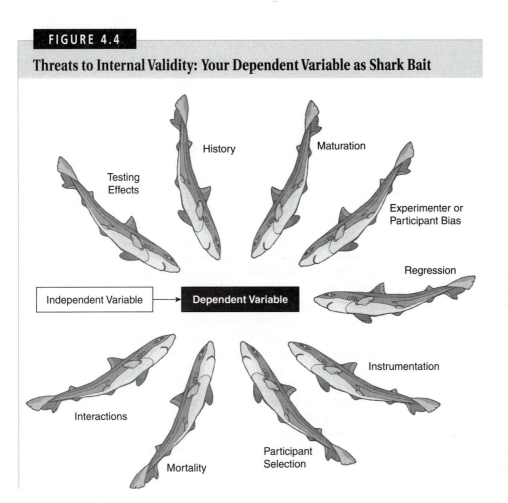

FIGURE 4.4

Threats to Internal Validity: Your Dependent Variable as Shark Bait

examining two levels (pretest/posttest) of the IV (treatment program). The researcher wants to know if there is a significant difference between language scores before and after treatment, presumably to validate the treatment regimen as effective. One example involves children, the other involves adults, but the designs of the studies are identical with pre- and posttests. Using the design notation introduced previously, the design appears in Figure 4.5.

Is this study a between subjects or within subjects design? If you checked out the arrow, you will have concluded that it is a within subjects, or repeated measures design. Our first example of the **maturation threat** involves a study with children as participants. Take as an example a researcher interested in examining the effectiveness of a language treatment program on children who were eighteen months of age. The researcher finds ten children with language impairment, gathers a language sample as a

FIGURE 4.5

Pretest/Posttest Study of Language Treatment

IV = Treatment Program
DV = Language Ability

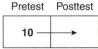

Pretest   Posttest

10

pretest of their communication ability, and then enrolls them in a language treatment program for six months. At the end of the treatment program, the researcher gathers a posttreatment language sample and finds that the children had increased their language ability in terms of length and complexity over the six-month treatment period, concluding that the treatment program was a success. The threat of maturation rears its ugly head because at eighteen months of age, a six-month treatment program represents a quarter of each participant's time on the planet. We also know that children develop or mature in terms of language without the benefit of a treatment program. So how do we know that these ten children did not improve their language simply due to normal maturation and development? We do not. That maturation shark just took a big bite out of the dependent variable and represents a viable alternative explanation to the independent variable. If someone said that these children have changed due to normal maturation, this is just as good an explanation as their participation in a language treatment program. One way the researcher might have controlled for the maturation threat is by using a **control group** of similar children who did not receive the language program. If the children who received treatment had significantly larger gains compared to the ones who did not, this adds some credibility to the effects of the treatment program. If there is no difference between the groups, then the treatment program may provide no benefits beyond normal development. Our second example of a maturation threat involves adults who have suffered strokes with resulting aphasia. The design is identical to the study of children discussed previously and represented in Figure 4.5. A researcher enrolls ten patients in an aphasia treatment program for six months. Pretests and posttests on their language ability were taken before and after the treatment period. However, patient improvement in language ability is not necessarily the result of the aphasia treatment program. We know, for example, that a phenomenon called "spontaneous recovery" takes place typically within a year of the brain injury. During this period of spontaneous recovery, a patient will naturally make gains in motor ability, language skills, and other functions just due to the nervous system recovering from the neural insult. Any improvements in language ability may have been due to the treatment *or* may have been due to spontaneous recovery. Again, with no control group we do not know. We are faced with another plausible interpretation of the results that does not include the independent variable of "treatment program." If you look at that arrow in Figure 4.5 and ask yourself, "What else was going on in these participants while they were receiving language treatment?" you can easily see that maturation is a threat. Another point to notice is that maturation is mainly a threat when the experimental design is within subjects. Maturation would not be an issue if the participants were only measured once, but of course, you could not really study therapy without measuring partici-pants twice. That is why a control group that did not receive treatment is typically the way to answer the maturation threat. There are some problems inherent in using control groups which we will discuss later, but for now, we just want you to see how maturation, without a control group, can be a major threat.

Maturation is not just confined to development. In our second example, we clas-sified the influence from spontaneous recovery as a maturation threat. This has noth-ing to do with normal maturation and development and more to do with recovery of the nervous system after it is damaged. The notion of maturation has been extended over the years to include *any* internal changes that might occur in participants such as fatigue or lack of motivation. In Figure 4.6 we have a design of a study calculated to determine if certain types of cues from a clinician result in greater word retrieval by patients with aphasia. Ten participants are found who will undergo all levels of the IV (phonetic cue/function cue) to see which one results in more words retrieved (DV). In the phonetic cue condition the experimenter shows the patient a photograph of a car and if the person has trouble retrieving the word the clinician says /k/ which is the first sound in the word. This type of cue is given as the patient goes through fifty different pictures. In the second condition, a photograph is shown and if retrieval difficulties ensue the clinician gives a function cue such as "You drive it." Again, fifty pictures are used in this condition as in the phonetic cue condition. For this example, let's say that the phonetic cues were superior to the function cues in stimulating word retrieval. This would suggest one cue is more effective than the other. A canny research shark, how-ever, would wonder if the participants in the second condition could have been more fatigued after they had gone through the fifty pictures in the phonetic cue condition. If the function condition had a lower number of words retrieved, it is certainly plausible that it could have been due to fatigue. This represents an alternative explanation to the researcher's independent variable, and compromises the study.

Now, just when the research shark is feeling cocky, the researcher says, "Oh no, the participants could not have been more fatigued in the function cue condition because I *counterbalanced* the order of the conditions across participants." "What do you mean?" says the research shark. The researcher explains that every participant

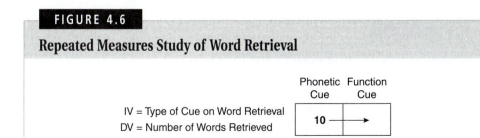

FIGURE 4.6

Repeated Measures Study of Word Retrieval

IV = Type of Cue on Word Retrieval
DV = Number of Words Retrieved

Phonetic Cue   Function Cue

10

had the cue conditions in a different order (1–2, 2–1, 1–2, 2–1, etc.) which takes fatigue, or the maturation threat, out of the picture. You cannot make a case that everyone was more tired for the function cue, because at least half of the participants had it first while they were still fresh and yet the phonetic cues were still more effective. Thus, the researcher is able to fend off the research shark. Touché. **Counterbalancing** is one of the mainstays of experimental design and it is especially important in within subjects designs in which participants are going to experience all levels of the IV. It is almost always a good strategy to counterbalance the order in which they experience multiple conditions so the threat of maturation is neutralized. One other point about designing a within subjects research project. Since within subjects designs involve repeated measurements of the participants, it is usually prudent to keep the intervals between these samples as close in time as possible. The longer the period of time between measurements, the more maturation effects can occur. In summary, the most effective allies of the researcher in dealing with maturation threats are 1) use of a control group, 2) counterbalancing of conditions, and 3) minimizing the amount of time between repeated measurements.

The History Threat

The threat of history refers to changes that occur over time due to influences *outside the participants* that could affect the dependent variable and act as alternative explanations to the independent variable. The **history threat** is every external influence that happens to participants between repeated measurements in a research project. Schiavetti and Metz (2002) provide an example of a researcher who wants to prove the effectiveness of a fluency training program for stuttering. Although not specified, we assume the researcher was conducting this program at a university speech and hearing clinic. The experimenter gathers pretherapy and posttherapy evaluations of disfluency in order to determine the effectiveness of the treatment program.

Let us assume that ten children with fluency disorders were in the study as in Figure 4.7. If the researcher finds that the posttest scores show significantly less disfluency than the pretest scores he or she would like to conclude that the treatment program is responsible for this gain. If it was determined, however, that some of the children had been receiving treatment for their disfluency from a local private practice or public school program at the same time that they participated in the university program, the study is confounded. The reduction in disfluency may have been due

FIGURE 4.7

Pretest/Posttest Study of Fluency Treatment

IV = Treatment Program
DV = Fluency

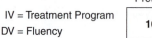

to the university program, the school or private clinic programs, or an interaction among the different therapies. This is not the same thing as maturation, because history involves something *outside* the participant (e.g., extra therapy) that could have intervened between the pretest and posttest. The extra therapy is just as valid an explanation for increases in fluency as the independent variable (university treatment program). If the researcher had used a control group of people who stutter, the study might have been salvaged. In a control group, the participants certainly could have availed themselves of treatment from other sources as did the group that received treatment from the university. However, if the group that received the university treatment program still had greater gains in fluency compared to the control group, it is most likely the result of the university program, since both groups had the potential to participate in additional forms of treatment.

In another study, a researcher is trying to see if anxiety level as measured by the palmar sweat index (PSI) changes in people who stutter under three conditions. The first condition is talking alone, the second condition is talking to one research assistant, and the third condition is giving a speech to a group of five research assistants. In Figure 4.8, you can see that this is a within subjects design, the IV is the number of listeners (3 levels), and the DV is the PSI. All ten participants experience all levels of the IV as the study progresses.

To illustrate the history threat in this example, let's say that the measurements of PSI were taken at weekly intervals over a three-week period. During this three-week period there was a major terrorist attack in the city where these participants reside. A terrorist attack is certainly an event *outside of the participants* and not analogous to development or fatigue as discussed in the section on maturation. Could a major terrorist attack affect a person's overall level of anxiety above and beyond the possible effects of number of listeners? Is this a reasonable alternative explanation for an increase in anxiety in condition three as compared to condition one? Many would call this a plausible competing explanation for anxiety increases in the later conditions, beyond the effects of the independent variable. Again, if the researcher used counterbalancing in the administration of the conditions, the effects of history could be somewhat counteracted. If the researcher found a steady increase in anxiety as the conditions moved from zero to one to five listeners even when these conditions were counterbalanced in their order of presentation, it suggests that the IV had some

FIGURE 4.8

Repeated Measures Study of Anxiety Level

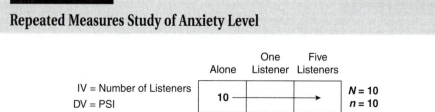

influence, regardless of the terrorist attack. Without counterbalancing, however, the researcher is defenseless. Therefore, just like controlling for maturation, the best ways to deal with the history threat are counterbalancing, short intervals between samples, and as in the first example, use of a control group.

The Threat of Testing Effects

The threat of testing effects on internal validity has also been referred to by a variety of terms such as **practice effects** (Schiavetti & Metz, 2002) and **reactive measures** (Campbell, 1957). Whenever a participant is exposed to *any* type of experience in the early part of a study, this exposure can conceivably have an influence on samples of behavior that are taken later in the experiment. Perhaps the best way to illustrate this is to provide a couple of examples:

• A researcher has developed a video for use in changing attitudes of school-age children toward vocal abuse. As part of the research project, the researcher administers a pretest and a posttest questionnaire (DV) to assess student attitudes toward pathological vocal behaviors (Figure 4.9). Many items in the questionnaire ask students to signal their agreement or disagreement with specific statements (e.g., "Frequent loud yelling can result in damage to your vocal cords.") The day after filling out the questionnaire, the participants are asked to view a thirty-minute video that focuses on vocal hygiene and avoiding pathological vocal behaviors. At the completion of the video presentation, the participants are again asked to fill out the questionnaire to assess their attitudes toward vocal abuse. The researcher now has a pre- and postvideo questionnaire and intends to measure changes in attitude toward vocal abuse by comparing the scores on the questionnaires taken before and after viewing the video. Any difference between the questionnaires would be viewed as a change in attitude. Since the video was interjected between the two questionnaire samples, the researcher feels that the video is responsible for any changes in attitude. Note that since the study was done over a short time period (2 days), the effects of maturation and history discussed earlier in the chapter are less likely. The results of the study showed that attitudes toward vocal abuse were significantly different between the pretest and posttest. The researcher now begins to market the video with advertisements indicating that the video has been shown to change the attitudes of school-age students toward vocal abuse. What could be wrong with this

---

FIGURE 4.9

Pretest/Posttest Study of Vocal Abuse Training Program

IV = Pretest/Posttest of Video Training
DV = Attitudes toward Vocal Abuse

Pretest	Posttest
10 →	

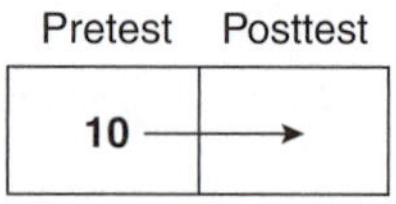

conclusion? First of all, the people buying the video are very different from the participants in the study in one important way. They have never been sensitized by a pretest (the prevideo questionnaire) as the participants in the study were. How do we know that the prevideo questionnaire did not actually serve to sensitize the students to vocal abuse and the subsequent viewing of the video really contributed very little to their change in attitude as measured on the postvideo questionnaire? Someone could make the argument that the pretest actually made the students think about vocal abuse, just by the content and wording of the questions, and their posttest scores were affected by this experience alone. We would suggest that this is a reasonable competing explanation and confounds the independent variable. Even if the video training did have some degree of effect on attitudes, people who purchase the video would never have any proof that the video training would have the same effect without the pretest.

• Another researcher wants to determine the effectiveness of a language training program with kindergarten-level children. No figure accompanies this one, because it is basically the same as other pretest-treatment-posttest designs discussed above. As in many studies of this type, children are selected because they earned low scores on some standardized test of language ability. After selection, the children participate in a two-week language treatment program. At the end of this short period of training, the participants are readministered the standardized language test to determine whether scores have changed, presumably as a result of the therapy program. It is very possible, however, that the experience of taking the pretest familiarized the child with the test format, the attentional requirements for successful performance, and even specific items on the test such that the second administration of the instrument (posttest) results in a higher score without any influence of the treatment program. If a researcher wanted to control for the possible effects of pretesting, the use of a control group (no therapy) would address this issue. If both the treatment group and the control group increased their scores on the posttest, then the treatment probably made little contribution. If the treatment group significantly outperformed the control group, then one might think that the therapy was effective beyond the threat of pretesting.

Schiavetti and Metz sum it up nicely by saying, "Any time pretreatment tests are used, the reader must ask whether posttreatment changes are due to treatment effects, testing effects or a combination of the two" (2002, p. 134)

The Statistical Regression Threat

The regression effect is a statistical fact of life because, in reality, pretest and posttest scores are not perfectly correlated (Anastasi, 1958; Thorndike, 1963). That is, there is no reason to believe that taking the same test or even a different form of the test a second time should result in exactly the same score. In each test administration there are elements of chance that affect the scores. As illustrated in Figure 4.10, **statistical regression** affects extreme scores in a predictable way. In this example, extreme scores would represent those in the "tail" of the normal distribution out

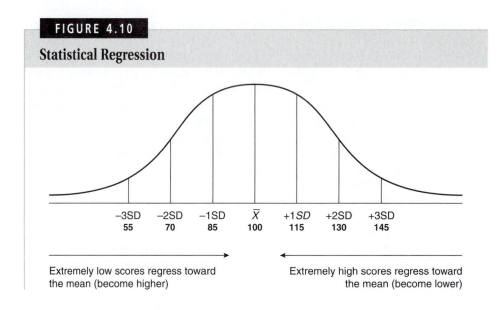

FIGURE 4.10

Statistical Regression

	−3SD	−2SD	−1SD	$\overline{X}$	+1SD	+2SD	+3SD
	55	70	85	100	115	130	145

Extremely low scores regress toward the mean (become higher)

Extremely high scores regress toward the mean (become lower)

past two to three standard deviations above or below the mean. (Note that *standard deviation* will be explained in Chapter 5.) In the figure, a person who scored 148 and then retook the test should probably expect to earn a lower score. That is, the extremely high score would "regress" toward the mean. Similarly, if a person earned a score of 55 on the test, a second administration of the instrument should result in a higher score. Think for a moment about therapy studies. In most cases, participants in treatment research are chosen due to their abnormally low scores on a particular measurement. For example, if you are looking for children with language disorders, you choose participants who earned scores on a language test that were low enough to qualify them as having "abnormal" language ability. A researcher who wanted to determine whether a language treatment program is effective might use the original test score as a pretest, then administer therapy, and administer the language test again as a posttest. Given statistical regression, one might expect that even without therapy, abnormally low scores (the pretest) would regress toward the mean (become higher) on the posttest. How then, can we control for the threat of statistical regression in this type of study? The answer is probably to use a control group that receives no treatment. This group would represent the possible effects of statistical regression and the treatment group would show the effects of treatment *plus* statistical regression. If the treatment group outperforms the control group, one might make a case that the treatment is effective beyond the threat of statistical regression. On the other hand, when no control group is used some shark can make the case that changes between the pre- and posttest are due to statistical regression, and this is a reasonable alternative explanation that competes with the independent variable.

The Experimenter/Participant Bias Threat

No one should be judge in his own cause.

Publilius Syrus, Roman mimographer, 1st Century BC

Earlier we used the metaphor of a fox watching the chickens to describe the possibility of a researcher having undue influence over his or her own experiment. The concept of **experimenter bias** is a subtle but significant threat to control for in the conduct of research. Ideally, researchers should want to avoid *even the appearance* of experimenter bias in their investigations. In reality, however, many studies are done without adequately controlling for this threat.

Experimenter's General Demeanor and Communication

There are several classical effects that an experimenter can have on the outcome of a study, believed by most authorities to be unintentional and not the type of scientific misconduct we discussed in an earlier chapter. One classical type of threat is the **Rosenthal effect,** sometimes called the *Pygmalion effect,* having to do with the experimenter setting up certain expectations on the part of participants, whether intentionally or unintentionally. In studying two groups of participants, an experimenter who has distinctly different ways of interacting and communicating with the two groups can set up different expectations between participants in the two groups. This differential way of interacting with the groups is the fault of the experimenter, not the participants. In a classic report, a researcher named Robert Rosenthal communicated to some teachers that the children in their classes were expected to undergo a spurt in their intellectual ability over the course of the coming school year whereas other teachers were not told this information. It was found that students in the classrooms of teachers expecting an intellectual growth spurt earned higher grades and even scored higher on cognitive tests administered during the school year. Rosenthal posited that perhaps the teachers treated students differently in this situation by paying more attention to them or teaching and testing them differently because of their expectations. Although this example was an intentional deception on the part of the researcher, scientists can also instill expectations in participants by their demeanor, communication style, and even nonverbal communication. If a researcher tells participants in a treatment group that they are really doing better and does not communicate this to control group members, it is possible that the treatment group could perform better just due to the experimenter's way of interacting with them and not due to the treatment. In most research projects it is standard procedure to attempt to minimize differences in how the experimenter interacts with groups under study. This is why all participants read the same information on the informed consent and why instructions for tasks given in the study are typically written ahead of time and read to the participants. No experimenter wants to inject error into a study just because of uncontrolled interaction styles. It is also good practice to interact with participants by using research assistants, who ideally are "blind" to the condition the participants represent. This "blinding" of the experimenter decreases the possible effects of experimenter bias. Figure 4.11 illustrates varying degrees of blinding used in science by depicting three principal players in a research project wearing opaque sunglasses.

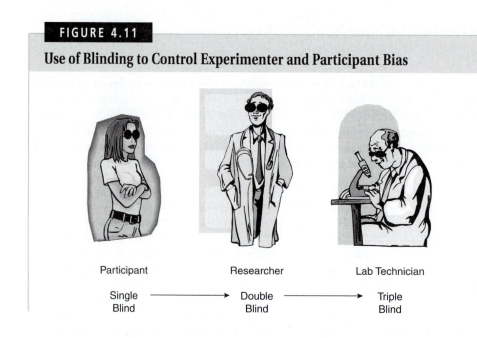

FIGURE 4.11

Use of Blinding to Control Experimenter and Participant Bias

Participant   Researcher   Lab Technician

Single ————————▶ Double ————————▶ Triple
Blind   Blind   Blind

A single blind study typically refers to a study in which the participant is not aware of the condition (control versus treatment) he or she is representing in an experiment. In a double blind study both the researcher and the participant are not aware of the condition. In this case the participants may be assigned numbers and randomly placed in a particular condition by someone other than the researcher, such as an assistant. In triple blinding, the participant is unaware of his or her condition, the experimenter is unaware of the participant's status, and the person scoring the participant's data (e.g., lab technician) does not know if the data being analyzed represent the experimental or control group. In a study that compared pretest and posttest scores, an experimenter who knew that a particular participant was in the treatment group might possibly interact differently during the posttest as compared to the pretest. A more friendly, calming researcher who gave the participants more encouragement during the posttest knowing they were in the treatment group could affect the outcome of the study. Ideally, the experimenter would delegate the administration of the posttest to a research assistant who was unaware whether the participant was in the control or the treatment group, which would reduce significantly the effects of experimenter bias. Blinding is an important way for researchers to maintain objectivity about their work. In practice, especially in smaller studies, blinding does not occur as much as it should. However, most medical studies routinely involve single and double blinding. Some issues with blinding sometimes make it difficult to implement. As mentioned earlier, participants must sign an informed consent before they are included in research. You can immediately see the conflict between keeping a participant unaware of which treatment he or she is receiving and the idea of disclosing relevant information about the study. Would the participant agree to take part knowing that he or she would be in the control group? Would a person really want to ingest sugar pills instead of a real medication to help their medical problem? Is it ethical to withhold treatment from certain groups while giving it to others? If the study is small, how can the experimenter possibly not know who is in the group with fluency disorders? After all, participants come in to the clinic and volunteer for the study and if the researcher is dealing with groups of ten, twenty, or thirty participants it is difficult to maintain blindness to their experimental grouping. These are all very thorny and important questions to ask and not everyone agrees on the best answers to them. In studies where there are thousands of participants at different experimental sites it is much easier to implement blinding in the conduct of a study.

Experimenter Gathering or Scoring of Experimental Data

Another example of experimenter bias involves how the data for the dependent variable are gathered and measured and by whom. In the following example the experimenter is interested in determining if children with attention deficit disorder (ADD) and those with normal attention differ in their language complexity. If you look at the design in Figure 4.12, you can see that it is a between subjects design with ten children in each group. The IV is attentional ability (ADD versus normal attention) and the DV is syntactic complexity as measured by the Developmental Sentence Score (DSS). The DSS is computed from a spontaneous language sample gathered in conversation. Now we return to the experimenter bias issue. If the researcher gathers the language samples and is aware whether each participant is in the ADD or normal attention group, it is possible that the researcher could influence the outcome of the study just by the way the samples are gathered. It is well known that language samples can be influenced by such things as the type of language used by the clinician, the types of stimuli used in gathering the sample, and even the topics of conversation. A researcher who inadvertently used more complex language while interacting with the children with normal attention and simpler language when talking to the children with ADD could affect the complexity of their language samples. Thus, even in gathering the data for a study it is possible for experimenter bias to affect the results. Now let's fast forward to a time when all the samples have been gathered. The computation of the DSS involves the scorer making many interpretations of point values to assign to parts of sentences. There is a certain amount of subjectivity to this process. Even in the segmentation of the language samples (deciding sentence boundaries in run-on sentences), there is some idiosyncratic decision making. A researcher who was aware of which language sample was from each group could possibly assign higher DSS point values to the normal attention group and lower values to the ADD group. It would also be possible to accept longer (more complex) utterances in one group and segment long utterances into two shorter (less complex) sentences in another group. Even if these decisions were made unconsciously, the experimenter could influence the outcome of the study by the language sampling style, how samples were segmented, and how samples were scored on the DSS. It should be easy to see that the gathering, segmentation, and scoring of data should be kept as far away from the researcher as possible. This can be done using research assistants and the

FIGURE 4.12

Between Subjects Study of Language Ability in Two Groups

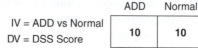

	ADD	Normal
IV = ADD vs Normal DV = DSS Score	10	10

"blinding" procedure referred to earlier. If a research assistant scored those language samples blind to the group the sample represented, experimenter bias is controlled. Using research assistants who were unaware of a child's group membership to gather language samples would control for bias in data gathering.

It can be seen from prior sections that an experimenter can potentially influence the outcome of a study by the expectations he or she might instill in participants and in the way data are gathered and analyzed. The following sections deal with biases that reside in participants, which can also have a powerful influence on the outcome of research.

The Hawthorne Effect

In the years from 1924 to 1933 some research at the Hawthorne plant of the Western Electric Company near Chicago focused on worker productivity under different conditions (lighting levels, rest breaks, pay, etc.). No matter which variable was manipulated, the result was an increase in worker productivity with an eventual return to baseline levels. A popular interpretation of this phenomenon was called the **Hawthorne effect** and centered on the idea that the behavior of the workers changed not due to the manipulation of the particular conditions (e.g., lighting) but rather just due to the fact that they were being closely studied (Mayo, 1933; Roethlisberger & Dickson, 1939). Draper defines the Hawthorne effect as:

> An experimental effect in the direction expected but not for the reason expected; i.e. a significant positive effect that turns out to have no causal basis in the theoretical motivation for the intervention, but is apparently due to the effect on the participants of knowing themselves to be studied in connection with the outcomes measured. (2005, p. 1)

It is not known exactly what participants are thinking when their behavior changes as the result of being studied in research. It is clear, however, that people who participate in research are not static systems; rather, they enter the study in a state of excitation or with specific attitudes and interpretations of the experimental situation. Many authorities, for instance, have questioned if there are differences between participants who volunteer for an investigation versus those who are randomly selected and solicited to take part in the study (Rosenthal & Rosnow, 1975). Perhaps volunteers are qualitatively different than nonvolunteers. Some researchers have noted that certain participants seem to behave as they believe the experimenter would want them to, or

The Instrumentation Threat

The **instrumentation threat** looms large in experimental design. Remember when we said that your study is only as good as your dependent variable? In many cases the dependent variable involves some sort of measurement by either a person or an electronic device. If the person is not well trained and the electronic device is shoddily built or uncalibrated, the dependent measure is not worth much to the scientist. But we are getting ahead of our story. First, we should take some time and explain what we mean by "instrumentation" and exactly how our research instruments can go awry. Figure 4.13 shows four types of "instruments" used in research. You might be surprised to see that not all of these instruments are machines or electronic devices and that in some cases people are used as instruments. Let us take a look at each category. Many research projects use electronic instruments to gather data on phenomena of interest. Whenever a researcher uses an audiometer, audiotape recorder, digital video recorder, computerized speech laboratory (CSL), or electroencephalograph (EEG), he or she is relying on an electronic instrument to gain information. At this point in time, most instruments are electronic in nature even if they used to be mechanical devices. For example a bathroom scale used to be a mechanical device with a circular dial and pointer but now have digital readouts with memory storage for each member of the family. Some can even compute the percent body fat of the user in addition to body weight. So it is with laboratory instruments. Several decades ago a standard piece of

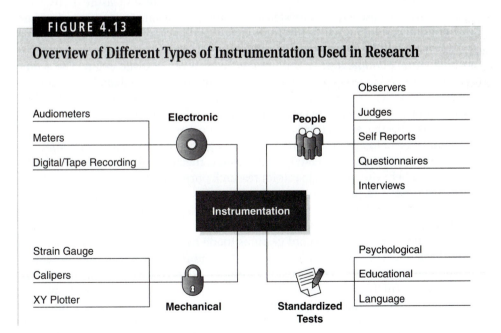

FIGURE 4.13

Overview of Different Types of Instrumentation Used in Research

laboratory equipment in speech-language pathology was the sound spectrograph, a device that analyzed the frequencies in a speech signal by burning a "spectrogram" on a piece of special paper attached to a rotating mechanical drum. Today, such instruments have been replaced by computer assisted devices that provide the same information outputted to a computer screen or laser printer. Electronic instruments are very common in communication disorders research.

Another category of instruments comprise mechanical devices, which are still in use despite the trend toward electronic replacements. A researcher measuring the size and shape of the articulators of different groups of participants might use calipers or some other sort of measuring device. Some researchers measuring strength of articulators (e.g., tongue strength) might use strain gauges or some other mechanical interface to obtain this measurement. A measurement of fine motor skill might involve having a participant place pegs into holes on a large board and determining how many pegs can be accurately placed by different groups under investigation. Reaction time might be measured by having the participant push a button or switch when a stimulus is presented. Some of these devices use mechanical components that interface with electronic devices.

Another category of instruments involves the use of standardized tests. Commonly with communication disorders participants are administered psychological, educational, or language tests to determine performance in these areas. Clearly, such tests do not involve electronic or mechanical instruments; the standardized test itself is an "instrument" that measures the construct of interest. Thus, a researcher interested in anxiety level can use psychological tests that provide a measure of this variable. Similarly, the researcher interested in reading level can administer a standardized reading test to determine a student's grade level in reading comprehension. In the area of language there are hundreds of standardized tests that tap semantic, syntactic, morphological, phonological, and pragmatic aspects of linguistic ability. The scores on these standardized instruments are really no different than a digital readout from an electronic device or a meter reading from a mechanical measurement. Remember, however, that standardized tests are administered and scored by humans, so they are not quite as objective as electrical or mechanical devices.

A final type of instrumentation involves using people to measure phenomena of interest. In some cases, we do not have electronic, mechanical, or standardized tests that measure behavior of participants for research purposes. Instead, we often employ humans as observers, judges, or respondents to gain information on phenomena. For example, the researcher interested in the gestural development of infants can neither use standardized tests nor mechanical or electronic measurements of such behaviors. Certainly if we want to record gestures made by infants, we must use an electronic device such as a digital video recorder to capture gestures; however, the actual measurement of gestures is really made by trained observers who count and analyze the movements of the participants. Often, researchers interested in vocal production use trained judges to rate vocal quality of participants. Although there are many instruments that can give us technical information on the human voice, some aspects still elude our computer-assisted measurements and human judges still are the gold standard for some judgments. In some cases, researchers are interested in self-reports from participants as measurements of internal states, opinions, and historical information. Use of such self-reports and interviews are a good example of how people can be used as instruments to gather relevant data. Finally, a large research literature exists on the use of questionnaires to gather information from people on a variety of issues. When people fill out questionnaires tapping their attitudes toward various issues or as they fill out rating forms indicating their agreement or disagreement with a particular statement, the participants are actually the instruments we are using to measure such constructs. The questionnaire is just a piece of paper, but it is the ratings by human participants that bring them alive and carry meaning. Thus, it can be seen that electronic, mechanical, human, and standardized test instruments can all be used to gather data for research in communication disorders. Although these four areas are clearly different, they also have much in common in terms of the ways they might allow error to affect research results, as we will discuss in later sections.

Common Steps in Using Instrumentation for Research

Figure 4.14 depicts six steps typically associated with using instruments in research. Although these steps are mostly associated with the use of equipment to gather data,

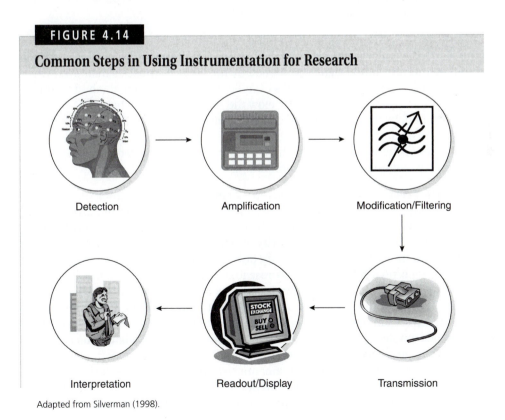

FIGURE 4.14

Common Steps in Using Instrumentation for Research

Detection

Amplification

Modification/Filtering

Interpretation

Readout/Display

Transmission

Adapted from Silverman (1998).

one can also apply them to using people and standardized tests. We will consider them one by one.

Detection.   A researcher who wants to study a particular phenomenon of interest must first detect when it occurs. In some cases, the object of the study is relatively obvious, such as a gesture, production of a certain linguistic element, or the participant's ability to produce a particular phoneme. In these cases, the researcher must preserve the behavior of interest and note its occurrence on some sort of coding sheet. If the behaviors are fleeting they can be preserved on audio or video long enough for a trained human judge to count and later interpret the behavior. In many cases, however, the object of study is not readily observable and must be detected using some sort of interface that will allow for later human analysis. For instance, a researcher interested in action potentials of specific muscles or certain frequencies of brainwave activity might use surface or needle electrodes to detect subtle signals that cannot be observed without specialized equipment. A researcher interested in analyzing the human voice must use a sensitive microphone to detect the vocal signal in enough detail for later analysis. Thus, the use of any type of "instrumentation" begins with some mechanism to detect the signal of interest. The detector can involve something as simple as human observation and counting or as complicated as the use of magnetic resonance imaging (MRI) technology.

Amplification.   After a signal is detected, in many cases it must be amplified or emphasized so that the researcher can evaluate it thoroughly. An obvious example would be the very subtle signals produced by the brain or muscles that, even when amplified, are registered in microvolts or millivolts. Without some method of amplification, these signals would be well below the sensation level of humans and could not be studied. In a sense, even behaviors that are easily observable may need to be emphasized or amplified to allow in-depth analysis. For example, a researcher studying gestures in children "amplifies" them by using a video recorder and playing them back in slow motion for detailed examination.

Modification/Filtering.   Many studies are not interested in examining the totality of a given phenomenon, but instead are designed to look at only certain aspects of an event. Take brain activity for example. The nervous system produces many frequencies and amplitudes of electrical activity at many different sites. A researcher may be interested in neural electrical activity only at specific sites (e.g., specific areas of the cerebral cortex). Additionally, the researcher might be focused only on certain bandwidths (e.g., alpha waves between 8 and 13 Hz) or specific time-linked electrical activity (e.g., auditory evoked potentials). In the latter example, the researcher may be interested in only one specific part of the auditory wave (e.g., P3). In order to reduce the complexity of these neural signals, the investigator might detect all brain activity through electrodes placed on the scalp. These signals are then amplified so that the researcher can see them for later analysis. In order to focus the investigation on the waveforms of interest, the researcher might put the amplified signal through some sort of filter that screens out unwanted signals and admits only the signal of interest. Thus, a scientist can filter out one band (e.g., 8–13 Hz) for analysis or several selected bands out of all the possible frequencies available. One might think that this only applies to physiological research; however, we can make an analogy from our prior example of studying gestures in children. Obviously, an infant makes many gestures and movements during play and interactions with his or her caregiver. A researcher, however, might only be interested in specific behaviors that are carefully operationally defined (e.g., pointing, reaching, showing, and giving.) These behaviors must be "filtered" out from the stream of movements produced by a child in a sampling session. Although the researcher watches the video record of a play sample in its entirety, only certain specific behaviors of interest are actually counted and analyzed. This is very similar to filtering out unwanted neurological activity in an electroencephalographic study.

Transmission.   We will operationally define transmission as moving the detected/amplified/modified signal to some sort of readout device (e.g., computer monitor, paper chart recorder, magnetic or digital audio/video recorder, or paper coding sheet filled out by observers). In many cases, the signal is transmitted via some sort of electronic cable to various types of readout devices. Some studies might transmit information to a readout device through wireless technology. Thus, the filter might be connected to a CRT monitor so the researcher can see a visual display of the signal being studied. In studying the development of gestural behaviors in children, the "readout device" might actually be a coding sheet with categories of gestural behavior. The gestural behaviors are transmitted to the coding sheet by a trained observer cataloging gestures from a video recording and writing down the type of gesture, time of occurrence, and duration on the coding sheet; no wires involved.

Readout/Display.   There are a variety of ways to display a signal of interest in a research project. Common displays include computer monitor, television, oscilloscope, strip chart recorder, X-Y plotter, printer, coding sheets, digital meter, analog meter, and many others. On each device the signal is displayed so that the researcher can ultimately record and store it, either on paper, magnetic recording tape, or digital media (diskettes, CD-ROM, DVD). Many of the readout devices mentioned must be calibrated in order to truly reflect the signal that is of interest to the researcher. In the case of meters, it is always good to put a known signal into the system to see if the meter registers it with a high degree of accuracy. It is always possible for a data storage system to lose a number in the process of saving the file, which could contribute error to the research project. Researchers should always check their readout mechanisms to ensure that they are displaying a true representation of a known signal. If human coders are being used to record behaviors, it is possible that the observer intended to check one box on the coding sheet but due to time constraints actually placed the check in the wrong box.

Interpretation.   In some studies, the final step in the montage of instrumentation is a computer. There are some signals that if examined individually as they occur do not mean as much as when the occurrences are evaluated over time after many trials. For instance, a researcher examining brain activity might be interested in differences in amplitude over several different sites on the cortex over a task that lasts five minutes or more. Thus, the occurrence of a single waveform may not be as important as thousands of waves summed over a longer period of time. Similarly, in examining a participant's vocal production just the computation of the fundamental frequency entails averaging waves that occur many times during a speaking task. It would be almost impossible for a researcher to carry out such analyses by hand, but a computer can be programmed to do them in a matter of seconds. In our example of the gestural study, the researcher is not particularly interested in the occurrence of a single gesture but more interested in the total number and proportion of gestures produced in a sampling session. This involves summing gestural productions over a sampling period, which can be done by a computer program once the gestural data have been input, or it can be accomplished manually by counting, cataloging, and using a calculator. Whatever method is used, most studies have some sort of step that involves summarizing the data for each participant so that it can be interpreted by the investigator.

Generic Sources of Error Related to Instrumentation

Each step in Figure 4.14 can contribute error into an experiment. That is, mistakes can be made in detection, amplification, modification/filtering, transmission, reading out, and interpretation. Such errors can be subsumed into a few basic categories, discussed in the following sections.

Quality of the Instrument.   The quality of the instruments is of paramount importance in gathering data for research. This applies to all steps in acquiring data from detection and amplification through filtering and interpretation. For example, the use of high-quality electrodes is important if a signal is to be detected adequately. Even if you have top flight equipment for the rest of your setup, cheap electrodes could jeopardize the whole project. If your amplifier is not of "research quality," how do you know if it is actually increasing the amplitude of the signal reliably for all participants? The same goes for filtering, transmission, readouts, and interpretation. A perfect signal sent to a defective mechanical meter will point to the wrong number. A good guideline is to stick with equipment designed by major companies for clinical and research use. If an audiologist decided to build a research audiometer by assembling it from parts purchased from a local electronics store, it would probably not be as well accepted in peer review as a device developed by a major manufacturer of audiometric equipment. With regard to use of standardized tests as instruments, it is always better to use a test that has been widely accepted by the clinical and research community rather than make up your own instrument. When choosing human judges to rate vocal quality it is better to select certified speech-language pathologists or highly trained graduate students as opposed to unsophisticated listeners who are less familiar with evaluating vocal quality.

Condition of the Instrument.   Perhaps it should go without saying that even high-quality equipment, if not in good repair, can threaten your study. For example, a researcher can purchase high-quality electrodes for an electroencephalographic study.

However, if a research assistant has stretched the electrode wires by handling them incorrectly, a potential problem has been created. It is possible that stretching the fine electrode wires can alter their impedance. As a result, signals passed through stretched electrodes may differ from signals of normal electrodes. This could be critical if an investigator was comparing brain activity from two different sites monitored by varying electrodes. Any differences in wave amplitudes found at these sites could simply be due to differences in electrode impedance and not brain activity. Similarly, if an amplifier rated as producing a certain level of amplification by the manufacturer is damaged, the researcher is not amplifying the signal of interest to the extent anticipated. Regarding use of standardized tests, the assumption is that the test administrator is familiar with the test and its administration and scoring for it to be considered valid. An untrained test administrator is no different than an amplifier that is not performing according to specifications. The bottom line is that all instruments should be checked to determine if they are in good working order prior to engaging in research.

Calibration.   The process of calibrating an instrument is simply a way of ensuring that the device is performing as it should according to specifications. Audiologists are intimately familiar with calibration because the audiometers they use must be calibrated on a regular basis to make sure that the devices are presenting auditory stimuli at a specific level. The whole field of audiology would be compromised if we thought we were presenting tones or speech at 30 decibels and it really was coming out of the speakers or earphones at 20 decibels. The estimation of hearing impairment would be wrong and the hearing aid prescribed for the person would be inappropriate if based on these data. Calibration is important in any study involving equipment and in the case where multiple pieces of equipment are linked together (e.g., amplifier, filter, readout) each step in the process should ideally be checked for proper calibration. One weak link and the whole study could be compromised. Calibration does not only apply to equipment but also to standardized tests and human judges. In the example of a person administering a standardized test without proper training, you can see that the unfamiliar administrator has not been properly "calibrated." In most cases, a person using a standardized test must read the manuals and give several test administrations to gain familiarity with giving the test as well as its scoring and interpretation. In some cases, test developers recommend attending a training course that allows administrators to become calibrated in using a particular test instrument. For example, intelligence testing requires specific coursework, supervised experience, and credentialing before a person is qualified to make judgments about an intelligence quotient (Flanagan & Harrison, 2005). In cases where judges are used to evaluate behaviors in research, some training is typically required prior to actually engaging in the investigation, essentially an exercise in calibration of the human judges often referred to as "reliability" in a research report. The bottom line is that most studies should address calibration and/or reliability issues in reports of the research.

Interpretive Skill.   When using any instrument, one thing is certain: You will always get a readout. Whether the readout is a meter reading, a test score, some digits on an

LCD display, some waveforms on a plotter, or a number of pointing behaviors on a data sheet, you will *always* have some sort of data. Data, however, are not necessarily evidence (Muma, 1998). Muma states:

> The distinctions between data and evidence are related to the distinctions between technicians and clinicians. Data are merely numbers open to any interpretation or dogma. It is relatively easy to compile data by using various simplistic checklists, developmental profiles, and simple, quick tests.... It is not ususual in the clinical fields to have a client's file filled with such data. (1998, p. 167)

In the field of intelligence testing, Flanagan and Harrison state:

> The classic description of the role of the assessment professional given by Matarazzo (1990) is still highly relevant today. Matarazzo argued that assessment is quite different from measurement, and that intellectual assessment in particular requires experienced examiners who carefully evaluate the match between the instruments and the examinee. (2005, p. 328)

Again, we can always obtain a score, but *what does that score mean*? It is one thing to report different amplitudes of brain activity under differing areas of the scalp; however, it is quite another thing to infer some level or type of "processing" that is allegedly going on in those locations. An acquaintance of ours compared learning about how the brain processes through EEG studies to learning about the game of football by putting a stethoscope on the roof of the Louisiana Superdome. Even if that analogy is a bit extreme, it does point out the big difference between measurement and interpretation. Even if a researcher uses high-quality instruments that are in good condition and well calibrated, the study can be easily nullified by improper interpretation of the data obtained.

The Participant Selection Threat

Earlier we talked about the threats of history and maturation to a research project. We made the point that such threats were especially troublesome when the same participants were being examined in several conditions over time in repeated measures (within subjects) designs. In such studies the actual composition of the participant group stays the same through the repeated measurements, and the researcher does not have to worry about their initial classifications changing over time (e.g., male/female, socioeconomic status, clinical disorder, etc.). However, when the study is "between subjects" or comparing completely different groups with one another, the threat of participant selection becomes highly significant. Take, for example, a study of children who represent Hispanic, white, and African American cultural groups (Figure 4.15). The researcher is interested in determining if there is a cultural difference in the mean length of utterance of three-year-old children from these groups. Since there are ten people in each group who will only be sampled once, and the researcher is interested in culture as the independent variable, it is very important that the three groups differ mainly by culture and not by some other extraneous variable. As we said earlier in this chapter, we want to rule out all other competing explanations for the results other than the independent variable. What are some possible competing explanations in this study? A partial list of variables having nothing to

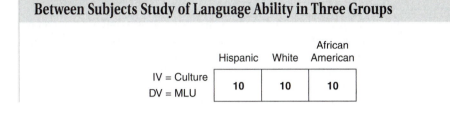

FIGURE 4.15

Between Subjects Study of Language Ability in Three Groups

	Hispanic	White	African American
IV = Culture DV = MLU	10	10	10

do with culture that could offer a competing explanation for groups having different MLU means include hearing loss, language ability, socioeconomic level, age, gender, family size, and bilingualism in the family. If the groups differed in any of these areas, a critic of the research could say these variables account just as well for MLU differences as cultural membership. Thus, the researcher would want to populate the three groups with participants screened for speech, hearing, and language disorders, having similar SES levels, genders, ages, family sizes, and bilingual status. How researchers ensure that participant selection for a between subjects investigation is not a threat to their study will be discussed in the following sections.

Establish Selection Criteria

One of the first lines of defense in a between subjects experimental design is for the researcher to develop very specific criteria for selection of participants. In the previous example, the researcher would want to "control for" hearing, speech-language disorder, SES, gender, age, family size, and the language spoken in the home. Only participants meeting the researcher's **selection criteria** would be allowed to participate in the study. In this way, alternative explanations for the results of the study that would compete with the independent variable (culture) are neutralized. Whenever you embark on a study using different groups, it is critical that you establish selection criteria for the people who participate. Obviously, you cannot control *everything* about your participants, but you can control variables that have relevance to the issue you are studying. For example, it may not be important to control for the religious affiliation of your groups in this study. There is no known relationship between religious affiliation and MLU that has been shown by prior research, so it is something that is not necessary to control for. Also, there is no logical argument one can make that suggests religion and MLU might be related. On the other hand, if someone can come up with research showing that MLU might be affected by the amount and frequency of adult-child shared book reading, then this would be an additional variable to control for in the above example. It all depends on what research has shown and what is logically likely to affect the results of the study.

Random Assignment

One of the most elegant notions in research design is randomization. Theoretically, if participants are truly assigned to groups using a table of **random assignment** or table of random numbers, and every participant has an equal chance to be assigned to any group, all relevant variables should be, from a statistical perspective, equally distributed among the groups. For example, if we were studying the effectiveness of two different types of language treatment against a control group that did not receive any treatment, it would be extremely important to pay attention to exactly how these groups were populated. We certainly would not want all the severe cases in one group and the mild cases in one of the other groups. In this study we could establish some general selection criteria in terms of range of language test scores and language sample data that would make a participant eligible for participation in the study. Once we have a relatively homogeneous group of children with language impairment, then we need to assign them to one of three groups (e.g., Treatment A, Treatment B, and No Treatment). Theoretically, if we randomly assigned these children to the groups, then all relevant variables including error variance would be distributed fairly equally among the three groups (e.g., gender, severity, SES, etc.) Of course, the groups should be checked after they are constituted to confirm that one of them is not unreasonably out of line with the others, but in most cases they will be remarkably similar even though there is a probability that the groups could be different due to chance. Random assignment also contributes to the objectivity of the scientific method because a researcher cannot be accused of populating the groups with participants whom he or she thinks might perform a particular way. If, for example, one of the types of language treatment involves child-directed play and the other involves drill, a researcher could unconsciously place a very distractible child in the play treatment group instead of the drill group. Conversely, if children are randomly assigned to groups, the experimenter is taken out of the equation.

Matching

Another method of equating groups in a between subjects design involves intentional **matching** of participants on relevant variables across the groups. Thus, a researcher might constitute the first group and assemble data on their relevant characteristics. Then in populating the other groups involved in the study, the researcher would specifically look for participants that "matched" those in the initial group on relevant variables. As you can guess, the more groups the researcher includes in the study, the more difficult it is to find participants who match the selection criteria (Kerlinger and Lee, 2000).

We should remember that matching is limited in other ways. For example, we can only match for so many variables, and even if we are successful in matching for intelligence, language ability, and socioeconomic status, we may create a mismatch on other variables such as gender, culture, or school achievement. Thus, in cases where matching is selected as a method for controlling extraneous variance, Kerlinger and Lee (2000) strongly recommend the use of randomization in addition to matching in assigning participants to groups. One other disadvantage to matching is addressed by Bordens and Abbott:

> Matched designs require you to use somewhat modified versions of the inferential statistics you would use in an unmatched, completely randomized design. These statistics for matched

groups are somewhat less powerful than their unmatched equivalents. This means they are less able to discriminate any effect of the independent variable from the effect of uncontrolled, extraneous variables. (2002, p. 262)

Of course, the ultimate matching procedure is to use a within subjects or repeated measures design in which each participant is self-matched. Unfortunately, many experimental questions cannot be answered with such designs, and we must control for variance in between subjects studies as best we can.

Including Extraneous Variables in Your Design and Using Statistics as Control

Kerlinger and Lee (2000) suggest that another way to control variance in a study is to include the extraneous variable in your design as another independent variable. If, for example, you are wondering if socioeconomic level could be an uncontrolled source of variance that may be of some interest in your experiment, you can add SES as another independent variable and actually evaluate the amount of variance that is accounted for by this factor. In this way, you control SES while formally evaluating another potentially important source of variation. An additional way to control variance is through the statistical method you choose to analyze your data. An example of such a statistic is the *analysis of covariance,* which is a statistic specifically designed to compensate for groups that are unequal on certain characteristics at the outset of the study. We will be discussing such statistical methods in a later chapter.

Group Summary Information

No matter which of the above methods a researcher has used to control variance in participants, it is always helpful to consumers of research if the investigator summarizes in the form of a table or chart the relevant characteristics of the different groups involved in the study. Even if the researcher could not control for every variable prior to participant selection, it is good to be able to demonstrate after the fact that the groups are more similar than different on relevant variables. If the groups were, in fact, different on certain characteristics it could help the investigator or consumers to account for research findings that may not be in line with prior studies. As a consumer or producer of research you should always zero in on the characteristics of participants in studies that compare groups.

The Mortality Threat

The final threat to internal validity is **mortality** or the attrition of participants during the course of an investigation. Attrition or mortality refers to the withdrawal of participants from a study before it can be completed. Recall that the informed consent indicates that a participant can withdraw from a study at any time, and some take advantage of this option. Participating in a research project may sound intriguing at the outset, but as the study progresses the person can become frustrated with scheduling problems, feel increased stress, or become fatigued. Other participants may be required to relocate due to job changes or family issues. Some participants may have to withdraw in the face of illness, death, or other family emergencies. How can mortality affect a study in progress? First, you will remember that a good researcher has spent considerable time populating groups. Especially in between subjects designs, participants have been randomly assigned to groups to compensate for unwanted sources of variance. If participants from certain groups withdraw, it affects the randomization of the groups; they are no longer randomly assigned. Second, when people from certain groups drop out of the study, you have to wonder about the type of person that remains versus the people who withdrew. Are the people who stayed in the study qualitatively different than those who chose not to participate? If one group has more dropouts than the others, what does this say about that particular condition? A final concern is that mortality can result in unequal numbers of participants across groups. The researcher may have started with twenty people in each group and after attrition may be left with groups of different sizes. This can have an effect on the types of statistical methods available to the researcher, since some statistics work the best with equal numbers of participants in each group.

Threats to External Validity

The discussion of internal validity concerned how well an investigation was controlled to compensate for extraneous sources of variance. Doctoral students often refer to studies with impressive experimental designs and strong internal validity as being "tight," as in tightly controlled. External validity refers to the generalizability of the results of a study or how the findings can be applied to the "real world." Many investigations are designed so that the results might be applied to clinical populations or situations beyond the laboratory setting. In such cases, it is important that the investigation study a population similar to the one to which findings will be applied. Also, it is critical that the methods used in the research reflect tasks and measurements that are common in the real world. If these conditions are met, the study is said to have strong external validity because the results can be applied to populations outside the laboratory setting. Not every study, however, has a goal of high external validity as defined here. Mook (1983) indicates that it is not necessarily true that all researchers are attempting to produce results that apply to situations in the real world. For example, it is possible that a researcher may be investigating a highly theoretical problem and merely wants to determine if a particular chemical reaction takes place under highly controlled laboratory conditions. In this case, he or she may not care how the reaction may or may not occur in the natural environment because the focus is on its occurrence in the laboratory setting. For the most part, however, researchers are concerned with both internal and external validity. Researchers are always being asked how their work affects the world at large, and most scientists like to be able to say that there are practical implications that flow from their research.

> In all science, error precedes the truth, and it is better it should go first than last.
>
> Hugh Walpole (1884–1941)

Figure 4.16 shows those persistent research sharks again coming after someone's investigation. This time, instead of threatening to attack the internal validity of the research, they are cruising in search of threats to external validity. We will briefly discuss each threat to external validity.

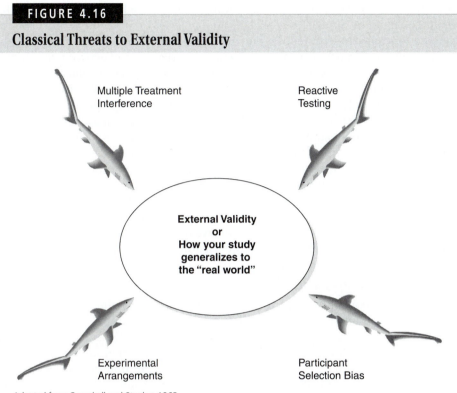

FIGURE 4.16

Classical Threats to External Validity

Multiple Treatment Interference

Reactive Testing

External Validity
or
How your study
generalizes to
the "real world"

Experimental Arrangements

Participant Selection Bias

Adapted from Campbell and Stanley, 1963.

Participant Selection Bias

Earlier we made the case that participant selection and how groups were populated can have a major effect on internal validity. This is also true with external validity. As we think of external validity or the generalizability of a study, one of the most important questions might be "Were the participants in the investigation similar to the population to which the results can be generalized?" In a tightly controlled study of stuttering and brain activity, a researcher at a university may have recruited participants very specifically to control for sources of error (internal validity). For example, a participant in the stuttering group may have had to meet the following criteria: (1) current college student, (2) male, (3) right-handed, (4) no history of head injury, (5) no recent history of treatment for stuttering, (6) a particular severity level of stuttering (severe) based on a diagnostic test, and (7) white. Given these criteria, the researcher recruits the participants and completes the study of their brain activity. To whom can these results be generalized? Since the participants were college students, the age range would probably be in the early 20s. The results could not be generalized to children or older adults. The educational level and socioeconomic level, which is partially determined by educational achievement, would be fairly restricted, and the results could not be applied to other educational levels or SES groups. Since the researcher controlled for handedness and history of brain injury, the results would not apply to left-handed people or those who had experienced a concussion in a sports injury. Controlling for history of treatment would make the results not applicable to any person who stutters who had experienced therapy. Since the severity levels were limited to severe difficulties, the findings would not relate to any person with a mild or moderate impairment. Finally, controlling for cultural group and gender would make the results only relevant to white males who stutter. It is easy to see from this example that the external validity of this study would be weakened based on the stringent selection of participants (**participant selection bias**). Consumers and producers of research should carefully consider if implications from a particular study are limited due to the characteristics of the people who were studied. One of the major errors made by researchers is studying normally developing individuals and then talking about clinical implications for people who have disorders. It is a giant leap to apply research results from a normal population to a group with impairments.

Experimental Arrangements

Research can be done in a variety of places ranging from the natural environment to strictly controlled laboratory conditions; external validity can be especially threatened by the latter. If a study is conducted in a highly controlled environment using artificial tasks and stimuli, it will be difficult to generalize the results of the experiment to the real world. In audiology, for example, it is not unusual for researchers to test auditory processing disorder in a sound-treated chamber using tests that are highly controlled. Keith describes some of the specific test procedures that might be used by clinicians and researchers:

> In regard to audiologic test procedures, low redundancy speech refers to such tests as filtered words and auditory figure ground (speech-in-noise) testing. Monaural testing is conducted using earphones, with the signal heard in one ear at a time. Dichotic testing is conducted by presenting different acoustic stimuli with simultaneous onset and offset times by earphone to the two ears. Dichotic stimuli include consonant-vowel syllables, digits, monosyllable words, two syllable words (spondees), and sentences. Binaural interaction procedures are conducted by presenting different stimuli simultaneously to the two ears, with interaction between the stimuli resulting in comprehension of a complete message (e.g., binaural fusion tests), or comprehension depending on changes in masking conditions (e.g., masking level difference test). (1999, p. 341)

Given such tests, a consumer of research must ask how the test environment, tasks, and stimuli compare to language processing in the natural environment. Most children with auditory processing disorders operate in homes and classrooms without the benefit of a sound-treated booth or calibrated earphones. The stimuli that they typically process consist of oral and written material presented in a context that provides visual cues in addition to auditory information. The information they process is usually meaningful language presented in the context of discourse and not unrelated material that may not be semantically relevant (e.g., syllables, digits, single words).

Information in the real world is not presented in only one ear or heard dichotically with two different words presented simultaneously to each ear. The point here is that laboratory research on auditory processing is limited in its external validity. It is a big step from the laboratory to the classroom, and there is no guarantee that a child who has difficulty processing artificial stimuli in a sound booth will have trouble in the classroom. Generally, the more artificial the **experimental arrangements** (e.g., setting, stimuli, tasks), the less external validity will be associated with a study. On a more general level, just the effect of participating in an experiment, being observed, or coming to a laboratory setting can make participants act differently than they ordinarily would in the natural environment. Researchers must be very careful about generalizing laboratory results to more natural conditions.

Reactive Testing

Campbell and Stanley (1963) made the important point over forty years ago that anything we do in an experiment can "sensitize" participants in particular ways. By this they meant that any test or task given to participants can influence their performance on later parts of an experiment. We discussed this point earlier in the present chapter in covering the threat of testing effects on internal validity. In our earlier example we presented a study in which a researcher had developed a video that was calculated to reduce vocal abuse. In that study, the participants were given a questionnaire dealing with their feelings about vocal abuse, then they watched the video, and finally they were given the questionnaire again to determine if the video had changed their attitudes toward vocal abuse. If the results of this study showed that the video was responsible for helping to change attitudes toward vocal abuse, the researcher might decide to market the product for widespread use. In advertising, the researcher might say something like "This video has been shown to help in changing attitudes toward vocal abuse." The problem from an external validity perspective is that anyone who purchases the video will not have the benefit of experiencing the questionnaire beforehand. We do not know if the attitude change in the study was due to the previewing questionnaire, the video, or a combination of the two. We cannot generalize the use of the video to people who have not experienced the questionnaire, thus compromising external validity. Any experience that we give participants such as filling out forms, pretests, counseling, and interactions with the researcher during the experiment can sensitize them and potentially influence their performance during the study (**reactive testing**). These events will not be experienced by those who were not participants in the experiment and thus, we must be very careful in our generalizations to other populations who have not experienced the research paradigm.

Multiple Treatment Interactions

Probably the critical difference between reactive testing and multiple treatment interactions is the length and intensity of exposure to the sensitizing event. In pretesting, a questionnaire may not take a lot of time to complete, and there is certainly no intent on the part of the researcher to alter participant attitudes by administering the instrument. In a study in which different treatments are compared, the intensity and duration of the treatments are typically greater than in clinical practice and the experimenter has the intent to affect participants by administering the treatment. As an example, a researcher is attempting to determine which of two treatments for stuttering is most effective in a within subjects design. In the study, twenty participants who stutter are administered two treatment conditions: (1) wearing a delayed auditory feedback (DAF) device, and (2) wearing a masking noise device. Even if the researcher counterbalances the conditions, all participants will have experienced both treatment regimens. If one treatment method (e.g., DAF) results in lower disfluency rates, ten of the twenty participants that experienced that condition would have experienced the masking condition first due to counterbalancing. Thus, one cannot say that DAF treatment done *without experiencing the masking treatment first* would have produced the same results for participants who received the DAF first. Half the group received two treatments, but the other half received only one. Certainly, when a researcher recommends one of these treatments over the other to people who had not experienced both treatments, the external validity is threatened. Any time multiple treatments are given in an experiment, it is problematic to generalize one of those treatments to a general population who will only receive one rather than multiple treatments.

The Linkage between Internal and External Validity

If you have not already guessed it, there is an important linkage between internal and external validity. As internal validity increases, external validity tends to decrease. We have said that it is very important to make the design of a study "tight" or high in internal validity. However, it is possible to control yourself right out of business in doing research. For example, a study that involves participants that are selected by very rigid criteria (gender, age, site of lesion, socioeconomic level, culture) and has them perform tasks using very complex laboratory equipment will have a high level of internal validity. The external validity, however, will be low because the results may not apply to participants not meeting the selection profile in more natural situations not involving the artificial tasks performed in the laboratory setting. Conversely, if we design a study that allows a wide variety of participants (different ages, genders, cultures, sites of lesion, socioeconomic levels), the results may apply to a diverse group, but we have not controlled for many sources of error in the study and the internal validity is low. Thus, as internal validity goes up, external validity goes down. How do researchers resolve this dilemma? Most scientists would agree that if internal validity is compromised so much that the independent variable is no longer the plausible explanation for changes in the dependent variable, the study is probably not worth doing. We should make internal validity as strong as possible without making the study so limited that it does not have some generalizability. Another consideration is the purpose behind doing the research. If it is the purpose of the investigator is to do research that has applied value, some compromises in internal validity can be made in the interest of increasing external validity. But again, if internal validity is compromised beyond a certain level, the study is hopelessly flawed.

Consumers and producers of research should always be mindful of internal and external validity in research. When evaluating research in our professional literature, we should be "sharky" about considering whether the results of a study have credibility. In most cases, a thorough and critical evaluation of the threats to internal and external validity is the key to determining the quality of research.

Research: The Art and Science of Compromise

All our science, measured against reality, is primitive and childlike—and yet, it is the most precious thing we have.

Albert Einstein (1879–1955)

The best scientist is open to experience and begins with romance—The idea that anything is possible.

Ray Bradbury

It may seem curious that even though scientists know about all the possible threats to internal and external validity, we still can commonly find research that is somehow scientifically flawed. After all, if we know about all these threats, why can't we design studies that are ironclad and impervious to criticism? As Figure 4.17 indicates, the answer lies somewhere at the borderline where the conceptually "ideal study" meets the "real world." It would not be too difficult to sit in one's office and design an investigation that is nearly perfect. The problems would arise when the scientist attempted to actually conduct the study given the limitations of the real world. In hopes of communicating how this process transpires, we submit to you the story of a thesis student named Joann. Joann and her thesis advisor were interested in studying word retrieval in patients with Broca's aphasia. In the confines of the advisor's office the two

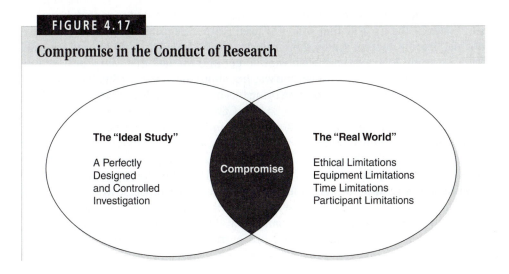

FIGURE 4.17

Compromise in the Conduct of Research

The "Ideal Study"

A Perfectly
Designed
and Controlled
Investigation

Compromise

The "Real World"

Ethical Limitations
Equipment Limitations
Time Limitations
Participant Limitations

researchers devised a plan that was fairly tight in internal validity. They wanted to find twenty patients with Broca's aphasia and twenty matched normal language participants and compare them on word retrieval ability. The group with aphasia would be between the ages of 50 and 70, equally balanced with males and females. All patients would have normal hearing, normal vision (corrected), a college education, and be of middle socioeconomic class. The brain damage of each patient would be confirmed by an MRI and only Broca's area would be affected. Only patients whose brain injury had occurred between one and three years ago would be recruited into the study. This would avoid the early part of spontaneous recovery in the first year and eliminate patients who had lived with their aphasia for extended periods of time such as a decade or more. All patients would have no history of language therapy and would score within one standard deviation of one another on two tests of aphasia. Patients would be living at home and not in a long-term care facility. Most of you can already see that these criteria are extremely strict but also that they might control for unwanted sources of variance. So here goes Joann, idealistic and full of energy skipping down to the newspaper office to place a classified ad announcing her study. She obviously could not use any of the patients receiving treatment in the university clinic, because they had been in therapy. As two weeks slid by, Joann received only one response to her advertisement. It was from a woman who had experienced her Cerebral Vascular Accident (CVA) five years before. This was clearly not within the three-year time window of the initial experimental design, but the clock was ticking and Joann only had a year left to complete her study. Sheepishly, she went down the hall to her advisor's office and asked if they could modify the initial selection criteria to one to five years post-onset. Joann was elated when the advisor approved of this change. During their first meeting, Joann and Mrs. Cardwell (her one and only participant) filled out consent forms and other paperwork associated with the study. During the hearing screening Joann noticed that Mrs. Cardwell wore a hearing aid which she said helps her a little bit in some situations. "You don't have normal hearing?" said Joann incredulously and excused herself for a moment to consult her advisor. She told the advisor that Mrs. Cardwell wore a hearing aid and did not have normal hearing as required by their criteria. Again, the advisor told her to proceed with the study. Joann did not even want to get into the fact that Mrs. Cardwell was wearing thick spectacles; however she was not about to whip out a Snellen Chart and screen her vision. She would not even bring this up with the advisor. Several days later after sending a release of information to Mrs. Cardwell's physician, a report arrived at the university documenting the brain damage in Joann's lone participant. Unfortunately, no MRI had been done and there was only a cryptic notation about a thrombosis of the middle cerebral artery. That was it. Nothing about Broca's area, no multicolored MRI printout, or any detailed neurological workup. Joann was rapidly wearing a new path in the carpet leading to the advisor's office. It was decided that they should run Mrs. Cardwell anyway, even with no MRI results, because this may be a problem with other patients. Joann then discovered that Mrs. C had only attended two years of college and did not earn a degree. The advisor and Joann hypothesized that there probably was not a big difference between someone with two years of college and a degree holder, so they opted to relax their educational criteria. It was also revealed that Mrs. C had received some language therapy while in a rehabilitation hospital during the first few months after her stroke. The research team decided that most patients would have experienced this, so the "no therapy" criterion had to be relaxed along with the other variables. Joann decided to enlarge her recruitment area to places within a one-hundred-mile radius around the university. She burned up a lot of gasoline and time searching for the ideal participant, but with each new person she was introduced to yet another compromise. Well, you get the idea. Joann had to compromise her selection standards quite a bit for her first participant, and it did not get any better as other participants were identified. Some of them had more severe hearing losses than Mrs. C. Others had "slight" visual field difficulties, but were allowed in the study. Joann was now down to a high school diploma as the entry level for her study. Socioeconomic level was totally thrown out because of availability of participants. None of the participants had an MRI in their record. Some of them had damage to other areas of the brain in addition to Broca's area. At least half of the participants lived in assisted living or long-term care facilities and not at home as required by the selection criteria. In case it has not occurred to you, we have not even touched upon the epic drama involved in finding the normal language participants who were supposed to be matched to the group with aphasia. Think of how difficult it would be to find a normal language person who matched each one of the patients with brain injury on socioeconomic level, age, gender, culture, hearing level, and educational achievement. Joann had to make many compromises, but she finally ended up with ten patients with aphasia and ten normal language individuals who were "in the ballpark" as far as their similarity. Certainly the age range was wider, the documentation of brain injury was less precise, the education level broader, and many other variables less precisely controlled. All of these variables were well described in Joann's thesis so readers would know exactly what kinds of participants were studied in her research. In the process of completing her thesis, Joann learned a lot about research and how compromise is necessary when facing the realities of actually doing a study. There is always a part in the written version of any study entitled something like "Limitations of the present research." In this section, Joann lamented some of the variables she could not completely control for and recommended that future studies tighten the selection criteria a bit more. But the choice was between doing the study with the participants who were available or not doing the research at all. To a much lesser degree, every research project goes like this. We start out with an ideal design and have to make compromises in the face of limitations put upon us by ethics, equipment, time, and participants. This is why there will *always* be some degree of error in research and something for research sharks to dream of. Most of the time those errors are not intentional but a product of compromise. Yet scientists continue to do research, even knowing that their studies cannot be perfect when affected by the limitations of the practical world. Research sharks should remember that criticism is fairly easy, but the real challenge is actually doing the science.

Summary

The design of a study is critically important to being able to answer the research question posed by the scientist. Ideally, a study must control for all threats to internal validity so that the independent variable can be the only explanation for changes in the dependent variable. Also, most researchers design their studies so that the results are applicable to people and situations in the real world (external validity). This chapter has discussed threats to internal and external validity that must be controlled by the researcher to make research scientifically sound. Unfortunately, there is a reciprocal relationship between internal and external validity such that as one increases, the other decreases. Researchers are always seeking a balance between the two and weighing the effects of various compromises they must make in conducting an investigation. This chapter is especially important for consumers of research as they critically evaluate articles in the professional literature, because a major part of any critical analysis is determining if the researcher has controlled for threats to internal and external validity. If a study has not done a good job of controlling for threats, its findings are of limited use to consumers.

LEARNING ACTIVITIES

1. In a between subjects design with a communication disordered group of your choice and a normal communication group, list the variables you would control for in terms of participant selection.
2. Find a table of random numbers and assign numbers to a group of one hundred hypothetical participants (1–100). Then use the table of random numbers to choose a population of fifty participants for a hypothetical study.
3. Develop a counterbalancing schedule for three conditions in a within subjects design where you have an N of ten participants.
4. Find three research articles that use electronic instrumentation. Summarize how they specify the instruments used and controlled for instrumentation threats.
5. Find three research articles and evaluate the use of single or double blinding in these studies.

CHAPTER 5

Levels of Measurement and Distribution of Scores

The only man who behaved sensibly was my tailor; he took my measurement anew every time he saw me, while all the rest went on with their old measurements and expected them to fit me.

—George Bernard Shaw (1856–1950)

One foot is short; one inch is long.

—Qu Yuan, Chinese poet and patriot (340–278 BC)

One accurate measurement is worth a thousand expert opinions.

—Admiral Grace Hopper (1906–1992)

Measure twice, cut once.

—Old carpenter's adage

Measurement is one of the most prominent concepts of science and it forms the basis for statistical analysis. In this chapter we introduce the basic concepts of measurement and organizing data for more detailed analysis. The types of data (e.g., nominal, ordinal, interval, ratio) gathered in a research project dictate to a large degree what statistical analyses are available. Furthermore, the distribution of the scores obtained in terms of measures of central tendency and variability will also have implications for which statistic is appropriate to use in analyzing the results of a study. Because this chapter is the first to delve into statistical concepts, we will approach the topic simply and methodically while providing many examples.

LEARNING OBJECTIVES

This chapter will enable readers to:

- List and understand the four levels of measurement (nominal, ordinal, interval, and ratio) used in research.
- Understand basic measures of central tendency (mode, median, mean).
- Understand the shape of a distribution and its importance in data analysis.
- Understand the difference between normal and abnormal distributions.

- List and understand measures of variability such as the range, variance, and standard deviation.
- Be able to list the assumptions of parametric and nonparametric statistics.
- Understand the rationale for data transformation in research.

Kerlinger and Lee (2000, p. 625) define measurement using a quote from Stevens (1951): "Measurement is the assignment of numerals to objects or events according to rules." Although this definition is short, it elegantly describes the process without undue verbiage. As stated in previous chapters, one step in the scientific method is to somehow quantify phenomena that are the objects of research investigation. Assigning numbers to phenomena, however, is a relatively easy process. We can take any measurement we wish and convert it into a number. As Lord (1953) illustrated, we can refer to football players by numbers on their jerseys, but the numbers signify nothing more meaningful than putting the athletes' names on their backs. Adding up the numbers on the jerseys and arriving at an average would be a meaningless exercise. We could continue this folly by using some sort of statistical analysis on the numbers and talk about the outcome of our research. But, as we said before, the results of such research would be meaningless since football jersey numbers do not really measure anything important. As Bordens and Abbott point out, "the numbers resulting from measurement are just numbers and a statistical analysis does not 'care' how the numbers were derived or where they came from" (2002, p. 129). Since statistics do not care, the researcher and research consumer must. We should be aware of the different types of measurements taken in science and the types of statistical analyses that can be appropriately done on them.

Levels of Measurement: What Kind of Data Does Your Dependent Variable Represent?

Most textbooks dealing with research methods contain a section on **levels of measurement.** Stevens (1946) postulated that there were four basic types of scales that can be ordered in terms of how much information they provide about the objects or events being measured. Figure 5.1 illustrates the four classical scales in an additive model with each successive scale building on the one before. We will discuss each level briefly and attempt to illustrate why levels of measurement are critically important to researchers in terms of the type of statistical analyses available to them.

Nominal Data

Nominal data are concerned with dividing objects or events into distinct groups that typically do not overlap. Examples include dividing people by gender (male/female), political party (Republican/Democrat/independent), or communication disorder (voice, fluency, phonology, language). In nominal measurement we assume that the groups do not overlap and that once we have made an assignment the object or event represents a group that is distinct from other groups. For example, we can group students by their declared major in college (audiology or speech-language pathology) as revealed on their transcript. We can assign an arbitrary number to each major (SLP = 1/AUD = 2) in order to quantify a student's area of study. Note that there would be no order to the groups; one group is not "better" or "higher" than another. The groups merely differ in their majors. It is also easy to see that doing mathematical operations on these numbers would tell us nothing. The result of adding, subtracting,

FIGURE 5.1

Levels of Measurement in Research

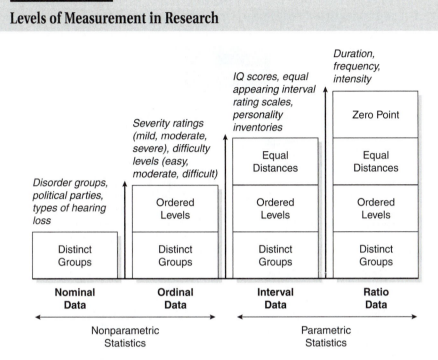

multiplying, or dividing the numbers would be meaningless. Figure 5.2 shows that a researcher with nominal data is confined to certain statistical methods, depending on the number of groups being studied and whether or not the measurements are repeated on a group (repeated samples/within subjects) or represent independent samples (between subjects). Statistics such as the McNemar test, chi-square test, and Cochran Q are designed to be used with nominal data and are typically not used on other levels of measurement. Do not worry that you are unfamiliar with these statistical methods at this point. We are only mentioning them to illustrate an important issue: *The type of measurement a researcher selects in research plays a critical role in determining which statistical methods are available for use in data analysis.*

Ordinal Data

The step up to **ordinal data** illustrated in Figure 5.1 adds the criterion of "ordered levels" to the data. Whereas there is no order in ranking people by gender or college major, there is an order when the values on the scale represent points along a continuum. When we say that a disorder is mild, moderate, or severe, we are implying that these three points on a scale do have an order of severity. Figure 5.3 illustrates the process of using a rule to assign ordinal values to individuals. Although the three

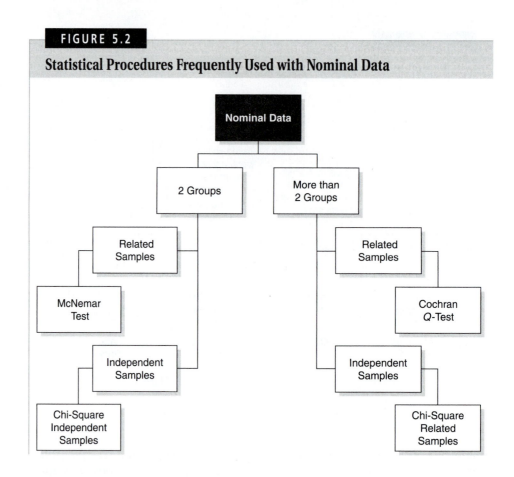

FIGURE 5.2

Statistical Procedures Frequently Used with Nominal Data

labeled points on the scale do imply an order, they do not refer to quantities that are absolute such as height or weight; they simply denote an order to the numbers. Similarly, the distance between the ordered points on an ordinal scale may not be consistent in reality, as illustrated in Figure 5.3. That is, the difference between mild and moderate may be more dramatic than the difference between moderate and severe. Figure 5.4 shows statistical methods designed for use with ordinal scales and makes the point once again that the type of measurement a researcher uses has a direct effect on the kinds of statistical analyses that should be used.

Interval Data

The step up to **interval data** means that the distances between the points on a scale are known and are fairly consistent. Typical examples of interval scales are intelligence quotients and scores on standardized tests of personality, language, educational achievement, or some other similar attribute. We assume that the difference

Ordinal Scales May Seem to Have Equal Intervals to a Researcher, but Intervals May Differ in Reality

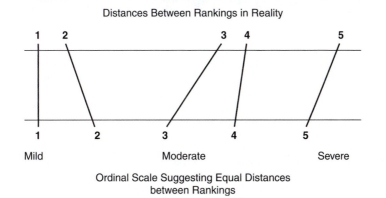

Distances Between Rankings in Reality

Mild   Moderate   Severe

Ordinal Scale Suggesting Equal Distances
between Rankings

Statistical Procedures Frequently Used with Ordinal Data

Ordinal Data

2 Groups

More than
2 Groups

Related
Samples

Wilcoxon
Matched Pairs
Signed Ranks Test

Independent
Samples

Mann-Whitney
U Test

Related
Samples

Friedman
ANOVA2

Independent
Samples

Kruskal Wallis
ANOVA1

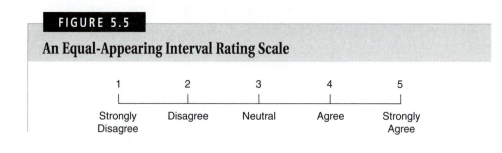

FIGURE 5.5

An Equal-Appearing Interval Rating Scale

in IQ between 90 and 100 is similar to a ten-point difference anywhere along the intelligence scale. Researchers may also use "equal appearing interval" scales on which judges are asked to rate specific attributes or degree of agreement with some statement. For instance, a scale such as that depicted in Figure 5.5 suggests equal distances between intervals. That is, the distance between "agree" and "strongly agree" is the same as that between "disagree" and "strongly disagree." In studies using such rating scales many statements may be rated, and the specific ratings may be averaged across participants. One point to note about interval scales, however, is that there is no absolute zero point, although some scales have a relative zero point that is not the same as an absolute zero point. For example, an absolute zero point suggests an absence of the quality being measured; a zero on a bathroom scale means the absence of weight. On the other hand, a zero on a subtest of some aspect of personality such as aggression does not mean the absence of aggression. A zero on an IQ test does not mean a total absence of intelligence. Similarly, a person with an IQ of 120 is not twice as intelligent as another person with an IQ of 60. Data from interval scales can be analyzed with the same statistical methods used for ratio data, discussed next.

Ratio Data

The final step in levels of measurement, **Ratio data,** adds an absolute zero point. It embodies distinct groupings, ordered levels, equal distances between levels, and an absolute zero. As a result, the researcher using ratio data can compare points along the scale in absolute terms. For example, let us again discuss weight. We cannot study the concept of weight unless we can turn it into some quantifiable term that can be measured. Weight obviously has an absolute zero point that represents the absence of any weight placed on a scale. It is possible to assign a numeral to a series of participants by having them step on a digital scale that provides a number representing each person's weight. In this example, the construct of "weight" is defined by the numeral displayed on the digital scale. This also represents the "numeral" referred to earlier in this chapter in the definition of measurement. The "rule" for assigning numerals to participants would be having each person step on the scale and then assigning them whatever number appears on the digital readout. Unlike other levels of measurement, use of ratio scales allows us to conclude that a person who weighs

200 pounds is twice as heavy as one who weighs 100 pounds. We cannot do this with any other scale because they lack an absolute zero point. Figure 5.6 shows the statistical analyses that are typically used with interval and ratio data.

We have tried to make the point that one of the first steps scientists and consumers of research should take is to consider the level of measurement used in a particular study, mainly because the type of data used in an investigation directly affects the kinds of statistical procedures appropriate for analyzing the results of the study. As indicated in the definition of measurement at the beginning of this chapter, every investigation assigns numbers to phenomena of interest using some sort of rule-based process. Consumers of research should be interested not only in the types of numerals assigned but in the process used to assign them. We should think about what the numbers really represent, and this goes back to our previous discussion of validity and reliability. It is *always* possible to come up with numbers and to assign the numbers to objects and events we are studying, but numbers in and of themselves mean nothing. The devil, as they say, is in the details.

FIGURE 5.6

Frequently Used Statistical Methods with Interval or Ratio Data

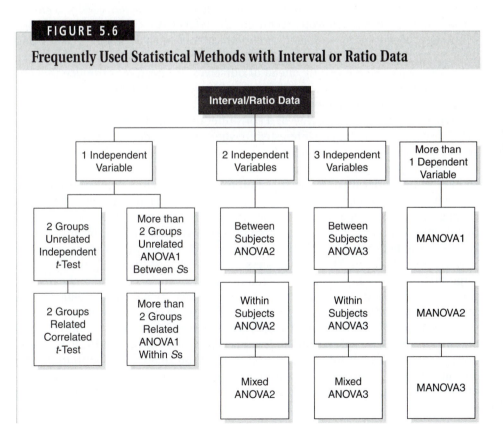

The Shape of the Distribution and Its Importance in Research

Nobody realizes that some people expend tremendous energy merely to be normal.
                                                            Albert Camus (1913–1960)

Normal is not something to aspire to, it's something to get away from.
                                                            Jodie Foster, actress

The perfect normal person is rare in our civilization.
                                            Karen Horney, American psychiatrist (1885–1952)

I don't care to belong to a club that accepts people like me as members.
                                                            Groucho Marx (1890–1977)

As evidenced by these quotes, the notion of "normality" in real life is controversial. Although many of us may strive to be perceived as normal, some people do all they can to escape this designation. In research, however, a **normal distribution** of scores in a research project is highly desirable and usually viewed as a thing of beauty. This is because the most powerful statistical methods are designed for use on data that are normally distributed. For example, a colleague of ours, Lawrence Molt, is known for saying "If you're skewed, you're screwed." He refers to the fact that abnormal distributions may not be appropriately analyzed with our most desirable statistics, and we are forced instead to choose among what some researchers feel are less-effective alternatives. But we are getting ahead of ourselves. We need to introduce this important concept clearly and carefully because the rest of the book depends on your understanding the information.

Whether you are a researcher or a consumer of research, one of the first pieces of information you should be interested in when you consider an experiment is the general performance of the groups of participants under study. By this we mean that the scores of participants will represent a particular range of performance, and the scores can be represented in a distribution based on their frequency of occurrence and actual value. In most studies, the quantity of numerical data generated by even small groups of participants will be so enormous that the researcher simply cannot make sense of it unless it is characterized by overall performance of the group. After all, the researcher probably embarked on the study in the first place to investigate the performance of groups. Thus, the process of reducing one's data to group trends is important just from the perspective of understanding what was found in the investigation. The distribution of scores is also important because it is a major determinant of the kinds of statistical methods the researcher can use in analyzing the data.

The shape of a distribution of scores is basically determined by examining two parameters: **measures of central tendency** and **measures of variability.** If you know both of these pieces of information, you can see the shape of a distribution. The plotting of central tendency measures has a lot to do with frequency of occurrence of individual numbers. When we look at a distribution, the height of the distribution on the "*Y* axis" depicts how many participants earned that score on the dependent variable. The "*X* axis" typically represents the actual score, as in a test score. Often, distributions are depicted using a bar graph or histogram. Thus, in Figure 5.7 you can see that fifty people earned a score of 50, forty people earned a score of 40, and so on. The higher the bar on the *Y* axis, the more participants earned a particular score on the *X* axis. The histogram in this figure mirrors the famous "normal distribution" in which most people earned a central score (50) and fewer people earned either high (90) or low (10) scores. This "bell-shaped" curve is traditionally associated with a normal distribution, in which most individuals earn scores in the center of the distribution and fewer participants earn extreme scores that are very high or very low. When large numbers of participants earn low scores, as in Figure 5.8, the distribution is **positively skewed.** If there are large numbers of participants earning high scores as shown in Figure 5.9, the distribution is **negatively skewed.** We will refine this definition in the next section after discussing the specifics of measures of central tendency.

Measures of Central Tendency

There are three measures of central tendency typically mentioned in research books. These measures ideally reflect the center point of a distribution of scores; however, as you will see some do it better than others.

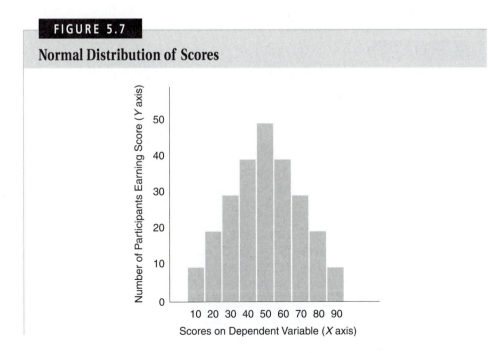

FIGURE 5.7

Normal Distribution of Scores

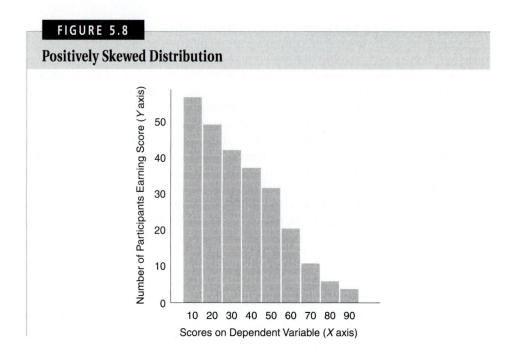

FIGURE 5.8

Positively Skewed Distribution

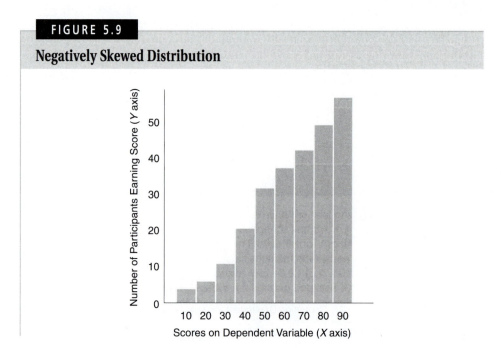

FIGURE 5.9

Negatively Skewed Distribution

The Mode

The **mode** is classically described as the most frequent score in a distribution. As a result, no confusing calculations are involved, just a process of finding which score occurs most often. For example, look at a data set from ten participants: 3, 4, 4, 5, 4, 10, 9, 1, 8, 2. The most frequently occurring score, and thus the mode, is 4. If we put these scores in numerical order (1, 2, 3, 4, 4, 4, 5, 8, 9, 10) one can see that the modal score of 4 is near the center of the distribution, sandwiched between three numbers on one side and four numbers on the other. So, in this example, the mode of 4 generally represents the "center" of the distribution. Unfortunately, the following distribution also has a mode of 4: 120, 300, 1023, 4, 10, 4, 2000, 4, 3000, 1500. If the mode is really the "center" of a distribution, it is certainly not shown when we order these numbers: 4, 4, 4, 10, 120, 300, 1023, 1500, 2000, 3000. If anything, 4 represents the lower end of the distribution and anything but the center. Yet if someone reported that the two groups of scores had the same mode, one might jump to the conclusion that the two distributions are identical or at least similar when in fact they are dramatically different from one another. One problem with the mode is that it does not take into account the other scores in the distribution. As in the previous examples, the mode can represent the center point of a distribution of scores, but it also can have very little to do with central tendency. This is one reason why we do not see the mode used much in research reports as a reliable measure of central tendency. Some distributions have two modes in which two numbers are tied for which is the most frequently occurring. Perhaps there are four 12s and four 20s in a distribution. In this case there are two modes and the distribution is bimodal.

The Median

The **median** represents the middlemost score in an ordered distribution. In research articles, it is sometimes represented by the abbreviation MDN. To determine the median of a distribution the researcher must place the scores in order from low to high or vice versa. The scores are then counted and the halfway point in the scores represents the median. Let us find the median in the following data set: 1, 3, 5, 7, 9, 9, 10, 12, 13. In this example we have nine ordered numbers in the data set and the halfway point is reached at the fifth number, which is 9. At this point, 50 percent of the data are above and 50 percent are below. This works conveniently when you have an odd number of scores. In cases where there are an even number of scores, some researchers take the two middle scores and average them to arrive at a median (Bordens & Abbott, 2002). There are more complicated methods of determining the median with even numbers, but the basic idea is to interpolate some value between the two middle numbers. Again, however, the median can be deceiving as a measure of central tendency. Take for example the following series of numbers: 1, 3, 5, 70, 80, 300, 500, 800, 1000. Although the median would be 80, it is easy to see that this value would not really represent the central tendency of the actual series of numbers. There are more large numbers than small numbers in this distribution, and the intervals between large numbers are much greater than between small numbers. Thus, although the median takes other numbers in the distribution into account, which is an improvement on the mode, some distortion is still possible.

The Mean

The **mean** is the arithmetic average of a numerical distribution.

$$\bar{X} = \frac{\Sigma X}{N}$$

The formula shows how the mean is calculated. Note first of all that the symbol for mean is an X with a bar over it. In articles that you read, the mean will usually be depicted as the $\bar{X}$ or sometimes an M. The Σ sign represents summation notation and simply means that you add up values. The X (without the bar) represents a score or number in a distribution. Finally, the N represents the total number of scores in the distribution. All of this mysterious mathematical coding simply translates as follows: To find the mean of a distribution you add up all the scores and divide by the total number of scores. It is easy to see that the mean, as a measure of central tendency, does the best job of taking into account the values of all scores in a distribution. It is not just looking for the most frequent score (mode) or the middlemost score (median) but is actually taking into account the individual values of the scores. That being said, the mean is also susceptible to considerable error. Look at these numbers: 1, 1, 2, 3, 5, 50. If you add these up, the total is 62. Then, as in the above formula, you divide by the number of scores (5). The mean for this distribution is 12.4. As you look at this distribution, it is easy to see that one of the scores is quite different from all the others. All of the scores were in single digits except for the 50, which is an example of a value called an **outlier,** meaning that it represents an unusually different score from the rest of the distribution. Outliers can be either abnormally high or abnormally low scores. The problem with outliers is that they affect the mean. For example, if you remove the 50 from the distribution and replaced it with a 5 (1, 1, 2, 3, 5, 5), which is more in tune with the other scores, the mean would only be 3.4 instead of 12.4. Outliers can either make the mean higher or lower depending on whether the score is abnormally high or low. Thus, you can see that the mean can be unduly influenced by outliers and may not really reflect the central tendency of the distribution. Nevertheless, the mean is the most common measure of central tendency used in research, and you will encounter it often as a research consumer or producer. Every study using groups should provide some measure of central tendency so that the performance of each group can be characterized and compared to other groups.

Relationships of Measures of Central Tendency in Normal and Abnormal Distributions

In the normal distribution depicted in Figure 5.7 you can see that there are some outliers scoring 10 and 90 but there are far more scores in the center of the distribution. If a distribution is normal, the mean, median and mode will all reflect fairly similar values in the center (Figure 5.10). When a distribution is either positively or negatively skewed as shown in Figures 5.8 and 5.9, the three measures of central tendency will no longer represent the same values. For example, in a positively skewed distribution such as Figure 5.11, the mean is higher than the median and mode. This suggests that the mean will be an overestimate of the true center of the distribution. Likewise, in

Relationships of Mean, Median, and Mode in a Normal Distribution

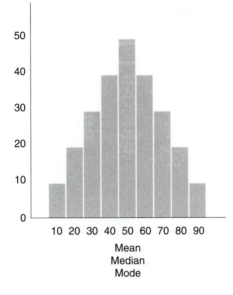

**Relationships of Mean, Median, and Mode in a Positively
Skewed Distribution**

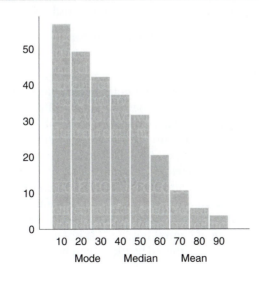

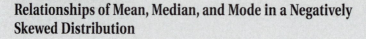

FIGURE 5.12

Relationships of Mean, Median, and Mode in a Negatively Skewed Distribution

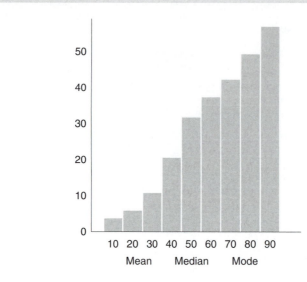

a negatively skewed distribution such as Figure 5.12, the mean is lower than the median and mode and underestimates the center point of the distribution. Thus, the use of the mean is ideal when distributions are fairly normal, but when they are skewed, some authorities suggest using the median instead (Bordens & Abbott, 2002).

Type of Data and Its Effect on Selection of Central Tendency Measures

Earlier we discussed the importance of level of measurement or type of data a researcher gathers in selecting statistical methods. Recall that a study can use nominal, ordinal, interval, or ratio data. These types of data all differ in terms of how scores relate to one another. In nominal data, categories are totally discrete, and we cannot even add up scores in any meaningful way. In ordinal data, scores are ordered, but there is no zero point or meaningful distance between scores. Only in the cases of interval and ratio data are scores related to some arbitrary or absolute zero point and have some equality in the distances between adjacent numbers. Table 5.1 depicts the effects of types of data on selection of central tendency measurements. Thus, although the mean is the central tendency measurement preferred by most researchers, the choice of a measure of central tendency is not an arbitrary one. It is largely determined by the type of data gathered by the researcher and the way those data are distributed.

TABLE 5.1		
Level of Measurement and Central Tendency Measures		
Level of Measurement	**Central Tendency Measure**	**Reason**
Nominal Data	Mode	Scores not meaningfully related on a scale (e.g., political party, gender)
Ordinal Data	Mode, Median	Distance between scores is unknown and the mean is sensitive to distances between scores.
Interval/Ratio Data	Mean, Median (if distribution is abnormal)	Scores have arbitrary or absolute zero point and equal distances between values.

Measures of Variability

As researchers or scientific consumers we need two basic pieces of information about groups studied in an investigation. One basic element is the measure of central tendency discussed above. The second piece of the puzzle is some measurement of variability or the spread of scores in the distribution. Together, these measures of central tendency and variability are known as **summary statistics** or *descriptive statistics*. It is critical for a researcher to report summary statistics so that consumers of research and other scientists can determine, among other things, if the correct statistical methods have been used.

The Range

A very general way of describing variability in a sample of scores is to report the **range** of values from low to high. For example, a researcher might say that "the group had a mean of 25 (range = 3–30)." This means that the lowest score was 3 and the highest was 30. Other researchers depict the range by using the formula of subtracting the lowest from the highest score. In the previous example the range would be 27. The range, by itself, is not particularly sensitive to how scores are distributed. Take for example the following distribution: 3, 22, 24, 25, 28, 30. The range of these scores, as in the previous illustration, is 3–30, but it is clear that most of the scores are toward the higher end of that continuum. It is also apparent that the range is unduly influenced by extreme scores (outliers) such as the 3. In actuality, the 3 was not a big player in this distribution, but the higher numbers certainly were. Most researchers that report ranges in their articles will also provide other, more meaningful, measures of variability.

The Variance

The **variance** is a measure that is usually not directly reported in the research literature. As we stated at the beginning, this book is not meant to be a text about statistical methods. There are many books that do a fine job of teaching students how to compute various statistical procedures. One of the most straightforward books on this topic is by Bruning and Kintz (1997). In the present text, however, we want students to have a conceptual understanding of what some of the statistics do, not necessarily how to compute them. In reality, the actual computation of statistics requires little more than adding, subtracting, multiplying, and dividing. The problem is that there is *lots* of adding, subtracting, multiplying, and dividing, so much that it is far easier to let computer programs handle calculations for you. They are faster with much less error, such as occurs with punching the wrong keys on a calculator. It is not until you get into very complicated algorithms involving multiple variables that the math gets to be a challenge. At any rate, you will not have to deal with it in this book. Below, you will see the formula for computing the variance in a group of scores. On the surface it may look daunting, but it is exactly as we said previously—just a bunch of adding, subtracting, multiplying, and dividing. The S^2 is a symbol many people use for variance, but as we said earlier, the variance is hardly ever directly reported in research articles. When we discussed the mean, we introduced the summation sign, so you should be familiar with that. The X represents an individual score, and the $\bar{X}$ represents the mean. So, the top of the formula just says that you take each score and subtract from it the mean, square the result, and add up the squared values. This quantity is divided by the total number of scores minus 1. That will give you the variance.

$$S^2 = \frac{\Sigma(X - \bar{X})^2}{N - 1}$$

For example:

Score (X)	$(X - \bar{X})$	$(X - \bar{X})^2$
1	2.57	6.60
3	0.57	0.32
5	1.43	2.04
2	1.57	2.46
7	3.43	11.67
6	2.43	5.83
1	2.57	6.60

Σ 25   35.61
$\bar{X}$ 25/7 = 3.57

$$S^2 = \frac{35.61}{6} = 5.93$$

Note that the mean of the seven numbers is 3.57. Look at what we did with the first score of 1. We took the mean and subtracted it from each of the scores (1 – 3.57 = 2.57, etc.) getting rid of any plus or minus signs. Then we squared these subtracted amounts (2.57 × 2.57 = 6.60, etc.). We added up the squared scores and got a total of 35.61. Finally we divided the total of the squared scores by $N - 1$ which is 6. Our variance is 5.93. Add, subtract, multiply, and divide. As mentioned above, the variance is not typically reported as a measurement of variability in research articles. The most commonly reported measure of variability is the standard deviation.

The Standard Deviation

The formula for computing the **standard deviation** (SD) is presented in the box below. If you are thinking that this formula looks familiar, you are absolutely correct. The only thing different about this formula from the one used to compute the variance is the square root symbol. That is right; the standard deviation is simply the square root of the variance. Another way to look at it is that the variance is the standard deviation squared.

$$SD = S = \sqrt{\frac{\Sigma(X - \bar{X})^2}{N-1}}$$

The standard deviation gives us a lot of information about the variability in a distribution. Figure 5.13 shows that in a normal distribution, variability is fairly predictable from a statistical perspective. For instance, the scores in the example distribution ranged from 50 to 150. For purposes of this illustration let us say that the mean is 100 and the standard deviation is 15. If the distribution is normal, 68 percent of the participants would earn scores between 85 and 115, which is plus or minus one standard deviation (15) from the mean of 100. Going two standard deviations above and below the mean you would find that 95 percent of the participants would earn scores between 70 and 130 in a normal distribution. If you go three standard deviations away from the mean you could account for the scoring of 99 percent of the participants in the group. Earlier we mentioned outliers in a distribution, generally considered to be those who scored more than two standard deviations above or below the mean and would representing about 5 percent of the group in the distribution.

Generally, the larger the standard deviation, the more variability in the group being investigated. The term used to refer to the general shape of a distribution near the mean is **kurtosis.** Groups with large standard deviations will typically have a low, wide curve called a **platykurtic** distribution. Groups with very small standard deviations will have a high, narrow curve called a **leptokurtic** distribution. A normal distribution, as in Figure 5.13, is known as **mesokurtic.**

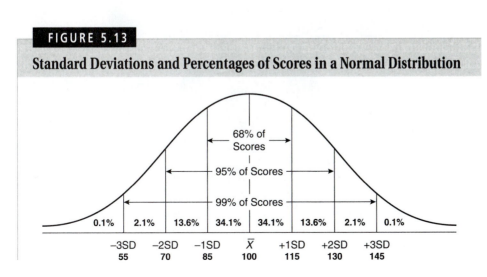

FIGURE 5.13

Standard Deviations and Percentages of Scores in a Normal Distribution

Assumptions of Parametric and Nonparametric Statistics

One common method of categorizing statistical methods is to distinguish between parametric and nonparametric procedures. **Parametric statistics** are inferential mathematical procedures ideally designed to analyze groups that have normal distributions. **Nonparametric statistics** are often called "distribution free" statistics and do not assume that data represent a normal distribution. One reason that we have spent some time talking about central tendency, variability, skewness, and kurtosis is that the shape of a distribution dictates to some extent the statistical method a researcher can use to analyze data. Figure 5.14 shows a researcher's arrival at a fork in the road. Presumably the researcher must decide which road to take in analyzing his or her data. We would like to take a moment to briefly discuss some of the critical variables that will help in the decision to turn right or left on this empirical expressway.

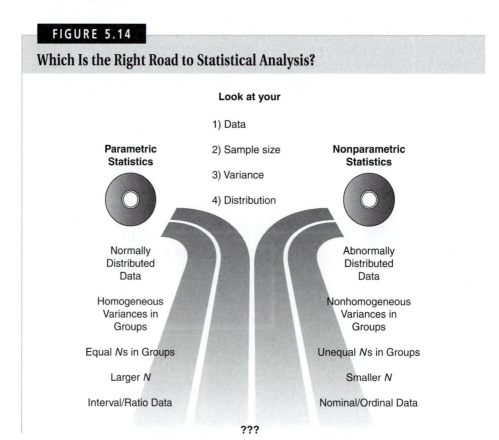

FIGURE 5.14

Which Is the Right Road to Statistical Analysis?

Look at your

1) Data

2) Sample size

3) Variance

4) Distribution

Parametric Statistics

Nonparametric Statistics

Normally Distributed Data	Abnormally Distributed Data
Homogeneous Variances in Groups	Nonhomogeneous Variances in Groups
Equal Ns in Groups	Unequal Ns in Groups
Larger N	Smaller N
Interval/Ratio Data	Nominal/Ordinal Data

???

Type of Data

We have already indicated that the level of measurement to a large degree dictates the choice of statistical methods. Generally, nonparametric statistics are used for nominal and ordinal data, and parametric statistics are used for interval and ratio data. One reason for this is that there are equal intervals and a zero point in interval or ratio data that are not present in nominal or ordinal data. Remember, we said earlier that a measurement such as the mean is not necessarily even appropriate for nominal or ordinal data, and the mean is one of the major determiners (along with the standard deviation) of a distribution. Thus, one may not even be able to have a "traditional" distribution when using nominal or ordinal data. This immediately eliminates parametric statistics from consideration because they require not only a distribution, but one that is fairly mesokurtic or normal.

Number of Participants

The number of participants or N of a group is another, perhaps indirect, determiner of what type of statistic can be used to analyze data. Long ago, Sir Ronald Fisher (1928) found that as the number of participants in a group increases, the distribution becomes more normal. Thus, if one has a small number of participants, there is an increased likelihood that the distribution of the group will not be a normal one. Researchers therefore tend to use nonparametric statistics when they have small numbers of participants, not only because parametric statistics work better with larger Ns but also because there is a good chance that a small group will be sporting an abnormal distribution. The issue of the size of a group also gets us into the issue of "statistical power" which we will talk about in a later chapter. Suffice it to say at this point that if you do not have enough participants, you may not be able to detect a significant difference between groups or lack thereof.

Normal Distribution

As mentioned in an earlier section, parametric statistics assume that groups to be analyzed exhibit a normal distribution. If a group deviates significantly from normality, many statisticians say that we should use nonparametric statistics, which do not assume a normal distribution. For reasons that we will discuss later, this is perhaps one of the most "violated" assumptions of parametric statistics. So far, the researcher has considered the type of data, the number of participants, and the type of distribution exhibited by the studied group in deciding whether to head down the parametric or the nonparametric avenue. There is one more consideration.

Homogeneity of Variance

We know that you are familiar with variance because we provided the formula and an example earlier in this chapter. The variance is the standard deviation squared and indicates how much variation occurs in the scores within a group. **Homogeneity of variance** implies that there is some similarity between groups in terms of variation. Another way to put it is to say that "similarity of variance" is an important variable in deciding whether to use parametric or nonparametric statistics. Let us look at two different groups. Group 1 has a mean of 50 and a standard deviation (SD) of 5. Group two has a mean of 70 and an SD of 20. Which group has the largest variance? First, to find the variance, you would have to square the SD. That means group 1 would have a variance of 25 and group 2 would have a variance of 400. Do we have homogeneity of variance? Probably not. The means are different by twenty points, but group 2 has much more variability than group 1. Actually, there are some specific tests that can help a researcher to determine if variances between groups are significantly different or not. Statistical procedures such as Bartlett's, Cochran's C, Levene's Test and Hartley's F-Maximum Test (Winer, 1971) can tell a researcher if variances are not homogeneous. If variances are grossly dissimilar, most researchers will elect to use nonparametric statistics, because the parametric statistics assume homogeneity of variance.

Differing Views of Assumptions

The previous sections have discussed the assumptions underlying the use of parametric statistics. One would think that knowledge of these assumptions would basically govern the selection of a statistical analysis technique. After all, who would want to use an inappropriate statistic for analyzing their data? Unfortunately, selection and use of parametric statistics is not always a simple issue, and there is disagreement among statisticians about when they can be used. It is beyond the scope of the present text to discuss all the nuances of the arguments among experts; however, the following quote from Kerlinger and Lee puts it in a nutshell:

> The problem of assumptions is difficult . . . Some statisticians . . . consider the violation of assumptions a serious matter. . . . Others believe that F- and t-test[s] . . . operate well even under assumption violations, provided the violations are not gross and multiple. (2000, p. 415)

Winer (1971), for example, found that even when within group variances differed by a ratio of 3:1, there was not significant bias to a parametric statistic called the analysis of variance. Most authorities suggest that, when possible, researchers should try to use parametric statistics (Kerlinger & Lee, 2000; Bordens & Abbott, 2002). There are two major reasons for this suggestion. First, parametric statistics are viewed by most statisticians as more powerful than nonparametric tests. Second, there are simply no nonparametric equivalents for some of the more complex parametric statistics that analyze multiple independent and dependent variables. Thus, our perspective is that most researchers should try to use parametric statistics even though there is some violation in the basic assumptions. However, if there are gross violations of multiple assumptions, nonparametric statistics should clearly be chosen.

Transforming Data

We have already said that parametric statistics are robust and can absorb some abuse in that they tend to perform correctly even though some basic assumptions have not been fully met. For example, researchers who have not grossly violated the assumptions of parametric statistics may find that they have distributions across their groups that lack homogeneity of variance. The researcher may decide to take advantage of the robustness of parametric statistics and run a parametric statistical analysis. On the other hand, the results of a test of homogeneity of variance (e.g., Levene's, Cochran's, Hartley's, Bartlett's) may show that the variances are significantly different, and a researcher may feel uncomfortable using a parametric statistic with such data. In such a case, one other option that some researchers select is to transform their data into a different metric or measurement scale to increase homogeneity of variance. Then they conduct the statistical analysis on the transformed data. Transforming data does not really change the relationships among the groups because most transformations simply add or subtract a constant to each score or take the square root or logarithm of each score. The effect of many **data transformations** is to make the means independent of the variances (Bland & Altman, 1996). This most often reduces the heterogeneity in variances, as in the following example:

	Group 1 Scores	Group 2 Scores	Group 1 Transformed Scores	Group 2 Transformed Scores
	1	12	1	3.46
	3	2	1.73	1.41
	5	9	2.23	3
	7	20	2.64	4.47
	2	15	1.41	3.87
Mean	3.6	11.6	1.80	3.24
SD	2.408	6.73	0.6495	1.158
S^2	12.96	45.29	0.4218	1.3409

This example shows the changes in variances when each score is subjected to a square root transformation (each score is changed to its square root). Notice that the variance of the untransformed scores of group 1 was 12.96 and the untransformed variance of group 2 was 45.29. Those variances are pretty far apart. When you look at the variances of the two groups after the square root transformation they are much closer (0.4218 versus 1.3409). Also, note that the means are in a similar relationship to one another in that group 1 is lower than group 2. Basically, this transformation keeps the numbers in the same basic relationship but reduces the differences in the variances by making the range of numbers smaller. Most researchers who transform data use the transformed version of the scores just in the statistical analysis and still report the untransformed means and standard deviations in their research report. On the surface, this may seem like "massaging" the data or something that smacks of scientific misconduct. Let us assure you that this is not the case and that data transformation is a fairly common procedure generally accepted by researchers. Bland and Altman state: "Some people ask whether the use of a transformation is cheating. There is no reason why the 'natural' scale should be the only, or indeed the best, way to present measurements" (1996, p. 770). It is beyond the scope of this chapter to go into the subtle aspects of data transformation, but you should know that the most commonly used transformations are square roots, logarithms, reciprocals, and arc sines (Ferguson, 1971). Researchers make decisions on the type of transformation they use based on the type of abnormality in their data (e.g., positive skews) or the types of scores they have to analyze. For example, the arc sine transformation is most often recommended for percentage or proportional data.

In upcoming chapters we will introduce you to various parametric and nonparametric methods of comparing groups to determine if there are significant differences. The information covered in the present chapter should give you a basis on which to build when considering these more complex procedures. It should be clear to you at this point, however, that the choice of a statistical procedure is intimately related to the type of data to be analyzed and how those data are distributed within and between groups. That is enough to know at this point.

Summary

The type of data that a researcher gathers and the normality of the distribution are significant determinants of which statistical analysis to use in answering the empirical question under study. Parametric statistics are best suited for interval or ratio data that are normally distributed with homogeneity of variance among the groups being studied. Nonparametric statistics are more appropriate for small numbers of participants, abnormal distributions, and differing variances. Researchers must always consider their summary statistics before selecting a statistical analysis and consumers of research must examine how data are distributed to determine whether the correct statistic was used.

LEARNING ACTIVITIES

1. Find three research articles and determine the dependent variable. Next, try to figure out what type of data the dependent variable represents (nominal, ordinal, etc.).

2. Find three research articles that compare groups. Look at their summary statistics to see if the standard deviations of the groups they are comparing suggest homogeneity of variance.

3. Roll some dice fifty times and record your results. Compute the mean and standard deviation. Draw a histogram of the results and see if the distribution is normal.

4. Find a study that uses one of the nonparametric statistics mentioned in the figures for nominal or ordinal data. What kind of data do they have in terms of level of measurement for their dependent variable.

5. Find a free program on the Internet that computes summary (descriptive) statistics and input the data from your dice rolling experiment. Do the answers agree?

CHAPTER 6

An Introduction to Hypothesis Testing with Inferential Statistics

Statistics are no substitute for judgment.

—Henry Clay, politician/lawyer (1777–1852)

Statistics is the art of lying by means of figures.

—Wilhelm Stekel, Austrian psychoanalyst (1868–1940)

There are three kinds of lies: lies, damned lies, and statistics.

—Benjamin Disraeli (1804–1881)

Statistics are like a bikini. What they reveal is suggestive, but what they conceal is vital.

—Aaron Levenstein (1911–1986)

This chapter presents the theoretical and practical bases for using statistics in research. Although the material is more technical than prior chapters, it is necessary to learn it if you are going to have a conceptual understanding of statistical reports typically seen in our field. We try to present the material in a straightforward manner without distorting too much the concepts we are discussing.

LEARNING OBJECTIVES

This chapter will enable readers to:

- Become familiar with the concepts of probability and confidence level.
- Understand the process of hypothesis testing and terms such as null hypothesis and alternative hypotheses.
- Understand how calculated values from a statistical procedure are compared to critical values from a table to determine statistical significance.

- Understand how decisions about rejection of the null hypothesis are made.
- Explain Type I and Type II errors and how to control for them.
- Understand statistical power and the results of a power analysis.
- Explain the difference between statistical and practical significance and the use of effect size measurements in determining this difference.

Probability and Level of Confidence

There are entire textbooks devoted to a discussion of probability; we will only discuss it briefly and superficially in the present chapter. It is, however, a critical concept that scientists consider in evaluating the results of an experiment. Analysis of probability tells the researcher if results are likely to be "real" or simply due to chance and sampling error. Scientists, like anyone else, want to have confidence that their findings are not merely a product of luck but instead reflect the effect of the independent variable on the dependent variable. So how does a researcher develop confidence in empirical findings?

First, let's discuss the notion of confidence in a nonstatistical way. We have all seen hallways constructed with floor tiles that are about one foot square. Imagine someone marking off with some red tape a three-foot section of tiles going wall to wall across the hallway. One day as you walk down the hall, you come to the red line and someone tells you that you cannot step on the three courses of tiles between the red pieces of tape. You decide to take a step back and simply jump over the three-foot section of tile. For most people, this is not a big jump. After all, it is approximately the length of three pieces of printer paper put lengthwise end to end. You have to think about it and position yourself well to make the jump, but it is easily accomplished. Most people would not be nervous about making this jump across the three tiles. After all, even if you miss, the consequence is nothing more than stepping on some forbidden tiles. Now picture if you will that the three-foot space between the tiles is not occupied by floor tiles but is rather a large chasm across the hallway that is over 500 feet deep and filled at the bottom with boiling lava. You peer into the crevice and know that if you fell into it you would certainly be dead. The red tape is still there and the distance to jump is only three feet, but the stakes are considerably higher. Most people would think long and hard about making such a jump. One slip on the tile or miscalculation in the jump could result in catastrophe. Many people would not even try to make the jump just because of the small probability of falling into the abyss.

We bring up this example to show how one's level of confidence influences making the jump. With no gaping chasm a person is fairly confident, but faced with the abyss there is a much lower level of confidence. Now picture a researcher faced with some numerical results. As an example, let's say that a researcher comes up with the finding that a group of males has a mean score on a vocabulary test of 88 and a group of females has a mean score of 95 on the same test. At first glance, it appears that females have better vocabulary scores than males. On reflection, the researcher might wonder if this difference occurred simply due to luck. After all, we know that the samples of males and females could have been selected in such a way that females scored higher due to chance or sampling error. The researcher in writing up the results in an article will be staking a professional reputation on saying that females have better vocabulary scores. When the researcher presents the results at a national conference, someone may call the results into question, resulting in embarrassment. Going public with these results is the scientific counterpart of looking into that lava-filled chasm; one's reputation is on the line. The researcher might wonder, "How much confidence do I have that these results are 'real' and not simply due to chance?" "If I did this study over again, would I come up with similar findings?" Ideally, researchers want the results to be due to their independent variable rather than chance. So they are very interested in the question. "What is the probability that these results are due to chance instead of my IV?"

In order to address this issue, statisticians have provided a mechanism to tell researchers the probability that their results might be due to chance so that they know how much confidence they should have in their findings. Later chapters will provide examples of the various statistical tests seen in the literature that address this issue. For now, however, let's go back to the tape in the hallway. If we told you that the probability was 80 times out of 100 that you might fall into the chasm, would you jump? Most people would say, "No way!" How about if we told you that the odds were 50 out of 100? Most folks would still not take the chance. Do the odds of falling 1 time out of 100 sound better? Would anyone take the challenge if we said that only 1 time out of 10,000 attempts you would fall into the crevice? We bet there would be a few takers. See, its all about your level of confidence. Remember, researchers are not searching for absolute certainty, so they might be perfectly happy poised on the edge of that chasm in the hallway if they knew they had only a 1 in 10,000 chance of falling, which represents a high level of confidence. Most scientists would feel that is about as close to a guarantee as you are going to get. Interestingly, the statistics used in hypothesis testing can give the researcher a pretty good idea of the probability that the results of an experiment were due to chance or likely due to the effects of the independent variable. These statistics describe the level of confidence a researcher can have in the results of an experiment. The next sections will briefly outline how this is done.

The Process of Hypothesis Testing

Our discussion of probability and confidence levels illustrated a question asked by every researcher who performs an experiment: "What is the probability that my results could be due to chance?" Another way to pose this question is "How much confidence can I have that my findings are not due to chance?" The answer to these questions comes from a process that has been around for decades. Kerlinger and Lee talk about the statistical aspects of this process as follows:

> Statistics can be reduced to one major purpose: to aid in inference making. . . . Statistics says, in effect, "The inference you have drawn is correct at such-and-such a level of significance. You may act as though your hypothesis were true, remembering that there is such-and-such a probability that it is untrue." (2000, p. 260)

When researchers talk about the process of hypothesis testing and making inferences from analyses of their data, there are several prototypical steps that are always discussed. The number of steps involved in this process varies depending on whether the author collapses various functions together in a single step or keeps each function separate. For example, Kerlinger & Lee (2000) discuss five steps involved in hypothesis testing while Huck (2004) discusses various scenarios of hypothesis testing that range from six to nine steps. The difference in the number of steps is because some authors combine several steps into one in their formulation of hypothesis testing. In all the formulations, however, the same major components are involved regardless of the number of steps illustrated by the author. We will go over each step in more detail below so that you can see the overall process.

In Figure 6.1 we use six steps in hypothesis testing and illustrate how the process would unfold when comparing two groups using a statistic called a *t*-test. Let us say that a researcher is interested in determining if children with conductive hearing loss have poorer metalinguistic skills than children with normal hearing. We will walk through the steps one by one and explain some important characteristics of each part in the hypothesis testing process.

State the Null and Alternative Hypotheses

The first step in hypothesis testing is to clearly state the null hypothesis and the **alternative hypotheses** related to the experiment. We briefly illustrated the concept of the null hypothesis in Chapter 2 and indicated that even when researchers do not make "formal" hypothesis statements, they are always implied. The null hypothesis is a numerical representation of the occurrence of a variable in a population. Sometimes this relationship is written like this: $H_0: \mu_1 = \mu_2$. The symbol μ stands for the mean of a large population. Remember in research we take a sample from this large population and the mean of our sample is depicted as X with a bar over it. In the null hypothesis statement above it indicates that the means of two large populations are equal. For example, children with conductive hearing loss (CHL) and children with normal hearing (NH) will have equal means on a particular variable of interest (e.g., metalinguistics). Some statisticians write the null hypothesis as $H_0: \mu_1 - \mu_2 = 0$, meaning again that there is no difference between population means. When a researcher makes a conjectural statement about how an experiment may turn out, it is called a substantive or alternative hypothesis. An example of a substantial or alternative hypothesis might be: Children with NH will have higher scores on a test of metalinguistics than children with CHL. This hypothesis must be tested against something for comparison, and this is where the null hypothesis comes in. For this question, the null hypothesis would say "$H_0:$ μ metalinguistic scores for children with CHL = μ metalinguistic scores for children with NH" *or* "μ metalinguistic scores for children with CHL – μ metalinguistic scores for children with NH = 0." The substantive or alternative hypothesis would be "$H_1:$ μ metalinguistic scores for children with NH > μ metalinguistic scores for children with CHL." Technically, there should be another substantive hypothesis which would state "$H_2:$ μ metalinguistic scores for children with NH < μ metalinguistic scores for children with CHL." The researcher's favorite hypothesis might be H_1 but it needs to be tested against H_0 before it can be supported. It is not typical for researchers to be pulling for the null hypothesis in their investigations.

Set the Alpha Level or Significance Level to Use in Evaluating Hypotheses

Bordens and Abbott say that part of hypothesis testing is determining if sample means represent the same population or different populations.

TABLE 6.1

Different Ways to Look at Statistical Significance

Probability Alpha Level	For Repeated Replications of Study, How Many Results Would Be Due to Chance?	How Much Confidence Can You Have That Results Are Due to the IV and Not to Chance? (as percentage)	Should You Reject the Null Hypothesis?	How Difficult Is It to Obtain Statistical Significance?	How Stringent is the Alpha Level?	How High is the Level of Confidence?
$p = .60$	$\frac{60}{100}$	40	Do not reject H_0	Easier to obtain a significant difference	Not stringent	Very low
$p = .30$	$\frac{30}{100}$	70	Do not reject H_0	↕	↕	↕
$p = .10$	$\frac{10}{100}$	90	Do not reject H_0			
$p = .05$	$\frac{5}{100}$	95	Reject H_0			
$p = .01$	$\frac{1}{100}$	99	Reject H_0			
$p = .001$	$\frac{1}{1000}$	99.90	Reject H_0			
$p = .0001$	$\frac{1}{10,000}$	99.99	Reject H_0	Difficult to obtain a significant difference	Very stringent	Very high

significant. Over the years most researchers have viewed the .05 alpha level as being the acceptable probability level for statistical significance in most studies and therefore any probability level less than .05 (e.g., .03, .01, .001, .0001) results in statistical significance. For a study that is preliminary or exploratory in nature some scientists might use the .10 alpha level as the cutoff for statistical significance, but this is rarely seen in most fields and most often viewed as only an indicator that the issue under study should be investigated more thoroughly. The higher alpha levels are set, the easier it becomes to obtain statistical significance. So if a researcher set the alpha level at .20, it is easier to get a statistically significant result than if it was set at .01. Researchers often refer to this as the **stringency of the alpha level.** That is, lower alpha levels are more "stringent" than higher alpha levels because it is usually more difficult to get a statistically significant result at .01 than it is at .10 (see column 6 of Table 6.1). In our study of metalinguistic ability in children with CHL and NH, we should probably set $p < .05$ as our alpha level, since that is a traditional and noncontroversial probability level for this type of research. Now that we have talked about how the researcher sets the alpha level as a benchmark for deciding whether or not to reject the null hypothesis, we need to explore some fundamentals in how the actual hypothesis testing process works.

Gather Data from a Research Sample

We stated earlier that hypotheses were concerned with a "population" that may be an idealized and essentially unmeasurable group whose mean is represented by the symbol μ. We could never measure *all* children with conductive hearing loss or *all* children with normal hearing. These are the populations we are trying to investigate, but testing them all is impossible. Thus, the researcher is in the position of having to take a "sample" of children with CHL and children with NH with the hope that they will adequately represent their respective populations. After analyzing the sample data the researcher can "infer" a relationship or difference in the population from looking at the performance of the samples. This is why statistical analyses are often referred to as inferential statistics. A good researcher will take much care in sampling a particular population so that the sample is a representative one. Procedures such as random sampling, matching, and controlling for participant variables such as geographical residence, ethnicity, race, intelligence, language ability, gender, age, and so on help to insure that the sample drawn for research will represent the population the scientist wants to investigate. Huck wisely says that "it is the quality of the sample (rather than its size) that makes statistical inference work" (2004, p. 119). So for our investigation of metalinguistic ability in children with CHL and NH, the researcher assembles a group of one hundred children, one group of fifty with conductive hearing loss and one group of fifty with normal hearing. Of course, we assume that the researcher has controlled for all threats to internal and external validity in designing the study and selecting participants as we discussed in Chapter 4. For this study the single independent variable is group (CHL versus NH). The dependent variable is the score on the Analysis of the Language of Learning (ALL), which is a test of metalinguistic ability (Blodgett & Cooper, 1987). The researcher, having gathered sample data and scored the ALL for the participants in both groups, will probably generate some summary statistics such as means and standard deviations (as discussed in Chapter 5) to see how the groups performed in relation to one another. After crunching the numbers, the researcher finds that the children with conductive hearing loss had a mean score of 75 on the ALL and the group of children with normal hearing had a mean score of 90 on the same test. The standard deviations were 5.3 for the CHL group and 4.9 for the NH group. The researcher's initial tendency is to start crowing about how children with NH are better at metalinguistics than children with CHL, but let's not be too hasty. First of all, it is altogether possible that the groups performed fifteen points apart simply due to chance or sampling error. Remember, error is ubiquitous in science. How is the researcher to know whether the fifteen-point difference in the sample reflects a true difference in the population being studied? Of course the researcher could simply *say* that one group scored higher than the other and it was not due to chance, but that is just an opinion. However, someone else might disagree and say that the difference was due to sampling error. So who is correct? There is a way that the researcher can prove beyond a reasonable doubt that the difference was real, which is where the statistics come into the process. By performing a relatively simple statistical analysis it is possible to determine the probability that the difference between groups was due to the independent variable (the hearing status of the groups). Further, the statistical analysis can tell us if the observed difference in the samples was due to chance and the likelihood that the groups really represented the same population in metalinguistic performance. To understand this more fully we must move on to the next stage in hypothesis testing.

Compute a Test Statistic on Sample Data to Obtain a Calculated Value

There are many test statistics that researchers use to determine whether or not to reject a null hypothesis. For example, some statistical tests evaluate differences between or among independent groups (*t*-test, analysis of variance, Mann-Whitney *U* test, etc.). In the study of metalinguistic ability in children with CHL and NH we have two independent groups that take a metalinguistic test; we want to compare the performance of these two groups. The groups are "independent" because they are made up of different children (you cannot be hearing impaired and have normal hearing at the same time). We listed many statistical tests in Chapter 5 when we talked about levels of measurement and how this relates to the types of statistics that could be used in analysis of data. If you look back at Figure 5.2 you will see that with nominal data, you can statistically compare two independent groups using the chi-square test. If you look back at Figure 5.4, you will see that with ordinal data, you can statistically compare two related groups using the Wilcoxon matched pairs signed ranks test. If you examine Figure 5.6, you will see that two independent groups can be compared using the independent *t*-test and more than two groups can be compared using the analysis of variance. A researcher interested in evaluating whether variables are related or correlated with one another can use test statistics that specialize in answering this question (e.g., Pearson product-moment correlation coefficient, Spearman rank order correlation). Later chapters will cover the major test statistics more thoroughly in terms of how to interpret them. For example, Chapter 7 includes a more detailed discussion of the *t*-test, which we know you are looking forward to. For now, however, we will focus on very general aspects of the *t*-test just to illustrate the process of hypothesis testing. In our metalinguistic study, we have placed the sample data into the statistical formula for the *t*-test, which outputs a statistic called the **calculated *t*** whose value is usually a number with two decimal places such as 2.81, 0.21, or 4.99. Obviously, "calculated" *t* is known by that name because the researcher *calculates* the *t* value by placing sample data into the statistical formula. Generally, the higher the *t* value, the more likely there is a significant difference between groups, but to know for certain, the researcher must compare the calculated value of *t* to what is called a "critical value of *t*." We will discuss the critical value of *t* in the following section; however for now, we will focus on how the calculated value of *t* is applied to our metalinguistic study. For purposes of illustration let's say that our calculated *t* value was 2.89. In order to know if this value is significant we must compare it to the critical value of *t*.

Compare Calculated Value of Test Statistic to the Critical Value to Determine Statistical Significance

Critical values of test statistics such as the *t*-test, analysis of variance, or correlation coefficients have historically been found in statistical tables. The researcher looks at a table of critical values with his or her calculated value in hand to determine if the calculated value exceeds the critical value. If it does, the difference between groups is "significant" or beyond chance. The **critical value** of a test statistic changes with the stringency of the alpha (probability) level set by the researcher and another factor called the degrees of freedom, which we will consider in a later chapter. For now, however, let us just consider the alpha level. For example, critical values for the *t* statistic change as seen in Box 6.2.

You can see that as the probability level becomes more stringent, the critical value becomes larger. This is important, because the calculated value of *t* must exceed the critical value of *t* for a particular alpha level to result in statistical significance. Thus, in Box 6.2 the calculated *t* value of 2.89 easily exceeds the critical values for the alpha levels of .50, .10, .05 and .01, but it does not exceed the critical value for .001. Therefore the difference between the two groups is significant at $p = .01$. This means that only one time out of one hundred would such a group difference between means be due to chance. This is a fairly high level of confidence that the sample data represent a difference in the populations studied, and the researcher will most likely infer that the populations are truly different. Contemporary researchers typically do not have to consult tables of critical values anymore because computer software programs that run test statistics usually print out the calculated value of the test statistic and the specific probability value as well. Thus, there is no real need to look up critical values since exact probability levels are provided in the analysis. This means that a researcher who has used the *t*-test might obtain computer output of a calculated *t* such as $t = 2.89$, $p = .01$. This means that the calculated value of *t* (2.89) is "significant" at the .01 level of confidence. As we stated earlier in our discussion of alpha levels, this

BOX 6.2

Appropriate Critical Values of t *for Different Alpha Levels at 98 Degrees of Freedom to Determine Statistical Significance of Calculated* t

Calculated t must exceed the critical value for statistical significance at a particular alpha level

Alpha Level	$p = .50$	$p = .10$	$p = .05$	$p = .01$	$p = .001$
Critical Value of t	.677	1.658	1.980	2.617	3.73

Calculated value of $t = 2.89$.

The calculated value of 2.89 exceeds the critical value of 2.61 at the $p = .01$ level so the difference between groups is significant at $p = .01$.

The calculated value of 2.89 does not exceed the critical value of 3.73 at the $p = .001$ level, so the difference between groups is not significant at $p = .001$.

suggests that the difference between means would be due to chance only one time out of one hundred.

Making a Decision about Hypotheses

The results of a test statistic (in this case, a t-test) indicate that this difference was statistically significant and that the p value is $p = .01$. This brings us to the fourth column in Table 6.1. In our earlier discussion of hypothesis testing we indicated that a researcher does statistical analyses on samples to determine whether or not to reject the null hypothesis. In cases where the probability level is less than .05 researchers typically reject the null hypothesis. If the null hypothesis is rejected it means that one of the alternative or substantive hypotheses has been accepted or that the difference observed in the sample means is highly likely to reflect a difference in the population means. Note that in Table 6.1 the null hypothesis is not rejected with alpha levels above $p = .05$. This means that the samples evaluated probably represent the same general population and are not significantly different. In our study of metalinguistics in children with and without hearing impairment mentioned previously you will recall that the hearing-impaired group earned a mean score of 75 and the normal hearing group scored 90 on the same test. If this difference on a t-test was significant at the .01 level, it means that once in one hundred times would the result be due to chance. It also means that the hearing-impaired group probably represents a different population with regard to metalinguistic ability as compared to the normal hearing group. In this case the researcher would reject the null hypothesis. Obviously, the closer the mean scores of the samples are to one another (e.g., 75 versus 80), the more likely it is that the difference will not be statistically significant and that the two groups really represent the same general population. In such a case the null hypothesis is not rejected.

We should also mention that there are two major ways in which alternative hypotheses are stated, and they carry statistical analysis implications. First, if a researcher predicts that the data will move in a particular direction, it is known as a directional hypothesis. This might be used by a company that makes an improvement on an already successful product. If the goal was to measure how much the improvement increased sales, the company might use a directional hypothesis stating that the improved product will result in increased sales, and they just want to determine how much the sales increase. In this case they might analyze these data from the **directional hypothesis** by only consider one of the "tails" of the null hypothesis distribution in their statistical analysis. This is known as a **one-tailed test.** A second way of considering an alternative hypothesis is from a nondirectional standpoint. In this case, the researchers do not make directional predictions as mentioned above but realize that the data could show movement suggesting an increase or decrease. It is simply unknown. As a result, the researcher may elect a **two-tailed test** that takes into consideration both tails of the null hypothesis distribution. As a research consumer you should know that it is highly unusual to find one-tailed tests of significance in the literature because such tests should be used only in cases where there is very strong logical or theoretical support for a directional hypothesis. As a result you will almost always see two-tailed tests of significance in the literature.

Errors in Hypothesis Testing

We wish that the process of hypothesis testing was as easy as we have illustrated, but there are some other issues to consider. Without going into too much detail on this topic, we must talk a bit about phenomena known as "Type I" and "Type II" errors. Almost every textbook on statistics illustrates Type I and Type II errors by introducing a table or figure that displays various decisions made about the null hypothesis. Figure 6.2 shows that a researcher can either reject the null hypothesis or fail to reject the null hypothesis. In reality the null hypothesis can be true or false, so there are two major types of errors a researcher can make. A **Type I error** is one in which the researcher concludes that there is a significant difference when in reality there is no significant difference. In our metalinguistic study, the researcher could commit a Type I error by saying that children with CHL and NH are significantly different in their metalinguistic ability when in fact they really represent the same population and are not different. You may have already thought of this, but the stringency of the alpha level set by the researcher can somewhat control the probability of committing a Type I error. That is, if the researcher sets the alpha level at $p = .01$, there is only one chance out of one hundred that the groups scored differently due to chance. On the other hand, if we set the alpha level at .20, our chances are twenty out of one hundred that any difference could be due to chance. So, the more stringent the alpha level, the less likely we would be to commit a Type I error.

It is important to mention here that inferential statistics are meant to be computed only once on a set of sample data; if you do a statistical analysis multiple times, you increase the probability of committing a Type I error somewhere in your calculations

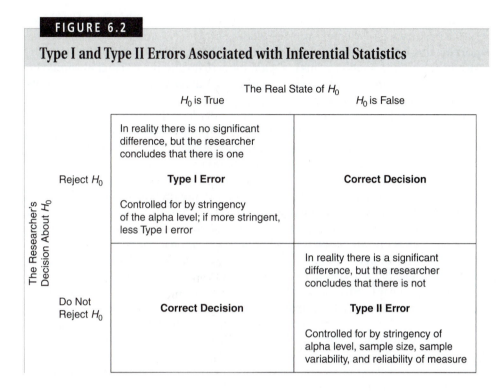

FIGURE 6.2

Type I and Type II Errors Associated with Inferential Statistics

The Real State of H_0

	H_0 is True	H_0 is False
Reject H_0	In reality there is no significant difference, but the researcher concludes that there is one **Type I Error** Controlled for by stringency of the alpha level; if more stringent, less Type I error	**Correct Decision**
Do Not Reject H_0	**Correct Decision**	In reality there is a significant difference, but the researcher concludes that there is not **Type II Error** Controlled for by stringency of alpha level, sample size, sample variability, and reliability of measure

The Researcher's Decision About H_0

(Huck, 2004). For example in our study of children with conductive hearing loss and normal hearing one *t*-test would be done on the scores from the ALL metalinguistic test. But lets say we are also interested in determining if these children differ in the mean length of utterance (MLU) calculated from a language sample and also their language complexity as measured by Developmental Sentence Analysis. Now we are up to three *t*-tests on these children and we have increased the risk of committing a Type I error. According to Huck:

> When researchers use the hypothesis testing procedure multiple times, an adjustment must be made somewhere in the process to account for the fact that at least one Type I error some-where in the set of results increases rapidly as the number of tests increases. Although there are different ways to effect such an adjustment, the most popular method is to change the level of significance used in conjunction with the statistical assessment of each H_0. (2004, p. 197)

One of the most popular methods of making this adjustment, the **Bonferroni proce-dure,** is to divide the alpha level you have set by the number of times the hypothesis is tested. So in our metalinguistic example, we have set an alpha level of $p < .05$ and we have done three *t*-tests: one for the score on the ALL, one for the MLU, and one for Developmental Sentence Analysis. Thus, we can make an adjustment to say that our new alpha level for significance is $p = .016$ (.05/3). You can see that the more times the hypothesis is tested, the more stringent the alpha level will become in order to prevent the occurrence of a Type I error. In reading articles, you might see a researcher report making the Bonferroni adjustment or the **Dunn-Sidak modification** to compensate for multiple analyses. This is a good thing to do and the researcher should be commended. Researchers who perform multiple analyses without such adjustments quickly get the attention of the research shark.

Type II errors involve the researcher coming to the conclusion that there is no significant difference when in fact there is a significant difference. In the metalinguistic study, we would commit a **Type II error** if we concluded that the children with CHL and NH were not significantly different with regard to metalinguistic ability when in fact they were different. Obviously, the alpha level is involved in committing Type II errors in that less stringent alpha levels would allow the researcher to detect significant differences if they are present. Unfortunately, raising the alpha level to detect a significant difference increases your probability of committing a Type I error. Thus, it is a balancing act in which the researcher must set alpha levels stringent enough to avoid a Type I error but not so stringent that a real difference could not be detected by the statistical testing. A researcher who set an alpha level of $p = .0001$ would no doubt miss some significant differences at the .001, .01, and .05 levels of significance. With Type II errors there are other variables that influence error occurrence. For example, sample size can affect the occurrence of Type II errors in that too small a sample may not have the statistical power to detect a significant difference. Doing a study with eight participants in each group might show no significant difference when one really exists, whereas if twenty participants in each group might allow a significant difference to be detected. But bigger is not always better as we will discuss later in this chapter when we discuss the difference between statistical and practical or clinical significance.

We mentioned above that Type II errors are influenced by variables that go beyond the alpha level. We will devote some time to generally explaining these variables because they are important in the interpretation of any statistical analysis.

Statistical Power

Bordens and Abbott state:

> You want your statistics to detect differences in your data that are inconsistent with the null hypothesis. The power of a statistical test is its ability to detect these differences. Put in statistical terms, power is a statistic's ability to correctly reject the null hypothesis. . . . A powerful statistic is more sensitive to differences in your data than a less powerful one. (2002, p. 408)

Batavia (2001) uses a metaphor of likening statistical power to entering a darkened room containing objects that you cannot see. By slowly turning a dimmer switch to gradually illuminate the room (increasing power), you begin to see the objects it contains. Thus, if you do not have enough statistical power it is possible that you will miss the discovery of a significant difference or significant relationship just as you would fail to see objects in a dimly lit room. Some researchers do an a priori **power analysis** to determine the sample size necessary to result in increased **statistical power.** Jacob Cohen (1983) wrote an entire book on power analysis and has developed formulas for determining if a study has adequate power to avoid committing a Type II error. Essentially, the power calculation includes variables such as amount of error variance, sample size, effect size, and the alpha level associated with the investigation. Other researchers (Gravetter & Wallnau, 2000; Keppel, 1982) have also discussed methods of determining the sample size of an investigation so that it has enough power to detect existing differences. Basically, the power analysis results in a number between 0 and 1 that reflects statistical power, with a result closer to 1.0 indicating more power in the statistical analysis and one closer to 0 indicating less power in the analysis. Thus, some researchers (e.g., Huck, 2004) suggest that a power analysis resulting in a value of .80 or more probably has sufficient power to detect significant findings. If a research article reports the results of a power analysis, the guideline of .80 is a general indicator that the study had enough power to avoid a Type II error and detect a significant difference. This means that you would have eighty chances out of one hundred of finding a significant result if it existed. It has probably occurred to you to ask "Why would a researcher do a study knowing it has inadequate power?" Actually, it is possible to determine the sample size required a priori by using a variety of available tables and computer programs that specialize in power analysis. However, many researchers do not perform preliminary power analyses, and it is only in the past few decades that post hoc estimates of power using Cohen's suggestions have begun to appear in the behavioral sciences literature. It has been noted for years that most research in the behavioral sciences has lacked adequate statistical power, specifically in the fields of psychology (Sedlmeier & Gigerenzer, 1989) and education (Deng, 2005). An examination of power analyses in the field of communication disorders has shown that as far back as thirty years ago it was noted that many research reports lacked appropriate statistical power (Kroll & Chase, 1975). Jones, Gebski, Onslow and Packman (2002) investigated statistical power in the area of stuttering research and determined that much of it was "underpowered." They state:

> A program of underpowered research is quite likely to replicate erroneous null findings. Underpowered research is a wasteful use of research resources that have little chance of detecting an effect. Further—in the social sciences at least—such research is unethical because it exposes human participants to inconvenience, discomfort, and/or risk without justifiable benefits. (p. 253)

Authors who want to avoid problems with statistical power can compute sample size requirements a priori to determine how many participants they will need to ensure that a Type II error will not be probable. There are many resources on the Internet that offer power analyses at little or no cost (Pezzullo, 2006; Buchner, Faul, & Erdfelder, 1996; Brown, 1993; Dupont & Plummer, 1990). Another strategy is to access large databases or collaborate with other researchers so that sample size will be adequate. Finally, it is important to note that in some areas it may not be possible to have enough statistical power. Researchers investigating unusual groups of participants simply may not be able to find enough of them to develop adequate power. The researcher, however, can at least acknowledge this fact in the research report.

As mentioned, one way of increasing statistical power is to increase the sample size in the experiment. It is possible that performing the study with more participants will allow the researcher to detect significant differences that are really present. Increasing the sample size too much, however, will allow the researcher to find significant differences that are statistically significant but unimportant on a practical level (Cohen, 1965). For instance, if we did a study using 10,000 participants and had them rate two different types of ice cream on a seven-point scale, the study might result in a significant difference between the two types of ice cream with one brand earning a mean rating of 5.3 and the other brand a mean rating of 5.7. It is altogether possible that the difference between these two means would be statistically significant even though the ratings are less than four-tenths of one rating point apart. Yet the researcher could say that one type of ice cream is "significantly" better than the other. However, in tasting the two desserts, it is possible that the 10,000 participants really did not find them to be different on a practical level, certainly not enough to decide to purchase one over the other. Perhaps, if we did this study with fifty participants, the difference would not have been statistically significant. The lesson here is that more is not always better. We need enough of a sample size to have adequate statistical power but not so many participants that we find statistically significant differences that are meaningless on a practical level.

Statistical and Practical Significance

One of the present authors recalls the following scenario taking place during his doctoral program:

> Frank came running down the hallway with a twenty-foot-long fanfold computer printout fluttering behind him. He was yelling, "I've got significance!" He brought the results of his dissertation into the graduate assistant's workroom and we all began to ponder the printout. Frank had found that there was a significant difference between two groups in terms of intelligence. One group (articulation disordered) had a mean of 102 and the other (normal articulation) had a mean of 110. The *t*-test showed that the difference between the groups was significant at $p < .01$, so the finding was beyond chance. If Frank had done the study over again one hundred times, ninety-nine of those times he would probably find the same basic result, that group B was higher than group A. After a long pause, one of the doctoral students asked the questions on everyone's mind: "I know you got significance, but do you really think that 8 points difference in IQ is *important*? What would a person with a 110 IQ be able to do that a person with a 102 could not do? How would these people appear to be different in real life? Aren't both of these IQ scores within normal limits and, in fact, above average? What is the clinical implication of this difference?" Unfortunately for Frank, these questions illustrated the painful difference between statistical and practical significance.

Typically, when a researcher finds a difference between groups, or a correlation between variables, he or she first asks whether the finding is statistically significant. The second step should be to then ask whether the difference is significant on a practical level. Failure to take this second step makes the interpretation of the research incomplete. Yet it has been the norm over the past fifty years to just report statistical significance and pay little or no attention to **practical significance.** One way to measure practical significance is by computing "effect size" (discussed in the following section). After reviewing ASHA research journals, Meline and Wang state:

> Inclusion of effect size in quantitative research reports increased from 5 reports with effect size in 1990 to 1994 to 120 reports in 1999–2003. Nonetheless, effect size was reported less than 30% of the time when inferential statistics were used, and only half of those reports included an interpretation of effect size. (2004, p. 202)

There is clearly a trend toward recognizing the importance of practical significance and it is especially important in conducting evidence-based practice. Our most prestigious journals now require investigators to report some measurement of effect size in their research articles. This is good for the researcher and especially good for the consumer of research. Now we will consider some measurements of effect size that you should look for as you read research articles. If the researcher only reports statistical significance and has no measurement of practical significance (effect size), research sharks become restless.

Effect Size and Practical Significance

One of the first notions that should occur to you is that the practical significance of a particular difference or correlation can be interpreted in many ways depending on the biases of the researcher, theoretical formulations, and practical issues. Lets take intelligence as an example. We know that IQ has a mean of 100 and a standard deviation of 15 in the general population. That is, the average person has an IQ of 100 and someone who is one standard deviation above the mean has an IQ of 115. A person who is two standard deviations above the mean has an IQ of 130. In the previous example Frank found a statistically significant difference between groups with IQs of 102 and 110 (8 points). Most people would not suggest that eight points worth of IQ would make a big difference in how these groups performed most tasks. But what if the difference had been thirty points? Would you think that a person two standard deviations above another person in intelligence could approach tasks differently? Although it is still a matter of opinion, many people would tend to think that thirty IQ points is a substantial enough difference to be "important." Most people would leave it up to the experts in psychology to actually make the judgment. This illustrates an important point. The practical importance of a difference is largely determined by looking at previous research, theory, and practical measurements conducted by experts in the particular field of research. Huck (2004) talks about two types of **effect size.** One type is shown by the researcher who, prior to conducting the study, actually specifies the differences between groups considered to be practically significant. In the previous example using IQ, the researcher might say that twenty points on an intelligence test would be "important" in terms of practical abilities. Of course, this is just the opinion of the researcher, but it should be based on a thorough review of related research, theory, and clinical practice. According to Huck this a priori determination of effect size is "a judgment call as to the dividing line between trivial and important findings" (2004, p. 201). The other type of effect size is actually computed from data gathered in an experiment. We will spend some time on these calculated effect sizes.

According to Meline & Wang, "Effect size is a metric that estimates the size of a treatment effect. Unlike tests of statistical significance, effect size metrics are unaffected by sample size" (2004, p. 204). There are many statistical measures of effect size (Kirk, 1996; Becker, 2000a) and the choice of metrics is somewhat dependent on the design of the experiment. Some effect size computations are for comparing two unrelated groups and some are for comparing two related groups. Other effect size computations are for use with the analysis of variance, and yet others are used with correlational data. Probably the most cited statistician with regard to effect size is Jacob Cohen (1983). Cohen developed a measurement for computing effect size between two independent groups called **Cohen's d.** Cohen's d is a relatively straight-forward computation that originally represented the difference between two means divided by the standard deviation of either group if the variances of both groups were homogeneous. Rosnow and Rosenthal (1996) and others recommend the use of "pooled" standard deviations which are arrived at by squaring the SDs, adding them, computing their average, and taking the square root of this value. Other methods of computing effect size use the information from the t-test to arrive at a value of d. **Hedge's g** is an effect size measurement that can be computed using information from the t-test or analysis of variance. Cohen's d can be used to compute Hedge's g, which shows that the two measures are intimately related. **Glass's delta** (Δ) is another effect size measure that uses the difference between means divided by the standard deviation of the control group in a study. Thus, there are many ways to compute effect size between groups and most of the differences tend to be in the denominator of the equation (pooled versus nonpooled, ANOVA data, t-test data, etc.). In many ways the effect size statistics mentioned above are highly related to one another and are merely different ways of looking at the magnitude of the mean differences. As mentioned earlier, Cohen's d appears to be the most popular and can be used to compute most other measurements of effect size so we will use it as our prime example.

The interpretation of Cohen's d can be considered in several ways. First, the d can be related to a distribution or to the two distributions being compared. Remember, we are comparing two means, and each one of them has a distribution associated with it. Table 6.2 depicts Cohen's d as it relates to other measurements. We will explain each relationship in the table. The first column contains Cohen's d, which was computed by taking the difference between group means and dividing them by the pooled standard deviations. The table only goes up to an effect size of 2.0, but you should be aware that effect sizes can exceed this number. Most textbooks only illustrate Cohen's d up to 2.0 because most research does not exceed this value. The second column tells us the number of standard deviations separating the two group means. Note that an effect size of 1.0 suggests that the two group means are separated by one standard deviation. Likewise an effect size of 2.0 means the groups are separated by two standard

TABLE 6.2

Relationships between Cohen's *d* Statistic, the Normal Distribution, and Pearson's *r*

Effect Size Using Cohen's *d*	Standard Deviations Separating Group Means	Percentage of Overlap of Group Distributions	Percent Chance of Predicting Group Membership from a Participant's Score	Pearson's *r*	r^2
2.0	2.0	19	84	.707	.500
1.8	1.8	23	82	.669	.448
1.6	1.6	27	79	.625	.390
1.4	1.4	32	76	.573	.329
1.2	1.2	38	73	.514	.265
1.0	1.0	45	69	.447	.200
0.8	0.8	53	66	.371	.138
0.6	0.6	62	62	.287	.083
0.4	0.4	73	58	.196	.038
0.2	0.2	85	54	.100	.010
0.0	0.0	100	50	.000	.000

Adapted from Becker, 2000a; Meline & Paradiso, 2003.

deviations. Figure 6.3 shows three distributions in different relationships. Think of distribution A as being one group and distribution B as being another group. Note that we have raised distribution A slightly so that you can see the SD lines of distribution B.

The top picture in Figure 6.3 shows that the two groups have identical means, their effect size is 0.0, and the two means are 0.0 standard deviations apart. If you look at the third column of Table 6.2, you can see that the two distributions overlap 100 percent. The middle picture in Figure 6.3 shows the mean for group A as one standard deviation higher than the mean for group B. The Cohen's *d* is 1.0 and the overlap of the distributions is 45 percent. In the bottom illustration, the Cohen's *d* is 2.0, suggesting that the mean for group A is two standard deviations above the mean for group B and these distributions overlap only 19 percent. Thus, you can see that the higher Cohen's *d* becomes, the greater the difference between the group means on the distribution and the less overlap there is in the two curves. The fourth column in Table 6.2 shows the chance of predicting group membership from a participant's score. Obviously, this would suggest that the farther apart the group means are, the more likely you would be to guess group membership. Note that at an effect size of 2.0, you have an 84 percent chance of correctly guessing a participant's group just from knowing his or her score. The fifth column of Table 6.2 requires a bit of explaining since we have not yet talked about specific statistical methods. Becker (2000a) illustrates how the effect size correlation can be computed with values from the *t*-test, analysis of variance, Cohen's *d,* or Hedge's *g.* When we interpret the Pearson *r* statistic, it is useful to square the value of *r* to arrive at r^2. The *r* squared is used to estimate the

FIGURE 6.3

Means of Two Group Distributions Illustrate Effect Size

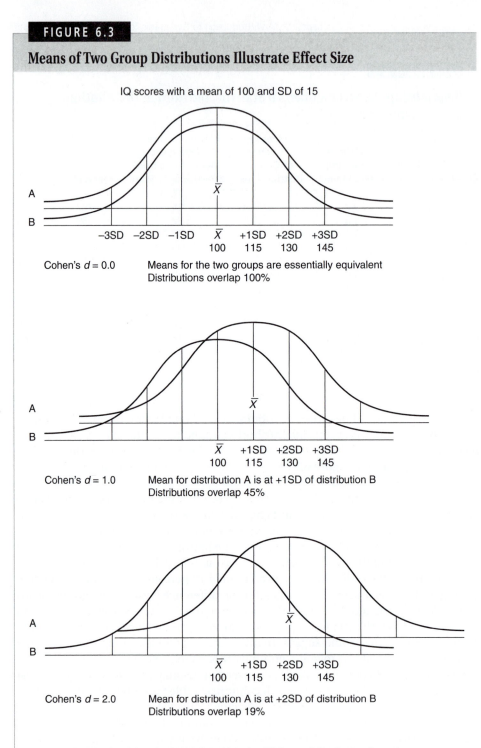

IQ scores with a mean of 100 and SD of 15

A

B

−3SD −2SD −1SD $\bar{X}$ +1SD +2SD +3SD
100   115   130   145

Cohen's d = 0.0   Means for the two groups are essentially equivalent
Distributions overlap 100%

A

B

$\bar{X}$ +1SD +2SD +3SD
100   115   130   145

Cohen's d = 1.0   Mean for distribution A is at +1SD of distribution B
Distributions overlap 45%

A

B

$\bar{X}$ +1SD +2SD +3SD
100   115   130   145

Cohen's d = 2.0   Mean for distribution A is at +2SD of distribution B
Distributions overlap 19%

Note: Distribution A is raised slightly so that the SD lines of distribution B can be seen.

amount of variance in the dependent variable that is accounted for by membership in the groups comprising the independent variable. Thus, with an effect size of 2.0, this translates into an r squared of .50, which suggests that 50 percent of the variance in the dependent variable can be accounted for by group membership. Obviously, this still leaves a lot of variation unaccounted for, but group membership is a big factor in accounting for test scores.

Of course, when Cohen developed his effect size measurements he knew that researchers would ask for an explanation of how to relate the d statistic to the size of an effect. Cohen knew that practical significance (effect size) should ultimately be based on an evaluation of specific research and theory in a particular field of study. Since the behavioral sciences are so diverse, it is probably not possible to "etch in stone" values of d that represent small, medium, and large effects, since these would change somewhat based on a specific area of investigation. But reluctantly, Cohen did suggest general standards of his d statistic for representing small ($d = .20$), medium ($d = .50$), and large ($d = .80$) effect sizes. We must always remember, however, that an effect size of .80 represents eight-tenths of one standard deviation difference. For some variables this may be practically significant, but for other variables it may require much more difference between means to be important on a clinical level. Thompson helps to put this into perspective:

> It should also be noted that Cohen (1988) provided rules of thumb for characterizing what effect sizes are small, medium, or large, as regards his impressions of the typicality of effects in the social sciences generally. However, he emphasized that the interpretation of effects requires the researcher to think more narrowly in terms of a specific area of inquiry. And the evaluation of effect sizes inherently requires an explicit researcher's personal value judgment regarding the practical or clinical importance of the effects. Finally, it must be emphasized that if we mindlessly invoke Cohen's rules of thumb, contrary to his strong admonitions, in place of the equally mindless consultation of p value cutoffs such as .05 and .01, we are merely electing to be thoughtless in a new metric. (2000, p. 3)

Earlier we stated that measures of effect size depend somewhat on the design of the experiment. So far, we have talked about comparing two independent groups and have said that we can use Cohen's d, Hedges g, Glass's delta, or account for variance using r squared. With correlated groups, or studies using repeated measures on the same participants, you still can use Cohen's d, but there is some controversy about using pooled standard deviations in the denominator. Becker (2000a) recommends using the original standard deviations instead of pooled values or data from t-tests or analyses of variance. There are many fine resources on the Internet that compute all of the above effect size measures if you input the means, standard deviations, and numbers of participants (Becker, 2000b; Lyons & Morris, 2007; Walker, 2006).

There are two other effect size measures often used in more complex experimental designs using the analysis of variance. We will not go into those designs here, but we will mention the effect size measurements that are recommended. One popular measure is eta squared which is symbolized as η^2 and it is interpreted as the proportion of variance in the dependent variable that can be attributed to the independent variable under investigation. Thus, if a research report states that there was a significant difference between three groups ($F = 9.67$; $\eta^2 = .40$). The eta squared is analogous to the r squared mentioned earlier and thus can be interpreted as the percentage of variance accounted for in the dependent variable by knowing about the independent or grouping variable. A final popular effect size measure for more complex group designs is omega squared which is symbolized by ω^2. This is interpreted similarly to eta squared in accounting for variance. Cohen recommends different criteria in the interpretation of effect size for eta and omega squared. Rather than the .20, .50, and .80 that were recommended for small, medium, and large effect sizes using Cohen's d, he recommends the following for eta and omega squared: small effect size is less than .06, medium effect size is .06 to .15, and large effect size is greater than .15.

The Null Hypothesis Revisited

You may not have noticed, but we were very careful in how we worded the decision-making process engaged in by the researcher when it comes to the null hypothesis. We stated that the researcher either rejects the null hypothesis in the case of a significant difference or fails to reject the null hypothesis when no significant difference is found in an analysis. Why do we not say "accept the null hypothesis" when we find no significant differences? Some researchers who find no significant differences between groups try to make the case that the groups are identical. That is, if we found no significance between CHL and NH children in our metalinguistic study, we might try to assert that the groups are actually the same in their metalinguistic ability. Why should we not try to do this? According to Kerlinger and Lee:

> Regardless of the results, it is only possible to "fail to reject" H_0 or "reject" H_0; one can never "accept" H_0. To "accept" H_0 would require repeating the study an infinite number of times, and getting exactly zero each time. . . . The status of H_0 is akin to the defendant in a trial who is deemed to be "innocent" until proved "guilty." If the trial results in a verdict of "not guilty," this does not mean the defendant is "innocent." (2000, p. 281)

Studies are designed to evaluate the alternative hypothesis against the standard of a null hypothesis; they are not designed to prove the null hypothesis. Thus, it is very difficult to prove lack of a difference just because a researcher fails to obtain statistical significance.

There are some other reasons that we cannot conclude that there is absolutely no difference between groups when we do not find a significant difference statistically. Remember when we were talking about statistical power, determined in part by effect size, alpha level, and sample size? We indicated that if the power in a study was not sufficient, the researcher may not be able to detect a significant difference in the sample data. In such a case a researcher would not reject the null hypothesis, but it would be inappropriate to conclude that the groups were identical. In fact, in this instance the groups could have really been significantly different, but the researcher simply did not detect the difference.

Huck (2004) brings up the issue of the reliability of the test instrument in finding differences between groups. In some studies a researcher who uses a dependent variable that does not have high reliability may find that groups are not significantly different. If the researcher had used a more reliable test instrument, he or she may have actually found a significant difference. Thus, if you read an article that finds no significant differences between groups it is important to examine the reliability of the measurement that was used to compare the groups before suggesting that the two groups are identical.

A final reason that it is difficult to conclude that lack of statistical significance is tantamount to two groups being equal has to do with alpha levels. You will recall that $p < .05$ is a common alpha level set for statistical significance. You should also remember that this alpha level is arbitrary, even though it has a tradition of being accepted by researchers as the "cutoff" for statistical significance. But think about it. Can you really say that a researcher who finds $p = .06$ is not looking at a possible difference that may be important? How about $p = .07$? Some researchers try to finesse their findings by saying that their results "approached significance" even though they did not attain a significant difference in relation to the alpha level they had set before the study. There is certainly some truth to the idea that a difference that was not significant at $p = .06$ is probably not the same as a difference that was not significant at $p = .90$. The point here is that a researcher cannot conclude that groups are "identical" or have "no difference" just because an alpha level less than .05 was not attained. There may, in fact, be a difference there if it were measured differently with perhaps a larger group of participants. Hypothesis testing is more about accepting the alternative hypothesis than about saying that groups are identical because we accept the null hypothesis.

In this chapter we have endeavored to communicate the process of hypothesis testing to consumers of research in communication disorders. It is important for you to be aware of how researchers try to infer the answers to questions by evaluating the results of statistical analyses. It is also important to realize that the whole process of using inferential statistics is based on the quality of the sample, the statistical power of the study, controlling for Type I and Type II errors, and determining the practical significance of findings through a consideration of effect size measures. Subsequent chapters will go into a bit more detail on commonly used statistical methods in communication disorders.

Summary

Researchers want to know that the results of their experiments did not occur simply by chance and sampling error. Quantitative methods have been developed for calculating the probability that results of a study were due to chance or a finding in which we can have confidence. In this chapter we discussed the process by which researchers make this determination by testing hypotheses. Since there is the possibility of error in scientific experiments the occurrence of Type I and Type II errors is always a consideration for researchers and consumers of research. Similarly, we should all be aware that an investigation must have adequate power to detect relevant findings. Researchers and consumers must always consider the difference between statistical and practical significance by looking at measures of effect size in published research.

LEARNING ACTIVITIES

1. Choose three research articles from the past five years and look for any mention of power analysis in these articles. What did you find?

2. Choose three research articles from the past five years and look for any mention of effect size in these articles. What did you find?

3. Find three articles that compare groups of participants and do not mention effect size. Examine the means of the groups to see how different they actually are. In the discussion section, does the researcher try to make the case that an actually small difference in reality is important because it is statistically significant?

4. Use the websites mentioned in this chapter for power analysis or run an Internet search using "power analysis" as a search phrase and determine how many participants you would need to conduct a hypothetical study.

CHAPTER 7

Common Statistical Analyses for Finding Differences among Two or More Groups or Conditions on One Independent Variable

Statistical thinking will one day be as necessary a qualification for efficient citizenship as the ability to read and write.

—H. G. Wells (1866–1946)

Do not put faith in what statistics say until you have carefully considered what they do not say.

—William W. Watt

A judicious man uses statistics not to get knowledge, but to save himself from having ignorance foisted upon him.

—Thomas Carlyle (1795–1881)

While a man is an insoluble puzzle, in the aggregate he becomes a mathematical certainty. You can, for example, never foretell what any one man will do, but you can say with precision what an average number will be up to. Individuals vary, but percentages remain constant. So says the statistician.

—Sir Arthur Conan Doyle (1859–1930)

One common theme of this chapter is a focus on statistics that allow us to find significant differences between two groups or among more than two groups. This focus will be restricted to studies having one independent variable (factor). Chapter 8 will cover analyses that help us to evaluate experimental designs with more than one independent variable. The first half of the chapter deals with between subjects designs and statistics and the second half covers within subjects designs and statistics. Finally, most of the chapter illustrates only univariate statistical methods. **Univariate statistics** are used to study only one dependent variable, such as reaction time, anxiety, or speech discrimination score. Univariate statistics can examine only one dependent variable at a time. At the end of the chapter we introduce you to **multivariate statistics,** which can examine more than one dependent variable simultaneously in an analysis. But, let's not get ahead of ourselves. We should start at the beginning.

LEARNING OBJECTIVES

This chapter will enable readers to:

- Understand the conceptual aspects of statistical analysis.
- Understand the use and output of the independent *t*-test, ANOVA1, and various parametric techniques to determine significant differences on one independent variable in between subjects designs.

- Understand the use and output of the correlated *t*-test, ANOVA1, and various parametric techniques to determine significant differences on one independent variable in within subjects designs.
- Understand how the MANOVA differs from the ANOVA.

Conceptual and Mechanical Aspects of Statistical Analysis

The present author recalls his study of statistics in graduate school. First, many theoretical and mechanical aspects were discussed in classes, followed by more detailed examinations of many different statistical procedures, most of which were designed to measure differences and correlations between height and weight, income levels, achievement test scores, or some other variables not really related to the study of communication disorders. We had to learn how to compute a statistical test, such as the t-test, to determine, for example, whether males and females differed significantly on their IQ scores. Learning the formulas and mathematical gymnastics associated with analyses of variance, regression, Mann-Whitney U tests, Pearson product-moment correlations, and many others is certainly possible if you are study hard and have a good memory. The problem, however, is that this type of information is not like fine wine; it does not improve with time. Soon, all those formulas you learned so diligently to pass tests in statistics courses will all run together, ultimately turn into electricity, and pass through the top of your cranium, disappearing into the ether. It is like the old adage: use it or lose it. To this day, the present authors still have to go back to textbooks or notes and relearn a statistical analysis that we have not actually used in research for a period of years. It is not uncommon for faculty members at almost every university to routinely rely on each other for help or use statistical consultants for advice on quantitative methods. It is important to emphasize that such faculty members do not have poor memories and are not simply dim bulbs in the academic chandelier. It is just that specific methods of statistical analysis are not something that one can remember for a long period of time unless one teaches the information or uses it repeatedly in research. Of course, there may be a small group of people who find themselves thinking about the mechanical details of statistical analysis even though they do not teach such material or do research. Such people are probably on their own unique cosmic frequency and are best left alone.

It was stated in the preface to this book that we would be taking a "conceptual approach" to discussing statistics. Some of you might have wondered, "What exactly is a conceptual approach to talking about statistics?" We would like to spend a bit of time discussing this issue. First of all, when we decided to write this text, we did not want it to be another in the legion of books on statistical methods. There are literally hundreds of books and software programs that teach students how to compute various statistical tests (Harris, 1998; Hopkins, 1996; Howell, 1995, Winer, Brown, & Michels, 1991; Box, Hunter, & Hunter, 1978; Dixon & Massey, 1983; Glass & Hopkins, 1996; Hays, 1988; Kachigan, 1986). They are loaded with formulas, dropdown menus, spreadsheets, and arcane symbols that most students find intimidating or, at best, uninteresting. Obviously, there is a place for such books for those who want to understand all the details of crunching numbers. It is especially necessary to study such textbooks if you will be expected to produce research as part of your job. However, when the audience is largely made up of research consumers such as students and practitioners in audiology or speech-language pathology, it is not necessary to focus on the mathematical aspects of statistics. Such things can be learned, but will soon be forgotten. It is much more important for consumers of research to understand what statistics do, when they are appropriately used, and what the statistical output means in the results section of an article or professional presentation.

Let's use a medical analogy. Most people know that it is important to measure blood cholesterol levels, especially as a person becomes older. Some of the specific numbers that we are interested in are the levels of "good" cholesterol, the levels of "bad" cholesterol, and the total cholesterol levels. Although we do not know the details of how these lab tests are performed, we can look at the output with our doctor and determine if we have healthy cholesterol levels and if we need to make changes in our diet or lifestyle. These numbers represent a *conceptual* understanding of blood cholesterol and allow us to determine along with our physician if we need to address a potential health problem. You can see that the physician orders the tests done by a lab technician who follows a consistent procedure in obtaining blood, subjecting it to various analyses requested by the doctor. Certainly the doctor could learn how the lab tests are done and perform them personally, but physicians seem to be satisfied with a conceptual understanding of the laboratory results. The doctor has never seen your blood or analyzed it but has a pretty good idea about your cholesterol situation just by requesting the appropriate tests and examining their output. The most important aspects for physicians and patients are conceptual. What kinds of tests should be done to answer questions about my cholesterol? What do the numbers generated by the lab test mean? What are the implications for any changes in diet or lifestyle?

It is a similar issue with statistics. We do not need to dwell on the formulas for computing various statistical measurements when, for consumers, the most important questions are conceptual in nature, such as: What kind of statistic will answer the research question? What do the numbers mean that are reported in the research results? What are the clinical implications of the research findings? Figure 7.1 illustrates some selected conceptual and mechanical aspects of statistical analysis. The box on the left is concerned with conceptual aspects of selecting a statistical analysis procedure. One of the first considerations in selecting an analysis procedure is to return to the research question asked by the investigator. As we indicated in Chapter 3, scientists spend a good amount of effort in crafting an answerable research question. The question may be "Do people with severe stuttering and people with mild stuttering differ in their general level of anxiety as measured by galvanic skin response?" The research question implies that the analysis method selected be appropriate for determining significant differences between two groups. On the other hand, if the research question was "Is there a significant relationship between stuttering severity and anxiety as measured with galvanic skin response?" then another type of statistic focusing on relationships such as a correlation would be appropriate. Thus, the research question to a large degree dictates the general type of statistical analysis to be used in an investigation. Another consideration that we raised in Chapter 5 dealt with levels of measurement. We made the case that different types of data (nominal, ordinal, interval, ratio) carried with them implications for statistical analysis. Thus, if

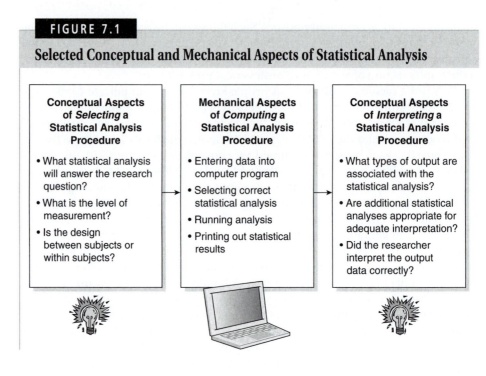

FIGURE 7.1

Selected Conceptual and Mechanical Aspects of Statistical Analysis

Conceptual Aspects of *Selecting* a Statistical Analysis Procedure	**Mechanical Aspects of *Computing* a Statistical Analysis Procedure**	**Conceptual Aspects of *Interpreting* a Statistical Analysis Procedure**
• What statistical analysis will answer the research question? • What is the level of measurement? • Is the design between subjects or within subjects?	• Entering data into computer program • Selecting correct statistical analysis • Running analysis • Printing out statistical results	• What types of output are associated with the statistical analysis? • Are additional statistical analyses appropriate for adequate interpretation? • Did the researcher interpret the output data correctly?

one used interval or ratio data and wanted to compare two independent groups, an independent *t*-test would be the statistic of choice. On the other hand, if one used ordinal data and was comparing two independent groups perhaps a Mann-Whitney *U* test would be more appropriate.

A third general consideration in selecting a statistical analysis is whether the design of the experiment is within subjects or between subjects. Statistics are computed in slightly different manners depending on whether participants are sampled only one time (between subjects) or are sampled multiple times (within subjects). Thus, we have two types of *t*-tests, one to be used in between subjects designs (independent *t*-test) and one to be used in within subjects designs (correlated *t*-test). The three variables mentioned (research question, level of measurement, between or within subjects design) are major determinants of which statistical analysis to select in an experiment. There may be some other more subtle factors in decision making depending on an individual type of investigation, but we will only consider the major factors here.

In the center block of Figure 7.1 we illustrate the mechanical aspects of computing a statistical analysis. The first aspect of performing an analysis is to input the data from each participant into a computer program. Depending on the software program used, the researcher will be required to input data into a spreadsheet or provide individual scores when prompted by the program. Data may be entered and organized in different ways depending on the statistical analysis performed. Obviously, it is important for the researcher to double-check the data entered so that typographical errors do not affect the results. When the data are entered the researcher must then select the correct statistical analysis, typically from a menu of options. For example, the menu may provide choices from a wide variety of statistical methods (e.g., independent *t*-test, correlated *t*-test, analysis of variance, etc.). The investigator must select the correct analysis for the research question, level of measurement, and between/within subjects design of the study. It is possible to make a grave error just by selecting the wrong analysis from the software program. For instance, let's say the investigator enters the data on the spreadsheet for a between subjects experiment and wants to compare two groups. If the researcher selects correlated *t*-test instead of independent *t*-test the analysis will still run and results will be printed. The problem, however, is that the analysis is wrong and may indicate a significant difference when there really is no difference between the groups. A careful investigator will examine every possible source of error in conducting statistical analysis. The good thing about computer-based analyses is that mathematical errors due to mistakes in adding, subtracting, multiplying, and dividing should not occur as in doing analyses by hand. Errors, however, can still occur in entering data and in the selection of a statistical analysis. When the researcher enters the data and selects the appropriate statistical analysis, he or she simply clicks an onscreen button and the statistical analysis is typically completed in a few seconds. For those of us who had the experience of spending hours computing these analyses by hand, seeing such rapid results is still a source of amazement.

The final block in Figure 7.1 concerns the conceptual aspects of interpreting a statistical analysis procedure. First of all, a consumer of research must know what kinds of output are associated with a statistical analysis. For example, reading a research report of a study that used an independent *t*-test, the reader should expect to see the calculated *t* value from a *t*-test with degrees of freedom and the probability value. Similarly, if the study used a correlation coefficient, the consumer should expect to see the Pearson *r* value, a plus or minus sign indicating the direction of the relationship, and a probability value. We will be talking specifically about such matters as we discuss individual statistical methods, but the point is that consumers of research should know what kinds of information to expect in the results section of a research report. A second aspect of interpreting a statistical analysis is to ask whether additional types of analyses are required in order to make sense of the results. In Chapter 6 we discussed the importance of statistical power and effect sizes to help determine the likelihood of committing a Type II error and to assess the practical significance of a result. Thus, in the *t*-test example above, we might expect the researcher to address the issue of statistical power with some sort of coefficient (e.g.,.80) and to report effect size using Cohen's *d* or some other measure. All the pieces of the puzzle need to be provided before a consumer or producer of research can interpret the results of an investigation. A final aspect of interpreting a statistical analysis procedure is to determine if the researcher "went beyond" the data analysis in discussing the results. As an example, a researcher finds a significant difference between two groups on a *t*-test. The Cohen's *d* statistic reveals that the effect size was small, yet the researcher expounds in the discussion section of the article about the importance and clinical implications of the statistically significant difference. This is one way that a researcher can go beyond the statistical analysis. Perhaps it would have been more appropriate to say that although the groups were statistically different, the practical significance suggests that the difference may not be clinically important. Another example of going beyond one's data involves extrapolating the results of a study to groups that were never investigated. For instance, a researcher may find that normally developing children produce longer utterances when participating in conversation than in a language sample elicited through picture description. Even though a statistical analysis may show a significant difference between conversational and picture sample elicitation in normally developing children, the researcher would be going beyond the data to suggest that this same difference would be found in children with language impairment. Consumers of research must know the types of output associated with commonly used statistical analyses, additional analyses that may be appropriate, and how the results can be reasonably interpreted. In the next few chapters we will discuss the more commonly encountered statistical analyses and highlight the conceptual aspects of the issues portrayed in Figure 7.1.

A Review of Basic Experimental Designs

The first part of the present chapter is concerned with studies that compare two or more different groups on one independent variable. If we returned to the notation and terminology introduced in Chapter 4, the studies in the first part of the present chapter would be "between subjects" investigations in which each participant would experience only one level of the IV. Just to refresh your memory, this study appears in Figure 7.2. Note there is no arrow between the cells so we know there are twenty different participants in each group (between subjects). The IV is "group," which has two levels (normal speaking/mild articulation disorder). This means that the normal speakers do not experience being articulation disordered and vice versa. The

---

FIGURE 7.2

Between Subjects Study with Two Groups

	Normal speaking five year olds	Five year olds with mild articulation disorders
$N = 40$ $n = 20$	20	20

DV = Number of /puh/ syllables produced in a ten-second speech motor task
IV = Group (Normal speaking/Mild articulation disorder)

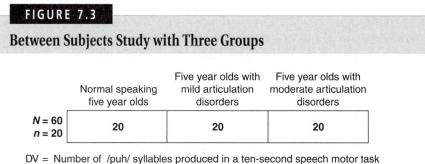

FIGURE 7.3

Between Subjects Study with Three Groups

	Normal speaking five year olds	Five year olds with mild articulation disorders	Five year olds with moderate articulation disorders
N = 60 n = 20	20	20	20

DV = Number of /puh/ syllables produced in a ten-second speech motor task
IV = Group (Normal speaking/Mild articulation disorder/Moderate articulation disorder)

investigator wants to determine if children with mild articulation disorders differ from normals in the number of times they can produce the syllable /puh/ in a ten-second period (dependent variable). Probably the researcher's favored hypothesis is that the group with articulation disorders will be slower than the normal speaking group in producing the syllables. As we said in the last chapter, however, the researcher must compare the result against the null hypothesis to determine if any difference exists between the groups. So this study shows one example of an investigation that compares two different groups on one IV. The researcher could also qualify the study for inclusion in this chapter by investigating the problem as in Figure 7.3, which simply adds another group or "level" to the IV. Remember, the chapter title said we are considering studies that compare *two or more* groups on one IV. The researcher could also do the investigation as in Figure 7.4.

The researcher could keep adding groups (within reason) and the study would still only have one independent variable. The only thing that would change would be the *number of levels* of the IV. In this chapter, however, we are going to use the three

FIGURE 7.4

Between Subjects Study with Four Groups

	Normal speaking five year olds	Five year olds with mild articulation disorders	Five year olds with moderate articulation disorders	Five year olds with severe articulation disorders
N = 80 n = 20	20	20	20	20

DV = Number of /puh/ syllables produced in a ten-second speech motor task
IV = Group (Normal speaking/Mild articulation disorder/Moderate articulation disorder/ Severe articulation disorder)

studies mentioned to introduce the notion of comparing different groups in a research project. For the design with only two groups, we will use the *t*-test and for the designs having more than two groups we will introduce the analysis of variance (ANOVA). We will also discuss some nonparametric statistical methods that can be used for comparing different groups in research when nominal or ordinal data are used.

Putting in the Summary Statistics

In Chapter 5 we indicated that one of the first things a researcher does after gathering and analyzing data is to combine the scores of participants in each group using summary statistics (e.g., means and standard deviations). Let us go back to the study of the two groups mentioned at the beginning of the chapter. When you look at that study as illustrated in Figure 7.2, you know certain specific information. For example, you know how many participants are in each group, the total number of participants, the identity of each group (normal/articulation disordered), the independent variable, and the dependent variable. Nothing in Figure 7.2 tells you how the groups performed on the syllable production task. Let us add some summary statistics in Figure 7.5.

The means tell us that the twenty normal speaking children had an average of forty/puh/ syllables in a ten-second period, whereas the twenty children with mild articulation disorders averaged thirty-five. The standard deviations are fairly close, so we probably have homogeneity of variance. Why do we care about homogeneity of variance again? We care because homogeneity of variance is a basic assumption for using parametric statistics. In this case the standard deviations are only one number apart. Now another question about level of measurement: What kind of data do syllable repetitions represent? Since the participants could vary from zero repetitions to many of them in a ten-second period, the numbers probably represent interval or ratio data.

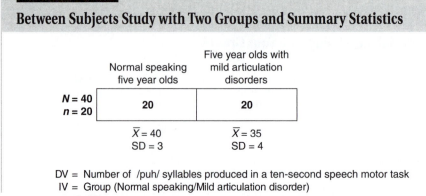

FIGURE 7.5

Between Subjects Study with Two Groups and Summary Statistics

	Normal speaking five year olds	Five year olds with mild articulation disorders
$N = 40$ $n = 20$	20	20
	$\bar{X} = 40$ SD = 3	$\bar{X} = 35$ SD = 4

DV = Number of /puh/ syllables produced in a ten-second speech motor task
IV = Group (Normal speaking/Mild articulation disorder)

They are clearly not nominal or ordinal since they are on a scale with equal intervals and even a zero point. But why do we care about the type of data and level of measurement? We care because the type of data helps to determine which statistical methods (parametric or nonparametric) we can use in analysis. See, we told you that material on summary statistics and the normal distribution would come back to haunt you.

The example in Figure 7.5 now adds to the information that the researcher knows about the investigation. Not only does he or she know about numbers of participants, groups, IV, DV, but also knows about the average performance of each group on the dependent variable (number of syllables produced) and the variability of performance in each group. From examining the summary statistics in Figure 7.5, the researcher might say that the normally speaking children produced more syllables in a ten-second time period than those with mild articulation disorders. In fact, they produced an average of five more syllables than the articulation disordered group. At this point a nonscientist might be content to say that children with articulation disorders are slower in the syllable repetition task than the normal speakers. The scientist, however, would approach this issue differently. Recall in Chapter 2 we said that scientists deal in "probabilistic knowledge." This means that they do not say things are true or false or slower or faster, because they know that error exists in the world and in their own investigations. What if those children with mild articulation disorders got a lower mean syllable repetition rate just due to chance or sampling error? Could the investigator have selected twenty motorically slow children with articulation disorders that do not really represent the total population of children with that disorder? Could the investigator have selected twenty normal speakers just by chance who were unusually fast in their motor ability and do not really represent the motor abilities of the total population of normal speakers? If we did this study over again, would we come up with similar results? These are questions that would bother a scientist, but maybe not a layperson. As we indicated in Chapter 6, the process of hypothesis testing can tell a scientist whether any difference between groups was likely due to chance or if it represents a "significant" difference. In fact, in our illustration of hypothesis testing in Chapter 6 we used the t-test, which is a statistical procedure used in determining whether the difference between means of two groups is statistically significant. Now we will focus on some specific statistical tests that can determine whether the two groups are significantly different.

Between Subjects Analyses: Independent t-Test, ANOVA1 (Between Subjects), and Selected Nonparametric Tests

The Independent t-Test

W. S. Gossett was a statistician and chemist who was employed by the Guinness Brewery in Dublin. Part of Gossett's job was to develop a procedure that would monitor the similarity of yeast content between batches of Guinness and an ideal standard for the brewery. Gossett developed the t-test to make this comparison and determine if a batch differed significantly from the industry standard. Although the brewery did not allow Gossett to publish his research on the *t*-test in an identifiable way, he did publish the procedure under the name "Student" and to this day the procedure is often referred to as Student's *t*-test.

Assumptions of the Analysis

Every statistical analysis procedure is based on certain assumptions that must be met for appropriate use. If these assumptions are not met, or are violated, the results of the statistical analysis are suspect. We mentioned in Chapter 5 that both parametric and nonparametric statistics have assumptions. Interestingly, parametric statistics generally tend to be more "robust" than nonparametric statistics. This means that some of their assumptions can be violated to some degree and the results will still be valid. The independent *t*-test is a parametric statistic and thus has the following assumptions:

1. The level of measurement should be continuous in nature (interval or ratio) as opposed to discrete (nominal or ordinal).
2. The data should approximate a normal distribution.
3. The samples should be drawn randomly from the populations of interest such that every participant has an equal chance of being selected for the study.
4. The two samples should represent a between subjects design in that they are independent of each other. This means that the samples should not represent repeated measurements on the same participants, use of twins, or extraordinary matching of two groups such that they are artificially made to be highly similar.
5. The variances of the two samples should be homogeneous. We do not want one group to be normally distributed and the other group to be highly skewed positively or negatively. We also do not want one group to have a large variance while the other group has a small amount of variation.

Probably the most violated of these assumptions concerns random selection. In many cases, especially in communication disorders, we must study participants who are available for investigation. As mentioned, however, the *t*-test is a robust statistic and can tolerate a bit of abuse in terms of violating assumptions.

The Research Question

The independent *t*-test is designed to evaluate whether two independent groups are significantly different on one dependent variable. Thus, any study that is comparing independent groups on interval or ratio data can be considered.

The Output

Consumers of research should expect specific output from the independent *t*-test in order to interpret the results of an investigation:

1. *The calculated* t *value.* The independent *t*-test calculates the *t* value, which, as stated in Chapter 6, the computer compares to a "critical value" of *t*. If the calculated value exceeds the critical value, the difference between the groups is significant, or beyond chance. In research reports you will rarely see a critical value of *t*, but you should always see the calculated value. The *t* value is typically in a format such as 2.14,

8.19, 0.22. Typically, the higher the calculated t value, the more likely it is to exceed any critical value and result in statistical significance.

2. *The probability.* The results section of an article always reports the probability that two groups may be different. Remember that comparing the calculated t value to the critical value allows us to determine if a difference is significant at a particular alpha level such as .05 or .01. Thus, if the statistical analysis prints out the probability level or tells us that we exceed a particular alpha level, knowing the critical value is not necessary. Probability is typically reported as an exact figure ($p = .032$) or as a cutoff level ($p < .05$ or $p > .05$). With the exact probability, if the p is less than .05 the difference is typically regarded as "significant" or beyond chance. In the case of a probability cutoff such as $p < .05$, we know that the difference is significant, but we do not know the exact probability value; however if we have set our alpha level at $p < .05$, and the actual p value is less than .05, some researchers opt to just report that the difference was significant at $p < .05$. More commonly, however, exact probabilities are used in the research literature.

3. *Degrees of freedom.* **Degrees of freedom,** typically abbreviated as df, is a rather slippery concept that is usually presented in introductory statistics courses (Howell, 1992; Jaccard & Becker, 1997). Perhaps the simplest explanation of df is from Kerlinger (1973, p. 168), who describes df as "the latitude of variation a statistical problem has." He goes on to say that

> there are no degrees of freedom when two numbers must sum to 100 and one of them, say 40, is given. Once 40 or 45 or any other number is given. . . . The remaining number has no freedom to vary.

Schiavetti and Metz state:

> In a most basic sense, df indicate the number of values in a set of data that are free to vary once certain characteristics of the data are known. Generally, if the mean or the sum of a set of scores is known, then the df are equal to the number of scores in each distribution minus 1 ($df = N - 1$). (2006, p. 187)

It is important to note that degrees of freedom are computed somewhat differently depending on the statistical analysis used. That is, the degrees of freedom for a t-test of independent samples differ from the df for a within subjects t-test. Generally, it is true that as the degrees of freedom value increases, the critical value for the t statistic decreases, so it is easier to obtain statistical significance. With the independent t-test the df being $N - 2$ also illustrates the importance of sample size in research. The larger the sample size, the larger the degrees of freedom. Likewise, the concept of degrees of freedom takes on a slightly different meaning for other statistical procedures such as analyses of variance, correlations, and regression analyses. Freedom to vary has a lot to do with numbers of participants and their scores, but it also is involved with the number of independent variables in an experimental design. We will discuss this in more detail when we talk about later analyses.

So what should consumers be looking for in terms of degrees of freedom for the independent t-test? First of all, it is conventional for researchers to report the degrees of freedom used in their analyses in the results sections of their articles. Thus, we should always expect to see the df noted in studies that use specific statistical analyses. We will be alerting you to such instances in this and later chapters. In the case of the independent *t*-test, the degrees of freedom will always be $N - 2$. Note that the large *N* represents the total number of observations in the study. For example, in the study illustrated in Figure 7.5, the *N* or total number of participants is 40. Therefore, the degrees of freedom would be $40 - 2 = 38$. In fairly simple analyses such as the independent *t*-test, it is not difficult for the consumer of research to determine if the degrees of freedom make sense in the results section of an article. Just remember $N - 2$.

4. *Effect size.* You should recall our discussion of clinical or practical significance (effect size) in Chapter 6. In that discussion, we indicated that increasingly more journals are requiring authors to provide effect size measurements when reporting statistical results. Reporting a Cohen's *d* value or eta or omega squared allows consumers to relate the results of a statistically significant *t*-test or ANOVA to meaningful or practical differences. Therefore, consumers of research literature (research sharks) should expect some effect size measurement to be reported in a research article and be critical of reports that omit such data.

5. *Putting the calculated* t, *degrees of freedom, probability, and effect size together.* A researcher can report the results of an independent *t*-test in several ways, but the elements usually include calculated *t*, degrees of freedom, probability, and effect size. In cases of no significant difference, as in the current example, there is no need to include effect sizes, mainly because the difference between means may be due to chance. For example, a researcher may report the results of the study illustrated in Figure 7.5 in three different ways, as shown in Box 7.1.

BOX 7.1

Two Independent Groups Analyzed by a t-Test

The children with normal articulation had a mean of 40 (SD = 3) productions of the /puh/ syllable in a ten-second period whereas the group with mild articulation disorders had a mean of 35 (SD = 4).

a. The results of an independent *t*-test revealed that this difference was not significant ($t = 1.12$; df = 38; $p = .14$).
b. The results of an independent t-test revealed that this difference was not significant ($t = 1.12$; df = 38; $p > .05$).
c. The table shows the means and standard deviations for both groups and the results of an independent *t*-test. The groups were not significantly different on the syllable repetition task.

Normal Articulation	Mild Articulation Disorder	*t*	*p*
40 (SD = 3)	35 (SD = 4)	1.12 (df = 38)	.14

You can see several components present in Box 7.1. First, the researcher mentions the summary statistics (means and standard deviations) in order to provide a context for how each group performed. Second, the researcher reports the difference between the means to not be statistically significant. We give several examples of how a researcher might talk about the results of the independent t-test. Even though we do not know the "critical value" of t, we do know that the calculated value of t needs to exceed this value for the difference to be significant at a particular alpha level such as $p < .05$. Example (a) gives the exact probability level ($p = .14$). It is greater than .05, so we know that the difference was not significant. In example (b) the researcher tells us that the difference was not significant because the probability was greater than the traditional alpha level of .05 ($p > .05$). It does not really matter what the actual p value was, just that it exceeded our desired alpha level for significance. It could be $p = .14$ or $p = .39$ or $p = .07$, but it just does not make the cut for a significant difference at $p < .05$. In example (c) the researcher uses a table to portray the same information presented in example (a). You should be able to see that a consumer given the summary statistics, the calculated t value, the degrees of freedom, and the probability is in a good position to evaluate the results of an independent t-test, even if he or she is unable to physically calculate one.

The One-Factor Analysis of Variance (Between Subjects)

Sir Ronald Aylmer Fisher was born in 1890 in London and became a well-known authority in genetics, biology, and statistics. In fact, Fisher was instrumental in developing the **analysis of variance (ANOVA)** in 1919 while working as a statistician at the Rothamsted Agricultural Experiment Station in the United Kingdom. The analysis of variance we will discuss in this section is known by a variety of names: *one-way analysis of variance, ANOVA1*, or *one-factor analysis of variance*. They all basically suggest that we are analyzing one independent variable, which can have multiple levels. The example in Figure 7.6 has added a level to the study used to illustrate the independent t-test in the previous section. Now we still have one independent variable, but it has three levels instead of two.

FIGURE 7.6

Between Subjects Study with Three Groups and Summary Statistics

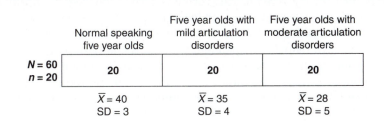

	Normal speaking five year olds	Five year olds with mild articulation disorders	Five year olds with moderate articulation disorders
$N = 60$ $n = 20$	20	20	20
	$\bar{X} = 40$ SD = 3	$\bar{X} = 35$ SD = 4	$\bar{X} = 28$ SD = 5

DV = Number of /puh/ syllables produced in a ten-second speech motor task
IV = Group (Normal speaking/Mild articulation disorder/Moderate articulation disorder)

Assumptions of the Analysis

The following assumptions are essentially identical to those underlying the *t*-test. This is because the ANOVA is an extension of the *t*-test and they are both parametric statistics.

1. The level of measurement should be continuous in nature (interval or ratio) as opposed to discrete (nominal or ordinal).
2. The data should approximate a normal distribution. We do not want one group to be normally distributed and the other groups to be highly skewed positively or negatively.
3. The samples should be drawn randomly from the populations of interest such that every participant has an equal chance of being selected for the study.
4. The samples should represent a between subjects design in that they are independent of each other. This means that the samples should not represent repeated measurements on the same participants.
5. The variances of the samples are homogeneous. We also do not want one group to have a large variance and the other groups to have a small amount of variation.

The Research Question

The one-factor analysis of variance (ANOVA1) is used to determine if there are significant differences among *more than two* groups. The ANOVA1 can be used to find differences among groups (e.g., 3, 4, 5, 6, and even more if the sample size is sufficient). You might be wondering why we do not just perform a bunch of *t*-tests on the three groups. If we did that, we would have to do three different *t*-tests: normal versus mild, normal versus moderate, mild versus moderate. The *t*-test is the most widely used statistic for finding differences between two groups, but it should not be used repeatedly on more than two groups. One of the assumptions of such statistics is that they are designed to be robust for one analysis, but if you keep using them, all bets are off (Huck, 2004). You will recall in Chapter 6 that the chance of a Type II error is increased by using a statistical analysis over and over again on the same data. This is why in Chapter 6 we discussed the Bonferroni adjustment, which makes the alpha level more stringent depending on how many dependent variables are being compared by a statistical analysis. Thus, a research question answered by the ANOVA can be illustrated by the data in Figure 7.6, which extends the two-group study considered in our *t*-test example. Notice that we have added a group to the *t*-test example, which now includes normal articulation, mild articulation disorder, and moderate articulation disorder groups. Our single independent variable is still "group," but we have three levels of grouping instead of two. Our research question might be "Are there significant differences in syllable repetition (DV) among the three groups labeled normal articulation, mild articulation disorder, and moderate articulation disorder?"

The Output

The output of an ANOVA1 includes many numbers that are summarized in an analysis of variance summary table, including the source, the sum of squares, the mean

TABLE 7.1

ANOVA Summary Table

Source	Sum of Squares	df	Mean Square	F	p
Group	567	2	28	28.60	<.001
Error	565	57	3.5		
Total	1132	59	9.91		

square, the degrees of freedom, the *F*-ratio and the probability. Table 7.1 illustrates an ANOVA1 summary table.

The source indicates the source variance evaluated in the analysis, the most important component being the analysis of variance between groups—normal, mild articulation, and moderate articulation as illustrated in Figure 7.6 previously. The other sources are the error term, which represents the variance within groups, and the total variance, which is the variance for between and within groups. The sums of squares represent the sum of the squared deviations from the mean and is a measure of variability in the sample. The degrees of freedom vary depending on the type of ANOVA being performed; in the case above, group has 2 degrees of freedom, representing the number of groups minus one. The total degrees of freedom in this analysis are $N-1$, which would be 59 since we have 60 participants in our example. Since the degrees of freedom must total 59 and the degrees of freedom for groups equal 2, the error degrees of freedom must be 57 to add up to 59. The mean squares are obtained by dividing the sums of squares by their corresponding degrees of freedom. The *F*-ratio is obtained by dividing the mean square for group by the mean square for error (283.5/9.91). The researcher can then look up the critical value for *F* in an *F* table. In this case he or she would find the critical value for a table with 2 and 57 degrees of freedom and see whether it is exceeded by the calculated *F*-ratio. For our example, the *F* table shows that our *F*-ratio has to exceed 7.76 to be significant at the $p = .001$ level and we certainly have passed that value with an *F* of 28.6. As a consumer of research, however, you will rarely see an ANOVA summary table in an article. This is partially due to space limitations in journals that restrict the use of lengthy tables that really do not add important information to the results section of an article. Analysis of variance summary tables are most often seen in theses and dissertations, since these are learning experiences for students and there are no space limitations as in published research articles. Thus, the following outputs are a minimum requirement for an ANOVA1 that you will encounter in the literature:

1. *The calculated F-ratio.* Just as in the *t*-test in which you calculate the value of *t* and compare it to a critical value of *t*, a similar operation occurs in the ANOVA1. In the analysis of variance the calculated value is called the *F*-ratio, and it is compared to a critical value of *F* in a table or the comparison is done by a computer program just as in the *t*-test. The calculated *F* is similar in format to the *t* in that it will usually appear

as a one- or two-digit number with two decimal places (e.g., 12.33, 3.12, 0.91). Again, the calculated F must exceed the critical value of F in order for a significant difference among groups to be found. In most articles, the researcher will not only state the F-ratio but also the degrees of freedom used to look up the critical value. In the case of our example on articulation disorders the author might say, "The groups were significantly different on the syllable repetition task ($F = 28.6$; df = 2,57; $p < .001$).

2. *Probability.* Just as in the independent t-test, a probability level is reported so that the researcher can determine if any differences among the groups are due to chance or if they are statistically significant according to the alpha level set prior to the experiment. Thus, if the F-ratio is significant at $p = .02$ that means that there is a difference among the three groups that has occurred beyond chance. We do not want to gloss over a very important point here. We just said that if a researcher gets a significant F-ratio at $p = .02$ it means that a statistically significant difference exists *among* the groups. It does not, however, tell us *which of the three groups* are, in fact, significantly different. Look again at the means presented in Figure 7.6. The mean for the normal group is 40, the mean for the mild group is 35, and the mean for the moderate group is 28. Clearly, the normal articulation group scored highest and the moderate group scored with the lowest number of syllables produced. A significant F-ratio tells us that somewhere among these three means there is *at least one* statistically significant difference. There could also be *more than one* difference among the groups. The obvious groups to be significantly different are the normals, with a mean of 40, and the moderates, with a mean of 28. This difference is pretty much guaranteed to be statistically significant. If there is a significant difference among the three groups, it is surely between these two means that are most different from one another. But the researcher must ask, "What about the difference between 40 and 35, or the difference between 35 and 28?" It is very possible that the significant F-ratio has revealed that all of the groups are significantly different from one another. This is why a procedure called **post hoc means comparison testing** is always used with statistics like the ANOVA that compare more than two groups.

3. *Post hoc means comparison.* Remember that the F-ratio tells us if we have at least one statistically significant difference among the three groups. Now the researcher must do some detective work to determine *where* the significant differences are. Obviously, with three groups you can have the following possible comparisons, any or all of which could be significantly different: group 1/group 2; group 1/group 3; group 2/group 3. The post hoc test examines all possible differences among groups and tells the researcher which ones are significant. We know that *at least one* will be significant because of the significant F-ratio, but there may be more. There are many versions of post hoc tests used to make this determination. Figure 7.7 shows some common post hoc tests, which vary in terms of how "liberal" or "conservative" they are. That is, a conservative post hoc test will find fewer significant differences among groups. For example, the means of groups will probably have to be farther apart to show a significant difference on a conservative test such as the Scheffé. On the other hand, a more liberal test such as Fisher's LSD might find more significant differences among groups, even those whose means are not that far apart. Most researchers tend to use either more conservative post hoc tests or those in the middle of the

---

FIGURE 7.7

Post Hoc Means Comparison Tests

Scheffé	Conservative
Tukey	
Newman-Keuls	
Duncan's Multiple Range	
Fisher's LSD	Liberal

---

conservative–liberal continuum because they do not want to find differences that may simply be a product of their choice of post hoc measurements.

4. *Effect size.* As in the *t*-test, a measure of effect size such as Cohen's *d* provides an indication of practical or clinical significance.

As illustrated in the Box 7.2, a researcher can report the results of an ANOVA1 in several ways. Example (a) provides information on the analysis of variance in

---

BOX 7.2

Output of ANOVA 1 with Three Groups

The children with normal articulation had a mean of 40 (SD = 3) productions of the /puh/ syllable in a ten-second period, the mild articulation disorder group had a mean of 35 (SD = 4), and the group with moderate articulation disorders had a mean of 28 (SD = 5).

a. The results of a one-way analysis of variance revealed that the groups differed significantly ($F = 28.60$; df = 2, 57; $p = .0001$). This represents a large effect size ($d = 2.00$). Post hoc means comparison using the Newman-Keuls procedure revealed that the normally developing group and the moderately disordered group were significantly different. The mildly articulation disordered group did not differ significantly from either the normal or moderate group.

b. The table shows the means and standard deviations for the three groups and the results of an ANOVA1. The groups were significantly different on the syllable repetition task and this represents a large effect size ($d = 2.00$).

Normal Articulation	Mild Articulation Disorder	Moderate Articulation Disorder	F	p
40 (SD = 3)	35 (SD = 4)	28 (SD = 5)	28.60 (df = 2, 57)	.0001

Post hoc testing using the Newman-Keuls procedure showed that the normally developing group and the moderately disordered group were significantly different. The mild articulation disorder group did not differ significantly from either the normal or moderate group.

paragraph form. Note that the critical components are named in this paragraph: the *F*-ratio, degrees of freedom, probability, effect size, and the results of post hoc testing. In example (b) the means and standard deviations, *F*-ratio, probability, and results of post hoc testing are illustrated by using a table and text.

All right, let's see if you have the concept of factors and levels as they are dealt with by the one-way analysis of variance. In Figure 7.8 we add one more group that represents children with severe articulation disorders. Remember, we still have only one IV (factor), which is group, but we now have four levels of that IV representing the four levels of articulation ability. We still have only one DV, which is the number of syllables produced in a ten-second period.

When we perform an ANOVA1 on these groups we will have the same types of output that we obtained in the study with three groups. Our results might look like those illustrated in Box 7.3. Note that we obtained a significant *F* at the $p = .01$ level. This means that we have at least one significant difference among the four groups. Our post hoc testing must compare the means of all groups with each other. This means that we need to compare normal/mild, normal/moderate, normal/severe, mild/moderate, mild/severe, and moderate/severe for a total of six comparisons. It turned out that only the underlined ones above were significantly different according to the post hoc test. You might have noticed that this time we elected to use the Scheffe instead of the Newman-Keuls. It gives us the same information, but it is just a more conservative test.

Nonparametric Analyses of Two or More Groups on One IV (Between Subjects)

We mentioned earlier in the chapter that the use of parametric statistics such as the *t*-test and analysis of variance depends on the data meeting specific assumptions. Sometimes, however, the data in a study do not meet the assumptions. For example,

---

FIGURE 7.8

ANOVA1 on Four Groups

	Normal speaking five year olds	Five year olds with mild articulation disorders	Five year olds with moderate articulation disorders	Five year olds with severe articulation disorders
$N = 80$ $n = 20$	20	20	20	20
	$\bar{X} = 40$ SD = 3	$\bar{X} = 35$ SD = 4	$\bar{X} = 28$ SD = 5	$\bar{X} = 20$ SD = 5

DV = Number of /puh/ syllables produced in a ten-second speech motor task
IV = Group (Normal speaking/Mild articulation disorder/Moderate articulation disorder/ Severe articulation disorder)

Output of ANOVA1 with Four Groups

The children with normal articulation had a mean of 40 (SD = 3) productions of the /puh/ syllable in a ten-second period, the mild articulation disorder group had a mean of 35 (SD = 4), the group with moderate articulation disorders had a mean of 28 (SD = 5), and the severe articulation disorder group had a mean of 20 (SD = 5).

a. The results of a one-way analysis of variance revealed that the groups differed significantly ($F = 4.66$; df = 3, 77; $p = .01$). This represents a large effect size ($d = .85$). Post hoc means comparison using the Scheffé procedure revealed that the normally developing group and mildly disordered group were not significantly different. There was a significant difference between the moderately disordered group and the severely disordered group. The moderate and severe groups were significantly different from both the normal and mild groups.

b. The table shows the means and standard deviations for the three groups and the results of an ANOVA1. The groups were significantly different on the syllable repetition task and the effect size is large ($d = .85$).

Normal Articulation	Mild Articulation Disorder	Moderate Articulation Disorder	Severe Articulation Disorder	F	p
40 (SD = 3)	35 (SD = 4)	28 (SD = 5)	20 (SD = 5)	4.66 (df = 3, 77)	.01

Post hoc means comparison using the Scheffé procedure revealed that the normally developing group and mildly disordered group were significantly different. There were significant differences between the moderately disordered group and the severely disordered group. The moderate and severe groups were significantly different from the normal and mild groups.

the level of measurement might be nominal or ordinal, the data may not be normally distributed, or the variances may not be homogeneous. In such cases, the researcher is not necessarily out of the data analysis business. Nonparametric statistics may be an option for occasions when assumptions of parametric statistics are not met (Gibbons, 1976; Gibbons, 1985; Siegel, 1956). Nonparametric statistics are "distribution free" and therefore do not have rigid requirements for normality or homogeneity of variance. We mentioned earlier that overall, nonparametric statistics are not considered by most researchers to be as powerful as parametric procedures. In general, this is probably true. However, in cases where assumptions of parametric statistics have been violated, the nonparametric route may actually be more appropriate (Huck, 2004). It is probably better to use a nonparametric statistic instead of a parametric procedure whose assumptions have not been met. We will not be spending as much time discussing nonparametric procedures, mainly because they are not seen in the literature as much as parametric analyses. It is important, however, for consumers of research to at least know the most common nonparametric analyses and the types of output they provide so that readers of research literature will be able to interpret the results of an investigation using such procedures.

In this section we will mention only nonparametric statistics used to analyze differences between two or more independent groups. Such procedures might be used as a substitute for an independent t-test or ANOVA1 between subjects. Although many nonparametric statistics have been developed over the years, we will only mention in this section a few of them that are the most widely used and likely to be seen by consumers of research.

Finding Differences between Two Independent Groups

Mann-Whitney U Test. This analysis is sometimes called the Mann-Whitney-Wilcoxon or the Wilcoxon rank-sum test. The most important thing to know about the U test is that it is used to determine whether there is a significant difference between two independent groups. It is typically used with ordinal data but might also be used when assumptions of parametric statistics are violated (e.g., homogeneity of variance). As suggested in its name, the statistic produces a calculated value known as U, using the same general process as the t-test in producing a calculated t value. Also similar to the t-test procedure, the calculated U is compared to a table of critical values for U to determine whether the difference is significant.

Chi Square Test for Two Independent Samples. The chi-square test is used for nominal data to determine whether there is a significant difference between two independent groups. It is usually recommended if the sample size includes more than twenty participants. As suggested in the name, the statistical analysis yields a number called chi square, symbolized as χ^2. The calculated value of chi square is then compared to a table of critical values for χ^2 to determine whether the two groups are significantly different.

Fisher Exact Probability Test. The Fisher is used in a similar fashion to the chi-square for nominal data in which N is less than twenty participants. The Fisher produces a calculated value D, which is compared to a critical value table to determine significant differences.

Finding Differences among Three or More Independent Groups

Chi-Square Test for K Independent Samples. This test works similarly to the chi-square test for two independent samples. The major difference is that it can analyze for differences among more than two groups when the level of measurement is nominal. The interpretation is the same as the chi-square for independent samples.

Kruskal-Wallis One-Way Analysis of Variance. The Kruskal-Wallis is analogous to the ANOVA1 but can be used with ordinal data and does not require homogeneity of variance. The statistical analysis calculates a value H, which is compared to a table to determine whether it exceeds a critical value for significant differences.

Within Subjects Analyses: Correlated t-Test, ANOVA1 (Within Subjects), and Selected Nonparametric Tests

The prior section dealt with statistics that determine if means are significantly different between two or among more than two independent groups (between subjects) on one independent variable. The present section examines the same types of procedures used on repeated measurements (within subjects) on a single independent variable. Our explanations will be less detailed because these procedures are analogous to the between subjects statistics.

The Correlated t-Test

A researcher wants to determine if two distinct types of hearing instrument microphones differ in the way they might affect speech discrimination ability in participants who wear hearing aids. The researcher would like to compare these two types of microphones on the same individuals. Although he or she could design the study as between subjects giving one group microphone 1 and the other group microphone 2, as you know, there are many difficulties with using this type of design to answer the research question. First of all, the researcher would have to make sure the two groups are equivalent on hearing impairment, types of hearing aids, age, and many other variables. It would be very difficult to populate two groups of different people and yet control for all of the threats to internal validity from differential subject selection. Conducting the study using a within subjects design would simplify things quite a bit. First of all, you only need to find one group of participants who would act as their own controls as they used the two types of microphones. Also, from a practical point of view, it is impressive if the researcher can show that the speech discrimination of the same individuals seem to be affected by the type of microphone used. Of course, the within subjects design is susceptible to its own threats to internal validity, which mainly have to do with order effects, history, maturation, and sensitizing the participants through multiple exposures. However, if the researcher counterbalances the conditions, and they are close together in time, these threats can be sufficiently counteracted. Figure 7.9 shows the within subjects design comparing the two types of microphones on speech discrimination. Notice that there are twenty participants who experience both levels of the independent variable as indicated by the arrow. The means for each microphone condition are provided without standard deviations, but let us assume that the variances among conditions are homogeneous.

The **correlated t-test** is known by a variety of names such as *t-test for dependent samples, t-test for repeated samples,* and *t-test for paired samples.* These names suggest a couple of important distinctions. First of all, samples can be related to one another

FIGURE 7.9

Repeated Measures Study with Two Conditions

IV = Type of Hearing Aid
Microphone (1, 2)
DV = Speech Discrimination %

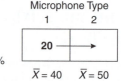

in a number of different ways. For example, repeated measurements on the same participants as in the example just discussed clearly makes the two samples related. Another example, however, comes from studies that investigate twins in two groups. Some say that the biological similarities of twin pairs, creates a situation much like studying the same people twice. A final example comes from studies that populate two groups so heavily matched on a host of variables such as exact age, gender, SES, race, intelligence and other factors that they are almost "the same" people. At any rate, the correlated *t*-test is used to examine within subjects designs, most commonly when repeated measurements are taken on a single group of people.

Assumptions of the Analysis

The assumptions of the correlated *t*-test are similar to those mentioned earlier in this chapter for the independent *t*-test: interval or ratio data, a normal distribution, random selection of participants, homogeneous variances, and a within subjects design.

The Research Question

The correlated *t*-test is designed to evaluate whether two related groups are significantly different on one dependent variable. Thus, any study comparing twins, extraordinarily matched groups, or repeated measurements on the same participants on interval or ratio data can be considered. The most common scenario involves repeated measurements on the same group of participants as in our example of the same people being given a speech discrimination test with two different microphones.

The Output

Consumers of research should expect specific output from the correlated *t*-test in order to interpret the results of an investigation. Fortunately, the output for the correlated *t*-test is identical to the independent *t*-test in terms of types of data to interpret:

1. *The calculated* t *value.* The correlated *t*-test calculates the *t* value, which the computer compares to a "critical value" of *t*. If the calculated value exceeds the critical value, the difference between the groups is significant, or beyond chance. As in the

independent t-test the t value is typically in a format such as 2.14, 8.19, 0.22. Typically, the higher the calculated t value, the more likely it is to exceed any critical value and result in significance.

2. *The probability.* The probability level is interpreted in exactly the same manner as the independent t-test. Thus, the statistical analysis prints out the probability level ($p = .032$) or tells us that we exceed a particular alpha level ($p < .05$ or $p > .05$).

3. *Degrees of freedom.* You may recall that the degrees of freedom for the independent t-test were $N - 2$. In the correlated t-test the degrees of freedom are equivalent to *the number of pairs of scores minus one.* Just as in the independent t-test it is conventional for researchers to report the degrees of freedom used in their analyses in the results sections of their articles. For the example on comparing two microphones and their effects on speech discrimination we have twenty participants who are sampled two times. Therefore we will have twenty pairs of scores. Participant 1 will have a discrimination score for microphone one and another discrimination score for microphone 2, constituting a pair of scores for that participant. Thus, the degrees of freedom would be $20 - 1 = 19$.

4. *Putting the calculated* t, *degrees of freedom, effect size, and probability together.* A researcher can report the results of a correlated t-test in several ways, but the elements of calculated t, degrees of freedom, and probability will always be there, just as in the independent t-test. For example, a researcher may report the results of the study as illustrated in Box 7.4. Again, several "required" components are present in the box, including summary statistics, the calculated t value, the degrees of freedom, and the probability. No effect size measurement was provided because there was no significant difference between the conditions.

BOX 7.4

Output of Correlated t-Test

The speech discrimination scores associated with the use of microphone 1 had a mean of 40 (SD = 3) whereas the discrimination scores of participants using microphone 2 had a mean of 50 (SD = 4).

a. The results of a correlated t-test revealed that this difference was not significant ($t = 1.01$; df = 19; $p = .33$).

b. The results of a correlated t-test revealed that this difference was not significant ($t = 1.01$; df = 19; $p > .05$).

c. The table shows the means and standard deviations for both groups and the results of an independent t-test. The groups were not significantly different on the syllable repetition task.

Microphone 1	Microphone 2	t	p
40 (SD = 3)	50 (SD = 4)	1.01 (df = 19)	.33

The One-Factor Analysis of Variance (Within Subjects)

The ANOVA1 for within subjects designs operates much like the one-way ANOVA for between subjects investigations. We will introduce the analysis by extending the study on microphones used to illustrate the correlated t-test. One day a different investigator reads the study comparing microphones 1 and 2 and was interested in the finding that the two microphones did not have a significant effect on speech discrimination. This new investigator had access to three different microphones and wanted to compare the results among all three instead of just comparing two. Remember, this is still a within subjects design in which all participants will experience each of the three different microphones. The proposed study is illustrated in Figure 7.10. Again, we have provided means for each microphone, and we assume the standard deviations are comparable.

Assumptions of the Analysis

The assumptions are essentially identical to those underlying the ANOVA1 for between subjects. This is because they are both parametric statistics. The within subjects ANOVA1 is an extension of the correlated t-test.

The Research Question

The one-factor analysis of variance (ANOVA1) for a within subjects design is used to determine whether there are significant differences among more than two conditions or tasks performed by the same participants. As in the ANOVA1 for between subjects, the within subjects analysis can be used to find differences among several conditions (e.g., 3, 4, 5, 6, and even more if the sample size is sufficient). Our research question might be "Are there significant differences in speech discrimination scores among participants using the three different types of microphones?"

The Output

The output of an ANOVA1 within subjects is similar to the output from an ANOVA1 between subjects. Thus, the following outputs are a minimum requirement for an ANOVA1 within subjects that you might encounter in the literature:

1. *The calculated F-ratio.* Just as in the ANOVA1 between subjects the calculated value is called the F-ratio, which is compared to a critical value of F in a table or the

---

FIGURE 7.10

Repeated Measures Study with Three Conditions

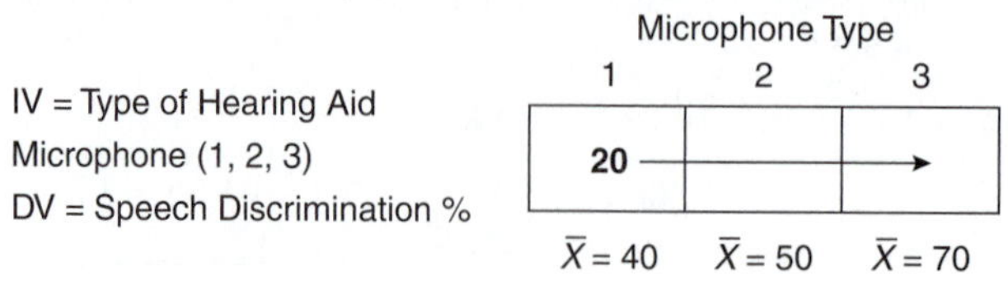

IV = Type of Hearing Aid
Microphone (1, 2, 3)
DV = Speech Discrimination %

Microphone Type
1   2   3

20

$\bar{X} = 40$ $\bar{X} = 50$ $\bar{X} = 70$

comparison is done by a computer program. Again, the calculated F is similar in format to the ANOVA1 between subjects in that it will usually appear as a one- or two-digit number with two decimal places (e.g., 12.33, 3.12, 0.91). The researcher will report the F-ratio and its associated degrees of freedom in the results section of the article.

2. *Probability.* A probability level is reported so that the researcher can determine whether any differences among the conditions are due to chance or if they are statistically significant according to the alpha level set prior to the experiment. Again, a significant F-ratio tells us that somewhere among these three means there is *at least one* statistically significant difference. There could also be *more than one* difference among the groups. But the researcher must ask, "What about the difference between means of 40 and 50, or the difference between the means of 50 and 70?" It is very possible that the significant F-ratio has revealed that all of the groups are significantly different from one another. Just as in the ANOVA1 between subjects, *post hoc means comparison testing* is always done to determine which specific conditions differ from one another.

3. *Post hoc means comparison.* The same group of post hoc tests referred to in Box 7.8 is used with the ANOVA1 within subjects to determine which of the repeated measurements differ significantly from one another.

4. *Effect size.* If a significant difference is found, consumers of research should expect the researcher to report an effect size measurement such as Cohen's d.

As illustrated in Box 7.5, a researcher can report the results of an ANOVA1 repeated measures in several ways, just as we illustrated with the between subjects version. Example (a) provides information on the analysis of variance in a paragraph. Note that the critical components are named in this paragraph: F-ratio, degrees of freedom, probability, and results of post hoc testing. In example (b) the means and standard deviations, F-ratio, probability, and results of post hoc testing are illustrated by using a table and text.

Adding another level to this study would produce a design that looks like the drawing in Figure 7.11. The output from this study would again be an extension of the results from the investigation of three microphones in Box 7.5 and would produce results such as those illustrated in Box 7.6. You should be getting more familiar and comfortable with reading such results after studying our examples. The results section of a research article is not as intimidating for consumers who know what to expect for a particular experimental design or statistical analysis method. After reading this chapter, you should find articles that have used a t-test or ANOVA1 more understandable than in the past.

Nonparametric Analyses of Two or More Groups on One IV (Within Subjects)

As discussed previously for independent groups, there are analogous nonparametric statistics designed to analyze differences between groups for within subjects designs. Again, we will only mention these briefly because consumers of research will not encounter nonparametric statistics nearly as often as the parametric ones discussed earlier.

Output of ANOVA1 Repeated Measures on Three Groups

The participants using microphone 1 had a mean of 40 on their speech discrimination score (SD = 10). When the participants used microphone 2 they had a mean of 50 (SD = 11) in speech discrimination. Microphone 3 resulted in a speech discrimination score of 70 (SD = 12).

a. The results of a repeated measures one-way analysis of variance revealed that the groups differed significantly ($F = 3.12$; df = 2, 57; $p = .02$). This represents a medium effect size ($d = 66.17$). Post hoc means comparison using the Newman-Keuls procedure revealed that microphones 1 and 2 were not significantly different; however, there were significant differences between microphones 2 and 3 and between microphones 1 and 3.

b. The table shows the means and standard deviations for the three microphone conditions and the results of a repeated measures ANOVA1. The groups were significantly different on the syllable repetition task.

Microphone 1	Microphone 2	Microphone 3	F	p
40 (SD = 10)	50 (SD = 11)	70 (SD = 12)	3.12 (df = 2, 57)	.02

This is a medium effect size ($d = 66.17$). Post hoc testing using the Newman-Keuls procedure showed that microphones 1 and 2 were not significantly different. There were significant differences between microphones 1 and 3 and between microphones 2 and 3.

Finding Differences between Two Related Samples

McNemar's Test.   McNemar's test is performed on nominal data to determine whether repeated measures on the same participants are different between two conditions, such as pre- and posttesting. The analysis actually yields a calculated chi-square statistic, which is compared to a table of critical values to determine if significant differences are present.

Repeated Measures Study with Four Conditions

IV = Type of Hearing Aid
Microphone (1, 2, 3, 4)
DV = Speech Discrimination %

Microphone Type

| 1 | 2 | 3 | 4 |

20 ——

$\bar{X} = 40$ $\bar{X} = 50$ $\bar{X} = 70$ $\bar{X} = 90$

BOX 7.6

Output of ANOVA1 Repeated Measures on Four Groups

The participants using microphone 1 had a mean of 40 on their speech discrimination score (SD = 10). When the participants used microphone 2 they had a mean of 50 (SD = 11) in speech discrimination. Microphone 3 resulted in a speech discrimination score of 70 (SD = 12), and microphone 4 had a mean discrimination score of 90 (SD = 11).

a. The results of a repeated measures one-way analysis of variance revealed that the groups differed significantly ($F = 3.12$; df = 2, 57; $p = .02$). This represents a large effect size ($d = 1.12$). Post hoc means comparison using the Newman-Keuls procedure revealed that microphones 1 and 2 were not significantly different; however, there were significant differences between microphones 2 and 3, 1 and 3, 1 and 4, 2 and 4, and 3 and 4.

b. The table shows the means and standard deviations for the four microphone conditions and the results of a repeated measures ANOVA1. The groups were significantly different on the syllable repetition task for large effect size ($d = 1.12$).

Mic 1	Mic 2	Mic 3	Mic 4	F	p
40	50	70	90	5.98	.01
(SD = 10)	(SD = 11)	(SD = 12)	(SD = 11)	(df = 3, 57)	

Post hoc testing using the Newman-Keuls procedure showed that microphones 1 and 2 were not significantly different. There were significant differences between microphones 1 and 3, 1 and 4, 2 and 3, 2 and 4, and 3 and 4.

Wilcoxon Matched Pairs Signed Ranks Test.   The Wilcoxon test is used on ordinal data to determine whether pairs of scores differ in direction and magnitude as in a pre- and posttreatment comparison. The calculated value z is compared to a table of critical values to determine whether the difference in conditions is statistically significant.

Finding Differences among Three or More Related Samples

Cochran Q test.   The Cochran Q test, which is an extension of the McNemar test mentioned previously, is used to determine significant differences between two related samples on nominal data. The Cochran Q extends the McNemar test to include an analysis of more than two samples. The analysis calculates a value for Q and this is compared to a critical value to determine whether significant differences exist.

Friedman Two-Way Analysis of Variance by Ranks.   The Friedman analysis is designed for ordinal data to determine whether more than two related samples differ significantly. The analysis calculates a value that Friedman calls χr^2, which is compared to a critical value to determine whether there are significant differences.

Multivariate Analysis of Variance (MANOVA)

Realizing that univariate statistics are difficult enough to comprehend, we approach a basic discussion of multivariate statistics with a certain degree of trepidation. If it is beyond the scope of the present text to adequately cover univariate statistics, it is certainly an impossible task to do justice to multivariate procedures, which are parametric statistics for finding differences among two or more groups or conditions on multiple dependent variables (between and within subjects). However, we would be remiss if we did not at least expose you in a general way to the world of multivariate analysis. You will recall that univariate statistics examine only a single dependent variable and how it may be affected by one or more independent variables. For example, we can take an independent variable of groups divided into one group with conductive hearing loss and another with sensorineural hearing loss and compare them on some dependent measure such as speech discrimination. For the analysis we could use a univariate statistic such as the independent t-test to determine whether any differences between groups are statistically significant. A major difference between univariate and multivariate statistics is that in the latter, the researcher can examine *more than one dependent variable simultaneously.* So, extending this example, a researcher might be interested not only in speech discrimination scores but also in two other dependent measures: a test measuring a person's ability to detect speech in noise and the results of a test of otoacoustic emissions. Now you might ask, "Why can't the researcher just analyze speech discrimination and be satisfied with that result?" Or you might ask, "Why can't the researcher just do three different univariate studies, one for each dependent variable?" The glib answer is that *life is multivariate.* Seldom does only one independent variable exclusively influence just one ability or dependent variable. The world is filled with multiple influences (IVs) that have profound single and interactive influences on multiple abilities (DVs). By analyzing data with multivariate methods we get a glimpse of the interrelatedness of influences and abilities. There are also several statistical answers to the questions posed above. First, as you already know, performing multiple univariate analyses on a bunch of individual dependent variables increases the chances of committing a Type I error and finding "significant differences" when there really are none. That is why we must use the Bonferroni adjustment if we perform multiple univariate analyses, whether they are t-tests or ANOVAs. The MANOVA, by using a linear combination of all the dependent variables in a "vector," can reduce many DVs to essentially only one DV as illustrated in Figure 7.12.

A second statistical reason to consider using a MANOVA is that the ANOVA misses possible correlations among the dependent variables by analyzing only one at a time. In fact, researchers using MANOVA are *encouraged* to select dependent variables that are likely to be correlated. Moreover, it is often said that the DVs *must* be correlated and it is ideal if this correlation is not just statistical but theoretical as well (Weinfurt, 1995). Finally, by using a MANOVA it is possible to obtain a significant multivariate difference between groups for several dependent variables combined when no significant differences may result from a series of univariate ANOVAs on the individual dependent

FIGURE 7.12

Differences between Univariate and Multivariate Analyses

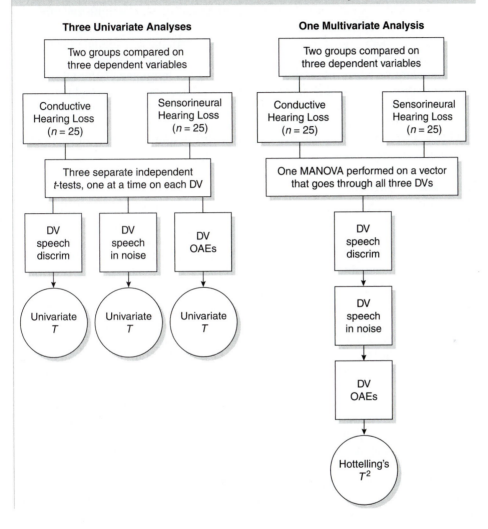

variables. A major strength of the MANOVA is this ability to determine group differences on several correlated dependent variables taken together as a construct.

Assumptions of MANOVA

1. Just as in univariate ANOVAs we assume that the data analyzed in a MANOVA consists of independent observations. Essentially, this means that the score of a particular participant in a study should not be influenced by other participants.

2. We assume in univariate statistics that all dependent variables are distributed normally; similarly in MANOVA we assume that the dependent variables *and their combinations* are normally distributed.

3. You probably remember that in univariate statistics we assume that our variances between groups are homogeneous. With MANOVA we assume that there is homogeneity of variance not only for each dependent variable considered individually, but also for "covariance matrices." This term refers to the shared variance between two dependent variables. So, essentially, we must have homogeneity for all DVs and all combinations of DVs. Such homogeneity of variance can be checked using Bartlett's chi-square test, which we referred to earlier, or Box's *M* test. Therefore, as consumers of research we might realistically expect a researcher who uses MANOVA to provide some proof that the multivariate normality assumption was not violated by reporting such test results.

The Research Question

Basically the research questions answered by MANOVA are the same as those addressed by the *t*-test and ANOVA1 in this chapter. A researcher would like to know whether there is a significant difference between two or more groups on one independent variable. With MANOVA, the dependent variables will be combined into a single vector and any differences between groups will be for all the dependent variables taken as a unit.

The Output

1. *Hotelling's T^2.* **Hotelling's T^2** is essentially a multivariate version of the calculated *t* in the univariate *t*-test. A significant T^2 indicates that there is a significant difference between two groups for the vector of all dependent variables under investigation.

2. *Univariate* t *values.* A researcher who obtains a significant T^2 is often encouraged to examine the results of univariate *t*-tests to determine which of the individual dependent variables contributed most to the significant multivariate effect. Thus, a printout might include the univariate *t* values for each individual dependent variable to allow for such a comparison.

3. *Probabilities.* Just as in univariate methods there will be a probability level associated with the Hotelling's *T* squared as well as with each of the univariate *t*-tests done to follow up the multivariate results.

The example provided in Figure 7.12 might result in the findings illustrated in Box 7.7. Note that the researcher first examines Hotelling's *T* squared to see if the three dependent variables taken as a unit significantly differentiate the two groups. Then univariate *t*-tests are used to determine which of the three variables made the most individual contributions to the difference.

Earlier in this chapter we illustrated how the ANOVA1 was an extension of the basic *t*-test and can be used when the researcher is studying more than two groups.

> ### BOX 7.7
>
> ### *Output of MANOVA1 on Two Groups*
>
> Two groups of participants were compared on speech discrimination scores, ability to process speech in noise, and otoacoustic emissions data. One group had conductive hearing loss and the other exhibited sensorineural hearing loss. The results of a multivariate analysis of variance (MANOVA) revealed a significant difference between the two groups on all three dependent measures taken as a unit (Hotelling's $T^2 = 9.56$; df = 3; $p = .001$). A series of univariate t-tests for each dependent variable individually showed that speech discrimination scores ($t = 5.98$; df = 48; $p = .001$) and speech in noise scores ($t = 4.67$; df = 48; $p = .009$) contributed to the difference more than otoacoustic emissions scores ($t = 2.03$; df = 48; $p = .042$).

It works in a similar manner for the MANOVA. The basic MANOVA for two groups illustrated in Box 7.7 utilizes Hotelling's T squared to determine whether the three dependent variables taken as a group differentiated the two groups of participants with hearing loss. Hotelling's T squared is the most common multivariate statistic for comparing two groups and is not typically used when more than two groups are being studied. This is very similar to the situation in which a t-test is used for two groups and an ANOVA1 is used for three groups. To study differences among three groups with multivariate statistics one would use a MANOVA1. There are a couple of important differences in the output of a MANOVA1. First, as stated, Hotelling's T squared is not typically used for three groups but rather one of several multivariate measurements such as **Wilk's Lambda, Roy's largest root,** or **Pillai's trace.** These measures are typically quite similar in the way they indicate what is basically a significant multivariate F-ratio and will typically come up with the same basic result. The most common measure used in the MANOVA is Wilk's Lambda (Λ); thus, we will use it in our examples. We mentioned previously that after obtaining a significant Hotelling's T squared, the researcher examines univariate t-tests to determine which of the dependent variables made the greatest contribution to the significant difference obtained. Similarly, when one obtains a significant Wilk's Lambda, the most common procedure is to look at univariate one-way ANOVAs containing F-ratios for each individual dependent variable to determine which ones made the most powerful contributions. As an example of output, let's expand the study of conductive and sensorineural hearing loss in Figure 7.12 to include another group of participants with mixed hearing loss. Again, we have just added a level to our independent variable of group and now have three groups to compare (Box 7.8). Whereas Hotelling's T squared is used for two groups, MANOVA1 is used for three or more groups and will output a Wilk's Lambda, degrees of freedom, and a probability level. Just as with univariate t-tests and ANOVA1s, MANOVA can be computed for both between and within subjects designs, and the outputs for both are similar.

BOX 7.8

Output of MANOVA1 on Three Groups

Three groups of participants with hearing loss (conductive, sensorineural, mixed) were compared on three dependent variables: speech discrimination score, speech in noise, and otoacoustic emissions. A multivariate analysis of variance (MANOVA1) was performed to determine if the three groups differed significantly on the three dependent measures. Results of the MANOVA1 showed that the three groups were significantly different on the three dependent variables taken as a unit (Wilk's Lambda = 3.89; df = 3; p = .001). Univariate F-ratios for the three dependent variables taken individually suggest that speech discrimination scores (F = 8.28; df = 2, 73; p = .001) and speech in noise scores (F = 6.34; df = 2, 73; p = .009) contributed to the difference more than otoacoustic emissions scores (F = 2.12; df = 2, 73; p = .049).

Summary

We started this chapter with a discussion of conceptual understanding of statistical methods. In our examples we spared you the mechanical aspects of statistical analysis, which, although critically important to researchers, are a bit less crucial to research consumers. The examples in the present chapter dealt with only one independent variable having two or more levels. Examples were given comparing two independent groups and two related groups that were analyzed using some form of t-test. Further examples were provided comparing three or four independent or related groups analyzed using some form of ANOVA1. We also presented nonparametric statistics that are analogous to the t-test and ANOVA1. Finally, we introduced the concept of multivariate statistics that analyze two or more groups on multiple dependent variables simultaneously. In the next chapter we will expand the ideas we have discussed to include two and three independent variables.

LEARNING ACTIVITIES

1. Find a research article that uses an independent t-test. See if you understand the design and results.

2. Find a research article that uses a correlated t-test. See if you understand the design and results.

3. Find a research article that uses an ANOVA1 between subjects. See if you understand the design and results.

4. Find a research article that uses an ANOVA1 within subjects. See if you understand the design and results.

5. Find a research article that uses one of the nonparametric procedures discussed in this chapter. Do you understand why they use the procedure?

6. Find an article that uses a post hoc means comparison test mentioned in this chapter.

CHAPTER 8

Studies That Analyze Differences in Groups Using Factorial Designs with More Than One Independent Variable—Between, Within, and Mixed

I gather, young man, that you wish to be a member of Parliament. The first lesson that you must learn is, when I call for statistics about the rate of infant mortality, what I want is proof that fewer babies died when I was prime minister than when anyone else was prime minister. That is a political statistic.

—Winston Churchill (1874–1965)

I always like to look on the optimistic side of life, but I am realistic enough to know that life is a complex matter.

—Walt Disney (1901–1966)

There is only one way in which a person acquires a new idea; by combination or association of two or more ideas he already has into a new juxtaposition in such a manner as to discover a relationship among them of which he was not previously aware.

—Francis A. Carter

To manage a system effectively, you might focus on the interactions of the parts rather than their behavior taken separately.

—Russell L. Ackoff

This chapter is concerned with factorial designs that allow us to compare groups with more than one independent variable. Thus far, we have only covered one independent variable, but you can easily see that in real life, and in real research, more than one variable comes into play when affecting the results of a study. While this chapter might stretch your synapses a bit, it is critical to understand factorial designs. They are probably the most common type of design used in scientific literature. We will try to ease into these designs in a logical way.

LEARNING OBJECTIVES

This chapter will enable readers to:

- Understand factorial designs in research and the difference between main effects and interaction effects.
- Understand between subjects, within subjects, and mixed factorial designs in research.

- Understand the differences and similarities between analysis of variance and analysis of covariance.
- Understand the basics of how MANOVA is extended into factorial designs.

The world would be a simple place indeed if it were univariate and just dealt with a single independent variable. But alas, things are never as simple as they seem nor as uncomplicated as we would prefer. In reality, many independent variables coalesce to influence our dependent variables and seldom can a single dependent variable account for the complexity of human behavior. Let's consider a hypothetical example. In this illustration we find some studies demonstrating that girls are ahead of boys in language development at age three. If we just believed that finding without asking any further questions, we would have "the truth" all tied up in a nice, tidy package. However, most people would not be prepared to say "the language development of girls is superior to boys at age three" without some qualifications. For instance, they might wonder if girls from lower socioeconomic levels would have language development that is more advanced than boys from the middle class. Others might ask about boys and girls from rural versus urban environments. Still others might ask about boys and girls from different family structures such as two-parent families versus single-parent families or those who spend a lot of time in daycare. People might ask about the measure of language that was taken on the boys and girls and if the measure encompassed all the areas of linguistic ability such as semantics, morphology, phonology, syntax, and pragmatics. Obviously, there are other questions to ask and these queries point out the fact that there are very few simple statements of "truth" that can be made without taking into account multiple variables. This is why researchers have developed techniques to analyze the effects of more than a single independent variable on a dependent variable. It would be easy to gather language development scores on a group of girls and a group of boys and do an independent t-test to find if they are significantly different. We know, however, that probably more goes into a child's language development than just gender alone. Researchers must go beyond examining single independent variables to see the effects of other influences on a dependent variable of interest.

Two-Factor ANOVA (Between Subjects)

You will recall that the ANOVA1 refers to a one-way or one-factor analysis of variance. It only examines the effect of a single independent variable on a dependent variable. The two-factor analysis of variance is sometimes referred to as an ANOVA2 or two-way analysis of variance. The reference to the number two highlights the fact that two independent variables are examined in this analysis. We can illustrate this using the example regarding boys and girls and language development at age three. You can see from Figure 8.1 that the group of fifty boys scored lower than the group of fifty girls on the language test that represented the dependent variable. The independent variable is gender, which has two levels (boys/girls). As you probably have already noticed, if we were only interested in gender, we could leave the design as it is in Figure 8.1 and just do an independent t-test to determine if boys and girls are different on their language scores. But what if a researcher wanted to find out if socioeconomic level also affected language development in boys and girls? To answer such a question would require another independent variable added to the experimental design. In

FIGURE 8.1

Comparing Two Groups

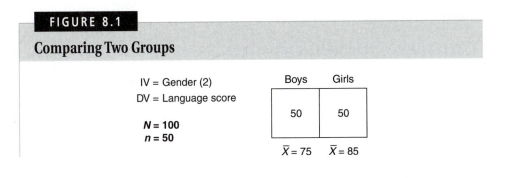

IV = Gender (2)
DV = Language score

N = 100
n = 50

Boys   Girls

| 50 | 50 |

$\bar{X} = 75$ $\bar{X} = 85$

Figure 8.2 below you can see we have added another IV to the design, which has two levels (low/middle).

We have created what is known as a **factorial design,** because it has two **factors** or independent variables. Factorial designs are often referred to by the number of IVs they contain, so our new example might be called a 2 × 2 factorial design. Factorial designs have a number of "cells" or boxes included in them representing each level of every independent variable. Thus the number of cells in a 2 × 2 factorial design is 4. In our example there is a cell for lower-SES boys, one for lower-SES girls, one for middle-SES boys, and one for middle-SES girls. It will ultimately be analyzed using a 2 × 2 ANOVA. When we say "2 × 2" we mean that there are two independent variables each having two levels. Two-way ANOVAs can take on many different appearances, as illustrated in Figure 8.3.

The important fact to remember is that they are called two-factor ANOVAs because they have two independent variables. The figure shows a 2 × 2 ANOVA, a 3 × 2 ANOVA, and a 3 × 3 ANOVA. Just having three or four **levels** to an independent variable does not increase the number of independent variables, only the number of levels of the independent variable. Later, when we talk about three-way ANOVAs, we will give examples of designs that are 2 × 2 × 2, which means there are three independent variables, each

FIGURE 8.2

ANOVA2 Between Subjects

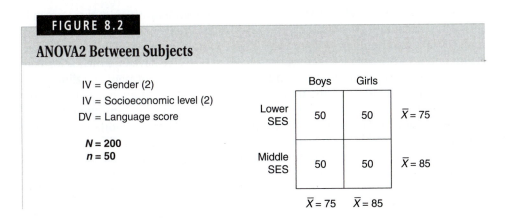

IV = Gender (2)
IV = Socioeconomic level (2)
DV = Language score

N = 200
n = 50

Boys   Girls

Lower SES | 50 | 50 | $\bar{X} = 75$

Middle SES | 50 | 50 | $\bar{X} = 85$

$\bar{X} = 75$ $\bar{X} = 85$

FIGURE 8.3

Types of Two-Factor Analyses of Variance

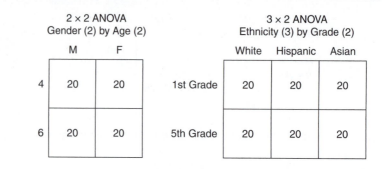

2 × 2 ANOVA
Gender (2) by Age (2)

	M	F
4	20	20
6	20	20

3 × 2 ANOVA
Ethnicity (3) by Grade (2)

	White	Hispanic	Asian
1st Grade	20	20	20
5th Grade	20	20	20

3 × 3 ANOVA
SES (3) by Hearing Loss (3)

	Lower SES	Middle SES	Higher SES
Conductive	20	20	20
Sensorineural	20	20	20
Mixed	20	20	20

with two levels. You can always know how many independent variables there are in a design by just counting the numbers (e.g., 2 × 2 is two IVs; 3 × 3 × 2 is three IVs).

Let's take another look at Figure 8.2, which was our example of language scores of girls and boys using a 2 × 2 factorial design. First of all, we have four means instead of two as in the earlier example (Figure 8.1). Two means represent the difference between boys and girls, and the other two means show the difference between the lower- and middle-SES levels. These four means are often called **marginal means,** partly because they are in the margins of the design. There is another important term used to refer to marginal means as they relate to the analysis of variance: **main effects.** In the Figure 8.2 design, there is the possibility of a main effect for gender and another main effect for SES. The term *main effect* simply refers to the possible difference between the levels of one of the independent variables. Thus, in this design we can have a significant main effect for gender if it turns out that the girls are better than boys on the language measure and the probability is less than .05. We could also have a significant main effect for SES if the lower-SES group does not score as well as the middle-SES group on the language test and the probability is less than .05. These main effects will be tested by the analysis of variance, and we will be told by its results if we have a significant main effect for age or a significant main effect for SES or both. We will also be told if we have a significant **interaction effect,** which is a combination of both gender and SES. We will wait until a later section to illustrate an interaction effect. For now, let's look at the output of the 2×2 ANOVA.

Output

1. *F-ratios.* You will recall from the last chapter that the ANOVA1 produces a single *F*-ratio used to determine whether there is a significant difference among three groups. If your *F* is significant in that case, you know that at least two of the three groups are significantly different. In the ANOVA2, the output produces *three F-ratios.* One *F*-ratio will be provided for each IV (the two main effects) and one for the inter-action effect. In our example we have two IVs (gender/SES). One *F*-ratio will represent the main effect for gender, and the other will represent the main effect for SES. That is, the ANOVA will tell us whether the boys and girls are significantly different (main effect for gender) as well as whether the SES groups are significantly different (main effect for SES). The third *F*-ratio will represent the interaction effect of gender × SES and tell us if some combination of these two variables was significant.

2. *Probabilities.* Just as in the ANOVA1 and the *t*-test, each *F*-ratio will be accompanied by a probability level. The *p* level means exactly the same thing as it did when we discussed it in the last chapter. Most of the time, researchers will regard their differences to be statistically significant if $p < .05$. This means that only five times out of a hundred will this difference be due to chance or sampling error.

3. *Degrees of freedom.* You will remember that df are provided in the *t*-test and ANOVA1 and are used to look up critical values of *t* and *F*. Degrees of freedom are also mentioned in the results sections of research articles involving the analysis of variance.

4. *Post hoc testing.* If post hoc tests are necessary to compare more than two means, these should be reported in the results section of the article.

5. *Effect size.* Just as effect size was an important indicator of practical significance for *t*-tests and one-factor ANOVAs, it is expected that it will also be reported in factorial designs.

A sample output from our ANOVA2 example as it might appear in the results section of an article is shown in Box 8.1. Bruning and Kintz (1997) provide good examples of the mathematical computations of most factorial designs discussed in this chapter, and any student interested in understanding such analyses is encouraged to consult this source. A gentle reminder about the hypothetical results presented in the text boxes. We know you will be tempted to skim over these examples or ignore them entirely. However, it is a goal of this textbook to expose you to how researchers might present the findings of their statistical analyses. When you can read through all of

BOX 8.1

Output from ANOVA2 Between Subjects

The means for the two gender groups and the two socioeconomic status groups were subjected to a two-way analysis of variance between subjects. The results of the ANOVA2 showed a significant main effect for gender ($F = 5.34$; df = 1, 196; $p = .041$) with the boys earning lower scores on the language measure ($\bar{X} = 75$) than the girls ($\bar{X} = 85$). There was also a significant main effect for SES ($F = 4.96$; df = 1,196; $p = .042$) with the lower-SES group ($\bar{X} = 75$) earning lower language scores than the middle-SES group ($\bar{X} = 85$). There was also a significant interaction effect ($F = 5.98$; df = 1, 196; $p = .03$). Results of the Newman-Keuls post hoc procedure showed that the mean on the language measure for the boys in the lower-SES group was lower than all other groups.

our results boxes and explain the results of a study to one of your classmates, you have mastered at least the basics required to understand the results of an experiment. Practice, as they say, makes perfect.

The results of this study as shown in the Box 8.1 clearly state that two significant main effects were found in the investigation. Boys' scores were significantly lower than girls' scores on the language measure, and lower-SES groups' scores were significantly lower than middle-SES groups' scores on the same measure. Now let's explore the meaning of the interaction effect, which was also statistically significant.

Interaction Effects

In Figure 8.4 below we have taken the $n = 50$ out of each cell and replaced them with the actual cell means on the language test earned by the four groups. For example, the lower-SES boys earned a mean of 65 on the language test. The lower-SES girls got a mean of 85, as did the middle-SES boys and girls. You should be able to see four cell means and four marginal means in the figure.

FIGURE 8.4

2 x 2 ANOVA with Cell Means

IV = Gender (2)
IV = Socioeconomic level (2)
DV = Language score

$N = 200$
$n = 50$

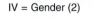

	Boys	Girls	
Lower SES	$\bar{X} = 65$	$\bar{X} = 85$	$\bar{X} = 75$
Middle SES	$\bar{X} = 85$	$\bar{X} = 85$	$\bar{X} = 85$
	$\bar{X} = 75$	$\bar{X} = 85$	

As we discussed in the previous section, the marginal means help us to interpret the main effects of the analysis of variance for gender and SES. The cell means help us to interpret any interaction effect that may have been found. You will recall that the ANOVA2 produces three F-ratios, one for each main effect and one for the interaction effect. In Box 8.1 we said that the ANOVA resulted in a significant main effect for gender ($F = 5.34$; df = 1, 196; $p = .041$), a significant main effect for SES ($F = 4.96$; df = 1,196; $p = .042$), and a significant interaction effect ($F = 5.98$; df = 1, 196; $p = .03$). The significant interaction effect means that some combination of the two independent variables of gender and SES came together to make a unique contribution to the results of the study. In other words, there is some unique combination of gender and SES that creates the real meaning in the results of this study. Therefore, we introduce an old adage associated with the analysis of variance that states: *In the presence of a significant interaction, significant main effects are uninterpretable.* Bordens and Abbott (2002, p. 400) say: "Consequently, you should avoid interpreting main effects when an interaction is present."

We will try to explain what this wise old axiom really means. First, let's take another look at the main effects. There was a significant main effect for gender indicating that girls scored higher than boys on the language test by ten points. But is this really true? Do all girls score higher than boys on the language test? If you look at the cell means, it is fairly clear that only in the lower-SES girls do score higher than boys. Girls and boys in the middle class have identical scores on the language test. Thus, it would be erroneous to say "Girls scored higher than boys." Looking at the other main effect for SES, you can see that the middle SES scored higher than the lower SES by ten points. Again, you have to ask yourself if this is really true. The cell means show that the only reason the marginal means for SES favored the middle class was because of the lower-SES boys. In fact, the lower and middle SES groups of girls scored identically. What the significant interaction effect tells us is that there is something special about being male and lower SES at the same time that affects the results of this study.

And now, back to the axiom. You should be able to see why a significant interaction makes it impossible to make general statements about gender or SES *independently* in this study. Those main effects cannot be interpreted as significant because, by themselves, they would distort the results of the investigation. Thus, when investigators obtain a significant interaction effect, most of their discussion surrounds the combination of the two independent variables on the data instead of dwelling on the main effects. The main effects still have to be reported in a research article; however, they should not be "interpreted" if there is a significant interaction effect. Some researchers report main effects first, followed by interaction effects, whereas others reverse this order because significant interactions are the most important.

If the analysis of variance results in an interaction effect, the researcher must perform post hoc analyses just as he or she did when an ANOVA1 with three groups resulted in a significant F-ratio. In our example, the researcher would have to compare the four cell means with one another to determine which cell was unique. It is fairly simple in the example to see that the lower-SES boys are the cell that stands out as different. It is not always this obvious, and the researcher will compare all four cells using one of the post hoc tests mentioned in Chapter 7 to find out the nature of the

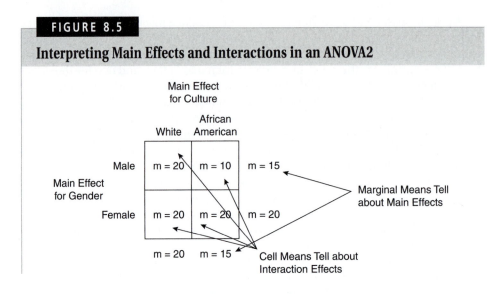

FIGURE 8.5

Interpreting Main Effects and Interactions in an ANOVA2

interaction effect. Figure 8.5 summarizes how to interpret main effects and interactions in a 2 × 2 ANOVA.

We have to give one more example to illustrate an important point about designs that have more than two levels to one or more of the independent variables. Lets add one more socioeconomic group to the design depicted in Figure 8.4 above. We already have lower and middle, so we will add higher SES to our social class independent variable. As you can see from Figure 8.6 we have created a 2 × 3 design. Each cell contains the *n* (50) and the mean for the cell on the language measure. As with the 2 × 2 design, we will have three *F*-ratios in our output: one for the gender main effect, one for the SES main effect, and one for the interaction effect of gender × SES.

You may remember that in our 2 × 2 design, we had to do post hoc tests for the significant interaction because we had to determine which of the four means in the four cells were significantly different from one another. We found that the mean for the lower-SES boys was significantly different from all the others. In the case of the design in Figure 8.6, we have a situation in which one of our independent variables has three levels and one has only two levels. If a main effect for gender is statistically significant, there is no need to perform a post hoc test because there are only two means under consideration (boys and girls). If, however, the main effect for SES is significant, the design in Figure 8.6 requires the researcher to do post hoc tests on the three SES levels to determine which of the three means are significantly different from one another. This is much the same situation as when you do an ANOVA1 with three levels. The significant *F*-ratio just indicates that there is a significant difference, but the post hoc test will help the researcher determine which of those three means are different.

The results shown in Box 8.2 demonstrate that we had two significant main effects and one significant interaction effect. You can see that we had to do post hoc

---

FIGURE 8.6

ANOVA2 Totally Between Subjects

IV = Gender (2)
IV = Socioeconomic level (2)
DV = Language score

$N = 300$
$n = 50$

	Boys	Girls	
Lower SES	50 $\bar{X} = 65$	50 $\bar{X} = 85$	$\bar{X} = 75$
Middle SES	50 $\bar{X} = 85$	50 $\bar{X} = 85$	$\bar{X} = 85$
Higher SES	50 $\bar{X} = 85$	50 $\bar{X} = 95$	$\bar{X} = 90$
	$\bar{X} = 82$	$\bar{X} = 88$	

---

testing on the main effect with three levels (SES) to see which groups were significantly different. We also had to do post hoc comparisons on the cell means because we got a significant interaction effect. In these results, there is something special about being a lower-SES male that contributes to scoring lower on the language measure. Likewise, there is something unique about being a higher-SES female that contributes to higher scores on the language measure. Although we got significant main effects, they do not tell the whole story about language performance in this study. The important result is in the interaction between SES and gender; any discussion of significant main effects would be inappropriate.

BOX 8.2

Output for 2 × 3 ANOVA Between Subjects

A between subjects 2 × 3 ANOVA was conducted on the language scores of children from three different socioeconomic levels. One factor was gender, with two levels (boys/girls), and the other factor was SES, with three levels (L/M/H). There was a significant main effect for gender ($F = 6.87$; df = 1,294; $p < .01$) with boys scoring lower than girls. There was also a significant main effect for SES ($F = 9.33$; df = 2,294; $p < .01$). A post hoc means comparison using the Tukey procedure showed that there were significant differences ($p < .01$) among all three of the SES groups, higher SES scoring the highest followed by middle and lower SES groups. The two-way interaction of gender × SES was also significant ($F = 6.71$; df = 2,294; $p < .01$). Post hoc comparisons revealed that the lower-SES boys were significantly ($p < .01$) lower on language scores as compared to all other groups and the higher SES girls were significantly higher on language scores compared to all other groups.

Two-Factor ANOVA (Within Subjects)

The same logic used in explaining the ANOVA2 between subjects can be implemented in illustrating the ANOVA2 within subjects. Remember that in the between subjects ANOVA2 each participant only experienced one level of each independent variable. Thus, the lower-SES boys only experienced being lower SES and male. In the ANOVA2 totally within subjects design, every participant experiences all levels of each independent variable. Let us say, for example, that we wanted to determine if people who stutter reduce or increase their disfluency under a number of different conditions. In this example we will use masking noise level as one IV (20 dB and 60 dB) and the grammatical complexity of a reading passage (simple and complex) as the other independent variable. Therefore, we have concocted a 2 × 2 design. Now we could do this study totally between subjects if we wanted to have four groups of participants each experiencing only one level of each independent variable. It would, however, be difficult to match the four groups for stuttering type and severity and other relevant attributes. Thus, we decide to do the study totally within subjects; each participant will experience every level of each independent variable. If you were a participant in this study you would read the simple passage with 20 dB of masking noise, the simple passage with 60 dB of masking noise, the complex passage with 20 dB of masking noise, and the complex passage with 60 dB of masking noise. Figure 8.7 illustrates what such a design would look like. The arrows that point to the right and downward suggest that the twenty participants will experience all of the conditions in the study. Of course the participants would be exposed to the four conditions in a counterbalanced order to control for the threats to internal validity associated with repeated measures designs such as order effects, practice, fatigue, and so on.

The output of the ANOVA2 within subjects design is essentially similar to the between subjects version. The researcher will end up with three *F*-ratios: one for the main effect of masking level, one for the main effect of grammatical complexity, and one for the interaction effect of masking × complexity. Just as in the between subjects design, if each IV has only two levels, no post hoc testing for main effects is necessary;

FIGURE 8.7

ANOVA2 Totally Within Subjects

IV = Masking level (2)
IV = Reading passage complexity (2)
DV = Percent disfluency

N = 20

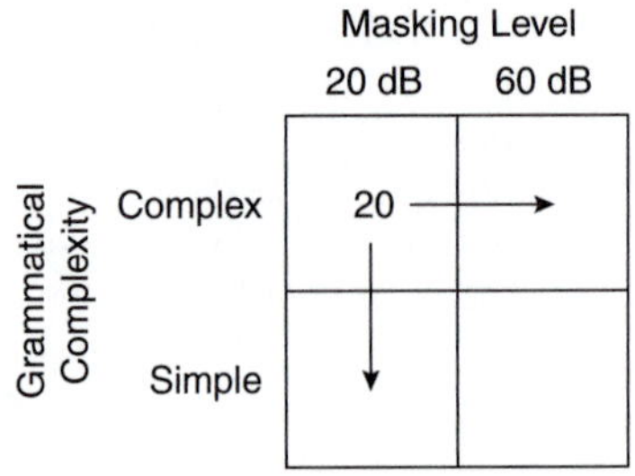

however, post hoc tests must be done in the presence of a significant interaction effect. The results of the study might look like the data in Box 8.3. Since each IV only had two levels and the interaction was not significant, there is no need for post hoc testing.

Three-Factor ANOVA (Between Subjects)

Most students are put off by the appearance of the ANOVA3 design because it looks somewhat like a prototype for a new condominium project with lots of apartments (cells) stacked on top of one another in a three dimensional arrangement. Figure 8.8

FIGURE 8.8

ANOVA3 Between Subjects (3 × 3 × 4)

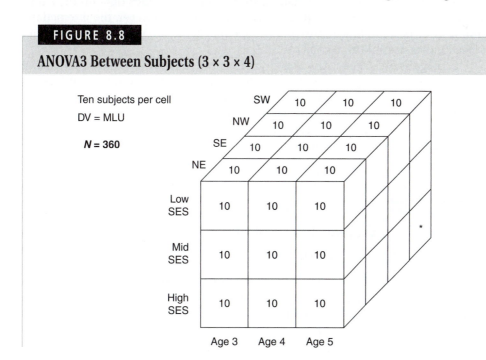

depicts a 3 × 3 × 4 ANOVA that is totally between subjects. From the three numbers in the factorial design we can see that there are three independent variables. One is geographical location with 4 levels (NE, SE, NW, SW), one is age (3, 4, 5), and the other is socioeconomic level (lower, middle, higher). The dependent variable is mean length of utterance. Remember that in the between subjects design, participants only experience one level of each independent variable, shown by how the cells are segregated with ten participants in each block. This means that we will have ten lower-SES three year olds from the northeast in one cell, and so on. See if you can find the cell that contains the higher-SES five year olds from the southwest. That's right, it is the cell on the bottom of the back row on the right side with the asterisk on it.

Output

The output of the ANOVA3 is a bit more complicated than the ANOVA2, but if you understand the logic of the F-ratios in the ANOVA2, you will have no trouble with this one.

1. *F-ratios.* You will recall that the ANOVA2 produced three F-ratios: one for the main effect for each independent variable and one for the interaction of the two independent variables. Our prior ANOVA2 example included a main effect for gender, a main effect for SES, and an interaction effect of gender × SES. In the ANOVA3 example above we have three independent variables of geographical location, age, and SES. Just as in the ANOVA2, we must have an F-ratio to represent a main effect for each of those independent variables, so that is three F-ratios right off the bat in the ANOVA3. Because we have three IVs in the ANOVA3, however, the interactions among those IVs are a little more complicated than in the ANOVA2. Box 8.4 shows all of the F-ratios possible in the ANOVA3.

2. *Degrees of freedom.* The degrees of freedom for an ANOVA3 are predictably more complicated than the simpler analyses of variance; however, some things remain the same. For instance, the degrees of freedom for each independent variable are the number of levels minus one. Thus, the df for geographical location in the previous example would be 3 because there are four levels. Similarly, the df for SES and age would be 2, since each of those variables has three levels. Regarding interactions,

---

BOX 8.4

The Seven F-ratios *Produced by the ANOVA3*

- Main effect of geographical location
- Main effect of age
- Main effect of SES
- Two-way interaction of geographical location × age
- Two-way interaction of geographical location × SES
- Two-way interaction of age × SES
- Three-way interaction of geographical location × age × SES

you just have to multiply the relevant variables to obtain the df for the two- and three-way interactions. Therefore the age × SES interaction would be 4 (two times two). The two-way interaction between geographical location and age would be 6 (three times two), and so on. The three-way interaction would also find degrees of freedom by multiplying all three factors (2 × 2 × 3 = 12).

   3. *Probability.* The probability will be computed for each of the three main effects and four interaction effects. Thus, there will be seven probability figures telling the researcher if any of the main effects or interactions are statistically significant.

   4. *Post hoc testing.* In the case of significant main effects (with more than two levels) and significant interaction effects, post hoc tests will be done to determine which levels are significantly different. The same post hoc tests used in ANOVA1 and ANOVA2 are used with the ANOVA3.

   5. *Effect sizes.* Just as with the ANOVA2, effect size measures can be reported for statistically significant main effects and interactions as a gauge of clinical or practical significance.

For the example of the 3 × 3 × 4 ANOVA, the results might look like the information depicted in Box 8.5. Note that three *F*-ratios are reported for the three main effects. Three more *F*-ratios are reported for the three **two-way interactions,** and one more *F*-ratio represents a **three-way interaction.** Post hoc tests need to be done on the significant main effects because there are three levels in each of them. Since the interaction of age × SES is significant, the post hoc test had to compare all cell means that combined different levels of age and SES, which means that the following comparisons had to be made: L3, L4, L5, M3, M4, M5, H3, H4, H5. Because the interaction was significant, it overrides the significant main effects in the interpretation of the findings.

BOX 8.5

Output for ANOVA3 Between Subjects

The data on mean length of utterance were subjected to a between subjects three-way analysis of variance. There were significant main effects for age ($F = 7.12$; df = 2, 324; $p = .01$) and SES ($F = 8.45$; df = 2, 324; $p = .01$). The main effect for geographical area was not significant ($F = 0.45$; df = 3, 324; $p = 0.98$). The two-way interaction of age × SES was significant ($F = 5.91$; df = 4, 324; $p = .02$) and the interactions of age × geographical region ($F = 0.89$; df = 6, 324; $p = 0.45$) and SES × geographical region ($F = 0.75$; df = 6, 324; $p = 0.39$) were not significant. Finally, the three-way interaction of age × SES × geographical region was not significant ($F = 1.11$; df = 12, 324; $p = 0.34$). Post hoc testing using the Newman-Keuls procedure revealed that the five year olds had significantly higher MLUs as compared to the three year olds ($p < .01$). For the main effect of SES, the higher-SES children had significantly higher MLUs compared to the lower-SES group ($p < .01$). The significant two-way interaction of age × SES was analyzed with the post hoc test and the three year old, lower-SES children had significantly lower MLUs as compared to all other age/SES groups ($p < .01$).

Three-Factor ANOVA (Within Subjects)

The three-factor ANOVA within subjects is similar to the between subjects version in terms of assumptions and output. The biggest difference is that each participant will experience all levels of the three independent variables. Figure 8.9 illustrates the three factor within subjects ANOVA using an example study of twenty patients with aphasia who have word retrieval problems. We want to determine if word retrieval is improved as we manipulate three different independent variables. The first is use of pictures or objects as stimuli to having the patient retrieve words. The second is use of words that are more difficult semantically (e.g., wrench) versus fairly easy (e.g., cup). The third independent variable is the cue that we use in trying to elicit the word. One cue would use a question ("What is this?"), and another cue would illustrate what function the object is associated with ("You tighten a nut with a _____"). A participant in this study using repeated measures on all three independent variables would experience the following eight conditions representing every combination of the different levels of the IVs: picture/difficult question, picture/easy question, picture/difficult function, picture/easy function, object/difficult question, object/easy question, object/difficult function and object/easy function. Again, as in any repeated measures study, these conditions would be experienced in a counterbalanced order to control for threats to internal validity. The beauty of the ANOVA3 within subjects, like any factorial design, is that it can tease out the individual and interactive effects of the independent variables on word retrieval to determine which individual or combination of variables results in the most effective naming, as shown by the sample results in Box 8.6.

FIGURE 8.9

ANOVA3 Within Subjects (2 × 2 × 2)

The same 20 subjects experience all levels of each IV

IV = Word difficulty
IV = Picture/Object
IV = Question/Function cue
DV = Word retrieval

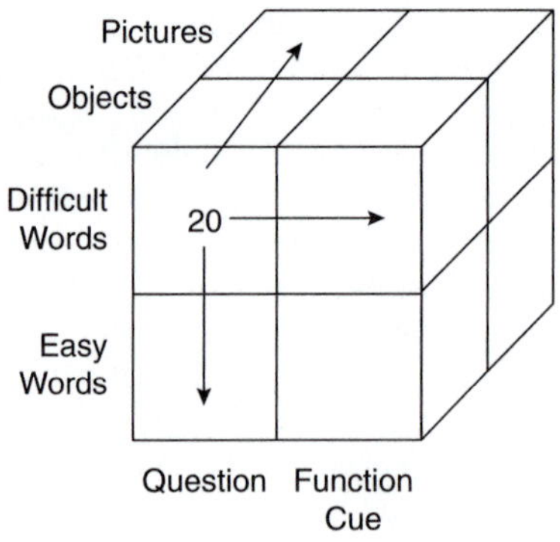

Pictures
Objects

Difficult Words   20

Easy Words

Question   Function
Cue

BOX 8.6

Output for ANOVA3 Within Subjects

The word retrieval data were subjected to a within subjects ANOVA3. The independent variables were stimulus type (picture/object), word difficulty (easy/difficult), and type of cue (question/function). There were significant main effects for word difficulty ($F = 9.11$; df = 1, 19; $p = .01$) and type of cue ($F = 7.32$; df = 1,19; $p = .02$). In these significant main effects the easy words were retrieved more often than difficult words and the function cue was superior to the question cue in facilitating word retrieval. The main effect for stimulus type was not significant ($F = 0.69$; df = 1,19; $p = .89$). Analysis of interaction effects revealed a significant interaction between word difficulty and type of cue ($F = 8.33$; df = 1,19; $p = .01$). The other two-way interactions, stimulus type and word difficulty ($F = 0.77$; df = 1,19; $p = .54$), as well as stimulus type and cue type ($F = 0.64$; df = 1,19; $p = .87$) were not significant. Similarly, the three-way interaction was also not significant ($F = 0.79$; df = 1,19; $p = .80$). Post hoc testing of the significant word difficulty × cue type interaction revealed that easy words elicited with the function cue were the most effectively retrieved compared to all other combinations of difficulty and cueing method.

Two-Factor Mixed ANOVA with Repeated Measures on One Factor

A "mixed" design typically refers to a factorial arrangement with mixed between sub-jects and within subjects variables in the study. In the ANOVA2 the only possibility for a mixed design is to have one factor between subjects and one factor within subjects. Figure 8.10 illustrates a design comparing children with normal language to children with specific language impairment on mean length of utterance while talking about pictures or objects during a language sample.

FIGURE 8.10

ANOVA2 Mixed Design with Repeated Measures

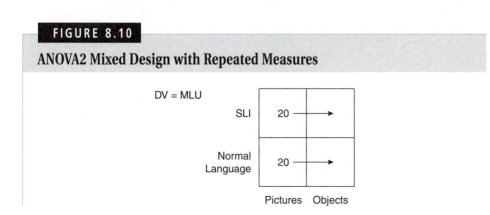

BOX 8.7

Output from a Mixed ANOVA2

Data were subjected to a mixed two-way ANOVA with language status (group) as the between subjects factor and stimulus type (picture/object) as the within subjects factor. The children with normal language abilities had a significantly higher MLU compared to the children with SLI ($F = 12.45$; df = 1,38; $p = .001$). The main effect for picture/object was not significant ($F = 1.12$; df = 1,39; $p = .27$) nor was the group × picture/object interaction ($F = 0.74$; df = 1,39; $p = .67$).

As you can see from the design, the between subjects variable is group (normal language or SLI). Obviously, a participant can only experience one level of the group independent variable since one cannot be both SLI and have normal language at the same time. The within subjects variable is whether pictures or objects were used as stimuli. As indicated by the arrows, the twenty participants in each group experience both levels of the picture/object factor, hopefully in a counterbalanced order to control for threats to internal validity with results shown in Box 8.7.

Three-Factor Mixed ANOVA with Repeated Measures on One Factor

Obviously in an ANOVA3 mixed design it is possible to have repeated measures on one factor or two factors. As long as there is some combination of between and within subjects independent variables it is still a mixed design. Our example of a mixed design in Figure 8.11 involves two between subjects factors and one within subjects

FIGURE 8.11

Mixed Design with Repeated Measures on One Factor (2 × 2 × 2)

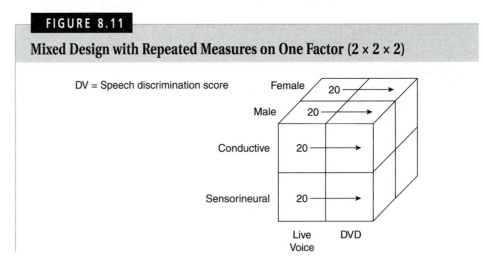

BOX 8.8

Output from a Mixed ANOVA3 with Repeated Measure on One Factor

The results of the speech discrimination test were subjected to a three-way analysis of variance with repeated measures on one factor. The two between subjects variables were gender (male/female) and type of hearing loss (conductive/sensorineural). The within subjects variable was presentation mode (live voice/DVD player). The main effect for type of hearing loss was significant with the sensorineural group scoring significantly lower than the conductive group ($F = 12.45$; df = 1,77; $p < .01$). The main effect for gender was not significant ($F = 0.44$; df = 1,77; $p > .05$). The main effect for presentation mode was significant with higher discrimination scores earned in the live voice condition ($F = 2.45$; df = 1,76; $p < .05$). The two-way interactions of gender × group ($F = 0.88$; df = 1,77; $p > .05$) and presentation mode × gender ($F = 0.66$; df = 1,76; $p > .05$) were not significant. The two-way interaction of group × presentation mode was significant ($F = 4.56$; df = 1,76; $p < .05$). The three-way interaction was not significant ($F = 0.34$; df = 1,76; $p > .05$.) Post hoc means comparison testing of the significant two-way interaction between hearing loss type and presentation mode using the Scheffé procedure revealed that the group with sensorineural hearing loss performed significantly ($p < .05$) better in the live voice condition as compared to all other combinations of hearing loss type and presentation mode.

---

factor. In this study we want to compare participants by gender (male/female) and type of hearing loss (conductive/sensorineural) as between subjects independent variables. Our within subjects factor is whether the discrimination test is presented via live voice or from a DVD recording. Thus, we have concocted a 2 × 2 × 2 mixed design. A participant in this study experiences every level of the within subjects variable, both live voice and DVD measures. The other independent variables are between subjects (gender and type of hearing loss) that cannot be experienced at more than one level of either variable. Some hypothetical results are presented in Box 8.8.

Three-Factor Mixed ANOVA with Repeated Measures on Two Factors

An example of a three-factor mixed design with repeated measures on two factors is presented in Figure 8.12. This study has one between subjects independent variable, which is severity of word finding problems in patients with aphasia (mild anomia/severe anomia). One of the within subjects factors is type of cue presented, investigating the efficacy of phonetic cues versus functional cues. An example phonetic cue is showing the patient a picture of a dog and if the patient has difficulty retrieving the word the investigator produces the first consonant sound by saying "d." The function cue is the investigator stating a function associated with the picture (by saying, "it barks.") The other within subjects factor is word familiarity. In this study the

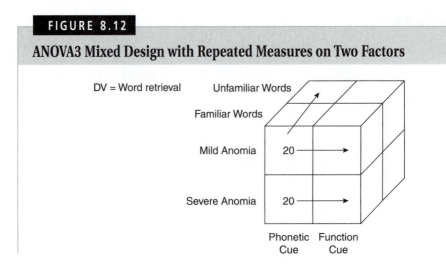

FIGURE 8.12

ANOVA3 Mixed Design with Repeated Measures on Two Factors

participants were allowed to look at a pile of pictures prior to the naming task so they would be "familiar" with the stimuli. Another pile of pictures were not presented to the participant prior to the word retrieval task and thus "unfamiliar." If participants in this study as a person having mild anomia experience four conditions: familiar words with function cues, familiar words with phonetic cues, unfamiliar words with function cues, and unfamiliar words with phonetic cues. The results are presented in Box 8.9.

BOX 8.9

Output from a Mixed ANOVA3 with Repeated Measures on Two Factors

In order to examine the effects of the independent variables an ANOVA3 with repeated measures on two factors was conducted. The between subjects factor was group (severe anomia/mild anomia). The within subjects factors were type of cue (phonetic/ function) and word familiarity (familiar/unfamiliar). There was a significant main effect for group ($F = 30.98$; 1,38; $p = .001$) with the mild anomic patients retrieving more words than the severe group. There was also a significant main effect for word familiarity ($F = 23.78$; df = 1, 114; $p = .001$) with the familiar words retrieved more effectively than the unfamiliar words. The main effect of cue type was not significant ($F = 0.78$; df = 1,114; $p = .46$). The two way interaction of group × familiarity was significant ($F = 14.56$; df = 1,114; $p = 001$). A Newman-Keuls post hoc means comparison showed that the severe anomic group retrieved significantly ($p < .01$) more words in the familiar word condition as compared to all other combinations of group and word familiarity. The other two-way interactions of group × cue ($F = 0.99$; df = 1,114; $p = .88$), word familiarity × cue ($F = 0.96$; df = 1,114, $p = .79$), and the three-way interaction ($F = 1.02$; df = 1,114; $p = .91$) were not significant.

Analysis of Covariance (ANCOVA)

The analysis of variance is perhaps the most widely used statistic in the research literature, and so we have devoted quite a few pages to discussing the most common experimental designs using the procedure. Although not used nearly as frequently as the ANOVA, the **analysis of covariance (ANCOVA)** is still used often enough to warrant the attention of a textbook for research consumers. This introductory text will not be able to go into too much detail about ANCOVA other than a flavor for what the analysis does. For the most part, ANCOVA operates similarly to the ANOVA, with the same underlying statistical assumptions as the ANOVA, plus a few additional ones such as independence of the covariate from the independent variable, homogeneity of regression slopes, and linearity (see Huck, 2004) that are beyond the scope of our text. Second, the ANCOVA can be used in experimental designs with one, two, or three factors, just like the ANOVA. Third, the ANCOVA produces F-ratios for main effects and interactions just as the ANOVA does. Fourth, the ANCOVA can be used in between subjects, within subjects, and mixed designs. Fifth, the ANCOVA is concerned with independent and dependent variables just like the ANOVA. Finally, the ANCOVA can use the same post hoc means comparison procedures (e.g. Newman-Keuls, Scheffé, etc.) as the ANOVA. At this point you are probably asking yourself, "With all these similarities, what makes the ANCOVA different?"

One factor differing analysis of covariance from traditional analysis of variance is the addition of another variable called a **covariate** to the independent and dependent variables. Actually, more than one covariate can be added to the equation; we'll start with one for simplicity in introducing the concept. A covariate is more similar to the dependent variable than the independent variable. By that we mean that the covariate shares a conceptual similarity with the dependent variable or in many cases the covariate actually *is* the dependent variable. Let's break the last sentence down and try to explain it more effectively. Say that a researcher is interested in two methods of training narratives (independent variable) for children with language disorders. The specific measurement (dependent variable) to be used is the length of their narratives in words on a posttest after the treatment period. The researcher finds a large pool of children with language disorders and randomly selects one hundred participants for the study. Each child is randomly assigned to one of the two training groups, with fifty children in each group. One of the first things the researcher does is administer a pretest requiring each child to produce a narrative to be used as a baseline of comparison for posttreatment narratives.

Let's say the initial pretest results looked like those in Table 8.1. It is easy to see that even though the researcher assigned the children randomly to the two treatment conditions, the group assigned to the control group had a higher pretest score in terms of number of words used in the narratives before the treatment. Any differences in the posttest scores must be considered in light of the initial differences between the groups in pretest scores. Obviously, we could just disregard the initial differences in the pretest scores and just do a one-way ANOVA on the dependent variable (posttreatment narrative scores). Since there is a difference of ten points

TABLE 8.1

Pretest/Posttest Design with Two Groups Differing at Baseline

Group	Mean Pretest Narrative Length	Mean Posttest Narrative Length
Control	35	60
Therapy	45	70

between the posttreatment scores of the groups, it may well result in a significant difference between the groups and the possible conclusion that the treatment was more effective than the control group. However, any researcher worth his or her salt would be bothered by the difference in the pretest narrative scores and want to do some damage control. One option would be to eliminate selected participants with high or low scores on the pretest and balance the groups on pretest scores. A problem with this is the researcher definitely compromising the random selection and random assignment having now tampered with it. Another problem is that by eliminating participants costs power and increases the probability of a Type II error. This is where analysis of covariance becomes effective. By using the ANCOVA the researcher compensates *statistically* for initial pretest differences without losing any participants or threatening the random assignment. The ANCOVA uses narrative scores on the pretest as a covariate. From a conceptual perspective, the analysis of covariance takes into account initial differences between the groups on the covariate (pretest) by adjusting scores on the dependent variable (posttest) downward for those scoring higher on the covariate versus upward for those scoring lower. The "adjusted mean" for the dependent variable takes into account initial differences on the pretest or covariate. You can see in Table 8.2 that the means on the posttest have been statistically adjusted based on the pretest performance of each group. The adjusted means are much closer together to preclude a statistically significant difference between the groups when analyzed with the ANCOVA. The analysis of covariance uses quite a complex process to achieve this balance that is beyond the scope of the present text

TABLE 8.2

ANCOVA Compensating for Pretest Group Differences

Group	Mean Pretest Narrative Length	Mean Posttest Narrative Length	Adjusted Posttest Means
Control	35	60	63
Therapy	45	70	66

to cover. For consumers of research, it is enough to know that the ANCOVA can be used to statistically compensate for initial differences in groups.

Output

The output associated with the ANCOVA is identical to the information provided for the analysis of variance. That is, you will see F-ratios, degrees of freedom, and probability levels for every main effect and interaction involved in the design. An ANCOVA2 will similarly have three Fs and an ANCOVA3 will have seven. Post hoc testing using the multiple comparison procedures discussed with the ANOVA (e.g., Newman-Keuls, Scheffé, etc.) are also used with the analysis of covariance. It is also common to see some measure of practical significance such as Cohen's d, eta squared, or omega squared.

Factorial Multivariate Analysis of Variance (MANOVA)

The details of the factorial multivariate analysis of variance are far too complex to cover in the present textbook. This section merely lets you know that factorial MANO-VAs are often used, interpreted as defining the effects of multiple independent variables on several dependent variables taken as a group. Remember that the univariate factorial ANOVAs discussed earlier in this chapter dealt with only a single dependent variable. In the last chapter we illustrated that the MANOVA can be used to compare two groups on multiple dependent variables using Hotelling's T^2. We also gave an example of MANOVA as an extension of the ANOVA1 in comparing three or more groups on one independent variable when measuring multiple dependent variables. The output of the MANOVA1 included a multivariate F-ratio in the form of Wilk's Lambda, Roy's largest root, or Pillai's trace, all used to tell us about significant differences among groups on all dependent variables taken as a group. The researcher then can use the results of univariate F-ratios to determine which dependent variables played the largest role in differentiating groups. There are also MANOVA counterparts for all factorial designs such as the ANOVA2 and ANOVA3 for between subjects, within subjects, and mixed designs such as those shown earlier in this chapter. The multivariate F-ratios (e.g., Wilk's Lambda) resulting from factorial MANOVAs represent main effects and interactions, just as the univariate F-ratios illustrated in designs using ANOVA2 and ANOVA3. A significant multivariate main effect, for instance, means that there was a significant difference for levels of an independent variable for all of the dependent variables taken as a group. Just as with the MANOVA1, univariate F-ratios are one of the options used to explore which dependent variables contribute most to the significant multivariate F-ratios.

Summary

We have attempted to show that the factorial designs presented in this chapter are merely extensions and combinations of the t-test and one-way ANOVA. The major difference is that additional independent variables were added to make the designs factorial in nature. We also tried to illustrate that factorial designs can be between subjects, within subjects, or mixed designs combining the two. Because of their ability to determine main effects and interactions among the different independent variables, factorial designs are probably among the most powerful in our literature. The factorial analysis of variance is no doubt the most common statistical method you will encounter in reading research articles. We hope that our relatively simplistic discussion of these methods will make you more able to interpret the results presented in articles.

LEARNING ACTIVITIES

1. Using the design notation presented in this chapter draw the following designs: 2×3 between subjects, 2×2 within subjects, $3 \times 3 \times 2$ between subjects, $3 \times 2 \times 2$ within subjects, 2×3 mixed, and $3 \times 3 \times 3$ mixed with repeated measures on one factor.

2. For the designs drawn in activity one, try to include independent and dependent variables that make sense for the studies.

3. For the designs created, think about which variables need to be controlled to have strong internal validity.

CHAPTER 9

Studies That Measure Relationships among Variables or Attempt Prediction

All science is concerned with the relationship of cause and effect. Each scientific discovery increases man's ability to predict the consequences of his actions and thus his ability to control future events.

—Lawrence J. Peters

There is only one way in which a person acquires a new idea; by combination or association of two or more ideas he already has into a new juxtaposition in such a manner as to discover a relationship among them of which he was not previously aware.

—Francis A. Carter

The invalid assumption that correlation implies cause is probably among the two or three most serious and common errors of human reasoning.

—Stephen Jay Gould (1941–2002)

It's tough to make predictions, especially about the future.

—Yogi Berra

The previous two chapters have dealt with finding significant differences among groups when they are compared on one or more dependent variables. The present chapter focuses on relationships among variables and the ability to predict performance on one variable from performance on another. So an important thing for you to do at the outset of this chapter is to put the notion of group differences out of your mind for a while and concentrate on how variables correlate with one another.

LEARNING OBJECTIVES

This chapter will enable readers to:

- Understand the basic nature of relationships expressed in research including direction, strength, significance, and importance.
- Be able to list nonparametric correlation procedures used to define relations among variables.
- Understand the purpose of a bivariate regression analysis.

- Be able to see how multivariate procedures for studying relationships and prediction extend from basic univariate techniques.
- Understand the purpose of doing a multiple regression, canonical correlation, discriminant analysis, and factor analysis in research.

The Nature of Relationships

A relationship between two variables can be characterized in a number of ways. Some of the most important characteristics of a relationship include the direction of the relationship, the strength of the relationship, and the significance of the relationship. We will discuss each of these in the following sections.

Direction of a Relationship

Figure 9.1 illustrates a **scattergram** of the typical positive relationship between chronological age in years and mean length of utterance (MLU) in normally developing children. You can see that there are fifteen data points on the scattergram, each representing a single child. Each data point is placed on the scattergram to represent *both* the score for MLU and chronological age. For example, the data point at the bottom left of the scattergram represents a child who is one year old and has an MLU of 1.0. We have drawn arrows from each axis so you can see how that data point stands for these values. All of the other data points on the scattergram represent the two scores for the other fourteen children in the sample. One thing to notice about the data points is that they kind of form a line that rises as the values move from left to right. We have drawn a solid line through the data points representing the **line of best fit** between all of the individual dots. Basically a scattergram like Figure 9.1 shows that as age increases, MLU also increases. It is known as a **positive relationship** because as the MLU value goes up, the age value goes up as well. It is sometimes best to think of a positive relationship as one in which the two variables move in the same direction, either up or down. You can see that it would be accurate to say that as age

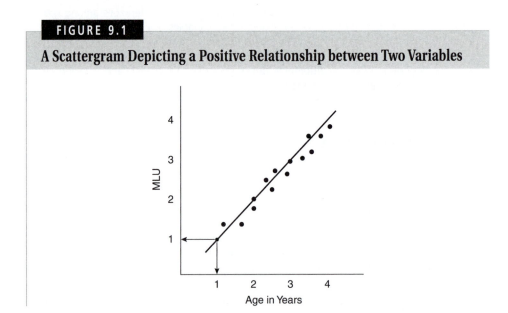

FIGURE 9.1

A Scattergram Depicting a Positive Relationship between Two Variables

FIGURE 9.2

A Scattergram Depicting a Negative Relationship between Two Variables

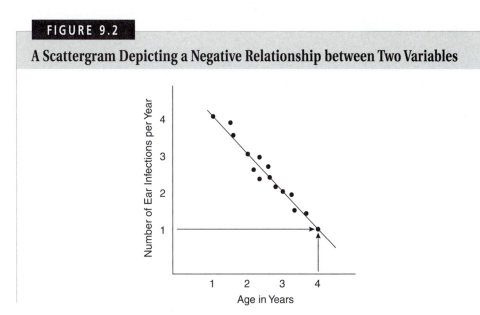

increases, MLU increases, but it would be just as true to suggest that as age decreases, MLU decreases. Even though in the latter statement age and MLU are going down, they are still moving in the same direction and it remains a "positive" relationship.

Figure 9.2 shows a scattergram depicting a **negative relationship** between two variables. This time we have age on one axis and the number of ear infections reported per year for fifteen children. You can see that the number of ear infections at age four is lower than the number of infections at age one. Again, each data point represents both age and the number of ear infections reported for each child. The line of best fit goes downward as you move from left to right on the scattergram, suggesting that as one variable goes up, the other variable goes down. They are moving in opposite directions. As age goes up, the number of ear infections goes down and as ear infections go up, age goes down.

The direction of a relationship is very important because it tells us how two variables change in relation to one another. In articles you will read about positive and negative relationships or correlations and they are really talking about whether variables move in the same direction or in opposite directions.

Strength of a Relationship

The scattergram can also reveal the strength of a relationship in addition to its direction. Strength of a relationship is illustrated by how close the data points are to the line of best fit. If they are tightly aligned along the line of best fit as in Figures 9.1 and 9.2, the relationship is strong. If the data points are arrayed as depicted in Figure 9.3, the relationship is weak or nonexistent. This scattergram shows the relationship between chronological age and number of siblings living with a particular child.

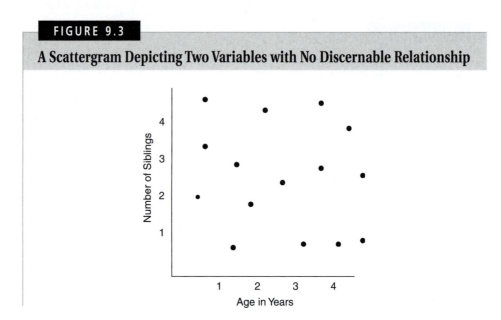

FIGURE 9.3

A Scattergram Depicting Two Variables with No Discernable Relationship

It is almost as if you cannot really have a line of best fit because the data points are nowhere near to forming a line that points in a particular direction. Just by looking at the individual data points, you can see that there are younger children with many siblings and older children with few. There does not seem to be a pattern that you can count on. Thus, one way to get a general idea about the strength of a relationship is to look at the density of the data points on a scattergram and see if the arrangement of the data points points to a positive or negative relationship. The greater the density of the data points and the more they form a line pointing either up or down, the stronger the relationship.

You might have already surmised that scrutinizing the arrangement of data points on a scattergram might be analogous to reading tea leaves in fortune telling. Obviously, different people could have varied opinions about the strength and direction of the data points while viewing a scattergram, and it might be difficult to obtain good agreement among these individuals. Fortunately for researchers, there are statistical methods that have been designed to characterize the strength as well as direction of the relationship between two variables. Probably the most common statistic for this purpose is the **Pearson product-moment correlation coefficient,** or Pearson r. It is called the Pearson r because the statistic generates a value called r, which is always somewhere between −1.00 and +1.00.

The basic assumptions for using the Pearson r are similar to those discussed when covering parametric statistics for analyzing differences between groups (e.g., normal distribution, homogeneity of variance, etc.) It is assumed that the Pearson r is computed on continuous data such as interval or ratio. The Pearson r assumes that the two variables you are examining have a **linear relationship** to one another. This means that a plot of the relationship forms a fairly straight line. An important issue is the presence of "outliers" that may dramatically affect the correlation coefficient. An outlier is a participant with an "extreme" score that appears to be unusual compared to the rest of the sample. If there appeared in Figure 9.1 a data point representing a four-year-old child with an MLU of 1.0, this clearly would reside far away from the line of best fit and be easily understood as an outlier. The presence on a scatterplot of scores on two variables of outliers not arrayed close to a line of best fit can throw off the correlation in terms of strength or direction. The effect of outliers is especially strong with a small sample.

Figure 9.4 illustrates the correlation coefficients produced by the Pearson for both positive and negative relationships. The zero point in the center of the graph represents no correlation between two variables. A scattergram of a zero correlation would resemble Figure 9.3. Note that as you move to the right or left from the zero point, the *r* coefficients become larger, either positively or negatively as they approach 1.00. The 1.00 indicates a "perfect" correlation between two variables. The more the *r* coefficient deviates from plus or minus 1.00 toward zero, the weaker the relationship between the two variables becomes. An important thing to remember is that the strength of the relationship is indicated by the value of the Pearson *r* coefficient. Thus, the closer to –1.00 or +1.00 the coefficient is, the stronger the relationship. Correlations closer to plus or minus 1.00 would produce scattergrams similar to Figures 9.1 and 9.2. This brings up the critical point that values of +1.00 and –1.00 have *exactly the same strength*. Positive correlations are not any stronger than negative ones. The plus and minus signs *only indicate the direction,* whereas the numerical coefficient of *r shows the strength* of the relationship. Thus, as we mentioned earlier, researchers

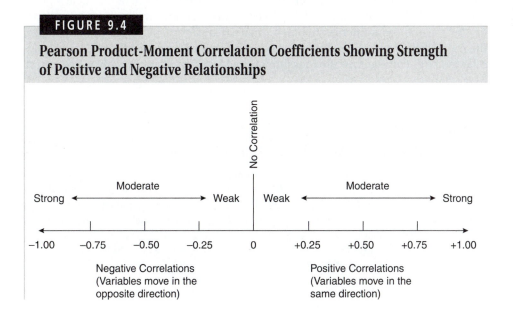

FIGURE 9.4

Pearson Product-Moment Correlation Coefficients Showing Strength of Positive and Negative Relationships

are not limited to pondering the density of data points on scattergrams to determine the strength of a relationship. The Pearson *r* will tell precisely the strength of the correlation that exists between two variables and whether the relationship is positive or negative.

Significance of a Relationship

Throughout many previous chapters we have extolled the virtues of probability levels in research. It is one thing to compute a *t* value or an *F* value, but it is quite another thing to know how much confidence you can have that the result was not due to chance or sampling error. The same situation exists with the Pearson *r* coefficient. Let's say you do the Pearson and come up with a result of +0.80. First of all, you should be able to tell that the correlation is a positive one in which the two variables are moving in the same direction. You should also know that the strength of the relationship is fairly high because it is relatively close to +1.00. It is certainly stronger than a coefficient of +0.35. When the Pearson product-moment correlation coefficient is computed by hand, you will be referred to statistical tables, just as you were when computing *t*-tests or ANOVAS to determine the probability level of your result. If your calculated value exceeds the critical value of *r* for your study at a specific probability level, you have a significant correlation. If you use a computer program to compute the *r*, it will print out the exact probability level. Thus, when you read an article that has used the Pearson *r* on two variables, the result might look like those in Box 9.1. Note that the direction, strength, and probability of the correlation are all provided in the explanation of the results.

Importance of a Relationship and Accounting for Variance

You may recall that in an earlier chapter we discussed the issue of practical significance. For studies that examine differences between groups, we presented a number of effect size measurements such as Cohen's *d* statistic. The larger the effect size, the more likely it is that the difference between groups is practically or clinically significant. With correlations, the measure of practical significance involves how much

---

BOX 9.1

Output of Pearson Product-Moment Correlation

The purpose of this investigation was to determine the relationship of intelligence quotients on the Stanford-Binet Test of Intelligence and the number of misarticulated phonemes they exhibited on the Goldman Fristoe Test of Articulation in children with cognitive impairment. The Pearson product-moment correlation coefficient between Stanford-Binet and Goldman Fristoe scores was −0.93 ($p < .001$). This suggests a strong and highly significant negative relationship between IQ and misarticulation showing that as IQ scores went down the number of misarticulations increased in this population.

variance we can account for by knowing about a relationship between two variables. In the example presented in Box 9.1 the Pearson r was −.93, significant beyond the $p < .001$ level of confidence. This, of course, means that the strong negative relationship between IQ and misarticulations would be found by chance only one out of one thousand times. Thus, we know that this relationship is negative, strong, and probably not due to chance or sampling error. To address the issue of practical significance, researchers are always interested in the **coefficient of determination** or r^2. If you square the value of r you will arrive at the coefficient of determination, telling you something about the practical significance of r. In our example, −.93 squared would be .8649. What this value tells the researcher is that approximately 86 percent of the variance in misarticulations in the population of people with mental retardation is accounted for by knowing a person's IQ score. This leaves about 14 percent of the variance unaccounted for by IQ. Obviously, there may be other factors accounting for misarticulations, such as motor skill, age, structural anomalies, and so on, but IQ seems to account for the majority of the variance in misarticulations. This relationship is illustrated in Figure 9.5. On the other hand, let's say that the Pearson r for this relationship was −.30 instead of −.93. If you square the −.30 you come up with a coefficient of determination of only .09, which means the relationship only accounts for 9 percent of the variance. That means that 91 percent of the variance in misarticulations remains unexplained and must be accounted for by other factors. Obviously, the more variance accounted for by a relationship, the more practical significance exists.

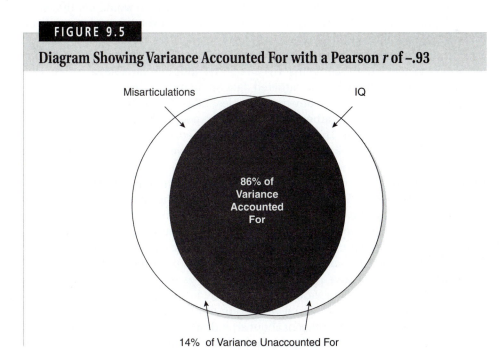

FIGURE 9.5

Diagram Showing Variance Accounted For with a Pearson r of −.93

Misarticulations

IQ

86% of Variance Accounted For

14% of Variance Unaccounted For

Accounting for variance also helps give an idea about the possible accuracy of predicting one variable value from another. For such a strong relationship as the one between IQ and misarticulations we would probably be fairly accurate in predicting number of misarticulations from knowing a person's IQ score. At least, we would be fairly accurate for groups of people and less accurate for any single individual. We could, for example, predict that a classroom of children whose mean IQ was 45 would probably have more misarticulations than a classroom of children with a mean IQ of 60. For Johnny Benson, whose IQ is 58, we could still make a prediction of fewer misarticulations but the accuracy of predicting for an individual would most likely be far less than for groups.

This brings us to an important point in considering correlations. You have no doubt heard the famous phrase "Correlation does not imply causation." This means that the two variables' movement in the same or different directions may not be caus- ally related. In the case of IQ and misarticulations, it would not be accurate to say that lower IQ *causes* misarticulations. There are many other factors in children with lower IQ that could relate to misarticulation. As mentioned previously, children with lower IQ could have poorer motor skills, significant language impairment, poorer pho- nological awareness, more structural abnormalities, more neurological issues, and so forth. IQ as a construct is just a "macrovariable" that encompasses many other factors that individually or in combination could be responsible for causing misarticulations. Another example concerns direction of causation. There is usually a big correlation between the appearance of umbrellas and the occurrence of rain. The more rain, the more umbrellas appear, constituting a positive correlation. We would bet that such a correlation would be statistically significant as well. However, it would certainly be inaccurate to say that umbrellas cause rain just because they are strongly correlated.

The Pearson *r* can be used to compare any two variables, given they represent in- terval or ratio data, but the comparisons can only be done two variables at a time. This means that a researcher who has gathered data on many variables can examine cor- relations with the Pearson *r* on any two variables. Table 9.1 illustrates a hypothetical example of many variables gathered in a university speech and hearing clinic regard- ing response to treatment. The table represents how correlations between variables can be depicted in a **correlation matrix.** Let us note several things about the matrix in Table 9.1. First of all, there are twelve variables related to clinical treatment, each assigned a number from one to twelve. To find out the correlation between any two of the variables you just find the cell in the matrix where they intersect. For example, if you wanted to find the correlation between client age and the number of sessions missed, you would put your finger on the sixth row and move to the right until you reach the seventh column. In this cell it tells you that the correlation between client age and number of sessions missed is –.86. From our prior discussion you should know that this is a negative relationship; as age goes up, the number of sessions missed tends to go down. You should also know that if you square the *r* value you find that age accounts for .7396 or about 74 percent of the variance in missed sessions. Maybe older clients are more diligent about attending treatment, or perhaps children tend to be sick more often. Also, notice that the correlation has two asterisks next to

TABLE 9.1

Correlation Matrix Showing Pearson Product-Moment Coefficients for Treatment Variables in a University Speech and Hearing Clinic

	1	2	3	4	5	6	7	8	9	10	11	12
1	1.00	.90**	.02	.22	.31	.16	.65	.35	.92***	.95***	.88***	.32
2		1.00	.05	.68	−.76*	.24	.20	.36	.89***	.91***	.82**	.78*
3			1.00	.02	.11	.14	−.68*	.20	.03	.92***	.10	.24
4				1.00	.65	.72	.59	.85**	.91***	.20	.85**	−.89***
5					1.00	−.78*	.43	−.88***	.38	.25	.94***	.31
6						1.00	−.86**	.25	.34	.10	.22	.23
7							1.00	−.84**	.95***	.20	.12	−.75*
8								1.00	−.56	.34	.85**	.98***
9									1.00	.21	.94***	.51
10										1.00	.12	.24
11											1.00	.92***
12												1.00

***Significant at < .001
**Significant at < .01
*Significant at < .05
1—Treatment Intensity (hrs/wk)
2—Severity of Communication Disorder Pre-Treatment
3—Client Annual Income Level
4—Number of Hours Clinician Experience
5—Severity of Communication Disorder Post-Treatment

6—Client Age
7—Number of Sessions Missed
8—Client Satisfaction Score
9—Number of Hours of Treatment for Dismissal
10—Dollars Spent on Treatment
11—Number of Additional Diagnoses
12—Supervisory Intensity (% time)

it in the matrix; this means that the correlation was significant at $p < .01$ or beyond chance. A researcher would say that this represents a significant negative correlation. Finally, notice what is left out. Half the matrix is blank. If we were to fill in the blank cells with correlations, it would be a mirror image of the completed portion of the matrix. In essence, the lower portion of the matrix would be redundant with the upper portion. Thus, in research articles that report correlations only the upper portion of the matrix is provided in a triangular shape. Also, along the "main diagonal" every correlation is 1.0, because any variable correlates perfectly with itself since the scores are identical. Research reports leave out not only the redundant part of the correlation matrix but the main diagonal as well. We will be returning to this correlation matrix later on in this chapter to illustrate some more advanced techniques of correlation and prediction.

Nonparametric Correlation Procedures

The Pearson product-moment correlation coefficient is for use with interval or ratio data. In an earlier chapter we indicated that the level of measurement represented by the data to be analyzed is critical to selecting a statistical analysis. If the data are not interval or ratio, the researcher will probably use a nonparametric or distribution-free

TABLE 9.2

Levels of Measurement in Nonparametric Statistics Used to Determine Relationships

Variable 1	Variable 2	Statistic
Ordinal	Ordinal or interval/ratio	Spearman rho
Ordinal	Ordinal	Kendall tau
Interval	Ordinal	Biserial correlation
Interval	Nominal	Point-biserial correlation
Nominal	Nominal	Phi coefficient

statistic to determine whether a relationship exists between two sets of variables. Table 9.2 shows five different nonparametric procedures and the types of data they are designed to analyze to determine if a relationship exists between two sets of variables. In the case of all of these methods, there is a way to determine if the relationship is statistically significant either by using another procedure such as a *t*-test or looking up the computed result in a table of critical values. We will briefly discuss each of these methods.

The **Spearman rho** correlation coefficient is used with two sets of rank-ordered data that are ordinal or higher in nature. For instance, if we wanted to determine whether teacher rankings of classroom performance are related to IQ, we could rank order the teacher rankings and rank order the IQ scores of the students in the class and determine whether there was a relationship between the two rankings. The **Kendall rank-order correlation** (symbolized with tau) examines the relationship between two sets of ranked ordinal variables and is often used as a substitute for the Spearman rho.

The **biserial correlation coefficient** is used when the researcher with both interval and ordinal data wants to examine their relationship. The biserial correlation computes a value known as r_b and a significance level can be determined using a version of the *t*-test. A related computation known as the **point biserial correlation** is used when one variable is continuous (interval data) and one variable is categorical (nominal data). It is calculated similarly to the Pearson *r*. The value that is computed in the point biserial correlation is r_{pb}. A final nonparametric relationship statistic is called the **phi coefficient** (Φ) used when both variables are nominal or dichotomous. A contingency table is constructed to show the relationships between the two categorical variables.

As in our earlier discussion of parametric and nonparametric statistics for studying group differences you can see that there are analogous procedures for examining relationships among variables. The determination of whether to use parametric or nonparametric statistics still revolves around the type of data to be analyzed (level of measurement) and the normality of the distribution. No matter which of the nonparametric procedures mentioned are used, the researcher will still be discussing how two variables relate to one another in terms of strength, direction, and significance.

Bivariate Regression Analysis: Prediction with a Single Independent and Dependent Variable

As stated in an earlier chapter, a major purpose of science is prediction. How can we use existing data to predict unknown information for groups of individuals? For instance, we know that there is a strong positive correlation between the pure tone average (PTA) of 500, 1000, and 2000 Hz and the speech recognition (reception) threshold (SRT) in speech audiometry (at least for people without functional, nonorganic hearing loss). In other words, the higher your PTA the higher your SRT. If, for example, we knew your score on the PTA, how could we predict your score on the SRT? The answer is to develop a regression equation in which the independent (predictor) variable is the PTA and the dependent (predicted) variable is the SRT. You would have to develop what is called a **regression equation** in order to make the prediction. The classical regression equation is $y' = a + b(x)$, with the y' representing the dependent variable or the score you are trying to predict, which in our example is the SRT. The x stands for the independent or predictor variable, which is the PTA. The a in the formula represents the "intercept," which is "where the regression line in the scatter diagram would, if extended to the left, intersect the ordinate" (Huck, 2004, p. 424). The a is also called a "constant" in that it is the same in the formula for all predictions. The b in the equation stands for the slope of the least squares regression line that minimizes the distances between observed and predicted individual scores. In essence, the regression line between the data points is described mathematically by the regression equation. Although it is beyond our purpose to further discuss regression, the important point to understand is that the equation allows the researcher to predict one score from another when data are plugged into the formula. If we put in the constants a and b from statistical computation and solve: $y' = 5.2 + .43(x)$ after inserting our known value for x, our result is the predicted value of y'.

Obviously, the predictions made from a regression equation are not perfect. Researchers interested in the efficiency of their predictions can address this by comparing the differences between predicted scores and actual scores. These differences are called **residuals,** and if the regression equation does a good job of predicting, the residuals will be low. Researchers can also compute the **standard error of the estimate,** which is also an indicator of the average amount of error in predictions made by the formula. Even the value of the Pearson r can tell the researcher how strongly two variables relate to one another; the r^2 would be an indication of the variance that might be accounted for in one variable by knowing about the other.

Let's use another example of **bivariate regression** that we will carry through in our later discussion of prediction. In this example, the director of a speech and hearing clinic would like to make predictions about client satisfaction with the services provided. Using bivariate regression, the director could input a piece of information about the client as an independent (predictor) variable and use the bivariate regression to predict the degree of client satisfaction on a rating scale questionnaire administered to all patrons of the clinic. The director has a lot of clinical data on the clients who come to the clinic for treatment. You will remember that Table 9.1 depicted a correlation matrix with such clinical variables earlier in this chapter. We will use those same variables to extend our discussion of correlation to bivariate regression. If the clinic director wanted to predict the dependent variable of client satisfaction score, one good strategy would be to examine correlations between the variables in Table 9.1 and client satisfaction. Clearly, the best bet at a potent predictor of client satisfaction would be a variable that has a high and significant correlation with this index and accounts for a significant amount of variance in client satisfaction. If you examine the matrix, you can see that there are three variables that have significant correlations with client satisfaction. First, the number of hours of clinical practicum experience the student clinician has accrued correlates positively (.85) with client satisfaction. The more practicum hours the student has, the more satisfied the clients seem to be. A second variable that significantly correlates with client satisfaction is the severity of the client's disorder posttreatment. The correlation here is a negative one (−.88), which suggests that the lower the severity at the time of dismissal, the higher the degree of client satisfaction. This probably suggests that the treatment worked to reduce severity below the level reported prior to receiving therapy, which is supported by the low correlation (.36) between satisfaction and severity level of the disorder *before* receiving treatment. The third variable correlated with client satisfaction is the number of treatment sessions missed. This also is a negative correlation (−.84), which suggests that the more sessions the client misses, the lower the degree of satisfaction with treatment. This is a good example of why correlations are not reliable indicators of cause and effect. It could very well be that clients missed sessions because they were not satisfied, or it could mean that they missed sessions and their lack of progress resulted in dissatisfaction. You simply cannot tell which one is the case. Now let's get back to the clinic director who wants to use bivariate regression to predict client satisfaction and must choose only one variable from the available data to use as a predictor. One strategy would be to choose the variable that is most highly and significantly correlated with the dependent variable of client satisfaction, which is severity of the disorder posttreatment, accounting for 77 percent of the variance in client satisfaction. If the director chose posttreatment severity as the independent variable and client satisfaction as the dependent variable a regression equation would have to be generated in which the "constants" are provided in the formula. Then the post-treatment severity score would be placed into the regression equation as the x and the predicted score (y') would be the satisfaction rating. In this way the director might be able to predict satisfaction ratings by examining severity ratings of clients at dismissal. The lower their severity rating, the higher their satisfaction rating should be. No doubt you are already thinking that, while interesting, it is not earthshaking to determine that if treatment is effective, clients will be more satisfied. Also, it is not particularly helpful for the director to only be able to predict client satisfaction when the treatment has concluded and the posttherapy severity rating becomes available. If another variable were accessible earlier in the treatment process, it might be possible to make efforts to improve client satisfaction as therapy progresses instead of waiting until the end of the process. We will be discussing some other options in the following sections.

Multivariate Procedures for Studying Relationships and Prediction

When we go beyond simple two-variable correlation and regression procedures like the Pearson r and bivariate regression, we are treading on very thin ice in terms of doing justice to the analyses we will discuss. The truth is, however, that you will encounter some of these analyses in the professional literature, and we feel that a basic understanding of what the methods are designed to accomplish will make these articles easier to digest. Thus, we will stick exclusively to a conceptual and very general treatment of these analyses knowing that there are hundreds of issues and exceptions that could be raised by statisticians (Anderson, 1984; Bartholomew, 1984; Cooley & Lohnes, 1971; Kim & Mueller, 1978; Morrison, 1990; Pedhazur, 1982; Ryan, 1997). Although we want to provide a sense of what can be accomplished with these procedures, we are not under any delusions about how difficult they are and how they can be misused and misinterpreted by both researchers and consumers.

The techniques mentioned below extend the Pearson r and bivariate regression procedures to encompass more variables. Figure 9.6 illustrates this expansion in a conceptual format so you can see the basic purposes of each analysis and how one builds on another.

Multiple Regression Analysis

The **multiple regression analysis** is an extension of the bivariate regression. Instead of having one independent variable to use in predicting the dependent variable, the researcher uses several independent variables to predict the value of a single dependent variable. The advantage of a multiple regression as compared to a bivariate regression is that the researcher can usually account for more variance in the dependent variable by increasing the number of predictors. For example, although it is possible to try to predict a student's graduate school grade point average with the single variable of his or her score on the Graduate Record Examination (GRE), as many students are already painfully aware, the GRE alone may not be an accurate predictor of their individual performance in graduate school; it may, however, be an accurate predictor for *groups* of graduate students. You have no doubt already concluded that it would be very difficult to find a single variable that would be an accurate predictor of almost any phenomenon. On the other hand, multiple predictors might increase the precision of your prediction considerably. For example, you might significantly increase the efficiency of your prediction of graduate school GPA if you used the student's undergraduate cumulative GPA, GRE score, GPA in the undergraduate major, and a composite score on a ten-point rating scale from faculty who recommend the student for acceptance. Using these four variables might make your prediction of graduate school GPA more effective than any single variable alone. In fact, it could be that using all five variables might account for 90 percent of the variance in graduate school GPA.

Conversely, you may be able to account for 85 percent of the variance in graduate school GPA by only knowing the two variables of undergraduate GPA in the major and

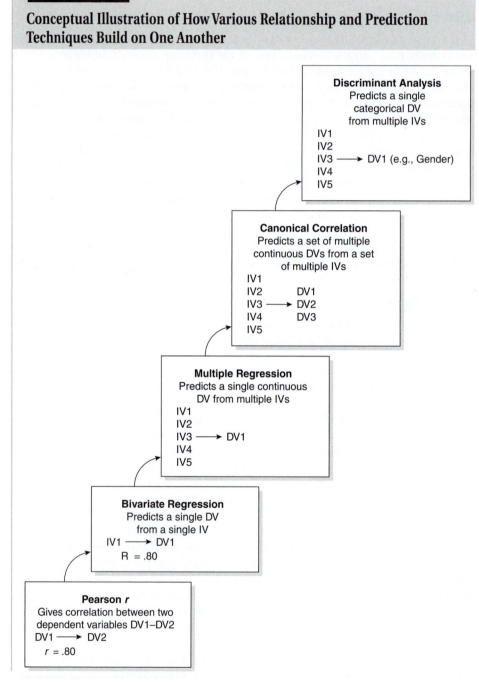

FIGURE 9.6

Conceptual Illustration of How Various Relationship and Prediction Techniques Build on One Another

Discriminant Analysis
Predicts a single
categorical DV
from multiple IVs
IV1
IV2
IV3 ⟶ DV1 (e.g., Gender)
IV4
IV5

Canonical Correlation
Predicts a set of multiple
continuous DVs from a set
of multiple IVs
IV1
IV2   DV1
IV3 ⟶ DV2
IV4   DV3
IV5

Multiple Regression
Predicts a single continuous
DV from multiple IVs
IV1
IV2
IV3 ⟶ DV1
IV4
IV5

Bivariate Regression
Predicts a single DV
from a single IV
IV1 ⟶ DV1
R = .80

Pearson *r*
Gives correlation between two
dependent variables DV1–DV2
DV1 ⟶ DV2
r = .80

GRE score. Anyone doing research on this issue would then have to ask the question: "Is it worth gathering data on all five variables in order to account for 90 percent of the variance in graduate GPA when you can account for 85 percent using only two variables? This illustrates an important notion in multiple regression: *We want to make the best predictions possible with the fewest variables.* It is always preferable for our predictions to be elegant and parsimonious rather than cumbersome and time-consuming. Gathering data on one hundred variables to make an accurate prediction would be neither elegant nor economical. If, on the other hand, we could make an accurate prediction about the same phenomenon with five variables, it would be a thing of beauty. Much research on educational, psychological, and medical issues uses multiple regression techniques to predict such things as academic success, response to treatment for depression, and risk of heart disease. All of these issues require gathering data on people and trying to predict present or future conditions. Typically the use of multiple predictors will be far more effective than a single predictor. Too many predictors, however, will be too cumbersome to be useful in the real world.

Multiple regression, like most procedures we have discussed, rests on a number of assumptions. We will mention some of these assumptions without too much detail to provide context for their use in research articles you might see typically while telling the reader that the assumptions have been met or controlled for in some manner. One assumption is that the relationship between the variables is *linear* in nature. If it is not linear or is curvilinear, the researcher will have to transform the data to increase linearity or not use the variable as a predictor.

Another important issue to deal with in many multivariate techniques is the presence of outliers. These participants with very extreme scores that can have a potent influence on the coefficients of many analyses we mention in this chapter. An outlier can have an extreme score on a single measurement or be a multivariate outlier in which the combined score for several variables is extreme. Sometimes outliers can be dealt with by data transformation, and in some cases all of the data from the offending participant can be removed from the analysis. In many research reports the researcher will discuss the presence of outliers and what was done to compensate for their appearance. We discussed the importance of a normal distribution in univariate statistics. This concept in multivariate statistics is called **homoscedasticity.** The researcher wants homoscedasticity and not heteroscedasticity. If the latter occurs, then data transformation may be required to normalize the data.

Another issue in multivariate analyses involves **multicollinearity,** a term used when variables are highly correlated with one another. In multiple regression, for example, you would not want to choose independent variables as predictors that were highly correlated with each other. In our example in Table 9.1, we could choose three variables that might predict client satisfaction ratings. If we chose intensity of treatment (hours per week), hours of therapy for dismissal, and dollars spent on therapy as independent variables to predict client satisfaction we probably would have a lot of multicollinearity. By looking at the correlation matrix you can see that the correlations among these three variables are all above .90, meaning they correlate strongly with one another. They may even be measuring the same thing. Therapy intensity involves number of hours per week scheduled, number of sessions prior to dismissal also involves hours of treatment, and dollars spent by the client pay for hours of treatment received. Thus, to prevent multicollinearity it is best to eliminate predictors highly correlated with one another because they will be redundant in accounting for variance in the dependent variable.

A final issue involves sample size. Although sample size varies with the statistic used, multivariate techniques discussed in this chapter usually involve larger numbers of participants, typically in the hundreds. With small samples, these techniques tend to be a lot less stable.

When a researcher uses multiple regression there are various ways that the independent variables are used to make predictions. The multiple regression equation is essentially an extension of the bivariate regression in which more constants and scores for independent variables (x) are systematically added. You can see from Figure 9.6 that the multiple regression is an extension of the bivariate regression in that there are multiple independent variables trying to predict a single dependent variable. Although it is not illustrated in Figure 9.6, the various types of multiple regression differ in part by the way the independent variables are entered into the regression analysis. For instance, in a **simultaneous multiple regression** (sometimes called a simple multiple regression) all of the predictor (independent) variables are entered together. In a **stepwise multiple regression** each predictor variable is entered one at a time depending on how much variance it accounts for or by the size of the Pearson r between the predictor variable and the dependent variable. In this way the researcher can see what the prediction is like for predictor variable 1 alone, then with predictor variables 1 and 2, then with predictor variables 1, 2 and 3, and so on. As variables are added in different combinations the researcher can see if the addition of a new predictor variable can improve the amount of variance (R^2) accounted for by the prediction model. For example, variable 1 may account for 30 percent of the variance in the dependent variable. The combination of variables 1 and 2 might increase the variance accounted for to 65 percent. The addition of variable 3 to the mix might only raise the variance accounted for to 66 percent and this might be viewed by the researcher as not very meaningful. If you can account for 65 percent of the variance with two variables, why add a third one that only contributes 1 percent to the prediction? When using stepwise regressions the researcher can opt to enter the variables in a forward stepwise regression, which adds one variable at a time depending on the strength of the correlation between the independent and dependent variable. This is done until all relevant variables have been added and as much variance as possible has been accounted for. Another method is the backward stepwise regression in which all variables are initially used in the prediction and then variables are removed to determine which ones make the greatest contribution to accounting for variance in the dependent variable. The point here is that the regression analysis will try to find the best combination of independent variables that leads to the best prediction of the dependent variable and accounts for the most variance with the fewest number of predictors.

Another type of regression is the **hierarchical multiple regression,** used by researchers to explore entering predictor variables in a particular way, usually based on some type of theoretical perspective. Often, they want to enter variables in such a way to "control for" the influence of one variable over another. Thus, in the hierarchical regression the variables are not necessarily entered in order by the strength of their correlation with the dependent variable or the amount of variance accounted for but more by the theoretical interest of the researcher. The goal, however, is still to identify the most efficient model to predict the dependent variable.

Returning to our example of the clinic director who wants to predict client satisfaction with the treatment experience, when we illustrated the bivariate regression, you could see that using only one independent variable to predict client satisfaction left something to be desired. We said in a prior chapter that "life is multivariate" and it is unrealistic to expect a single variable to effectively predict performance on another. In multiple regression, as we have stated above, we can use more than one variable as an independent variable and perhaps improve our ability to predict. You will recall that the strongest correlations with client satisfaction in Table 9.1 were posttherapy severity rating, number of practicum hours accrued by the student clinician, and the number of missed sessions. One approach to doing a multiple regression is to enter not only these variables but even some of the other ones that did not have high correlations with client satisfaction. It is possible that a variable may not have a strong relationship to the dependent variable individually, but it may have predictive value when combined with other variables. We could conceivably enter eleven predictors (independent variables) into the analysis in order to predict the dependent variable of client satisfaction although some may have to be eliminated because they are highly correlated with each other (multicollinearity). As mentioned above, there are many ways to approach the multiple regression in terms of entering independent variables into the prediction model. In some approaches, all variables are entered simultaneously. In other approaches variables are entered in various combinations determined by the amount of variance in the dependent variable they are likely to account for. At the end of the analysis, however, the researcher will be left with the most efficient regression model that uses the fewest independent variables to account for the most variance in the dependent variable. Some of this is done statistically, and some is done by the researcher making judgment calls on which variables make sense theoretically and account for sufficient variance in the dependent variable to justify their inclusion in the prediction model.

In our example posttreatment severity rating accounts for 65 percent of the variance by itself, but if you add the number of missed treatment sessions, the variance accounted for rises to 78 percent. The addition of number of practicum hours accrued by the student may only add another 1 percent to the prediction for a total of 79 percent. In this case, however, it might be the most elegant model to use posttreatment severity and missed sessions to make predictions about client satisfaction. The implication here is that the clinic may want to try and decrease missed sessions by use of counseling or incentives as early as possible in treatment. This, however, will not necessarily guarantee client satisfaction. Remember the old correlation-causation example given earlier. Clients could be missing sessions because they are already dissatisfied and hassling them about attendance may result in even lower satisfaction ratings. On the other hand, missed sessions may have an impact on treatment progress as reflected in severity level at dismissal. Probably an attempt at dealing with missed sessions early on in the treatment regimen is a good policy whether those sessions are a cause or an effect of client level of satisfaction. Regression is mostly about prediction, not cause and effect. This does not mean, however, that causal connections cannot be *initially hypothesized* from correlational or regression results. In many cases, correlations occur because one factor causes another; we just don't know if that is truly the case by just examining the results of a correlation or regression. There is a technique called **path analysis** in which causal relationships *are* the subject of interest, but it is beyond the scope of this chapter to discuss such procedures.

An important concept relating to multiple regression studies is the notion of **shrinkage.** According to Licht (2004) the multiple regression prediction model that you generate from the analysis is unique to the sample you have analyzed. This, of course, depends on factors like sample size and whether the sample was randomly selected or a sample of convenience. Even if you are describing accurate predictions for your sample, it is quite another thing to imply that these same predictions will be as strong or as valid for other samples, especially if the sample was not selected randomly or was small in number. One method of dealing with shrinkage is doing a cross-validation study that essentially replicates the original study and allows the researcher to compare the regression model across two different samples. A regression analysis generating the same or a similar model in a second sample with fairly equal predictive values between the two samples for each variable goes a long way to validate the prediction model. There are also some statistical formulas that are designed to deal with shrinkage, but we will not address those here.

Canonical Correlation Analysis

As seen in Figure 9.6, the **canonical correlation analysis** is an extension of the multiple regression analysis that attempts to use multiple independent variables to predict multiple dependent variables taken as a group. Let's say this time that our clinic director was an audiologist who wanted to not only determine client satisfaction but also clients who return to purchase additional hearing instruments or assistive listening devices or who make referrals to the clinic for acquaintances. In this case we have three things we want to predict as a construct: client satisfaction with services, future purchases, and referrals. We are not just interested in satisfied clients but those who do the other two things as well. We could set up a series of independent variables to act as predictors, not just of satisfaction, but of the three dependent variables taken as a group. The prediction model works similarly to multiple regression in that the analysis tries to find out the group of independent variables that result in the best prediction with the fewest number of variables. The difference is that they will be trying to predict the three dependent variables as a unit instead of just a single dependent variable.

Demorest and Erdman (1989) used canonical correlation to examine environmental and affective communication variables in participants who were hearing impaired. The instrument they used to examine the issue was the Communication Profile for the Hearing Impaired (CPHI) which assesses multiple domains related to hearing impairment, communication, the environment, and affective issues. Among the predictor variables were questionnaire items tapping the areas of communication need, communication environment, attitudes of others, and behaviors of others. The variables that they tried to predict were maladaptive behavior in the hearing-impaired client, verbal communication strategies, and nonverbal communication strategies. This was a complex study with many interesting results, among the most interesting of which was the relationship between the hearing-impaired client's perception of others as being understanding and supportive and the use of maladaptive behavior (withdrawing, pretending to understand, avoiding communication). The more the client perceives behaviors that suggest low understanding and support, the more maladaptive behaviors tend to occur. Another important facet of this study is the use of two samples comprising over four hundred hearing-impaired individuals with the second sample serving as a cross-validation mechanism for the investigation. The relationships they found in one sample were generally replicated in the second sample of participants, thus adding validity to their prediction model. Canonical correlation is a very complicated analysis and seldom encountered, but you should at least know that a mechanism exists for examining such issues.

Discriminant Analysis

Figure 9.6 illustrates discriminant analysis as using multiple independent variables to predict a single dichotomous variable such as membership in a group or some other categorical classification. Sometimes this analysis is called a **discriminant function analysis** because it computes and plots discriminant functions that are used to differentiate groups from one another. Discriminant analysis has been likened to both multivariate analysis of variance and multiple regression in terms of how it differentiates groups. Such an analysis might be used if a researcher wanted to predict two-year-old children who would spontaneously grow out of a language delay (e.g., late talkers) from those who would ultimately be diagnosed with language impairment. In this case, the researcher has two dichotomous groups that are defined by whether they achieved normal language development or not at three years of age. Obviously, you could take the two groups and measure whether or not they had a history of language disorder in the family. You could do a simple *t*-test between the groups comparing the number of family members reported with a history of language impairment. If you found a significant difference between the groups, you might use family history as a predictor to determine group membership at age 3. However, there may be many other predictor variables suggested by the existing literature. For example some of the following measures might be used as independent variables: number of consonants in the child's phonetic inventory, scores on a language comprehension measure, frequency and type of gestural communication, level of symbolic play, or number of relatives reported to have experienced language disorder. The discriminant function analysis will determine the best combination of predictor variables to place individuals in the appropriate group, in this case children with language disorders and those with normal language. After the analysis produces the best prediction model, it is customary to construct a table indicating correct versus incorrect predictions to give the researcher data on their proportion and how many false positives or negatives were generated by the prediction model. Correct predictions would place children with and without language impairment correctly in their groups. A false positive might place a normal language child in the disordered group, whereas a false negative might place a language-impaired child in the normal language group. This is similar to a procedure typically used to calculate sensitivity and specificity measures on standardized tests designed to identify clients with disorders (Haynes & Pindzola, 2008).

Liles, Duffy, Merritt, and Purcell (1995) used discriminant analysis to determine which combinations of language variables would be the best at predicting whether a child was the member of a language-disordered or language-normal grouping. This, as you can see, is a study that uses a number of linguistic variables to predict group membership, an ideal situation for the use of discriminant analysis. The results of the study showed the four linguistic variables that served as the best predictors of group membership were percent of grammatical T-units, percent of complete cohesive ties, mean number of subordinate clauses per T-unit, and mean number of words per subordinate clause. Among these predictors the percent of grammatical T-units and the percent of cohesive ties made the most contribution to accurate group prediction. It should also be noted that in this investigation the authors used data from three separate studies to aid in cross-validating their prediction model.

It is very important to note that discriminant analysis conducted on data that have already been collected is different than trying to predict group classifications on people in the future. Duarte-Silva and Stam (2004) differentiate between **descriptive discriminant analysis** and **predictive discriminant analysis.** Descriptive analysis would involve making predictions based on known groupings and trying to statistically account for group membership. Predictive (sometimes called prescriptive) analysis is concerned with making group designations for cases that have not yet been diagnosed or classified. You can see that there is a big difference between using discriminant analysis to account for known data versus using it to predict a person's group membership before they have been formally classified. Thus, if you read a descriptive discriminant analysis it might tell you some combinations of variables you might consider in predicting an unknown client's diagnostic group, but remember that the accuracy of the group classification in a descriptive study is tied to the sample of participants that were investigated in that research.

Factor Analysis

As do most of the techniques we have talked about in this chapter, **factor analysis** begins with correlations among variables. However, it examines many relationships shared by a large number of variables and tries to define the dimensions that these correlations have in common. In essence, the technique of factor analysis is designed to reveal underlying factors that make up a construct. For example, a general construct among speech-language pathologists working in the public school setting might be "job satisfaction." We could obtain satisfaction ratings from hundreds of public school SLPs to a variety of statements regarding their work setting, colleagues, benefits, and so forth, on a seven-point rating scale. For instance, we might ask them to rate the statement "I have enough time to get the job done" on a seven-point rating scale with 1 representing "strongly disagree" and 7 representing "strongly agree." We might have many statements for these SLPs to rate and we include them in the study because we think they relate to the overall construct of job satisfaction. This is exactly what was done by Pezzei and Oratio (1991) in research that asked a national sample of 281 public school SLPs to rate their agreement with thirty-four different statements related to their jobs, with the goal of measuring job satisfaction. It would have been easy to simply take the mean ratings of the thirty-four statements and come up with a measure of overall job satisfaction. That is, the researchers could have said that the mean rating of SLPs to statements about their job satisfaction was 6.2, which suggests strong job satisfaction on the seven-point scale. However, Pezzei and Oratio were not just interested in the overall score representing job satisfaction. They knew that many of the statements that the clinicians had to rate might represent different aspects of satisfaction. For instance, some of the statements had to do with benefits, some with colleagues, some with caseload, and so on. They wanted to find out not only about overall satisfaction but the subcomponents that contributed to or made up the general construct of job satisfaction. This was an ideal situation to use factor analytic techniques. When Pezzei and Oratio analyzed the clinician ratings, they found that the overall construct of job satisfaction in their study was represented by three underlying factors or components, the clinician's supervisor, the workload, and the coworkers the SLP spends time with in the workplace. These three factors were defined by thirteen of the initial thirty-four variables on the rating form that "loaded" on the three factors identified in the study. It turned out that these three factors accounted for 48 percent of the factor variance in job satisfaction. Obviously, there are additional determinants of job satisfaction, but it is important that three factors can account for about half of the variance in this construct. Thus, this example points out that the researchers could take a general concept such as job satisfaction and determine that it comprises three subcomponents of supervisor, workload, and coworkers. These researchers also went on to perform several multiple regression analyses to see if they could predict job satisfaction with a series of demographic or work setting variables they had gathered data on in addition to the rating scale. These were questions about level of education of the clinician, caseload size, and so forth. Interestingly they found that level of academic achievement (e.g., hours post–master's degree) and caseload size were the best predictors of job satisfaction in their investigation, accounting for over 90 percent of the variance in the prediction. This study illustrates how the factor analytic process can help to more clearly define the components that make up a larger construct and that these components can then be used to make predictions about variables of interest using a multiple regression analysis. Another example of how factor analysis can be used comes from the clinical supervision literature. Oratio (1976) in investigating the concept of "clinical competence" in speech-language pathology had clinical supervisors across the country rate the importance of statements gathered from clinical supervision forms used in university training programs to determine how important supervisors felt each item was as a contributor to clinical competence. Interestingly, the factor analysis determined that clinical competence had two major underlying factors: technical skill and interpersonal relationships. When you think about it, it makes a lot of sense that clinical competence would involve a variety of technical skills (knowledge base, experience, gathering data, making progress) as well as interpersonal variables (good relationship with client, positive attitude, likeability). The point here is that the general construct of clinical competence has some underlying factors that contribute to it and we would not know as much about these without factor analytic studies.

Sometimes factor analysis is used as part of a procedure to validate a standardized test. For example, a researcher may develop a standardized test to examine three underlying factors such as grammatical production, grammatical comprehension, and phonological awareness. If the test developer administered this test to hundreds of children, a factor analysis of the scores obtained on the individual test items should fall into three underlying factors: grammatical production, grammatical comprehension, and phonological awareness. If the factor analytic results show the presence of three underlying factors that are consistent with the intent of the test, this is another way to validate that the test actually examines what it intends to evaluate. On the other hand, if the factor analysis reveals only two factors such as a phonological awareness factor and a single grammatical factor that includes both comprehension and production, there is less support for the idea that language comprehension and production represent two separate components. Language comprehension and production may rely on a single underlying linguistic construct instead of the two postulated by the test developer. As an example of some factor analytic output let's assume that the analysis supported the original design of the test with grammar production, grammar comprehension, and phonological awareness. Remember, the researcher has administered a test to hundreds of children who have responded to individual test items that allegedly tap the three areas of the test design. The initial output that the researcher will want to examine is a correlation matrix similar to Table 9.1. This will tell the correlations between individual test items representing all of the domains of the test. Another type of output in factor analysis is a table of numbers called **eigenvalues** which are, in part, used to define the factor structure of the analysis. It is common to define factors based on eigenvalues of 1.0 or above. In other words, the factor analysis might indicate that there are six factors that have been discovered in the data, but only those with eigenvalues of 1.0 or above are used to define important underlying constructs. When the output from a factor analysis is printed the first factor always accounts for the most variance and successive factors account for less and less variance. Table 9.3 illustrates some typical output.

The data in Table 9.3 show that five factors were discovered by the analysis. Notice how each factor accounts for less variance. Also observe that only the first three factors had eigenvalues over 1.0. These three factors account for a total of 89 percent of the variance in the test questions. Among the types of output from a factor analysis is the **rotated factor matrix,** which helps to define the test items that "loaded" on each factor. These loadings range from 0 to 1.0 with higher values suggesting that the test items helped to define a particular factor. Take a look at Table 9.4 to see an example of factor loadings. In the box we will not put all of the items on the test, just enough to give you the basic idea.

TABLE 9.3

Output from Factor Analysis

Factors	Eigenvalue	Percentage of Variance Accounted for
1	2.63	37
2	2.10	30
3	1.69	22
4	0.52	6
5	0.33	5

Remember these are hypothetical data and we have tried to make this a very clear example. In reality, there is quite a bit of interpretation that goes into understanding the results of a factor analysis. In our example, however, we just want to try to make the general process clear to beginners. First, notice that we only have fifteen test items in the box, but on the real test there may have been several hundred. Remember that these test items dealt with grammar comprehension, grammar production, and phonological awareness. A second thing to notice is that in our limited example, certain test items loaded highly on specific factors. For example, test items 1 through 5 were high loaders on factor one, whereas test items 6 through 10 loaded highly on factor two. The final five test items had high loadings on factor three. In real results, the high loading would not necessarily be arranged so nicely, but might be

TABLE 9.4

Example of Factor Loadings

Test Items	Factor 1	Factor 2	Factor 3
1	**.88**	.22	.36
2	**.75**	.12	.02
3	**.95**	.32	.21
4	**.79**	.25	.15
5	**.94**	.33	.39
6	.22	**.98**	.12
7	.15	**.87**	.41
8	.25	**.79**	.32
9	.11	**.84**	.12
10	.22	**.93**	.26
11	.10	.22	**.94**
12	.25	.35	**.84**
13	.33	.29	**.78**
14	.15	.39	**.88**
15	.41	.25	**.91**

Note: Bold items note items that load heavily on factor.

scattered among all the lower-loading items. We just put the high loaders together so our illustration would be a bit easier to understand. It is the high-loading items that help to "define" a factor, and here is where the interpretive part comes into play. The researcher might see those first five items loading highly on factor one and wonder what they have in common. Perhaps these items were all test questions that dealt with comprehension of grammar. In this case, that would support the researcher's initial construction of the test as tapping comprehension as one of its domains. The researcher might then "label" this factor as "grammatical comprehension" as defined by these test items. The next group of five test items might all have to do with production of grammar, and the researcher might call this factor "grammatical production." Finally, if the third factor as defined by the last five items has to do with phonological awareness, the researcher might label this factor as "phonological awareness." Returning to our scenario in which we said that the factor analysis might only come up with two factors—one related to phonological awareness and one that combined grammatical comprehension and grammatical production. You can see that a factor including high loadings for both production and comprehension items might suggest a name something like "grammatical knowledge" to include both comprehension and production. At any rate, we hope that you can understand that factor analysis helps researchers to detect underlying constructs in data and is very useful in the exploration of certain questions.

Summary

Research that involves correlation and prediction is fairly common in the communication sciences and disorders literature. These types of studies are often used to validate theories and answer clinical questions revolving around diagnosis, prognosis, and response to treatment. Although the present chapter did not focus on the mathematical and statistical aspects of such research, we hope that students can at least gain an appreciation of the types of questions that can be answered by the different types of analyses.

LEARNING ACTIVITIES

1. Find a research article using the Pearson product-moment correlation coefficient and see if you understand the results.
2. Find a research article that uses multiple regression analysis and see if you understand which independent variables constitute the best prediction model for the dependent variable.
3. Think of an experimental design in which you might use a multiple regression. Define the

independent variables and the dependent variable that you would want to predict.
4. Think of an experimental design in which you might use a canonical correlation analysis. Define the independent and dependent variables.
5. For Activities 3 and 4 list the issues that you would need to address for internal validity in the studies.

CHAPTER 10

Single-Subject Experimental Designs in Clinical Fields

In the field of observation, chance only favors the prepared mind.
—Louis Pasteur (1822–1895)

Life is perpetual instruction in cause and effect.
—Ralph Waldo Emerson (1803–1822)

It is common error to infer that things which are consecutive in order of time have necessarily the relation of cause and effect.
—Jacob Bigelow

In previous chapters, we have discussed the use of group-experimental designs in intervention research in which two or more equally matched groups are used to assess the effectiveness of different treatments of communicative disorders. For example, the effectiveness of a specific protocol may be assessed by comparing the pre- and posttreatment mean performance of a treatment group to that of a control group (e.g., sham or no treatment). The comparison of pre- and posttreatment group means assesses the relative outcomes for a theoretically "average" patient, one receiving treatment and the other not. However, group designs are not the only way to conduct research in communication sciences and disorders. **Single-subject-design research** involves measuring the behavior of the same participant, serving as his or her own control, over time. When executed properly, these designs can contribute valuable information on the effectiveness of various treatments, applied singularly or in combination, in ameliorating communication disorders. In this chapter, we will discuss the characteristics of single-subject research, including various designs, scientific methodology, and statistical procedures. We will conclude the chapter with a discussion of the advantages and disadvantages of single-subject versus group designs and introduce a tool for critiquing this type of research.

LEARNING OBJECTIVES

This chapter will enable readers to:

- Differentiate between descriptive and experimental single-subject designs.
- Explain the difference between different types of experimental single-subject designs.
- State the important components in the scientific methodology in single-subject-design research.
- Compare and contrast single-subject-versus group-design research.
- Consider the use and limitations of statistical procedures in single-subject-design research.
- Critique single-subject-design research.

Characteristics of Single-Subject-Design Research

One way to learn about single-subject research is to discuss the fundamentals within the context of specific designs. The two major categories of designs are **descriptive** and **experimental**. Descriptive designs involve observing trends in patients' behavior over time without experimental manipulation. Alternatively, experimental designs observe patients' behavior before treatment, during treatment, and then after treatment and seek to establish causality between changes in the dependent variable and the treatment. We will discuss several such designs.

Descriptive Designs

Single-subject-design research involves observing behavior of an individual over time. The results of these studies are plotted on a graph with the behavior, or dependent variable, on the ordinate (*Y* axis) and time represented on the abscissa (*X* axis). The number of behaviors observed during discrete points in time is plotted and then contiguously connected to show trends in behavior, as shown in Figure 10.1.

The primary objective of single-subject-design research is to determine if treatment can influence behavior. Commonly used in the behavioral sciences (e.g., psychology) and in communication sciences and disorders, these designs are ideal for exploring questions such as, "Will training on specific communication strategies improve the conversational fluency of adult with sensorineural hearing loss?" or "Can a relaxation technique reduce the number of disfluencies experienced by a stutterer when delivering a presentation?" If done properly, single-subject-design research can provide convincing evidence for answering these questions.

Conventionally, letters (e.g., A, B, and C) have been used to denote the segments of single-subject-design studies (Silverman, 1998). Observing a behavior over time

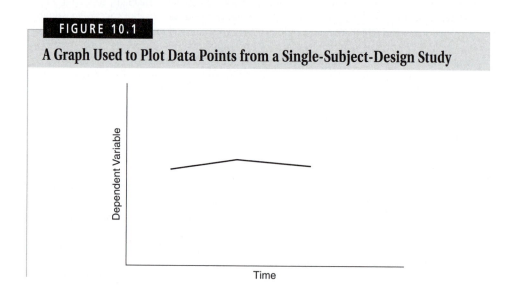

FIGURE 10.1

A Graph Used to Plot Data Points from a Single-Subject-Design Study

without any experimental manipulation of independent variables or changes in environmental conditions is an observational or baseline study called an A-only design. A-only designs are also known as "case studies" or "longitudinal diary studies" (Silverman, 1998). This segment provides information regarding the stability of a behavior over time, which can be increasing at different rates, changing in level, stable, highly variable, or slightly variable, as shown in Figure 10.2. For instance, the audiologist may engage in conversation with the participant to determine conversational fluency for several sessions in a row before teaching any strategies. Similarly, the speech-language pathologist may determine patients' number of disfluencies per minute when doing mock presentations over several days. Behaviors measured during baseline theoretically predict the future status of the behavior, assuming that no treatment is provided (McReynolds & Thompson, 1986). Before beginning the treatment phase of a study, it is best if these three requirements are fulfilled when experimenters have established (1) reliability through multiple measurements, (2) stability in measurement, and (3) opportunity for contrasting results (Hegde, 2003). Investigators must consistently measure the target behavior over a series of sessions to determine the reliability of performance. Ideally, the behavior or dependent variable should achieve **stability** or no more than 5 percent variability from interval to interval with no upward or downward trends of performance (Schiavetti & Metz, 2006). Attainment of stability is important because confounding variables (e.g., maturation or repeated testing) are present during all phases of a study (McReynolds & Kearns, 1983; Schiavetti & Metz, 2006). In addition, the proficiency of baseline performance

---

FIGURE 10.2

Possible Performance of the Dependent Variable over Time during the Baseline of a Single-Subject-Design Study

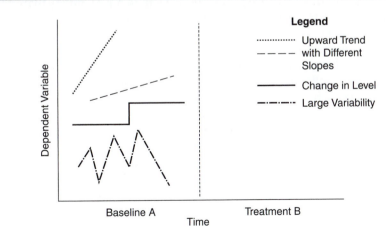

Legend

.... Upward Trend
— — — with Different Slopes

———— Change in Level

—·—·—· Large Variability

Baseline A   Treatment B
Time

Adapted from Schiavetti and Metz, 2006.

should not be too high or too low relative to criterion levels (e.g., treatment goals) to avoid ceiling effects (e.g., nowhere to go) or inappropriate levels of expectation for a patient (Hegde, 2003; McReynolds & Kearns, 1983).

More-complex designs require a more elaborate coding system. For example, the following letters denote different segments of a study:

- A = baseline
- B = first treatment
- C = second treatment that is different from the first

In addition, subscript numbers are used to indicate repetitions of segments (A_1, A_2, B_1, B_2, etc.) (Silverman, 1998). The B-only design is treatment-only and is frequently used in intervention protocols administered by audiologists and speech-language pathologists. However, changes in the behavior (i.e., dependent variable) cannot be attributed to treatment (i.e., independent variable). The A-B design is the classic "before-and-after" or case study design that includes baseline measures (i.e., A) and then application of an independent variable or treatment (i.e., B) (McReynolds & Kearns, 1983; Silverman, 1998). The A-B design is not experimental, but is slightly better than the treatment-only design in that the target behavior is measured before application of the treatment, but any changes in behavior also cannot be ascribed to manipulation of the independent variable. For example, some unaccounted-for factor other than the independent variable may have been responsible for changes in the dependent variable (McReynolds & Thompson, 1986).

Experimental Designs

Treatment–no treatment comparisons assess the question whether the treatment results in improved performance relative to no treatment. We will discuss three different designs: (1) withdrawal and reversal designs, (2) multiple-baseline designs, and (3) multiple-probe techniques (Kearns, 1986). The A-B-A (i.e., baseline-treatment-baseline) or baseline-treatment-withdrawal design is the simplest option that qualifies as an experimental study. The A segment serves as baseline, followed by a treatment segment, B. The removal of treatment or second baseline, A, allows experimenters to assess whether the treatment or independent variable was responsible for the change in status of the behavior or dependent variable. If it was, then the behavior should return to baseline levels of performance. Figure 10.3 depicts the results for such a design, in which the stability of a behavior is achieved in the baseline segment (i.e., A), increases with treatment (i.e., B), and then subsequently decreases during withdrawal or the second baseline (i.e., A). Therefore, it can be concluded that the treatment resulted in a change in behavior.

Other withdrawal designs include the B-A-B and the A-B-A-B. In the B-A-B design, the study begins with treatment and after stable performance at criterion levels has been achieved, the intervention is removed (e.g., A phase) to see if performance decreases and then increases again to past levels with reapplication of a second treatment phase (McReynolds & Kearns, 1983). The A-B-A-B withdrawal design is an extremely powerful design that includes measurement of behavior during a second

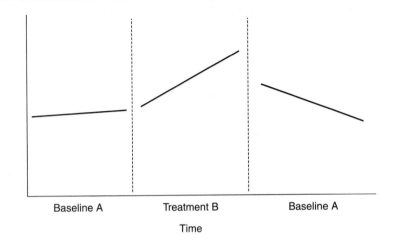

FIGURE 10.3

A Graph of the Results of an A-B-A Single-Subject-Design Study in Which the Dependent Variable Significantly Improved during Treatment and Decreased during the Second Baseline or Reversal

Baseline A Treatment B Baseline A

Time

withdrawal and treatment phase. If the dependent variable returns to pretreatment levels of performance during the second baseline, evidence is even stronger for causality between the treatment and changes in the target behavior. Other variations are the A-B-A and A-B-A-B **reversal designs** that, instead of removing treatment, apply the intervention to alternative and/or incompatible behavior(s) during the second baseline phase instead of the target behavior (Kearns, 1986).

Another type of A-B-A-B reversal design is returning the behavior in the second baseline (A) to levels observed during the first baseline (A) (Kearns, 1986). For example, Fisher, Ligon, Sobeks, and Roxe (2001) employed a full-reversal design (A-B-A-B) to assess the effect of body-fluid retention without dehydration on phonation threshold pressure, patient-perceived phonatory effort, and voice quality. Subjects were persons with end-stage renal disease requiring hemodialysis. Patients were assessed before dialysis during the first baseline (first A), after dialysis that removed bodily fluids through ultrafiltration during the first treatment (first B), and after fluid replacement during the second baseline (second A), which reversed the patients' states to levels observed during the first baseline. Patients were then assessed again after the second dialysis or second treatment (second B). The authors concluded that intracellular fluid removal without dehydration may result in a reduction of voice quality.

One major advantage of the treatment–no treatment designs is their simplicity for determining the effectiveness of an intervention. However, a disadvantage to this design is that many treatment effects for communicative disorders are longstanding and that the removal of treatment may not result in a return to baseline performance (e.g., learning a phoneme in articulation treatment) (Kearns, 1986). After all, the purpose of treatment is for amelioration of communicative disorders and dismissal from therapy. Another major disadvantage of withdrawal and reversal designs is that the removal of treatment can be viewed as unethical (Kearns, 1986). In other words, patients must relapse in order to demonstrate effectiveness.

Multiple-baseline single-subject designs offer other types of treatment–no treatment designs, but unlike some withdrawal and reversal designs, intervention need not be removed in order to establish the effectiveness of a therapy regimen. There are several types of multiple-baseline designs, including multiple baselines across behaviors, settings, subjects, and/or groups (McReynolds & Kearns, 1983). Important considerations for multiple-baseline designs are whether two functionally independent behaviors, compatible settings, or homogeneous participants can be identified for the studies (Kearns, 1986).

Multiple-baselines-across-behaviors designs test the effectiveness of a treatment in changing two functionally independent behaviors within the same subject. Figure 10.4 shows a graph of multiple-baselines for two behaviors in the same subject. Baseline measures are obtained on both behaviors simultaneously until stability is attained, at which time treatment is applied to behavior A while behavior measurement of baseline is continued on behavior B. When performance on behavior A has reached its criterion, treatment is initiated on behavior B and continues until a change occurs, demonstrating an effect on both behaviors (McReynolds & Kearns, 1983). For example, using a multiple-baseline-across-behaviors design, Casby (1992) assessed

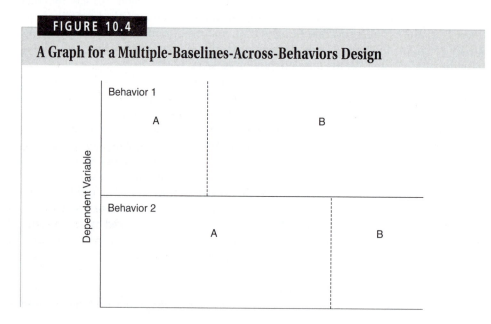

FIGURE 10.4

A Graph for a Multiple-Baselines-Across-Behaviors Design

the effect of an intervention on reducing the naming difficulties of an eleven-year-old boy. He demonstrated the effectiveness of the treatment protocol initially in reducing response time (behavior A) and then in the number of naming errors (behavior B). If no change is observed in behavior B, then neither the effectiveness of treatment for behavior A nor B can be claimed and the experiment has no more rigor than a simple A-B or before-and-after design (McReynolds & Kearns, 1983).

Multiple-baselines-across-subjects designs assess the effectiveness of an intervention on changing the same behavior(s) across a group of homogeneous subjects. For a period of time, all subjects are in baseline and then treatment is applied systematically to each subject as they successfully achieve their goal levels of performance. Palmer, Adams, Bourgeois, Durrant, and Rossi (1999) used a multiple-baselines-across-subjects design to assess the effectiveness of amplification in reducing caregiver-identified problem behaviors in patients with Alzheimer's disease and hearing impairment. Treatment compliance (i.e., number of hours hearing aids are worn each day), reduction of problem behaviors, and hearing handicap were measured in this study. Figure 10.5 shows occurrence frequency of several problem behaviors (e.g., searching, making negative statements, repeating questions, and so on) across baselines and during hearing aid treatment for subject 1. The study found that all eight participants were able to partake in the audiologic evaluation and hearing aid evaluation, and complied in wearing hearing aids for between five to fifteen hours per day, with several patients reducing the number of caregiver-identified problem behaviors.

Similarly, Ingham, Kligo, Ingham, Moglia, Belknap, and Sanchez (2001) used a multiple-baselines-across-subjects-and-tasks design to evaluate the efficacy of the Modifying Phonation Intervals (MPIs). MPI is a stuttering program that teaches patients to reduce the frequency of short phonation intervals across phases—that is, within-clinic speaking phases (establishment), beyond-clinic speaking phases (transfer), and systematic decreases in assessment occasions (maintenance)—and tasks—that is, reading, monologue, and telephone. Figure 10.6 illustrates the multiple-baselines-across-subjects component of the study. In addition, Figure 10.7 shows frequency of stuttering (i.e., stuttering events) and frequency of target range phonation intervals (TRPIs) for subject 1 during within-clinic test results measured during three-minute samples of reading, monologue, and telephone situations obtained three times each within the pretreatment (i.e., baseline) and establishment phases of the study and once during maintenance. Ingham and colleagues (2001) explained that the vertical broken line shows the point during the study when the MPI was introduced. The study ultimately found that participants continued their level of performance twelve months after completion of the maintenance segment of the investigation.

Multiple-baselines-across-settings designs evaluate the effectiveness of a treatment for a target behavior in the same subject(s) across treatment settings. In other words, baseline and treatment are applied in one setting, and when performance reaches its criterion, the target behavior is measured sequentially during baseline and treatment in other settings. Multiple-baselines-across-settings designs offer an opportunity to demonstrate generalization of achievement of criterion levels of

Results of a Multiple-Baselines-Across-Behaviors Study for a Single Subject

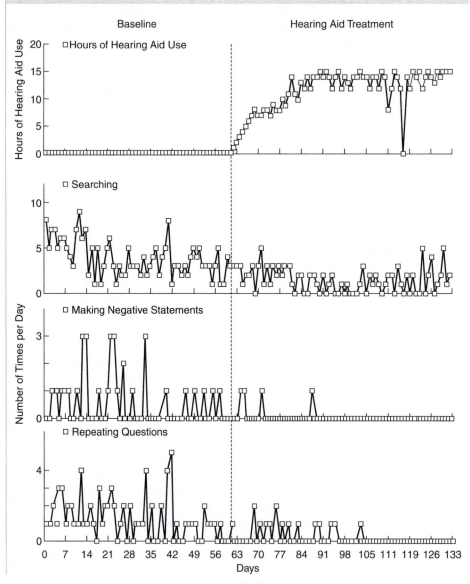

An Example of Multiple-Baselines-Across-Subjects Design

Individual participant findings are reported for percent syllables stuttered (%SS), stutter-free syllables spoken per minute (SFSPM), and naturalness ratings (Na, 1 = highly natural; 9 = highly unnatural) obtained from reading tests obtained at two-week intervals during baseline (pretreatment) and at the completion of MPI treatment for reading monologue, and telephone treatments steps during establishment. The broken vertical line indicates the end of baseline (progressively longer for each speaker) and the introduction of MPI treatment, illustrating the multiple-baselines-across-subjects design.

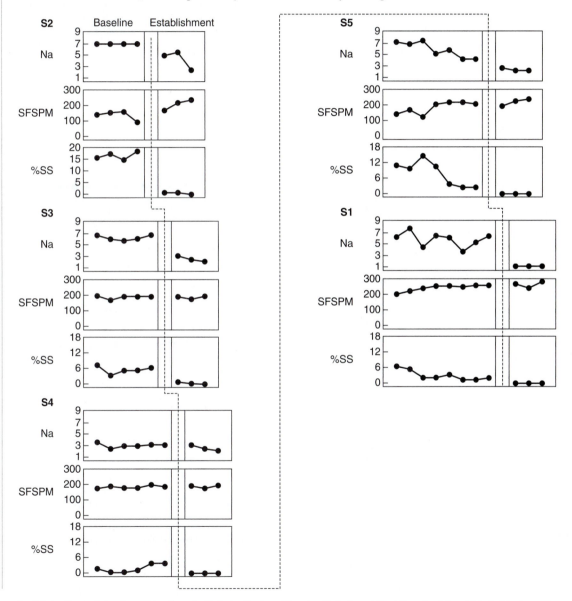

An Example of the Multiple-Baselines-Across-Tasks Aspect for Subject 1

Subject 1: Treatment process results as reflected in the measurement of the frequency of stuttering (stuttered events) and the frequency of target range phonation intervals (TRPIs) are shown for each speaker in a multiple-baseline experiment across speaking tasks. Each speaker's figure shows the within-clinic test results for three-minute samples in reading, monologue, and telephone during three occasions within the pretreatment and establishment phases and one occasion within the maintenance phase. Participants completed a different number of tests in each phase. Partial results are shown for pretreatment, the initial, middle, and final tests (P1, P2, P3, respectively): for establishment tests administered at the completion of reading monologue, and telephone TRPI treatment (E1, E2, E3, respectively); for maintenance, tests obtained at the second measurement occasion (M2), twelve weeks following the completion of transfer. The broken vertical line shows when MPI training was introduced for reading, then monologue, and finally telephone tests. The horizontal broken line in the establishment and maintenance phases shows the target frequency for the TRPIs.

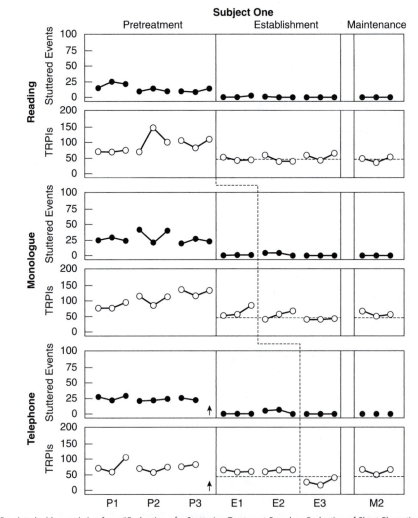

performance of the target behavior in different environments such as home, class-room, playground, and other relevant settings (Hegde, 2003).

The multiple-probe technique involves measuring performance of multiple functionally independent behaviors at continuous intervals. Dworkin, Abkarian, and Johns (1988) used a multiple-probe technique to demonstrate the effectiveness of a treatment regimen that began with simple oroneuromotor tasks progressing to syllables, words, and then to sentences. Treatment failed to show generalization to untreated behaviors; it was concluded that the intervention was effective for an adult with apraxia of speech. The multiple-probe technique is more time efficient than multiple-baselines-across-subjects designs that require simultaneously measuring the performance of behaviors currently under intervention in addition to others that have already and have yet to be treated.

Other Assessments

Component-assessment designs evaluate the degree to which individual components of a treatment package contribute to a change in behavior (Kearns, 1986). These studies can assess either reduction or additive effects of individual components of treatment packages. Kearns (1986) explained that these designs are similar to A-B-A design except that instead of using a reversal design, individual components are compared against the entire treatment package. A **reduction design** assesses the effectiveness of an entire treatment regimen (e.g., BC) against a single component (e.g., B) in an interaction design (e.g., BC-B-BC-B); an **additive design** evaluates the effectiveness of a treatment protocol (e.g., B) that is compared with an addition of another component (e.g., C) with the following component arrangement: B-BC-B-BC (Kearns, 1986).

Treatment-treatment designs investigate the relative effectiveness of two or more rapidly alternating treatments that are counterbalanced in their presentation to equally distribute possible influences of different clinicians, regimen order, and time of presentation (Kearns, 1986). Kim and Lombardino (1991) used an alternating-treatment design to investigate the relative effectiveness of script-based versus non-script-based treatments on the language comprehension of four children with mental retardation. Figure 10.8 shows the results for subject 1, who was trained to act out agent-action-object construction in the scripted condition (i.e., S) and action-object-location for the no script (NS) condition. The graphs show that the subject's performance reached criterion (i.e., 75 percent over three consecutive sessions) for the S condition within fifteen sessions but failed to reach criterion for NS conditions (Kim & Lombardino, 1991). Overall, S conditions were more effective in reaching criterion for language comprehension goals for three of four children. Another type of treatment-treatment design is the replicated crossover design; readers are referred to Kearns (1986) for further explanation.

Another sophisticated single-subject design is the **successive-level analysis** that assesses whether treatment results in the acquisition of successive steps as part of a chaining sequence of behaviors (Kearns, 1986). In communicative disorders, target behaviors in therapy are often addressed in hierarchical fashion that builds in

FIGURE 10.8

An Example of a Treatment-Treatment Design Showing (a) Script and Nonscript Training Data for a Single Subject and (b) Script and Nonscript Generalization Data for a Single Subject

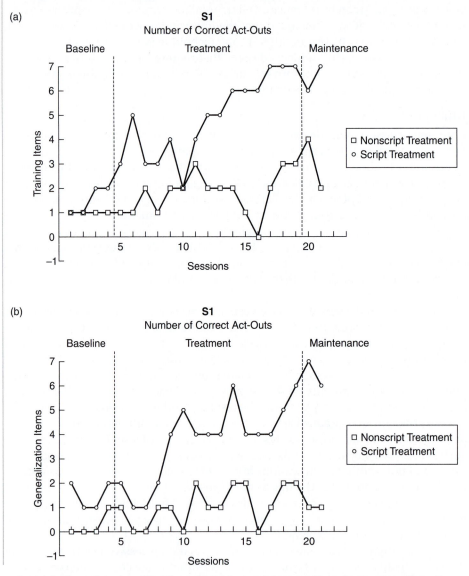

complexity (Kearns, 1986). Dworkin et al. (1988) used a successive-level analysis to-gether with a multiple-probe technique to assess the treatment effectiveness of a regimen that built in complexity from neuromotoric tasks, to syllables, words, and then sentences for an adult with apraxia. Figure 10.9 parts A through D shows the performance of the patient across behaviors of increasing complexity.

The **changing-criterion design,** another successive-level analysis, investigates the effectiveness of treatment with ever-increasing criterion levels of performance achieved on a gradually acquired behavior (Kearns, 1986). Warnes and Allen (2005) used a changing-criterion design to evaluate the effectiveness of surface electromyography (EMG) biofeedback to treat paradoxical vocal folds in a sixteen year old who attended therapy over a ten-week period. The dependent variable, the EMG data in microvolts (mV), is plotted on the ordinate and the treatment sessions on the abscissa of Figure 10.10. Two weeks of baseline and subsequent treatment were provided in a university biofeedback clinic. Treatment consisted of the patient viewing a visual representation of her muscle tension (i.e., EMG). Throughout the experiment, she was told to simply relax to reduce her tension to increasingly lower levels.

Scientific Methodology in Single-Subject-Design Research

McReynolds and Thompson (1986) stated that the scientific methodology of single-subject-design research comprised four key components: (1) operational specificity, (2) repeated measurement, (3) interobserver agreement, and (4) external validity.

Operational Specificity

In other chapters of this textbook, we have discussed factors important in group-design research. In both single-subject and group-design research, both the independent and dependent variables must be operationally and specifically defined so that others can replicate the study or correctly apply the treatment protocol to appropriate patients. The independent variable or treatment protocol must provide the who, what, where, when, and why of a treatment. McReynolds and Thompson (1986) stated that, at a minimum, the description should include instructions to the patient, visual/tactile stimuli, response time provided, parameters of the response, and the feedback given. For example, the previously mentioned study by Ingham and colleagues (2001) not only described the MPI program in general but also specifics about the program through all four phases: pretreatment, establishment, transfer, and maintenance.

Similarly, the dependent variable or **target behavior** must be operationally defined. Recall that the measurement of the target behavior is plotted using the ordinate of the graphic representation for results of a single-subject-design study. There are two main types of measures. **Direct measures** assess the actual manifestations of the communicative disorder (e.g., the number of disfluencies per minute, percent correct production of a phoneme) (McReynolds & Thompson, 1986). **Indirect measures** are those not directly observable or physiological in nature and are measured in

FIGURE 10.9

An Example of a Successive Level Analysis with a Multiple-Probe Technique

A. Bite-block activities: baseline and treatment sessions. b/m = beats per minute of metronome, and t/s = trials per treatment session. Absence of b/m indicates that the behavior was sampled without metronome pacing.

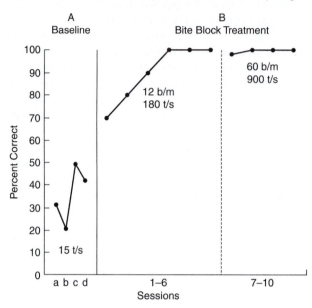

B. Alternate motion rates (AMR): baseline and treatment sessions. b/m = beats per minute of metronome, and t/s = trials per treatment session. Absence of b/m indicates that the behavior was sampled without metronome pacing.

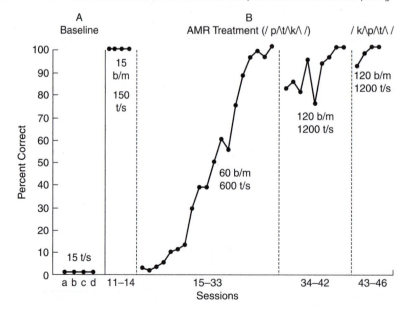

(Continued)

(Continued)

C. Isolated word activities: baseline and treatment sessions. b/m = beats per minute of metronome, and t/s = trials per treatment session. Absence of b/m indicates that the behavior was sampled without metronome pacing.

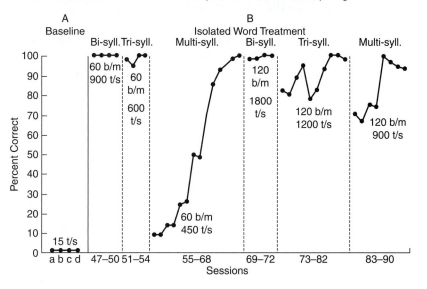

D. Unstressed and stressed sentence activities: baseline and treatment sessions. # refers to sentence number, b/m = beats per minute of metronome, and t/s = trials per treatment session. Absence of b/m indicates that the behavior was sampled without metronome pacing.

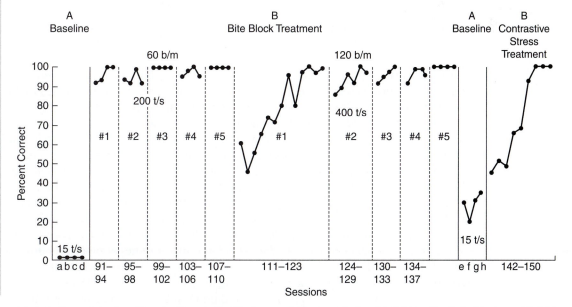

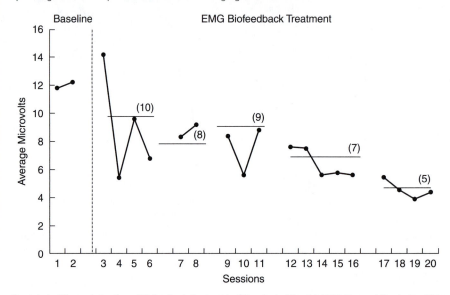

FIGURE 10.10

An Example of a Changing-Criterion Design with a Sixteen-Year-Old Subject

Average microvolts per session across baseline and treatment conditions. Horizontal lines and corresponding numbers in parentheses indicate changing criterion levels.

Reprinted with permission from "Biofeedback Treatment of Paradoxical Vocal Fold Motion and Respiratory Distress in an Adolescent Girl" by E. Warnes and K. D. Allen. *Journal of Applied Behavior Analysis,* 38, 529–532.

the laboratory setting (McReynolds & Thompson, 1986). For example, the previously mentioned study by Warnes and Allen (2005) involved an indirect dependent variable using surface EMG as the target behavior when measuring the deleterious effects of a paradoxical vocal fold in a sixteen-year-old adolescent female.

Several subtypes of direct measures have been well described by McReynolds and Thompson (1986). The most frequently used measure in communication sciences and disorders is **trial scoring,** in which the proportion of number of times a target behavior occurred per the number of opportunities is calculated as percent correct. Examples include percent correct production of a target phoneme or the percent correct identification of phonemes on a nonsense syllable test. One advantage of trial scoring is that it is particularly efficient for use in the intervention milieu. For example, clinician-researchers can elicit a relatively high number of target behaviors through use of stimuli in drill work. A disadvantage of trial scoring is that it may not be amenable for use in assessing behavior occurring in more naturalistic settings.

Several other direct measures are based on frequency of occurrence per unit of time. **Rate measures** are represented by the ratio of the number of times a target behavior occurred per period of time (e.g., the number of instances of secondary stuttering behaviors per minute). The number of behaviors may be counted during an hour-long session, which may be used to calculate the rate or average number of behaviors per minute by simply dividing the number of secondary stuttering behaviors occurring by sixty minutes. **Frequency measures** are the tally or number of times a behavior occurs during an observation period. The difference between rate and frequency measures is that the former seeks to determine the average number of times an event occurs per unit of time, whereas the latter is simply the number of times a behavior occurs that may or may not be linked to a specific period of time. For example, Palmer, Adams, Bourgeois, Durrant, and Rossi (1999) used frequency measures in assessing the effectiveness of amplification in reducing the number of negative behaviors per day. **Interval scoring** involves breaking an observation period into consecutive, equal segments of time and then counting occurrences of the target behavior during each portion. An example includes dividing an hour up into thirty-second segments and then counting the number of times a verb was used incorrectly. **Time sampling** involves sporadically observing target behaviors for specific periods of time during therapy, such as three one-minute intervals during a thirty-minute session. And finally, **duration measures** simply measure how long a particular behavior lasts; such measures are seldom used in communicative sciences and disorders.

Investigators must also determine the **criterion level of performance** of the dependent variable, which is the performance required for mastery of the particular goal and must be achieved over the course of at least two data-collection sessions. For example, a criterion level of performance may be achievement of 90 percent accuracy in the productions of /r/ during a story narrative over two consecutive sessions. Selection of an appropriate criterion level determines the effectiveness of a treatment. Therefore, the goal should be specific to the patient and to that of the communicative disorder.

We would like to illustrate the importance of specifying the who, what, where, when, and why of a single-subject-design study. The who, usually easy to establish, comprises the participant as well as experimenter and research assistants. An extremely important aspect of single-subject-design research is to provide a detailed description of the participant. For example, Dworkin and colleagues (1988), previously mentioned, provided an extremely detailed description of their subject with apraxia to include a copious medical history so that generalizations to similar patients could be made. Most articles using these designs provide a table with the participant's demographics, test scores, and other information so readers have a good idea for which type of patient the results may be generalized. The what is *conversational fluency*, which has been defined as how well an interaction flows. Good conversations are marked by partners equally giving and taking turns and conveying information. Equality means that conversational partners have the same length of speaking turn. Tye-Murray (2008) recommends the use of two indices in measuring the amount of speaking time per conversational partner: (1) *mean length of turn* (MLT) in words and (2) *mean length of turn ratio* (MLT ratio). The MLT is defined as the average number of words used by a person during a conversational turn. It is computed by counting the number of words used by a speaker within a conversation and then dividing by the number of speaking turns. The MLT ratio is simply the ratio of the patient's MLT to the conversational partner's MLT. Let's calculate these measures using the conversation exchange below:

> **Audiologist:** Where did you go on vacation this winter?
> **Patient:** We went to Breckenridge, Colorado, and stayed at a resort.
> **Audiologist:** Are you and your wife skiers?
> **Patient:** She is, but I'm not. I like to go for a hike.
> **Audiologist:** I can imagine that it gets pretty cold there during the winter.
> **Patient:** Oh yes! It averages about thirty-five degrees Fahrenheit with very low humidity.
> **Audiologist:** With the low humidity, she probably enjoys the powdery snow when she skis.
> **Patient:** Oh yes, my wife enjoys going there the best during winter ski season.

The first step in computing MLT is to count the total number of words used by each conversational partner. The second step is to count the number of conversational turns by each partner. The third step is to divide the total number of words by the number of conversational turns to compute the MLT for each speaker. Let's do the computations.

	Audiologist	Patient
Step 1: Count the number of words	39	47
Step 2: Count the number of turns	4	4
Step 3: Divide number of words by the number of turns	9.75	11.75

Therefore, the MLT for the audiologist is 9.75 words per turn versus 11.75 words per turn for the patient. The MLT ratio is computed by dividing the MLT of the audiologist by the MLT of the patient, yielding 1.2. What does MLT ratio mean? An MLT ratio of 1.0 signifies that the mean length of turn, in words, of the patient and the audiologist are approximately the same, exemplifying equal conversational turn time. A number less than one indicates that the MLT of the patient is, on average, less than the audiologist and represents a comparative proportion of MLT of the patient to the audiologist. For example, an MLT ratio of 0.8 means that, on the average, the patient's MLT is 80 percent of the audiologist's. Conversely, a number greater than 1 represents that, on the average, the patient's MLT is greater than the audiologist's. For example, an MLT ratio of 2.0 means that, on the average, the patient uses twice as many words per turn as the audiologist.

The where is the environment in which the behavior is to be measured; in our example, it is an interview room in a research laboratory. The when is during a data-collection session, and the why is to determine the effects of communication training on conversational fluency.

The resulting rubric appearing next can be used to operationally define the dependent variable to assist in framing the experimental question.

- Who: The participant, an adult with a sensorineural hearing loss; experimenter; and assistants
- What: Mean length of turn and mean length of turn ratio
- Where: In an interview room
- When: When involved in conversation with the investigator or research assistant
- Why: To determine the effectiveness of communication training

The rubric may be very useful in framing a specific experimental question. For example, the following research question specifies the who, what, where, when, and why of the study:

> Experimental question: What is the effectiveness of communication training in improving the conversational fluency (i.e., as measured by mean length of turn and mean length of turn ratio) of an adult with sensorineural hearing loss when interacting with the investigator or research assistant in an interview room?

Repeated Measurement, Interjudge Reliability, and External Validity

Repeated measurement means that participants' behaviors are assessed often and consistently over time. Care must be taken so that measurement of the dependent variable is made in the same way (e.g., by the same observer, at the same time of day, using the same stimuli, and so on) at fairly consistent intervals. After all, repeated measurement provides opportunities to observe behavior over time, assessing for trends, particularly during different segments or phases of a study (McReynolds & Thompson, 1986).

It is important in repeated measurement to observe intra- and interobserver reliability for both the dependent and independent variables providing four different types of consistency. **Interobserver reliability for the dependent variable** is the degree of agreement (e.g., percent) between the assessments of the same target behavior(s) in the same subject by two independent judges. For example, two observers judge the accuracy of a patient's production of the /k/ phoneme. Percent of interobserver reliability is then calculated using the equation [(Agreements + Disagreements)/Agreements] × 100. A high degree of interobserver reliability for the dependent variable means that two judges are consistent in their assessment of the dependent variable. A low degree of interobserver reliability may indicate that one or both of the observers need reinstruction or additional practice.

Intraobserver reliability for the dependent variable is the degree of agreement (e.g., percent) between the assessments of the same target behaviors in the same subject by the same judge made at two different times. For example, an observer may assess the accuracy of a patient's production of the phoneme /k/ in real time and then later while viewing a videotape recording of the same session. The same equation given for interobserver reliability is used to calculate the percent of intraobserver agreement for the dependent variable. A high degree of intraobserver reliability for the dependent variable means that the judge is consistent in assessing the dependent variable. A low degree of intraobserver reliability may mean that the clinician-researcher is inconsistent in his or her judgments of the dependent variable.

Assessment of the reliability of independent variable(s) is to ensure that treatment is applied consistently across sessions. **Interobserver reliability of the independent variable** is the degree to which two judges agree that treatment has been consistently applied when evaluating the same session. **Intraobserver reliability of the independent variable** is the degree of agreement between the evaluations of the application of treatment within the same session by the same judge. Assessment of reliability of the independent variable is a little more complex than it is for the dependent variable. McReynolds and Thompson (1986) stated that critical aspects of application of the independent variable are selected for assessment, such as the number of trials per session, reinforcement provided by the clinician, and so on. Readers are referred to McReynolds and Kearns (1983) for more detail.

Lastly, **external validity in single-subject-design research** is the degree with which the results of the study represent possible effects of treatment on behavior with specific patients in the real world. External validity is accomplished through the replication of the study by other investigators using the same methodology with similar patients. Therefore, the external validity is dependent on the internal validity of the study, particularly in the accurate description of the participants and experimental methodology.

Advantages and Disadvantages of Single-Subject versus Group-Design Research

Both single-subject and group-design research have advantages and disadvantages that must be carefully considered prior to electing a particular approach to answering an experimental question. Table 10.1 shows the relative advantages and disadvantages of both types of studies.

One advantage of single-subject-design research is its ease of use by clinician-researchers because recruitment requires only one participant. Similarly, clinician-researchers may conduct single-subject-design research across various subjects, behaviors, and settings. Because each participant serves as his or her own control, the effectiveness of a new voice therapy program can be determined for several patients with different profiles across different clinical settings. Moreover, the protocol can be applied for the remediation of different voice behaviors for each patient.

Alternatively, use of a group design can be problematic at several levels for the clinician-researcher. First, he or she would have to conduct a power analysis to determine the minimum number of subjects to recruit, usually no fewer than ten participants. Second, the number of voice behaviors to be considered would be limited. It may be difficult or nearly impossible to recruit a homogeneous group of participants with similar vocal pathologies that manifest in the same way such that one or two dependent variables are able to be identified for the entire sample. Therefore, group-design research frequently employs strict inclusion and exclusion criteria for

TABLE 10.1

Advantages and Disadvantages of Single-Subject versus Group Design Research

Single-Subject Designs

Advantages	Disadvantages
1. Ease of use by clinician-researchers	1. Difficulty in controlling for order/sequence effects
2. Employment across varied behaviors, subjects, and settings	2. Generalization to a population generally not possible
3. Flexibility in design before and during the experiment	3. Statistical procedures assessing reliability of data not well developed
4. Identification of "functional relationships" between variables	
5. Determination of factors that do/do not affect performance	
6. Exploration of intra- and intersubject variability	
7. Detection of individual differences	
8. Examination of individual responsiveness to treatment	
9. Application to participants with comorbidities or unusual forms of a disorder	

Group Designs

Advantages	Disadvantages
1. Execution of protocol no more than once per participant	1. Requirement of ten or more subjects
2. Ease in controlling sequence effects	2. Limitation of number of behaviors under consideration
3. Statistical power for making inferences between cause and effect	3. Application to excluded subjects or across service-delivery sites
4. Statistical procedures for assessing reliability well developed	4. Requirement of rigid experimental control in "ideal" conditions
5. Generalization from subject sample to population	5. Lack of flexibility in design during experiment
	6. Generalizations made to a theoretical "average" member of a particular population

Adapted from Connell and Thompson, 1986; Kearns, 1986; McReynolds and Thompson, 1986; Robey, 1999; Schiavetti and Metz, 2006; Silverman, 1998; Wambaugh, 1999.

participants for limited applications of treatment. In addition, rigid experimental controls mandate that members of both control and experimental groups must be measured on those parameters by the same investigators, at the same point in time, using the same instruments, and hopefully in the same ideal laboratory setting. These measures serve as the only baseline measures of performance prior to initiation of the treatment protocol. Unfortunately, a single pretreatment measure does not represent individual patients' performance over time. Some participants may be performing poorer than usual, whereas others may be less affected by their vocal pathologies on the day of measurement. However, some investigators believe that measuring participants' pretreatment behaviors only once is a convenient logistical advantage of group-design research. One advantage of single-subject-design research in this case is that the participant's performances are measured regularly, over time, such that the stability of performance can be obtained prior to initiation of treatment. Another advantage of single-subject-design research is the opportunity to examine individual responses to treatment that may reflect discrete learning styles for participants representing a particular diagnostic group or severity. This information is obscured in group studies.

Using a group design, all patients in the experimental group (i.e., receiving the voice therapy) would have to have the same treatment protocol administered at the same frequency, intensity, and duration, and ideally, in the same clinical setting. The experimental methodology cannot be altered for the duration of the study even if some aspect does not seem to be working well. In addition, some patients may not be able to complete the study and may drop out, which precludes determining the effectiveness of the therapy regimen.

These logistical issues and problems may make it particularly difficult for a single clinician-researcher to execute this study using a group design, particularly with little or no help. However, single-subject designs offer considerable flexibility in designing the study before and during an experiment. Because each participant serves as his or her own control, it is possible to modify aspects of treatment to suit the needs of the patient, particularly if a certain aspects of the treatment protocol are not successful. In this way, assessment of "functional relationships" between the independent variable (e.g., new voice therapy programs) and dependent variable (e.g., voice measures) help determine which factors do and do not affect performance. If the voice therapy program is being used on several patients, the clinical investigator can explore intra- and interparticipant variability in the detection of individual responsiveness to treatment. One methodological disadvantage of single-subject research is that the order or sequence of treatment phases may affect measurement of the target behavior over time. Using group-design research, however, it is easy to control for order-and-sequence effects by counterbalancing the order of treatment conditions across subjects.

Other advantages of group-design research, providing measures are taken to minimize bias, are statistical procedures for making inferences about cause and effect between applications of a treatment (i.e., independent variable) on participants' vocal behaviors (i.e., dependent variable). Moreover, the treatment effects can be generalized from the participant sample to the respective population of patients with voice disorders. In addition, the statistical procedures for assessing reliability are well developed. Conversely, the results of single-subject-design investigations are less able to generalize to a theoretical statistical average member of a population. In addition, unlike for group-design research, statistical procedures assessing the reliability of data are not well developed in single-subject design research. Clearly, the power of single-subject and group-design research lies in knowing when to use one approach versus the other.

When is it appropriate to use one design versus another? The next section of this textbook is devoted to evidence-based practice and the case is made for double-blinded, randomized, controlled clinical trials to serve as the gold standard for healthcare research. However, single-subject-design research can be used to test the effectiveness of treatments on a limited basis, serving as a precursor for conducting a clinical trial, particularly if experimental control was exercised in assessing differences in performance between baseline and treatment via a multiple-baselines design (ASHA, 2005). In addition, single-subject-design research may be very appropriate for intervention research involving patients who may have comorbidity or unusual forms of disorders that have been excluded from recruitment into traditional studies

(Frattali, 1998; Holland, Fromm, DeRuyter, & Stein, 1996). For example, Alzheimer's patients have not traditionally been considered to be suitable candidates for amplification due to their inability to participate in an audiologic evaluation and their incapability of using and caring for hearing aids (Palmer et al., 1999). Recall that Palmer and colleagues (1999) used a multiple-baselines single-subject design that demonstrated the effectiveness of amplification in reducing such behaviors of Alzheimer patients as negative statements, forgetfulness, and pacing, while increasing the likelihood of their participation in prosocial behaviors (e.g., interactions and conversations) and awareness of environmental sounds.

Statistical Procedures in Single-Subject-Design Research

One advantage of group-design research is the ability to use inferential statistics for hypothesis testing. How do experimenters know for certain whether trends in the dependent variable in a single-subject design are really significant? Are there any statistical procedures that may be used for this purpose? The use of statistics in single-subject-design research is somewhat controversial and most believe that simple observation of trends in the data is evidence enough regarding the effect of treatment on target behaviors. Trend or **slope** is the change in the dependent variable per unit of time, whether accelerating (i.e., increasing with time with respect to starting value), decelerating (i.e., decreasing with time), or having zeroceleration (i.e., no change with time) (Maxwell & Satake, 2005). Of course, errors can be made and some misinterpretations may occur due to distortions in plotting of data. For example, expanding units of measure on the ordinate may overemphasize changes in the dependent variable that may or may not be significant.

Some statistical procedures used in group-design research have been applied to single-subject designs. For example, *t*-tests and analysis of variance determine if the mean of the observations are significantly different between or among the segments of the single-subject-design study, with *t*-tests used to assess for significant differences between the means of the observations between two segments or phases. Analysis of variance or *F*-tests have been used to determine any significant differences between or among means of observations in more than two segments or phases. However, the use of these statistical tests requires the fulfillment of the following assumptions (Janosky, 1991):

- The observations within a segment or phase are normally distributed.
- The variances between or among segment(s) and phase(s) are equal.
- The observations within a phase or segment are independent.

The fact that data points or observations between and among segments of a single-subject-design study are serially dependent and highly correlated argues against the use of these statistical procedures (Janosky, 1991).

Other types of proposed statistical procedures include **curve fitting, time-series analysis, autoregressive integrated average technique, *C*-statistic,** and **nonparametric smoothing.** Curve fitting assigns observations within each segment to a curve and then assesses whether the slopes or the interfaces of the phases are significantly different. Although violating the assumptions of linearity and that the data points are independent observations of a nonrandom variable (Janosky, 1991), some statistical procedures used in single-subject-design research do not have to fulfill these requirements. For example, time-series analysis evaluates for differences between or among sequential measurements in different segments or phases that do not vary independently and tend to differ over time (Maxwell & Satake, 2005). Similarly, the **autoregressive integrated average technique** allows for statistical dependence among the observations that occur at different points in time, but both this and time-series analyses require between fifty and one hundred observations which may be impractical for studies in communicative disorders (Janosky, 1991; Maxwell & Satake, 2005). The characteristics, relative advantages, and disadvantages of the various statistical procedures used in single-subject-design research are beyond the scope of this chapter and readers are referred to Satake, Jargaroo, and Maxwell (2008).

Critiquing Single-Subject-Design Studies

A checklist for evaluating single-subject research that may either be used for designing a study or for critiquing an investigation published in a journal is given in Appendix 10A. The introduction of the article should include a rationale that is supported by the literature and is appropriate for single-subject-design research. For example, the purpose of the study should not be to assess the efficacy of management for an entire population of patients, but should focus on the effectiveness of an operationally defined treatment protocol for particular subject(s) who serve(s) as their own control(s). Moreover, the design should also be appropriate for the experimental question. Recall that in order to assess the effectiveness of a treatment on patient behavior, the design must at least consist of a baseline-treatment-baseline (i.e., A-B-A) design, the simplest level of experimental investigation. Researchers often use much more complex designs with multiple components. It is important to determine if the components of the study are arranged appropriately in relation to the purpose of the study. For example, a reduction design (e.g., BC-B-BC-B) should be used to in order to assess the relative effectiveness of an entire treatment regimen (e.g., BC) against a single component (e.g., B) (Kearns, 1986). Lastly, all the necessary components of the design should be assessed to determine that all the requirements for an experimental study have been fulfilled.

Assessment of the internal validity begins with determining if the subject(s) have been adequately described. Evaluation of the scientific method concerns whether the independent and dependent variables have been operationally defined in enough detail to permit accurate replication of the study. Moreover, dependent variables must be appropriate for the communicative disorder under consideration. What types of measures and respective criterion levels are most appropriate to be directly representative of the severity of a communication disorder and its responsiveness to treatment? Should direct or indirect measures have been used, and specifically, was the type of measure the *best* one that could have been considered? For example,

frequency counts (i.e., tallying the number of times a behavior occurred during a period of time) of correct productions of the consonant /k/ would not be appropriate
because the measure provides no indication of the percent correct production of the
target phoneme. In addition, the criterion levels for performance should be appropriate for the purposes of the study.

Adequate internal validity also requires that the effects of the independent variable have been isolated from confounding variables. For example, were the investigators absolutely sure that the participants were not receiving any other treatment
during the course of the study? Similarly, did the investigators ensure that the same
environmental variables were constant during baseline and treatment conditions?
All aspects of the experimental milieu must be consistent, especially during baseline
and treatment phases, to isolate the effects of the independent variable on the dependent variable. In addition, although multiple-baseline designs across behaviors,
subjects, or clinical settings offer ethical alternatives to the A-B-A design (i.e., patients
must relapse to establish treatment effectiveness), evaluators must ensure that these
designs have been implemented appropriately. That is, if the multiple-baselines-
across-behaviors design was used, the dependent variables must be functionally independent. Similarly, the multiple-baselines-across-subjects design requires that the
participants are a homogeneous group. Lastly, the multiple-baselines-across-settings
design requires implementation of the same experiment (e.g., treatment, target behaviors, and subjects) across settings.

Prior to initiating treatment, certain criteria must be met during the baseline
phase of the study. Both the reliability and stability of the dependent variable must be
demonstrated over a significant period of time, allowing opportunities for contrasting
results. Moreover, it is essential that observers are trained in the measurement of the
dependent variables and told that measures should be taken repeatedly and at regular
intervals with attention to consistency of the time of day, environmental conditions,
instructions, stimuli presented, and experimenter behavior. For example, teenagers
may have different levels of attentiveness that may affect the dependent variable if
measured in the morning for some sessions and during the afternoon for others. In
addition, the study should clearly indicate how both intra- and interobserver reliability were determined and that those measures were adequate for both independent
and dependent variables. Most single-subject-design studies in communication sciences and disorders include reliability in measurement of the dependent variable with
steady improvement in compliance. However, few studies report the reliability of the
independent variable(s). For example, Thompson (2006) reviewed the status of aphasia
research using single-subject designs and found an increase in the number of studies
including reliability assessment on dependent variables from only 22 percent in 1978
to 1987 to 64 percent in 2000 to 2005. However, results on reporting these data for independent variables totaled only 18 percent for studies published from 2000 to 2005.

Results should be clearly depicted and described. For example, graphs should be
easily read, including labels for the ordinate, abscissa, symbols, and so on. Because
the results of most single-subject research are analyzed through visual inspection,
the spacing of increments should not over- or underestimate trends in the data over

time. In addition, each graph should be introduced and described accurately within the text. Moreover, the use of any statistical procedures should be clearly justified with appropriate references. Lastly, reasonable explanations for and appropriate conclusions from the results should be provided in addition to suggestions for future research.

Summary

This chapter provided an introduction to single-subject-design research in communication sciences and disorders in which each subject serves as his or her own control. Characteristics of repeated measurement over time were discussed within the context of descriptive and experimental designs. Requirements for adequate internal validity were discussed using concrete examples. Appreciation for this type of research was reinforced through comparing and contrasting advantages and disadvantages of single-subject versus group designs. A checklist was provided for designing and critiquing single-subject designs.

LEARNING ACTIVITIES

1. Use the checklist provided in Appendix 10A to evaluate two single-subject-design studies found in the literature.

2. With a colleague, compare and contrast the use of a single-subject versus a group-design study to answer an experimental question.

REVIEW EXERCISES

1. *Types of Single-Subject Designs:* Please match the correct term with its definition below.

A. Multiple-baselines-across-behaviors designs
B. Changing-criterion designs
C. Multiple-probe techniques
D. Component-assessment designs
E. Successive-level analyses
F. Interaction-reduction designs
G. Multiple-baselines-across-subjects designs
H. Withdrawal designs
I. Multiple-baselines-across-settings designs
J. Interaction-additive designs

_____ Assess the effectiveness of an intervention on changing the same behavior across a group of homogeneous subjects

_____ Evaluate the degree to which individual components of a treatment package contribute to a change in behavior (Kearns, 1986)

_____ Assess the effectiveness of an entire treatment regimen (e.g., BC) against a single component (e.g., B) in an interaction design (e.g., BC-B-BC-B) (Kearns, 1986)

_____ Evaluate the effectiveness of a treatment protocol (e.g., B) compared with an addition of another component (e.g., C) with the following component arrangement: B-BC-B-BC (Kearns, 1986)

_____ Probe performance of behaviors at continuous intervals, which is more time efficient than a multiple-baseline design that involves measuring the performance of behaviors currently under intervention in addition to others that have already or have yet to be treated

_____ Assess whether treatment results in the acquisition of successive steps as part of a chaining sequence of behaviors (Kearns, 1986)

_____ Investigate the effectiveness of treatment with ever-increasing criterion levels of performance achieved on a gradually acquired behavior (Kearns, 1986)

_____ Test the effectiveness of a treatment in changing two functionally independent behaviors within the same subject

_____ Evaluate the effectiveness of a treatment in a target behavior in the same subject(s) across treatment settings

_____ Use in single-subject research having a baseline, treatment, and withdrawal phase (e.g., A-B-A) in which treatment is removed during the second baseline phase to see if patient behavior returns

to baseline performance levels, indicating effectiveness of the treatment

2. *Types of Measures:* Please match the following examples of dependent variables with the appropriate measure.

A. Frequency measures
B. Rate measures
C. Direct measures
D. Interval scoring
E. Trial scoring
F. Indirect measures

_____ Percent correct production of /r/

_____ The number of instances of secondary stuttering behaviors per minute

_____ The number of times an incorrect form of a verb is used during a session

_____ Blood pressure when experiencing tinnitus

_____ Frequency, rate, interval, and trial scoring

_____ Number of disfluencies per ten-second intervals

ANSWERS TO THE REVIEW EXERCISES

1. G, D, F, J, C, E, B, A, I, H
2. E, B, A, F, C, D

APPENDIX 10A

Checklist for Evaluating Single-Subject-Design Research

Citation: _____

_____

_____

Background Information, General Purpose, and Design

Have the results of a systematic review of the literature supported the rationale for the study?

Yes   No

Is single-subject design suitable for the purposes of the study?

Yes   No

Was the specific design selected the most appropriate for the experimental questions?

Yes   No

Were the components of the study arranged appropriately for inferring causality between the independent and the dependent variable (e.g., minimally an A-B-A design)?

Yes   No

Notes: _____

_____

_____

Internal Validity and Scientific Methodology

Was/were the subject(s) adequately described?

Yes   No

Dependent variable(s): Are the following conditions met?
- Was/were the measure(s) employed appropriate for the experimental question(s)?

Yes   No

- Was/were the criterion level(s) of performance appropriate for the purposes of the study?

Yes   No

Independent variable: Are sufficient details provided for the following?
- Instructions to the patient   Yes   No
- Visual/tactile stimuli   Yes   No
- Response time provided   Yes   No
- Parameters of the response   Yes   No
- Feedback given   Yes   No
- Other:_____   Yes   No

Have the effects of treatment been isolated from all other events that could influence the dependent variable?

Yes   No

Were environmental conditions similar during baseline and treatment conditions?

Yes   No

If a multiple-baselines-across-behaviors design was used, were the dependent variables functionally independent?

Yes   No

If a multiple-baselines-across-subjects design was used, were the subjects homogeneous?

Yes   No

If a multiple-baselines-across-settings design was used, were the experimental conditions consistent with the exception of the settings?

Yes   No

Were the following conditions for baseline met prior to application of the treatment?
- Reliability through multiple measurement   Yes   No
- Stability of measurement   Yes   No
- Opportunity for contrasting results   Yes   No

Were the following conditions for measurement of the dependent variable(s) met throughout the experiment?
- Adequate training of observers   Yes   No
- Repeated measurements at regular intervals   Yes   No
- Consistency of measurement regarding:
  - Time of day   Yes   No
  - Environmental conditions   Yes   No

• Instructions	Yes	No
• Stimuli presented	Yes	No
• Observer behavior	Yes	No
Interobserver reliability		
• Appropriate assessment	Yes	No
• Adequate reliability	Yes	No
Intraobserver reliability		
• Appropriate assessment	Yes	No
• Adequate reliability	Yes	No

Notes: _____

_____

_____

Results and Discussion

Are the results of the study clearly depicted?	Yes	No
Are the results of the study clearly described?	Yes	No
Were any statistical procedures appropriately used?	Yes	No
Were the results of the study adequately interpreted?	Yes	No
Are reasonable explanations provided for the results?	Yes	No

Notes: _____

_____

_____

Conclusions

Were the conclusions of the study appropriately stated considering the findings of the study?

Yes   No

Notes: _____

_____

_____

Adapted from McReynolds and Kearns, 1983; Kearns, 1986; and McReynolds and Thompson, 1986.

CHAPTER 11

Overview of Evidence-Based Practice

If the people who make the decisions are the people who will also bear the consequences of those decisions, perhaps better decisions will result.

—John Abrams

The deepest sin against the human mind is to believe things without evidence.

—Thomas H. Huxley (1825–1895)

Human nature constitutes a part of the evidence in every case.

—Elisha Potter

Do you ever wonder how a doctor decides the best course of treatment for you or a family member who has an illness? Most of the time, a patient is eager to take the medicine or have a procedure done to make them feel better. Fortunately, most often physicians' decisions regarding patient care are for minor illnesses, aches, and pains. However, the stakes become higher when a patient has a serious illness and a physician's decision can make the difference between life and death. At that point, patients become concerned about the basis on which a physician provides options and makes recommendations regarding the best treatment.

Up until about forty years ago, physicians' decisions were based on the "art of medicine" or "clinical judgment," accumulated from rigorous medical educations, knowledge and skills obtained via continuing education, articles read in professional journals, experiences, and input from colleagues when making decisions (Eddy, 2005). However, around 1970, a consensus began to emerge pointing at two major flaws in this system. First, physicians varied widely in the approaches to care even for those presenting with the same conditions, with some of those patients receiving inappropriate care (Eddy, 2005). Second, there was variation in what physicians were doing and what practices were supported by the scientific evidence (Eddy, 2005).

In addition, the efforts of some individuals stood out regarding the importance of considering scientific evidence in medical practice. In 1972, Charlie Cochrane wrote *Effectiveness and Efficiency: Random Reflections on Health Services,* advocating use of the best scientific evidence in clinical decision making. His influence was such that in the 1990s an international group focusing on these principles named itself the *Cochrane Collaboration,* an international nonprofit independent organization dedicated to making available up-to-date, accurate information, primarily in the form of systematic reviews about the effects of healthcare, to healthcare providers and patients around the world (Cochrane Collaboration, 2008). **Systematic reviews** are observational studies designed to retrieve and weigh the evidence from numerous sources regarding the efficacy of diagnostic tools, medical treatments, and nonmedical procedures for patients (Cochrane Collaboration, 2008). David Sackett, Gordon Guyatt, and colleagues at McMasters University were also very influential, developing the concept of and methodologies for **evidence-based medicine** (EBM). Sackett, Rosenberg, Gray, Haynes, and Richardson (1996) defined EBM as "the conscientious, explicit, and judicious use of current best evidence in making decisions about the care of individual patients."

At face value, it is difficult to disagree with EBM. Most people would agree that medicine should be based on sound scientific evidence. Physicians' decisions should be made on the results of sound research studies. Scientific evidence separates medicine from quackery, which was defined earlier as a special category of pseudoscience usually related to the medical profession. Every day though, the public is exposed to advertisements for unproven treatments of various medical conditions, such as the use of lemon oil on the scalp to prevent hair loss and wonder pills for dramatic weight loss without dieting. The old adage "Let the buyer beware" applies to those who purchase and use such remedies. However, the stakes are higher for patients diagnosed with life-threatening illnesses and their families seeking treatment. In these cases, scientific evidence is very helpful in clinical decision making.

Scientific evidence, however, is only one part of the equation. Medical research often employs special studies called double-blinded, randomized controlled clinical trials that utilize hundreds of participants and are rigorously designed to minimize bias, such that any differences in outcomes are due to the independent variable rather than any confounding factors. These studies provide statistics to assist physicians in trying to predict outcomes for individual patients, based on pathways of care. One criticism of clinical trials has been that that they fail to recruit a wide variety of participants, namely women and members of minority groups. It is important for physicians to remember that evidence is being applied to decide the fate of a single human being with his or her own unique set of needs, abilities, values, and preferences (ASHA, 2005).

How well do statistics apply to individual patients? How much should physicians rely on medical trial statistics and how should they be interpreted? How can physicians assist patients digest information they may read on the Internet? Some of these questions may be answered by considering the predicament of Stephen Jay Gould, an evolutionary biologist and professor at Harvard University who was diagnosed with incurable abdominal mesothelioma. Based on his experiences, he wrote an essay, *The Median Isn't the Message,* that tells an uplifting story of how statistics are simply estimates and that they are not the end all, be all for determining outcomes for individual patients. After his surgery, Dr. Gould was puzzled why his physicians did not provide any literature for him to read on his condition. Therefore, he was determined to learn as much as he could on his own. At Harvard's Countway Medical Library, he learned why his physicians did not immediately tell him about his disease when he found that the median survival rate was only eight months after diagnosis. He surmised that if he did not know anything about statistics, his conclusion would be that he only had eight months to live. Fortunately, he knew that an eight-month median meant that half of the patients lived longer but that the other half lived less than eight months. Unlike the mean, the median is not affected by outlier scores. So a median of eight months provided no indication longest survival past diagnosis. He also knew this statistic included all patients, regardless of age, general health, attitudes, and other characteristics that could affect the outcome. He took comfort that he was young, would receive the best medical treatment, and had a positive attitude. Dr. Gould exceeded the statistics and lived for twenty years beyond his diagnosis!

What can the medical profession and patients learn from Dr. Gould? One lesson is that scientific evidence is just one part of the picture and that statistics are tools to assist in clinical decision making. Another lesson is that statistics are based on theoretical averages, which may or may not necessarily generalize to a particular patient. A third lesson is that effective physicians realize that they are dealing with real people who should be their partners in pursuing positive outcomes. Many, many gifted physicians and surgeons have been labeled highly skillful in their clinical acumen but lacking in their bedside manner. Optimal patient care is achieved when scientific evidence blends with clinical expertise and consideration of patients as real people in clinical decision making. In the next section, we will discuss how EBM has influenced communication sciences and disorders.

LEARNING OBJECTIVES

This chapter will enable readers to:

- Define EBM and EBP.
- List the skills needed for EBP in communication sciences and disorders.

- Sequence the five-step process used in EBP.

Evidence-Based Practice in Communication Sciences and Disorders

As audiologists and speech pathologists, clinicians have long made decisions regarding the *best* diagnostic tools and treatment protocols to use with patients. What do we mean by *best*? Does *best* mean EBM? Yes, when referring only to scientific evidence. However, what course of action or decision is best depends on who is asking the question. For example, from a patient's perspective, the best diagnostic test is the least invasive and most accurate in determining the cause of their symptoms. The definition of *best* is similar for speech-language pathologists and audiologists in that they want a diagnostic tool that is accurate but also provides direction for treatment. From the standpoint of a hospital or speech and hearing clinic, "best" diagnostic tools are those that are safe and accurate and also billable. Thus, the definition of best practices shifts slightly from stakeholder to stakeholder, but they all focus on quality.

Who determines quality? Is it the American Academy of Audiology (AAA) or the American Speech-Language-Hearing Association (ASHA)? Both professional organizations have published **position statements, clinical practice guidelines,** and **preferred practice patterns.** Position statements are documents written by groups of experts that represent the official position of the professional organization on a timely topic related to professional issues or clinical practice (ASHA, 2007). Clinical practice guidelines are statements and recommendations developed by groups of experts to help clinicians and patients make clinical decisions (ASHA, 2007). Preferred practice patterns are statements that define universally applicable characteristics of specific clinical activities including definitions, professional roles, expected outcomes, clinical indications, clinical processes, setting and equipment specifications, and documentation (ASHA, 2007). For example, the preferred practice pattern for counseling specifies that audiologists (professional roles) should assist patients to develop appropriate goals (expected outcomes) as part of audiologic services (clinical indications). Moreover the clinical process of audiologic counseling includes disability screening and assessment, evaluation of counseling needs, provision of information, and use of strategies to modify patients' behavior and environment. The preferred practice patterns further mandate the development of coping mechanisms and systems for emotional support and development and coordination of patient self-help support groups.

All of these documents are available on the ASHA website to its members and those of the National Student Speech-Language-Hearing Association. However, do speech-language pathologists, audiologists, or students ever wonder on what basis these documents were formulated? Would clinicians be satisfied if they learned recognized leaders in the field simply had convened and held discussions to decide the best practices in communication sciences and disorders? Customarily, proposed documents are available for peer review and comment by the membership prior to adoption. Therefore, most of these documents are developed on the basis of expert opinion and consensus. Is expert opinion good enough? The answer may depend on who the experts are. If they are skilled clinicians, they may base their recommendations on their professional training and experiences of practices found to be effective with patients. However, clinical expertise is just one piece of the puzzle. If the experts are researchers, their recommendations may be based on scientific evidence, which also is just another piece of the puzzle. If the experts are patients and their family members, the recommendations are based on their values and preferences, another important piece of the puzzle. However, up until recently, most of these documents were based on clinical expertise, with little consideration of scientific evidence or patient preferences. Expert opinion alone is not sufficient for clinical decisions.

Readers may be wondering what good are these documents if they are based only on clinical expertise. Some may even be frustrated that there is no single source to consult for clinical decision making. So far, readers have been encouraged to evaluate research studies providing the scientific evidence for communication sciences and disorders. However, your critical thinking skills should not be left in your research design class, but should be applied to clinical practice. To understand EBP in communication sciences and disorders, readers must know what it is and the knowledge and skills required for its implementation.

What Is Evidence-Based Practice?

Communication sciences and disorders has been affected by the EBM movement along with other allied health professions. ASHA and AAA have embraced the concept and strategically moved toward its implementation at multiple levels through position statements, guidelines, and the creation of an *Evidence-Based Practice Compendium*. *Evidence-Based practice* (EBP) refers to an approach by which current high-quality research evidence is integrated with practitioner expertise, patient preferences, and patient values into the process of making clinical decisions (ASHA, 2005). Figure 11.1 shows the interaction of the three components of EBP.

ASHA's definition of EPB contains three important concepts and poses a question that requires explanation. The first important point is that clinical decision making should be based on *high-quality* research evidence. Fortunately, more often than

FIGURE 11.1

Interaction of the Three Components of Evidence-Based Practice

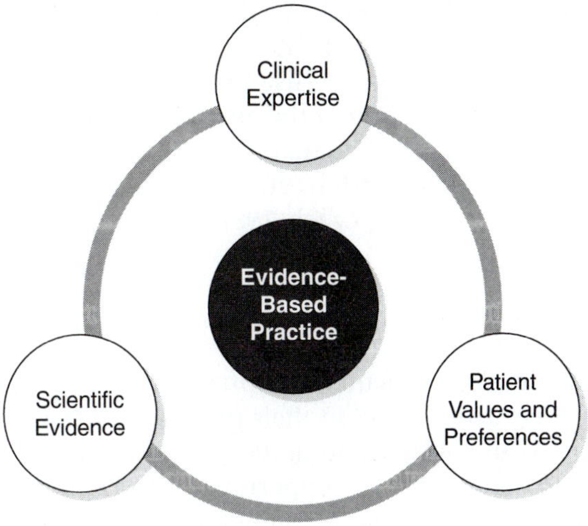

not, audiologists and speech-language pathologists seek out evidence rather than relying entirely on intuition to guide clinical practice (Plante, 2003). However, they may not know how to differentiate low- from high-quality research. High-quality research evidence can be defined in a number of ways. At the level of a single study, high-quality research evidence requires well-controlled experimental designs that eliminate potential sources of bias. EBP requires assessing the quality of studies on their own merit. By now, readers should be confident in their ability to critique the validity and reliability of studies in communication sciences and disorders. This ability will be strengthened as one becomes more familiar with EBP appraisal criteria. The second important concept is that sound research studies must be evaluated according to their **level of evidence.** Levels of evidence are hierarchies for categorizing the scientific rigor of research studies that determine how results should be used for EBP. Third, it must be underscored that clinical decision making is an interaction between scientific evidence, clinician expertise, and patient values and preferences, requiring specific knowledge and skills.

What Knowledge and Skills Are Required for Evidence-Based Practice?

What sorts of skills are required to do EBP? ASHA's *Evidence-Based Practice in Communication Disorders: Position Statement* (ASHA, 2005) lists six requisite EBP skills for audiologists and speech-language pathologists:

- *Skill 1.* "Recognize the needs, abilities, values, preferences, and interests of individuals and families to whom they provide clinical services, and integrate those factors along with best current research evidence and their clinical expertise in making clinical decisions."

Most audiologists and speech-language pathologists serve populations varying in age, ethnicity, and cultural background which requires **cross-cultural competence,** or the ability to understand the origin of one's bias (e.g., personal history) in order to establish a common ground with patients from diverse backgrounds (Hanson, 1997). Understanding patient and family needs, strengths, weaknesses, core values, and preferences for services is a prerequisite for clinicians prior to blending current research findings and their clinical expertise for decision making. Consideration of patient characteristics is prerequisite to the appropriate generalization of research findings to clinical situations. In addition, expertise in cross-cultural service delivery increases the likelihood that decisions are appropriate for both the patients' and mainstream cultures (Hanson, 1997; Lynch, 1997).

- *Skill 2.* "Acquire and maintain the knowledge and skills that are necessary to provide high-quality professional services, including knowledge and skills related to evidence-based practice."

Students need to develop the acumen for providing high-quality clinical services in addition to those needed for EBP in their professional training programs. Current practitioners have an obligation to update their knowledge and skills through continuing education and to seek out opportunities to learn about EBP. Moreover, academicians must update their course content to reflect current research findings in diagnosis and treatment that have been evaluated using EBP appraisal criteria. Didactic and clinical coursework should provide students with the opportunity to use EBP skills in classroom and clinical situations, respectively.

- *Skill 3.* "Evaluate prevention, screening, and diagnostic procedures, protocols, and measures to identify maximally informative and cost-effective diagnostic and screening tools, recognized appraisal criteria described in the evidence-based practice literature."

Students and practitioners must be able to use evidence-based appraisal criteria to select the prevention, screening, and diagnostic protocols that provide the greatest amount of information for the least resource expenditure. To do so they must clearly understand the nature of the study and then use the most appropriate appraisal criteria.

- *Skill 4.* "Evaluate the efficacy, effectiveness, and efficiency of clinical protocols for prevention, treatment, and enhancement using criteria recognized in the evidence-based practice literature."

In order to be able to evaluate the efficacy, effectiveness, and efficiency of prevention, treatment, and enhancement protocols using EBP criteria, it is important to know the definition of these terms. **Efficacy** is the degree to which interventions result in positive outcomes in ideal settings (ASHA, 2007). Ideal settings are often research laboratories or experimental conditions providing studies with a high degree of internal validity. EBP requires the ability to discern which findings are generalizable to real patients in a wide variety of service-delivery sites. **Effectiveness** is the extent to which treatments provide positive patient outcomes in real-world settings (ASHA, 2007). Results from studies conducted in actual clinical settings are common in communication sciences and disorders. **Efficiency** is the extent to which one treatment provides relatively better outcomes than other treatments, important when counseling patients on two or more treatment options.

• *Skill 5.* "Evaluate the quality of evidence appearing in any source or format, including journal articles, textbooks, continuing education offerings, newsletters, advertising, and Web-based products, prior to incorporating such evidence into clinical decision making."

Students and practitioners are exposed to a plethora of information in a variety of professional and non-professional formats and need the ability to evaluate information from various sources to use in clinical practice. Whether information in professors' lectures, assigned textbooks, websites, news stories, research articles, trade magazines, continuing education activities, products introduced in professional exhibits, or recommendations from colleagues, evaluative criteria used in EBP can be applied to all forms of information to improve service delivery and to assist patients and their families in clinical decision making. However, it is important to know that there are a wide variety of evaluative criteria that must be applied to the appropriate type of evidence. In addition, the validity and reliability of these sources varies, and clinicians should assist patients in being savvy consumers of scientific information.

• *Skill 6.* "Monitor and incorporate new and high-quality research evidence having implications for clinical practice."

More of a promise than new learning, the final skill is a commitment to keeping abreast of the latest technological advancements and cutting-edge research in the field, praising its validity, and the implementing any useful knowledge into clinical service delivery. Students and practitioners must also know which information resources provide the best evidence and how to search for it in an expeditious manner.

Many in the field of communication sciences and disorders have mixed emotions regarding EBP, not only because it represents a change in the status quo but also because it is surrounded by myths (Dollaghan, 2003). One myth is that it requires hours and hours of library research per month, particularly if clinicians are to stay abreast of *all* "cutting-edge" research (Dollaghan, 2003). However, Sackett believed that clinicians are likely to have no more than thirty minutes per week to devote to EBP. Most of the tasks listed in the position statement begin with the word *evaluate,* meaning that clinicians must be able to assess the validity and usefulness of scientific evidence. Valid evidence is that which is gleaned from the results of studies that have little or no source of bias, whereas useful information is that which is applicable to the patient and clinical scenario. As practitioners become experienced, they should be able to derive benefit from EBP in the time they have available.

Cox (2005) stated that EBP from the level of the clinician is accomplished one patient at a time and one issue at a time, involving a five-step process. The first step is to generate a focused, answerable clinical or research question, recognizing the variety of possible clinical questions going from prevention, screening, and diagnostics to intervention, prognosis, and cost effectiveness. The second step involves finding the best available scientific evidence that is both relevant to the clinical question and has the least amount of bias. Effective searches require knowledge of the databases that pertain to communication sciences and disorders and the skill for conducting strategic searches. The third step is to evaluate the validity, importance, and relevance of the scientific evidence. The fourth step is to make a recommendation after carefully weighing the scientific evidence, clinical expertise, and patient variables in making decisions in the clinical milieu. Because these decisions involve real patients, the fifth and final step is to evaluate the results and seek ways of improving the process for patients in the future.

Summary

Textbooks may provide foundational information regarding critiquing research studies. However, effective implementation of EBP requires some intangible skills such as clinical intuition and the ability to connect on a human level with patients and their families. These skills cannot be taught and are honed via clinical and life experiences. Therefore, it is paramount that readers keep in mind when reading the next few chapters on levels of evidence, crafting focused clinical questions and searching for evidence, evaluating identified scientific information, and putting all of the information together for clinical decision making that the information provided just covers one part of EBP. However, in Chapter 15 we blend all three aspects of EBP and apply its principles to a clinical scenario.

LEARNING ACTIVITIES

1. Reflect on your own clinical experiences involving making a decision. Did you use all three aspects of high-quality research evidence, clinical expertise, and patient values/preferences required for EBP?

2. Trace the steps that you typically use for clinical decision making. How does the process differ from that used in EBP?

REVIEW EXERCISES

1. *Sequencing:* Please sequence the following steps in EBP in the order in which they appear.
   A. Evaluating the evidence
   B. Grading the clinical recommendation
   C. Evaluating the process
   D. Finding the best available evidence
   E. Framing a focused clinical or research question

   _____ First
   _____ Second
   _____ Third
   _____ Fourth
   _____ Fifth

2. *Definitions:* Please define EBP.

ANSWERS TO THE REVIEW EXERCISES

1. E, D, A, B, C
2. EBP is an approach by which high-quality research is integrated with clinical expertise and patient values/preferences in clinical decision making.

CHAPTER 12

Levels of Evidence

There is no greater evidence of superior intelligence than to be surprised at nothing.
—Josh Billings (1818–1885)

Beautiful evidence follows a growing concern in my work: assessing the quality of evidence and of finding out the truth.
—Edward Tufte

Evidence can vary depending on the circumstances, the weather, and how long it has been hanging around.
—Pat Brown

The first step in learning about evidence-based practice (EBP) is to acknowledge that not all information accessed by audiologists and speech-language pathologists to aid in clinical decision making is equivalent in terms of scientific rigor. Is information from clinical practice guidelines of high scientific rigor? Some may feel that any information appearing in a textbook must be scientifically rigorous. Otherwise, why would it be published? Similarly, others may believe that information provided by clinical experts at continuing education activities must also be reliable and valid. Unfortunately, such information may not be based on sound scientific evidence and must be scrutinized prior to use in EBP. The purpose of this chapter is to introduce readers to the idea of ranking information according to its level of evidence or scientific rigor. The higher the level of evidence, the greater is the scientific rigor of the information. Readers will be introduced to the concept of "levels of evidence" and how this is applied for intervention and diagnostic studies in communication sciences and disorders. Moreover, particular attention will be focused on types of research that are relatively new to the professions, namely systematic reviews with meta-analysis and double-blinded, randomized controlled clinical trials.

LEARNING OBJECTIVES

This chapter will enable readers to:

- Discuss the concept of levels of evidence.
- Compare and contrast different levels of evidence.
- Acknowledge the levels of evidence for intervention and diagnostic studies in communication sciences and disorders.

- List the criteria for establishing hierarchies of rigor.
- Explain the nuances of types of research found at various levels of evidence.

Levels of Evidence

To understand levels of evidence, readers must recognize hierarchies appropriate for communication sciences and disorders and what constitutes scientific rigor.

What Hierarchy Is Appropriate for Communication Sciences and Disorders?

We have already defined levels of evidence as hierarchies for categorizing the scientific rigor of research studies. Levels of evidence are used across healthcare disciplines, from medicine to occupational therapy to physical therapy, to name a few. Not all healthcare professions use exactly the same hierarchy for levels of evidence. For example, some countries (e.g., the United Kingdom) use a national level of evidence. To make matters more confusing, different professions have adopted different hierarchies for levels of evidence. According to the Agency for Healthcare Research and Quality there are several dozen of these hierarchies, which may vary in the number of levels from as few as three to as many as eight (Robey, 2004), but most of the hierarchies basically have the same characteristics. First, all hierarchies use numbers, plus or minus signs, and/or letters to define the particular levels of evidence. The lower the number, the higher the scientific rigor. Hierarchies have been designed for different purposes and procedures and use differing criteria for rigor. For example, different hierarchies exist for measurement technologies, diagnosis, prognosis, safety, efficacy, and effectiveness, basing their rankings on such statistical criteria as magnitude of effect sizes, confidence intervals, number of results, consistency of results, sample size, or Type I and Type II error rates (Robey, 2004). Two hierarchies, one from the Scottish Intercollegiate Guidelines Network (Harbour & Miller, 2004; Scottish Intercollegiate Network, 2008) and the other from Oxford Centre for Evidence-Based Medicine (CEBM, www.cebm.net) are levels of evidence for intervention and diagnostic studies, respectively, and are shown in Tables 12.1 and 12.2. These rubrics are particularly detailed and are useful in evidence-based medicine.

In this textbook, we will use a hierarchy adapted from Cox (2005) for intervention studies and an adaptation of the CEBM version for diagnostic investigations. The hierarchy for intervention studies contains six levels and is shown in Table 12.3 (p. 308). Although systematic reviews are of the highest level of evidence, the individual studies contributing to the meta-analysis ultimately determine the level of rigor. The hierarchy for diagnostic studies contains five levels and is shown in Table 12.4 (p. 308).

What Criteria Are Used in Establishing Hierarchies of Scientific Rigor?

Before we discuss levels of evidence, we must consider five themes in the evidence ratings of scientific information (ASHA, 2004). The first theme is that the highest levels of rigor require independent confirmation and converging evidence (ASHA, 2004). In other words, clinical recommendations must be made based on more than the results of one or two studies. The highest levels of scientific rigor are reserved for studies that aggregate the results of several high-quality studies using special statistical

TABLE 12.1

Levels of Evidence According to the Scottish Intercollegiate Network

Level	Description
1++	High-quality meta-analyses, systematic reviews of randomized controlled trials (RCTs), or RCTs with a very low risk of bias
1+	Well-conducted meta-analyses, systematic reviews of RCTs, or RCTs with a low risk of bias
1−	Meta-analyses, systematic reviews or RCTs, or RCTs with a high risk of bias
2++	High-quality systematic reviews of case-control or cohort studies or high-quality case-control or cohort studies with a very low risk of confounding, bias, or chance, and a high probability that the relationship is causal
2+	Well-conducted case-control or cohort studies with a low risk of confounding, bias, or chance, and a moderate probability that the relationship is causal
2−	Case-control or cohort studies with a high risk of confounding, bias, or chance, and a significant risk that the relationship is not causal
3	Nonanalytic studies (e.g., case reports, case series)
4	Expert opinion

Adapted from Harbour and Miller, 2004; Scottish Intercollegiate Network, 2008.

procedures. In the previous chapter we noted that systematic reviews are observational studies designed to retrieve the evidence from numerous sources regarding the efficacy of diagnostic tools and nonmedical and medical treatments for patients. Systematic reviews often include conducting **meta-analyses,** or statistical procedures that combine the results of individual studies in order to weigh the evidence regarding the efficacy of a particular procedure or intervention. A second theme shows that the studies at the highest levels of evidence require careful prior planning to ensure

TABLE 12.2

Levels of Evidence for Diagnostic Studies According to the Centre for Evidence-Based Medicine

Level	Description
1a	Systematic review of homogeneous diagnostic studies based on randomized, controlled clinical trials
1b	Cohort studies that validate the index with a gold standard or very good reference standards
1c	Cohort studies that show absolute sensitivity or specificity
2a	Systematic reviews of homogeneous Level 2b or better diagnostic studies
2b	Exploratory cohort studies that collect data and use techniques such as regression analysis to determine which factors are "significant" using good reference standards
3a	Systematic reviews of Level 3b or better studies
3b	Nonconsecutive cohort studies without consistently applied reference standards
4	Case-control studies or superseded reference standards
5	Expert opinion

Adapted from CEBM, 2008.

TABLE 12.3

Levels of Evidence for Intervention Studies Suggested for Use in Communication Sciences and Disorders

Level	Description
I	Systematic reviews and meta-analyses of randomized clinical trials and other well-designed studies
II	Double-blinded, prospective, randomized, controlled clinical trials
III	Nonrandomized intervention studies
IV	Nonintervention studies:
	• Cohort studies
	• Case-control studies
	• Cross-sectional surveys
V	Case reports
VI	Expert opinion of respected authorities

Adapted from Cox, 2005.

high internal validity and random assignment of participants to treatment and control groups. The third theme illustrates that studies at the highest levels of evidence avoid subjectivity and bias through the double-blinding of experimenters and participants. In addition, high-quality studies avoid bias through inclusion of data points from all recruited participants, not just those who managed to complete the protocol or had positive outcomes, and through use of special statistical procedures. These are called **intention-to-treat analyses** and they are done using all participants recruited to avoid

TABLE 12.4

Levels of Evidence for Diagnostic Studies for Use in Communication Sciences and Disorders

Level	Description
I	Systematic reviews and meta-analyses of double-blinded prospective, randomized, controlled clinical trials of diagnostic studies High-quality cohort studies that:
	• Validate an index with a gold standard or very good reference test
	• Show absolute sensitivity or specificity
II	Systematic reviews of homogeneous Level 2 or better diagnostic studies Exploratory cohort studies using statistical procedures (e.g., regression analysis) to determine "significant" factors with use of adequate reference standards
III	Systematic reviews of Level 3 or better diagnostic studies Nonconsecutive cohort study without consistently applied reference standards
IV	Case-control studies or superseded reference standards
V	Expert opinion of respected authorities

Adapted from CEBM, 2008.

biasing results by only including the data of those who completed the experimental protocol. A fourth theme is that research at a high level of evidence should report both effect sizes and confidence intervals regarding the effectiveness of an intervention. As you learned in an earlier chapter, effect sizes are statistical calculations that estimate the clinical significance of a particular intervention. Confidence intervals are measures of the precision of the summary effect estimate that should be reported. A fifth theme is that studies at the highest levels of evidence should show relevance by recruiting samples of participants who accurately represent the intended population and should also demonstrate sufficient feasibility to permit replication. Throughout the rest of this chapter, we will highlight these five trends as they relate to the levels of evidence used to rank the scientific rigor of research in communication sciences and disorders. We will discuss criteria for evaluating various types of scientific evidence in Chapter 14.

Level I: Systematic Reviews of Well-Designed Clinical Studies

Level I of evidence includes meta-analysis of multiple well-designed clinical studies. To understand the purpose of a meta-analysis, readers must first know what a systematic review is, what it looks like, and characteristics of a good one.

What Is a Systematic Review?

The highest level of evidence includes systematic reviews complete with meta-analyses that aggregate the results from well-designed clinical studies. Meta-analyses use **secondary measurement methods** in which experimenters analyze data collected by other researchers. This strategy is different than **primary measurement methods** in which the experimenter collects and analyses the data. For example, Law, Garrett, and Nye (2003) completed a systematic review with a meta-analysis determining the efficacy of interventions for children with developmental speech and language delays and disorders. Their search found thirty-six articles that reported on thirty-three different trials. Only twenty-five studies provided sufficient information to use in the meta-analysis. On closer inspection, only thirteen of these were considered to be similar enough to be combined in the meta-analysis. The results of the meta-analysis indicated that speech and language therapy may possibly be effective for children with phonological or expressive vocabulary difficulties. However, the evidence was inconclusive regarding the effectiveness of treatment for children with expressive syntax difficulties. Moreover, there was a paucity of data supporting the effectiveness of intervention for children with receptive language difficulties. Intervention lasting greater than eight weeks was associated with positive clinical outcomes.

As stated in the previous section, systematic reviews are needed to validate research because causality between treatment and positive patient outcomes cannot be established on the basis of a single investigation. Systematic reviews may be done with or without meta-analyses and involve

- Assessing amassed evidence about targeted interventions from a foundation of clearly formulated questions

- Systematically using explicit methods to identify, select, critically appraise, and narrow down a vast body of literature to focus in on only the most relevant research pertaining to the topic
- Collecting, analyzing, aggregating, and interpreting data from pertinent studies to answer the question (Cochrane Collaboration, 2008)

Systematic reviews, with or without meta-analyses, are done for at least five reasons (McKibbon, Easy, & Marks, 1999). First, systematic reviews get to the "bottom line" of all studies involving a particular treatment or intervention. For example, Robey and Dalebout (1998) completed a meta-analysis of a few studies investigating the reduction of self-perceived hearing handicap measured by the *Hearing Handicap Inventory for the Elderly* (Ventry & Weinstein, 1982) and the *Hearing Performance Inventory* (Giolas, Owens, Lamb, & Schubert, 1979). They found that hearing aid treatment is effective when indexed as a reduction of patient-perceived hearing difficulty (Robey & Dalebout, 1998). Second, systematic reviews are undertaken to estimate the amount of benefit derived from a treatment or intervention. In the same study, Robey and Dalebout (1998) averaged the amount of benefit across studies to come up with an "effect size" or how much reduction in self-perceived hearing handicap can be expected based on a review of all studies. Third, systematic reviews combine the results from patients in clinically relevant subgroups across studies, thereby increasing statistical power. For instance, the results of many promising studies have low numbers of participant recruitment. However, a meta-analysis of the findings from several studies with small sample sizes can make a powerful statement regarding the effectiveness of a particular treatment. A fourth reason to do a systematic review is to resolve discrepancies among the findings of studies. Thus, a systematic review can settle discrepancies in findings among studies that demonstrate varying results in the effectiveness of interventions. Another reason to do a systematic review is to plan for future studies. For example, if a systematic review does not find support for a specific intervention, it is just as important as finding supportive evidence. The lack of good studies in a particular area demonstrates a need for future research.

What Does a Summary of a Systematic Review Look Like?

We have defined and provided rationales for undertaking a systematic review. To further understand how such reviews are used in research, please look at the summaries of systematic reviews in speech-language pathology and audiology provided in Figures 12.1 (pp. 311–312) and 12.2 (pp. 313–314).

What Are the Major Components of a Systematic Review?

Even though the examples in Figures 12.1 and 12.2 are only summaries, they demonstrate that all systematic reviews have the same basic parts. First, notice that the summary has a version in "plain language" that summarizes the overall results of the review in simple terms so that the findings may be understandable to all. The next part of the summary is the **structured abstract,** a style of abstract that emphasizes the critical elements of an investigation through the use of separate headings. Structured abstracts are particularly useful for EBP because they allow readers to quickly access

FIGURE 12.1

Summary of a Systematic Review in Speech-Language Pathology

Speech and language therapy versus placebo or no intervention for dysarthria in Parkinson's disease

Deane K H O, Whurr R, Playford E D, Ben-Shlomo Y, Clarke C E.

Plain language summary

This review will compare the benefits of speech and language therapy versus placebo (sham therapy) or no treatment for speech disorders in Parkinson's disease. Relevant trials were identified by electronic searches of 21 medical literature databases, various registers of clinical trials and an examination of the reference lists of identified studies and other reviews.

Only unblinded controlled trials were included in this review. These were studies where two groups of patients were compared, one group of patients had speech and language therapy, the other was untreated. The patients were assigned to each of the groups in a random fashion so as to reduce the potential for bias.

Three trials were found comparing speech and language therapy with an untreated group in 63 patients. The quality of the trials' methods was variable with all studies failing in at least one critical area. All three of the controlled trials reported a positive effect of speech and language therapy for speech disorders in Parkinson's disease. Many of the outcome measures examined appeared to improve by a clinically significant amount after therapy.

Considering the flaws in the studies' methods, the small number of patients examined, and the possibility that studies with a negative result were not published (publication bias), there is insufficient evidence to prove or disprove the benefit of speech and language therapy for the treatment of speech disorders in people with Parkinson's disease. However it should be unblinded that this lack of evidence does not mean lack of effect.

A large well designed placebo-controlled unblinded trial is needed to assess the effectiveness of speech and language therapy for speech disorders in Parkinson's disease. Outcome measures with particular relevance to patients should be chosen and the patients followed for at least 6 months to determine the duration of any improvement. As there does not appear to be a consensus as to the 'standard' form of speech and language therapy to use to treat dysarthria in Parkinson's disease, a survey of therapists is needed to determine what methods of speech and language therapy are currently being used by therapists to treat Parkinsonian dysarthria, and whether there is a consensus as to 'best-practice'. This could then be used to inform the design of the unblended controlled trial.

Abstract

Background

Dysarthria is a common manifestation of Parkinson's disease which increases in frequency and intensity with the progress of the disease (Streifler 1984). Up to 20% of Parkinsonian patients are referred for speech and language therapy (S&LT), its aim being to improve the intelligibility of the patient's speech.

(Continued)

FIGURE 12.1

(Continued)

Objectives

To compare the efficacy of speech and language therapy versus placebo or no interventions in patients with Parkinson's disease.

Search strategy

Relevant trials were identified by electronic searches of MEDLINE, EMBASE, CINAHL, ISI-SCI, AMED, MANTIS, REHABDATA, REHADAT, GEROLIT, Pascal, LILACS, MedCarib, JICST-Eplus, AIM, IMEMR, SIGLE, ISI-ISTP, DISSABS, Conference Papers Index, Aslib Index to Theses, the Cochrane Controlled Trials Register, the CentreWatch Clinical Trials listing service, the metaRegister of Controlled Trials, ClinicalTrials.gov, CRISP, PEDro, NIDRR and NRR; and examination of the reference lists of identified studies and other reviews.

Selection criteria

Only unblinded controlled trials (RCT) were included.

Data collection and analysis

Data were abstracted independently by KD and RW and differences settled by discussion.

Main results

Three unblinded controlled trials were found comparing speech and language therapy with placebo for speech disorders in Parkinson's disease. A total of 63 patients were examined.

The loudness of the patients' voices were increased by between 7–18%, depending on the speaking task being performed. It is likely that this is a clinically significant improvement. After six months the degree of improvement was reduced but was still statistically significant. Overall measures of dysarthria were measured in two trials and also improved. The clinical significance of these improvements was less clear cut as intelligibility of speech was not measured in any of these studies.

Authors' conclusions

Considering the small number of patients examined, the methodological flaws in many of the studies, and the possibility of publication bias, there is insufficient evidence to support or refute the efficacy of speech and language therapy for dysarthria in Parkinson's disease. A Delphi-style survey is needed to develop a consensus as to what is 'standard' S&LT for dysarthria in Parkinson's disease. Then a large well designed placebo-controlled RCT is needed to demonstrate speech and language therapy's effectiveness for dysarthria in Parkinson's disease. The trial should conform to CONSORT guidelines. Outcome measures with particular relevance to patients should be chosen and the patients followed for at least 6 months to determine the duration of any improvement.

critical elements of a study. Research in EBP is facilitated when searching for critical studies through electronic databases and journals highlighting key aspects of a study for quick review.

Structured abstracts for systematic review typically have the following sections: (1) Background, (2) Objectives, (3) Search Strategy, (4) Selection Criteria, (5) Data

FIGURE 12.2

Summary of a Systematic Review in Audiology

The Epley (canalith repositioning) maneuver for benign paroxysmal positional vertigo

Hilton M, Pinder D

Plain language summary

Benign paroxysmal positional vertigo (BPPV) is caused by a rapid change in head movement. The person feels they or their surroundings are moving or rotating. Common causes are head trauma or ear infection. BPPV can be caused by debris in the semicircular canal of the ear that continues to move after the head has stopped moving. This causes a sensation of ongoing movement that conflicts with other sensory information. The review of trials found the Epley maneuver (four specific movements of the head and body designed to move the debris out the ear canal) is safe and effective. More research is needed.

Abstract

Background

Benign paroxysmal positional vertigo (BPPV) is a syndrome characterized by short-lived episodes of vertigo in association with rapid changes in head position. It is a common cause of vertigo presenting to primary care and specialist otolaryngology clinics. Current treatment approaches include rehabilitative exercises and physical maneuvers including the Epley maneuver.

Objectives

To assess the effectiveness of the Epley maneuver compared to other treatments available for posterior canal benign paroxysmal positional vertigo, or no treatment.

Search strategy

The Cochrane Central Register of Controlled Trials (CENTRAL) (Cochrane Library Issue 1, 2004), MEDLINE (1966 to 2004), EMBASE (1974 to 2004) and reference lists of identified publications. Date of the most recent search was January 2004.

Selection criteria

Randomized trials of adults diagnosed with posterior canal BPPV (including a positive Dix-Hallpike test).

Comparisons sought:

Epley maneuver versus placebo Epley maneuver versus untreated controls
Epley maneuver versus other active treatment
Outcome measures that were considered include: frequency and severity of attacks of vertigo; proportion of patients improved by each intervention; and conversion of a "positive" Dix-Hallpike test to a "negative" Dix-Hallpike test

Data collection and analysis

Both reviewers independently extracted data and assessed trials for quality.

Main results

Fifteen trials were identified but twelve studies were excluded because of a high risk of bias, leaving three trials in the review. Trials were mainly excluded because of

(Continued)

FIGURE 12.2

(Continued)

inadequate concealment during unblended on, or failure to blind outcome assessors. The studies included in the review (Lynn 1995; Froehling 2000; Yimtae 2003) addressed the efficacy of the Epley maneuver against a sham maneuver or control group by comparing the proportion of participants in each group who had complete resolution of their symptoms, and who converted from a positive to negative Dix-Hallpike test. Individual and pooled data showed a statistically significant effect in favor of the Epley maneuver over controls. There were no serious adverse effects of treatment.

Authors' conclusions

There is some evidence that the Epley maneuver is a safe effective treatment for posterior canal BPPV, although this is based on the results of only three small unblinded controlled trials with relatively short follow up. There is no good evidence that the Epley maneuver provides a long term resolution of symptoms. There is no good evidence comparing the Epley maneuver with other physical, medical or surgical therapy for posterior canal BPPV.

Collection and Analysis, (6) Main Results, and (7) Authors' Conclusions. The Background section provides the context of the systematic review. For example, the background for the systematic review in speech-language pathology defines dysarthria as a manifestation of Parkinson's disease that gets worse with the disease process. The Objective states the aim of the systematic review. For example, the objective of the systematic review in audiology was to assess the effectiveness of the Epley maneuver compared to other treatments available for posterior canal benign paroxysmal positional vertigo or to no treatment at all. The Search Strategy is a section of a structured abstract that is unique to systematic reviews and specifies the databases and other methods used to find relevant studies. For example, for the speech-language pathology systematic review, the authors used electronic databases (e.g., MEDLINE, EMBASE, CINAHL, and so on) and the examination of the reference lists of identified studies and other reviews. We will discuss more about database search in the next chapter. In a full-length systematic review, the search strategy is described in sufficient detail that it is transparent or can easily be replicated, which is a characteristic of any well-written research methodology. Note that the search strategy of the audiology systematic review has the most recent date of search as January, 2004, illustrating a critical concept regarding systematic reviews. They are never finished! Once a systematic review is completed, it must be updated at regular intervals. Why is that? Well, the electronic databases are updated on a daily basis. The articles that show up today may not have been there yesterday. Another way to think about doing systematic reviews is that it is like raking leaves in early fall; just when you think you're done, a few more leaves fall from the tree. Therefore, the date of the search is a critical piece of information for a systematic review because it indicates the extent of update required for recovering relevant evidence.

The Criteria is the section of the structured abstract that states the components of studies being sought. For example, in both the speech-language pathology and audiology systematic reviews, the criteria sought for type of study was randomized, controlled clinical trials at Level I of evidence. Other traditional criteria mentioned may be the type of participant, intervention, or outcome measure. For instance, the audiology systematic review sought patients with benign paroxysmal positional vertigo (BPPV) who were treated with specific types of interventions compared in the studies. Members of a systematic review carefully analyze candidate studies that must satisfy specific criteria to be included in the systematic review. Studies that are included in the systematic review undergo a rigorous quality assessment. Systematic review teams must become research sharks to separate the high-quality investigations to be included from the lower-quality studies that must be excluded.

The Data Collection and Analysis section describes how the data were extracted from the study and how they were analyzed. Even though systematic reviews are not traditional research studies, researchers do collect data for their analysis by extraction. **Data extraction** involves carefully taking statistical results from studies included in the review that directly pertain to the research question posed in the systematic review. Extracted data are placed into tables according to specific outcome measures and questions. **Rev-Man 5.0 software** is a tool developed by the Cochrane Collaboration for documenting a systematic review in ways that facilitate the study, particularly for data management. Data analysis in systematic reviews may be qualitative or quantitative or both. **Qualitative analysis** involves analyzing how many studies showed certain results for various outcomes. For example, in the audiology systematic review, investigators assessed trends in the studies that showed the effect of the Epley procedure singly and in combinations with other treatments or with no treatments at all. **Quantitative analysis** involves applying statistical procedures of individual studies in a meta-analysis to determine the sum total effect of an intervention across different investigations. For instance, earlier we mentioned how Law et al. (2003) conducted a meta-analysis of the results of several studies to assess the efficacy of speech and language therapy for children with developmental speech and language delays and disorders.

Note that in the speech-language pathology and audiology systematic reviews, the initials of the authors who completed the data extraction are listed along with how reliability was determined and how disagreements were settled. Knowing who was involved in this important process provides the information on who to contact in case of questions by readers. The Main Results section describes what was found during the systematic review. For example, the audiology systematic review explained that although fifteen trials were identified, twelve of them were excluded due to potential bias or inappropriate concealment of the treatment, leaving three studies in the systematic review. Sometimes teams will report on the total number of participants in all included studies to increase the clinical or statistical findings of the systematic review. For instance, the speech-language pathology systematic review contained the data from sixty-three studies. The overall trends are reported regarding the experimental questions (qualitative) in addition to any meta-analyses (quantitative).

Finally, the Authors' Conclusions answer the experimental questions asked in the systematic review. In the audiology systematic review, it was concluded that there was some evidence that the Epley maneuver is a safe, effective treatment for BPPV, although this is based on the results of only three small randomized clinical trials with small sample sizes.

What Are Characteristics of Good Systematic Reviews?

Hearst, Grady, Barron, and Kerlikowske (2001) have formulated the characteristics of a good systematic review, as shown in Table 12.5. One positive characteristic of a good systematic review is a clear research question that describes the condition of interest, the population, the setting, the intervention and comparison treatment, and the outcome of interest (Hearst et al., 2001). For example, an audiologist might be interested in the effectiveness of hearing aids for elderly people living in assisted-living facilities. To formulate a clear research question, the condition of interest must be described. Obviously, the condition of interest is hearing loss, but there are several types of hearing loss. Therefore, the audiologist must state "sensorineural hearing loss" because conductive and mixed hearing loss can be ameliorated either completely or partially through medical management, not amplification. The next step is specifying the population and the setting. In this case, it is persons over sixty-five years of age who reside in assisted-living facilities. Next, the intervention and comparison treatments should be specified. The audiologist may be very specific about the types of hearing aids (e.g., analog or digital) and how they are worn (e.g., monaurally or binaurally). However, being too specific may limit the number of studies found in the search and retrieval process. Specifying comparison treatments are important for designing randomized,

---

TABLE 12.5

Characteristics of a Good Systematic Review

- Clear research question
- Comprehensive and unbiased search and retrieval process for studies
- Logically defined inclusion and exclusion criteria
- Clearly and uniformly presented information from studies:
  - Characteristics
  - Findings
  - Data
- Calculation of a summary estimate of effect sizes and confidence intervals for included studies, as appropriate
- Assessment
  - Heterogeneity of the findings
  - Potential publication bias
  - Subgroup and sensitivity analyses

Adapted from Hearst, Grady, Barron, and Kerlikowske, 2001.

controlled clinical trials. For example, Jerger, Chmiel, Florin, Pirozzolo, and Wilson (1996) conducted a randomized clinical trial assessing the effectiveness of hearing aids as compared to assistive listening devices and to using hearing aids plus assistive listening devices. We will be discussing the nuances of clinical trials later on in this chapter. However, a systematic review does not have to compare one intervention with another but may simply compare the use of hearing aids to a nonaided condition or pre- versus posttreatment comparison in the same subjects in studies using a within-subjects design. And finally, the audiologist must specify the outcome(s) of concern. For example, in elderly people, the reduction of the social and emotional impacts of hearing loss or hearing handicap is an important outcome. In summary, a well-formulated question for our scenario could be, "Among persons sixty-five years of age and over who live in assisted-living facilities, does use of hearing aids reduce hearing handicap as compared to not using hearing aids for sensorineural hearing loss?"

A second characteristic of a good systematic review is a comprehensive and unbiased search and retrieval process for studies, which requires three steps (Hearst et al., 2001). The first step is to generate search strings that are likely to yield a high retrieval of possible studies for inclusion in the systematic review. Using our scenario, search strings such as "geriatrics + hearing aids + assisted-living facilities" would yield relevant articles for review. The second step is to specify which databases to use in the search. For example, databases such as Medline, the Communication Sciences and Disorders Dome (ComDisDome), and so on are very appropriate databases for communication sciences and disorders (see Chapter 13). The third step is to determine how to search for studies that either have not or have yet to be published to avoid **publication bias,** the tendency of journals to only publish statistically significant findings. Review teams can identify sources of unpublished studies through conference proceedings, clinical trials, master's theses, and doctoral dissertations. The search for articles in issues of journals or for unpublished studies is known as **handsearching.** Another way of reducing bias and increasing the rigor of the search is to use independent reviewers to access the same databases with calculations of interjudge reliabilities for various stages of the search and retrieval process. Furthermore, good systematic reviews include a transparent search and retrieval process that is described in such a way that it could be replicated by almost anyone.

A third defining factor for a good systematic review is logically defined inclusion and exclusion criteria for studies that should directly reflect the clinical or research question being asked. **Inclusion criteria** are those characteristics a study must have in order to be included in a systematic review. For example, inclusion criteria for our scenario should specify condition of interest (sensorineural hearing loss), the population (persons sixty-five years of age and older), the setting (assisted-living facilities), the intervention (use of hearing aids), comparison treatment (pre–hearing aid status), and the outcome of interest (use of the *Hearing Handicap Inventory for the Elderly*). Another important inclusion criterion is the level of evidence of studies.

However, reviewers should not be overzealous in setting unrealistic standards for studies for inclusion in a systematic review. For example, communication sciences and disorders professionals may wish to limit their systematic review to Levels I and II of evidence. However, being too restrictive may severely limit the number of applicable studies included in their systematic review or recover no evidence at all. **Exclusion criteria** are characteristics that may eliminate a study from inclusion in a systematic review. An example of exclusion criteria may be poor experimental control. Good systematic reviews specify both the process and the outcome of the quality assessment of each and every study. Finally, good systematic reviews clearly state the exclusion criteria and reasons why certain studies were eliminated from the systematic review.

A fourth characteristic of a good systematic review is accurate and copious presentation of study characteristics, data, and findings. For example, the study characteristics reported should also reflect on the experimental question to include accurate portrayal of the condition of interest, the population and the setting, the intervention and comparison treatment, and the outcome of interest. The audiologist in our scenario should report specifics on the sample of participants in each study such as number, age, gender, degree of hearing loss, and so on. Furthermore, the data and findings should be reported accurately and completely in an unbiased manner. Use of independent judges to report these aspects of the same studies increases the validity and reliability of the summaries. Moreover, use of independent judges is particularly important when extracting the data and reporting the findings of studies. The types of data extracted from the studies include the results of statistical tests (e.g., F-ratios, degree of freedom, and probability levels) for computing treatment effects and confidence intervals.

Fifth, good systematic reviews will include meta-analyses of the results that provide **summary effect estimates** and **confidence intervals** (Hearst et al., 2001). A summary effect estimate is an average effect of all studies included in the meta-analysis weighted by the size of each contributing study (Hearst et al., 2001). In addition, a confidence interval or a measure of the precision of the summary effect estimate should be reported. We will discuss more about how to obtain these measures in the chapter on EBP research methodologies.

The sixth important characteristic of good systematic reviews is the assessment of (1) the heterogeneity of the findings, (2) subgroup and sensitivity analyses, and (3) publication bias (Hearst et al., 2001). A sound systematic review assesses for the homogeneity of the findings of individual studies that are included in a meta-analysis. Ideally, meta-analyses are conducted with studies that have similar study designs, participant samples, application of interventions, and so on such that they do not differ in clinically significant ways. Sensitivity analyses assess whether similar results are obtained whether or not certain controversial studies (e.g., presence of potentially confounding factors) are included in the systematic review. Testing for publication bias involves ensuring that unpublished studies are included in systematic reviews. Special procedures include the creation of **funnel plots,** or special graphs whose shape denotes presence or absence of publication bias.

Level II: Well-Designed Randomized Clinical Trials

Level II of evidence includes well-designed randomized, controlled clinical trials. In order to appreciate the rigor of clinical trials, readers must understand their role in healthcare, their relevance to communication sciences and disorders, and their characteristics as well as advantages and disadvantages.

What Is the Role of Clinical Trials in Healthcare?

When listening to the evening news, the average citizen may hear a story about clinical trials. The news story may report promising information about new medical treatments for serious illnesses or that a clinical trial had to be terminated due to unexpected risks for patients. However, most people do not know the role that clinical trials have in healthcare. Clinical trials are required for new treatments, such as drugs, to be approved for a specific population of patients through the Food and Drug Administration (FDA). However, FDA approval is not a blanket approval for a drug or treatment to be used ubiquitously. Clinical trials are required to assess the benefits and risks of a treatment on a particular group of patients who may have a different disease than the one for which the drug was originally approved. For example, even though the promising new drug Avastin has been approved for use in treating colorectal cancer, clinical trials are required to assess its efficacy for patients with other types of cancer. The FDA has specific guidelines for clinical trials conducted in the United States, which are available on their website. Generally, clinical trials are conducted in phases or stages so that no patient is exposed to unnecessary risk at any particular stage. Table 12.6 shows the different stages of a clinical trial.

In the preclinical phase of a clinical trial, experimentation is often done at the cellular level and tests hypotheses using animal models so that no harm is done to human participants. Phase I of clinical trials involves unblinded and uncontrolled studies in which the therapy is administrated to a few participants to assess its safety.

TABLE 12.6

Stages of Clinical Trials

Stage	Description
Preclinical	Studies in cell cultures and animals
I	Unblinded, uncontrolled studies in a few volunteers to test safety
II	Relatively small randomized, controlled, blinded trials to test tolerability and different intensity or dose of the intervention on surrogate outcomes
III	Relatively large randomized, controlled, blinded trials to test the effect of the therapy on clinical outcomes
IV	Large trials or observational studies conducted after the therapy has been approved by the FDA to assess the rate of serious side effects and evaluate additional therapeutic uses

From Grady, Cummings, and Hulley (2001). Designing an experiment: Clinical trials II. In S. B. Hulley et al. (Eds.), *Designing clinical research* (2nd ed., pp. 157–174). Lippincott, Williams, and Wilkins, p. 171. Reprinted by permission.

Phase II of clinical trials consists of relatively small randomized and controlled studies to test the tolerability of the therapy and appropriate dosage on **surrogate outcomes,** intended to capture the treatment effect on an important clinical endpoint but not directly measuring the main benefit of the intervention. For example, in high-stakes cancer chemotherapeutic clinical trials, the main clinical benefit is median survival time. However, over the short term, long-term survival time is not practical to measure or may not reflect responsiveness to therapy. Therefore, surrogate outcomes such as tumor markers in the blood (e.g., CA-19) that are strongly related to clinical endpoints (e.g., survivability) may be measured as indices of treatment effectiveness. Phase III clinical trials increase in size to relatively large randomized, controlled, blinded trials that measure the effectiveness of the therapy on clinical outcomes. Effective therapies are usually approved by the FDA after successful Phase III clinical trials. Phase IV involves large clinical trials or observational studies that assess the rate of serious side effects and test additional possible uses of therapies.

It should be clear from the previous paragraph that some clinical trials are very serious business. Clinical trial monitoring involves every aspect of the experiment (i.e., recruitment of participants, adherence to the study protocol, randomization, follow-up, and so on). In small studies, the experimenters do the monitoring. However, in large clinical trials, monitoring may be done by an independent group to avoid bias. Generally, clinical trials must be monitored for at least three ethical reasons. First, any harmful effects from therapies must be documented and addressed to prevent unnecessary harm to patients (Grady, Cummings, & Hulley, 2001). Second, if the therapy demonstrates early effectiveness, the trial should then be stopped to provide treatment to participants receiving the placebo (Grady et al., 2001). Third, if the trial clearly will not answer the experimental question, the study should then be terminated to avoid wasting valuable resources and patients' time and effort, not to mention exposure to unnecessary risks (Grady et al., 2001).

Monitoring rarely discovers effects so serious to result in the complete termination of a clinical trial. However, the Women's Health Initiative (WHI) clinical trial of estrogen plus progestin was stopped early because the risks of therapy to women exceeded its benefits (Heiss, Wallace, Anderson, Aragaki, Beresford, et al., 2008). More frequently, though, changes are made in the protocol to alleviate problems identified through a quality control process. For example, one treatment condition or "arm" of a clinical trial may be stopped. Similarly, use of a drug may be terminated and patients excused from a clinical trial due to unanticipated side effects. However, other arms investigating the effectiveness of less toxic drugs may continue on in the clinical trials. Monitoring may also result in changes in the recruitment of participants and adherence to the protocol. For example, a protocol may specify exact recruitment procedures to be used to enroll patients in a particular study. However, if insufficient patients are enrolled, the protocol should be amended to include additional sources for the identification of suitable patients. Similarly, if participants failed to adhere to the protocol, then patients should be contacted to determine the reason for failure so that changes can be made in the protocol (e.g., subsidizing transportation to and from the treatment facility).

How Relevant Are Clinical Trials to Communication Sciences and Disorders?

As mentioned above, clinical trials are most commonly seen in the field of medicine. However, they are relatively rare in communication sciences and disorders. It is important for students and practitioners to acknowledge and appreciate that clinical trials represent the "gold standard" in research. Other chapters have made the point that audiology and speech-language pathology may be "research light" professions. Every year, ASHA and AAA must lobby for continued reimbursement for the identification, diagnosis, and treatment of speech-language-hearing disorders. It is much easier to obtain reimbursement from third-party payers in the field of medicine. Communication sciences and disorders may not deal with life and death medical issues, but what we do does make an important difference in the lives of our patients and their families. Those medical disciplines that demonstrate the efficacy of their specialties through clinical trial research with evidence that is compelling and convincing will receive reimbursement for services and earn the respect of their patients.

As mentioned earlier, in the field of medicine, double-blinded prospective, randomized clinical trials (DBPRCT) represent the "gold standard" of evidence-based medicine (EBM). DBPRCTs are not popular in communication sciences and disorders research, and the question arises as to why this is. Are the researchers in our field remiss in their approach to EBP? Some authors suggest that it is difficult to apply DBPRCTs in the behavioral sciences as they are used in medical and pharmaceutical fields (Hegde, 2003; Pocock, 1983; Robey & Schultz, 1998). Several possible reasons are often given for why DBPRCTs might be more of a thorny problem in communication sciences and disorders (Hegde, 2003).

One difference between the medical research community and our field is the availability of large numbers of participants representing multiple centers. It is not unusual in medical research to have studies that include thousands of participants, sometimes even tens of thousands of people located across a broad geographical area. For example, the WHI estrogen plus progestin versus placebo clinical trial enrolled over 15,730 women recruited by forty different centers (Heiss et al., 2008). In our field, most research reports contain groups of less than twenty participants. Often, these participants come from a common geographical area and receive services at a single clinic or school system. A problem with small sample sizes is that statistical power suffers and results may not be generalizable.

Small sample sizes lead to other problems. In large medical studies, participants may be randomly selected from an even larger population to participate in the research. This means that variables such as geographical area, age, socioeconomic level, and other factors are represented in the participant group. If you only have fifteen people who stutter in a study, they may not represent the heterogeneity of the general population to which you want to generalize the results. Another byproduct of small sample sizes is difficulty in blinding the investigator to the identity of participants, creating experimenter bias. With small numbers of participants, it is also difficult to conceal from patients whether or not they are receiving treatment. With larger numbers of participants it is much easier to create a double-blind condition, just because an experimenter is not likely to know which group or condition a specific person might represent.

In medical and pharmaceutical research there are federal mandates preventing the use and marketing of medications that have not undergone clinical trials. There is no such legal basis in the behavioral sciences, so it is not uncommon for treatments to be used before they have received widespread testing. Because of government controls on medical and pharmaceutical treatment, billions of dollars are available each year to subsidize the development and field testing of new drugs and interventions. Although there is some funding available from the government for work in communication sciences and disorders, it is minute in comparison to medical research support.

Hegde (2003) indicated that the treatments used in medical research are much more straightforward than in the behavioral sciences. It is much easier to control dosages of medications and how they are administered than to control a behavioral therapy. Think how difficult it would be to train two clinicians to administer treatment in exactly the same way to two different clients with their own unique characteristics. It is much easier to dispense medications. Related to the difficulty of providing consistent treatment in the behavioral sciences is the measurability issue (Hegde, 2003). In medicine, laboratory tests are far more valid and reliable than behavioral measures that may include such dependent variables as analysis of language samples or scoring of client satisfaction questionnaires. In medicine, if your lab tests indicate blood chemistry has changed, it is a far more straightforward and possibly more meaningful indicator of change than indicating whether your satisfaction level has increased on a post–hearing aid treatment questionnaire.

Another difficulty with the types of interventions administered in behavioral sciences versus medical research is that behavioral treatments are far more labor intensive (Hegde, 2003). Whereas physiological changes may occur after only a few days of receiving a medication, behavioral changes may only be evidenced after weeks, months, or years of weekly treatment. Moreover, in medical research the treatment may be administered by a nurse or technician; for communication disorders the intervention must be administered by a specialist in audiology or speech-language pathology. This creates a very labor-intensive enterprise for behavioral sciences when compared to medical research.

A final difference between medical and behavioral research is that many conditions we deal with may be multiply affected by various bodily systems. Voice disorders, for example, may be affected by respiratory, phonatory, endocrine, neurological, and psychological systems. To complicate matters further, some of the disorders that we deal with in communication sciences have many different theoretical perspectives from which researchers approach treatment. In medicine, there is probably less diversity in theoretical bases for research.

Thus, given that DBPRCTs are no doubt the preferred method for approaching the development of effective treatments, some fields are disadvantaged in conducting such research. This does not mean that behavioral sciences should not strive to engage in DBPRCTs. It just means that it is more of a challenge for the behavioral sciences. These challenges have historically limited the number of large clinical trials in our field. Currently, however, we are seeing more Level I and II studies in the communication disorders literature and this is expected to increase with the growing emphasis on EBP.

Communication sciences and disorders cannot compete with medicine, but our professions can fare a lot better in comparison to our peers in the allied health professions. For example, nursing and physical therapy do quite well; we must do better! Being successful in the competition for healthcare dollars means learning as much about research design as possible, particularly about clinical trials. We should be able to answer the following questions: What are the characteristics of well-designed controlled clinical trials? How difficult are clinical trials to conduct in the field of communication sciences and disorders? What are the steps in conducting a clinical trial?

What Are the Characteristics and Related Advantages and Disadvantages of Well-Designed Clinical Trials?

Well-designed randomized, controlled clinical trials have three important characteristics: (1) double-blinding, (2) prospective execution, and (3) randomization. They are called **double-blinded prospective, randomized clinical trials** (DBPRCTs). What a mouthful! However, readers can best understand DBPRCTs by breaking down the phrase and analyzing the components. Double-blinding, which we explained in an earlier chapter, means that neither the experimenter nor the participant has knowledge of whether the treatment or intervention is administered or a placebo. The term prospective, randomized clinical trial (PRCT) signifies studies in which patients are (1) enrolled as participants prior to conducting the experiment, (2) randomly assigned to groups receiving either the treatment or a placebo, (3) measured after some period of time, and (4) compared for any statistically significant differences attributable to the treatment or intervention. Table 12.7 presents advantages and disadvantages of DBPRCTs and other experimental designs (Centre for Evidence-Based Medicine, 2007; Cummings, Grady, & Hulley, 2001; Cummings, Newman, & Hulley, 2001; Newman, Browner, Cummings, & Hulley, 2001). A major advantage of DBPRCTs is that by being doubled-blinded, as stated earlier, they eliminate both experimenter and participant bias. Experimenter bias is anything that the experimenter does that has measurable influence on the dependent variable that is not attributable to the independent variable. For example, a researcher who expects more speech recognition errors in noise for a participant wearing an analog hearing aid rather than a digital hearing aid may show an unconscious bias in recording behavior. **Participant bias** is anything that a participant does that has a measurable influence on the dependent variable that is not attributable to the independent variable. For example, participants who rate an expensive digital hearing aid as providing higher quality sound than a more inexpensive analog hearing aid may reason that if something costs more, it has to be better.

Bentler, Niebuhr, Johnson, and Flamme (2003) investigated whether the label attached to hearing aids would bias outcome measures toward newer high-technology hearing aids. **Outcome measures** are data collected to determine the benefit of

TABLE 12.7

Advantages and Disadvantages of Types of Research Designs

Type of Design	Advantages	Disadvantages
Randomized, controlled trials	• Double-blinding • Random distribution of confounding factors • Establishment of causality between independent and dependent variable(s)	• Difficult to design, execute, and complete • Poor external validity • Ethical issues • Time intensive
Cohort studies	• Smaller sample size than required by randomized, controlled trial • Shorter durations than randomized, controlled trials • Estimations of incidence • Time sequencing of predictor and outcome variables • Prospective or retrospective	• No randomization • Blinding difficult • Linkage to predictor variable may have confounding variables • Expensive to prospectively follow cohort over time
Case-control studies	• Relatively low cost • Shorter duration than randomized, controlled trials and cohort studies • Smaller sample size than randomized, controlled trials • Estimations of odd ratios • Ideal for rare diseases and disorders	• Sampling bias • No establishment of sequence of events • No estimations of incidence, prevalence, or relative risks • Reliance on memory or records
Cross-sectional studies	• Simpler than other designs • Relatively inexpensive • No loss to follow-up of participants • Several predictor or outcome variables possible • Estimations of prevalence and relative risk	• No establishment of causality • Only hints at associations • Susceptible to Neyman bias

Adapted from Centre for Evidence-Based Medicine, 2007; Cummings, Grady, and Hulley, 2001; Cummings, Newman, and Hulley, 2001; Newman, Browner, Cummings, and Hulley, 2001.

treatment. Bentler et al. (2003) matched two groups of participants for age, gender, previous hearing aid experience, and degree or configuration of hearing loss. One group of participants wore two digital hearing aids for one month each. The other group wore the same hearing aids but were told that they were wearing a digital hearing aid for one period and a "conventional hearing aid" during the other month. Outcomes measurement consisting of behavioral speech perception tasks and self-report measures were made at the beginning and end of each trial month. Bentler et al. (2003) found that labeling the hearing aid influenced the results on the outcome measures; the hearing aids were rated higher when labeled as digital rather than conventional. The results of this study indicated the need for "double-blinding" in investigating the effectiveness of high-technology digital hearing aids as compared to more conventional hearing aids.

Another advantage of DBPRCTs is that participants are randomly assigned to either control or treatment groups such that any confounding factors from sampling bias are equally distributed. **Random assignment** implies that each participant has a 50–50 chance of being assigned to receive a placebo or the treatment. Random assignment of participants reduces the **sampling bias** or the measurable influence on the dependent variable by assignment of participants to treatment or control groups that is not attributable to the independent variable. In other words, assignment of participants to treatment and control groups must be based on chance alone in order to establish causality in that any treatment effects are due to the manipulation of the independent variable rather than sampling bias.

Although considered the "gold standard" for scientific evidence, DBPRCTs have several disadvantages to consider prior to experimental implementation. First, DBPRCTs are very difficult to design, execute, and complete. For example, the largest hearing aid clinical trial required collaboration between the Department of Veteran Affairs (DVA), the largest healthcare system in the United States, and the National Institute of Deafness and Other Communication Disorders of the National Institutes of Health (NIDCD-NIH) in order to recruit hundreds of participants meeting specific criteria to provide the required statistical power for a large-scale clinical trial (Larson, Williams, Henderson, Luethke, Beck, et al., 2000). A second disadvantage to consider is that DBPRCTs describe outcomes for treatment variables often found in highly controlled situations, not those found in the real world. For example, outcomes of the NIDCD/VA hearing aid clinical trial limits generalization to clinical scenarios found specifically within the experimental protocol, not to all patients across service-delivery sites. Moreover, clinical trials research may pose some ethical dilemmas for researchers, clinicians, and their patients. For example, DBPRCTs require random assignment of participants to treatment and control groups, meaning that half will receive the new treatment and half will receive the placebo or conventional treatment. Is it ethical that some patients are prevented from receiving a treatment that will provide better hearing aid circuitry or, in a more extreme case, a new drug that may shrink or kill their tumors and save their lives?

Another disadvantage of clinical trials research is the requirement of a great deal of time to validate treatment regimens, thus delaying the introduction of treatments for use by society in general. For example, pancreatic cancer strikes five out of every 100,000 Americans, about 28,000 every year, which is approximately the same number who will die from the disease during the same time period. Pancreatic cancer is particularly lethal in that the condition often goes undiagnosed until the later stages of the disease process. In October 2001, scientists at Johns Hopkins University initiated a Phase II clinical trial assessing the effectiveness of a pancreatic cancer vaccine for patients who have had their tumors resected (i.e., removed via surgery) and had no clinical evidence of metastases (i.e., spreading of cancer outside of the pancreas). Unfortunately, only 10 percent of patients with pancreatic cancer meet these criteria and are eligible to receive the vaccination that may prevent the recurrence of the disease after surgery. Several more phases of the clinical trial are required before widespread use of the vaccine on patients who are dying now. Another problem with clinical trials is that optimal experimental circumstances are necessary to enable research in the "real world" involving all types of patients across a wide variety of afflictions, behaviors, and service-delivery sites (Johnson & Danhauer, 2002). Efficacy studies demonstrating benefit, improved quality of life, and a reduction of healthcare costs as a result of audiologic rehabilitative services are required prior to further reimbursement by third-party payers. The trial may not show a "real" benefit. For example, the NIDCD/VA hearing aid clinical trial was able to demonstrate that wide-dynamic-range compression is better than compression and peak-clipping analog hearing aids. Although the clinical trial provided important evidence regarding relative outcomes for various circuits in analog hearing aids, most of the hearing aids fit even at that time were much more sophisticated than the ones assessed, limiting the applicability of these findings.

In the medical profession, physicians must provide the best information available to patients so that they can make decisions about treatment. Patients diagnosed with cancer must make decisions about their options and need accurate information regarding treatment alternatives for ameliorating cancer along with data on safety and effect on quality of life. For example, patients with early stage breast cancer need to know that equally effective noninvasive treatments (e.g., brachytherapy or placement of radioactive seeds and external beam radiation) exist as an alternative to radical surgery (e.g., mastectomy) that statistically has a high cure rate but results in deformation and change in perceptions of body image. Physicians use levels of evidence in presenting information about the benefits and risks of various treatment options to patients. Similarly, communication sciences and disorders professionals should let the level of evidence guide their recommendations to patients and their families.

Research at the highest level of evidence ensures greater certainty when interpreting experimental results. This high degree of certainty is the result of double-blinding, randomization, and rigid experimental control in order to reduce any error in measurement of the dependent variable. The results of Levels I and II of evidence suggest *causality* between manipulation of independent variable(s) and the effect(s) on the dependent variable(s). In other words, causality assumes a cause-and-effect relationship between treatments and patient outcomes. Communication sciences and disorders professionals should not imply causality between treatment options and specific outcomes when counseling patients *unless* the assertion is supported by Levels I and II of evidence. Moreover, clinicians should avoid terms like "proven efficacy" when presenting treatment options to patients. *Proven* implies rather than suggests cause and effect and the term *efficacy* should only be used when discussing findings at Levels I and II of evidence. Most of the intervention research in our field is at Level III of evidence or lower (i.e., III, IV, and so on) that includes well-designed nonrandomized, controlled trials or quasi-experimental research that can only claim trends, associations, and estimates of connections between the independent and dependent variables. We will discuss how to present the results of evidence to patients in Chapter 15 on blending patient values/preferences, scientific evidence, and clinical expertise.

Level III: Nonrandomized Intervention Studies

Level III involves nonrandomized intervention studies or quasi-experimental research designs that do not randomly assign participants to treatment and control groups. Nonrandomized intervention studies assign participants largely on the basis of logistics or convenience. Failure to use random assignment runs the risk of sampling bias because confounding factors are not equally distributed between treatment and control groups. For example, researchers may want to investigate the effectiveness of a new treatment protocol against a standard treatment for increasing prosocial behaviors in children with autism-spectrum disorder. Comparing the pre- and postintervention performance of two **intact groups** (e.g., two groups of children at different schools) would be more feasible than randomly sampling and assigning the children to experimental and control groups. Therefore, quasi-experimental designs are those that are conducted in the real world rather than in ideal conditions.

Hegde (2003) presented several examples of quasi-experimental research designs including use of nonequivalent group designs, separate sample pretest/ posttest design, and time-series designs. Nonequivalent group designs utilize intact groups to serve as treatment and control that are compared pre- versus postmanagement. The design can be strengthened if the group receiving treatment is randomly selected. Using the above example, a researcher may randomly select one of two programs for children with autism-spectrum disorders at one of two schools to receive the new treatment protocol. Hegde (2003) advised that random selection of intact groups is superior to parents' self-selecting to participate in studies because families who volunteer for innovative treatments may be more motivated than those who do not, thereby biasing results. A weaker design, the separate sample pretest/posttest design, involves selecting two samples, measuring one group preintervention and then providing some treatment that does not relate to the independent variable. The second group, assumed to be equivalent, is administered the actual treatment and then is measured posttreatment. Comparisons are made between pre- and posttest measures but may be extremely biased if both groups are not equivalent. Finally, time-series design research involves measuring group(s) of subjects several times before administration of the treatment and then multiple times after intervention to provide an indication of the stability of results. There are many types of time-series studies and readers are referred to Campbell and Stanley (1963).

Level IV: Nonintervention Studies

Cohort studies, case-control studies, and *cross-sectional surveys* are known as observational studies because there is no manipulation of any variables. The advantages and disadvantages of the studies appear in Table 12.7.

Cohort Studies

Cohort studies follow a group of participants over time. There are multiple types of cohort studies (Cummings et al., 2001). **Prospective cohort studies** recruit a group of participants, measure predictor variables, identify potential confounders, and follow the cadre over time, measuring outcome variables (Cummings et al., 2001). Basically, these studies are initiated prior to the development of a pathological condition to assess who does and does not develop a disease based on one or more predictor variables (Frattali, 1998). Two general purposes of this design are to describe the **incidence** or analyze **associations** of risk factors (i.e., predictor variables) for a particular disease (e.g., outcome variables) or condition (Cummings et al., 2001; Newman, et al., 2001). Recall that incidence is the number of people who develop a particular condition during a specific period of time per the number of those at risk (e.g., the number of new cases of preschoolers diagnosed with autism this year). Associations are relationships between variables (e.g., predictor and outcome) that may range from no relation whatsoever to cause and effect. Generally, fewer subjects need to be recruited for shorter periods of time than DBRCTs. However, participants are not randomized and blinding is difficult in cohort studies. Another disadvantage of these studies is the cost of following the subjects over a long period of time.

In communication sciences and disorders, we can also use prospective cohort studies to assess the long-term outcomes of a disease or intervention on speech-language and hearing difficulties. For example, as part of the Nijmegen otitis media study, Grievink, Peters, van Bon, and Schilder (1993) tested the language outcomes of three groups (i.e., otitis media free, early bilateral otitis media with effusion, and recipients of pressure equalization tubes during preschool) of children seven years of age who had been screened via tympanometry at three-month intervals between their second and third birthdays. They found that even up to nine cases of otitis media did not result in negative language outcomes at age seven years. Similarly, the Childhood Development after Cochlear Implantation Study is a large multicenter prospective cohort study following 188 children with early cochlear implantation along with 91 children with normal hearing on measures of language, maternal sensitivity, cognition, and social development (Eisenberg, Fink, & Niparko, 2006). The study will help determine the benefits of early cochlear implantation through benchmark comparisons with a cohort of children with normal hearing.

Retrospective cohort studies recruit a group of participants, measure predictor variables from past data, and measure outcomes that occurred at a later date (Cummings et al., 2001). The major advantages of the retrospective cohort study over the design previously discussed are its lower cost and no need to follow participants over time. The major disadvantages of this design are the lack of control of sampling and quality of the selection of predictor variables (Cummings et al., 2001). A good example is Reefhuis, Honein, Whitney, Chamany, Mann, and colleagues (2003) who conducted a retrospective cohort study involving children who had received cochlear implants by age six years who either developed or did not develop bacterial meningitis in order to identify factors associated with the disease. They found that postimplantation bacterial meningitis was strongly associated with use of an implant with a positioner and the radiographic confirmation of inner ear malformation with cerebrospinal fluid leak. Due to the increased risk of developing bacterial meningitis, the study concluded that all children who are implanted should be vaccinated and monitored for bacterial infection. Other examples of cohort studies include *nested case-control and case-cohort studies* and *multiple cohort design*, but these designs are beyond the scope of this textbook and readers are referred to Cummings et al. (2001) for additional information.

Case-Control Studies

Case-control studies are retrospective investigations that seek to identify factors or predictor variables associated with a particular disorder or affliction. They are conducted after an outbreak of a disorder and involve identifying groups of subjects with and without the condition. Next, they measure the predictor variables and assess any significant differences between the groups to help determine causes or risk factors for a disease (Newman et al., 2001). For example, an investigator hypothesizes that excessive use of personal listening devices (PLDs) at certain levels and periods of time during the late teens and twenties is a risk factor for the development of sensorineural hearing loss. A case-control study is used to test the hypothesis and begins with identification of a sample of thirty-five year olds with no history of occupational noise exposure who have noise-induced hearing loss. A matched control group without noise-induced hearing loss is also found. Care is taken to ensure that both groups are matched as closely as possible on pertinent variables such as the presence of other high-risk factors and so on. Audiologic evaluation qualifies participants who do and do not have noise-induced hearing loss. Past history of PLD usage is gathered from both groups by the experimenter using a consistent questionnaire method. Odds ratios are calculated to determine the strength or association of PLD listening behaviors on the likelihood of developing nonoccupational noise-induced hearing loss.

Some advantages of case-control studies are their relatively low cost, short duration, small size, and capability to calculate odds ratios (i.e., relative probability of developing or not developing a disease). For example, participants are not followed over time to see if they develop a disease or condition in the future. The case-control design may be the only option for investigating rare diseases and disorders. Some disadvantages of this design are the possibility of bias in sampling and failure to establish a prospective sequence of events (i.e., risk factors present followed by development of the disease) for determining prevalence, incidence, or excessive risks. Moreover, these investigations rely on participants' recall or records to determine status on variables. Controlling for sampling and measurement bias are key issues in the evaluation of case-control studies. Table 12.7 lists advantages and disadvantages of case-control studies (Centre for Evidence-Based Medicine, 2007; Cummings et al., 2001; Newman et al., 2001).

Cross-Sectional Surveys

Cross-sectional studies involve assembling a sample of participants at one point in time to assess both predictor and outcome variables simultaneously to determine any associations or prevalence for particular diseases or disorders (Newman et al., 2001). **Prevalence** is the number of persons who have a disease as a function of the number of those at risk. For example, Pouryaghoub, Mehrdad, and Mohammadi

(2003) used a cross-sectional study to determine the prevalence of noise-induced hearing loss for smoking and nonsmoking workers at a food processing plant who were exposed to noise levels of at least 85 dB A. They found that the 63.4 percent of the workers who smoked has noise-induced hearing loss compared to only 16.4 percent for nonsmokers.

Cox, Alexander, and Gray (2005) used a multisite cross-sectional survey design to determine if patients whose hearing aids were provided at different service-delivery sites differed in significant ways. Participants served in private practice (PP) versus Veterans Administration Healthcare Systems (VA) settings completed self-report instruments pre- and post–hearing aid fitting. They found that the VA participants demonstrated higher prefitting expectations, more problems in the unaided condition, and better postfitting outcomes than their PP peers. The investigators caution against the practice of grouping hearing aid wearers served at different service-delivery sites.

Because all participants are assembled and assessed at one point in time, cross-sectional studies are relatively simple, inexpensive, and have no loss of subjects to follow-up. These studies are also ethically safe because no participant goes without treatment. Moreover, these studies are efficient because several outcomes may be assessed at one time. Also, their results may serve as a foundation for a cohort study, and as mentioned earlier, prevalence and relative risk rates may be determined. Alternatively, one major disadvantage of this design is the inability to establish causality between predictor and outcome variables. At most, only associations between variables may be assumed due to the high degree of sampling and **Neyman bias,** seen when variations in incidence may affect prevalence estimates (e.g., estimating prevalence when the sample is drawn from an increasingly at-risk population). Table 12.7 contains advantages and disadvantages of case-sectional studies (Centre for Evidence-Based Medicine, 2007; Cummings et al., 2001; Newman et al., 2001).

Level V: Case Reports

Case-study research investigates individual participants in detail and compares their profile to typical cases of a particular patient population. Chapter 10 discussed single-subject research, such as A-only (i.e., baseline only) or B-only (i.e., treatment only) types of case studies (McReynolds & Kearns, 1983). The A-only design with its baseline component is considered to be a longitudinal study in which a participants' behavior is observed in a natural environment (McReynolds & Kearns, 1983). The B-only design is considered to be an intervention case study in which a participant's response to treatment is described.

The major advantage of a case study approach is the opportunity to execute an in-depth analysis of participant(s) for a variety of purposes (McReynolds & Thompson, 1986; Silverman, 1998). Case studies may be used to challenge accepted notions in clinical practice. For example, Windsor, Doyle, and Siegel (1994) conducted a longitudinal case study of a woman spanning ages ten to twenty-six years who acquired spoken and written language with intervention, thus challenging the poor prognosis of patients with mutism secondary to autism spectrum disorder. Similarly, case studies can illustrate rare occurrences such as the development of dysphagia from Fores-tier syndrome (Aydin, Akdogan, Akkuzu, Kirbas, & Ozgirgin, 2006). In addition, case studies may be effective in developing clinical insights. For example, Martin, Jerger, Ulatowska, and Mehta (2006) report on how behavioral and electrophysiological test-ing in two different languages with comparison to the performance of a younger peer may be required to sort out auditory-based versus non-auditory-based (i.e., linguistic experience) processing disorders in an older bilingual patient. The major disadvan-tages of case studies are their subject selection, experimenter bias, and the generaliz-ability of results to larger populations.

Level VI: Expert Opinion of Respected Authorities

Expert opinion is at the lowest level of evidence because it is based on opinion rather than scientific evidence. In Chapter 11, we noted that before evidence-based medi-cine, physicians' decisions were based on the "art of medicine" or "clinical judgment." Physicians made decisions based on what had always been done. This does not work when there is disagreement in the field about "best practices" or those methods con-tradict scientific evidence. Therefore, about forty years ago, a shift from using only expert opinion to evidence-based medicine began. More recently, the field of com-munication sciences and disorders has made a similar transition to EBP.

Expert clinical opinion had been the standard method by which position state-ments, clinical practice guidelines, and preferred practice patterns (see Chapter 11 for definitions) were developed. Audiologists and speech-language pathologists from across the country have consulted such documents for clinical decision making. **Expert clinical opinion** involves the knowledge, skills, and experiences of recognized leaders in the professions who have established themselves through clinical work or scholarly activity. Customarily, a group of experts in a particular area of clinical practice would convene to create or update these types of documents for the American Acad-emy of Audiology and the American Speech-Language-Hearing Association. Typically, these groups consulted the literature to incorporate new findings but did not tradi-tionally evaluate the scientific evidence using EBP appraisal criteria. Recently, both AAA and ASHA have incorporated EBP principles into the development of these pro-fessional documents. We will be discussing this issue in greater detail in Chapter 15.

Continuing education is the acquisition of knowledge and skills via sanctioned events for practicing audiologists and speech-language pathologists. Expert opinion plays a major role in such events for audiologists and speech-language pathologists, who must attend a certain number hours of these activities in order to satisfy licen-sure and/or certification requirements. Customarily, continuing education activities are submitted to rigorous approval processes through AAA and ASHA, including scru-tiny of learning objectives linked to a time-ordered agenda and instructor biogra-phies. Although continuing education in communication disorders is based on expert opinion and not evaluated using EBP appraisal criteria as is required in continuing medical education, it is anticipated that this is likely to change as EBP is infused throughout professional activities in communication sciences and disorders.

Many of our graduate and professional training programs have also taught on the basis of expert opinion. University professors have had a tendency to develop class materials and then use them for many years, incorporating new information as needed. However, rarely is any of this information assessed using EBP appraisal criteria. In addition, didactic courses use textbooks written by experts in the field who may not have used EBP appraisal criteria in recommending best clinical practices. Moreover, clinical faculty demonstrate clinical procedures to their students that they have used and been successful with in the past. However, until recently, most have not taught students to blend scientific evidence, clinical expertise, and patient values and preferences for clinical decision making. These tendencies are currently changing due to the EBP mandate of the professions and commitment to educating future audiologists and speech-language pathologists.

General Characteristics and Rigor of Diagnostic Studies

Up until this point, we have presented some of the experimental designs at various levels of evidence for intervention studies not commonly encountered in our professions. Studies investigating the validity and reliability of screening and diagnostic instruments in communication sciences and disorders also vary in scientific rigor. The individual types of studies at the different levels of evidence will not be discussed separately here because several of the commonly used designs for screening and diagnostic topics are the same for intervention studies. Instead, the general principles of diagnostic studies are discussed first along with a short description of some of the important indications that bias has been minimized. This section concludes with a general discussion of the levels of evidence for diagnostic studies compared to those of intervention studies.

Newman, Browner, and Cummings (2001) stated that the usefulness of a screening or diagnostic test are determined by reproducibility (reliability) and accuracy (validity). Other important factors involve effects on clinical decision making, including costs, risks, acceptability of the test, and improvements in clinical outcomes. In communication sciences and disorders, few of our screening or diagnostic tests pose any risk of adverse effects to patients. Costs and resource allocation for test administration may be important factors. For example, the cost-benefit ratio is high when considering the cost of universal newborn hearing screening programs in relation to the number of babies actually diagnosed and treated for hearing loss. For our purposes, the current discussion focuses on assessing test reproducibility and accuracy.

A good screening tool or diagnostic test is one that achieves consistent results on the same patient(s) if repeated by the same healthcare practitioner using the same equipment in the same facility. Assessment of test reproducibility is best done by utilizing a cross-sectional design in which the same participants are tested in the same conditions. The analysis used in the assessment depends on whether the dependent variables are categorical (i.e., nominal or ordinal) or continuous (i.e., interval or ratio) data. For example, the use of open-set nonsense syllable tests such as the

Edgerton-Danhauer Nonsense Syllable Test (Edgerton & Danhauer, 1979) requiring patients to repeat consonant-vowel-consonant-vowel items in phonemes are scored as correct or incorrect (e.g., nominal data) using the four blanks that appear to the right of each CVCV item on the score sheet. Intra- (e.g., same judge transcribing the same responses at different times through videorecording) and interjudge reliability (e.g., different judges scoring the same responses at the same time) has been repeatedly verified in numerous investigations by determining the number of agreements (A), disagreements (D), and using the equations $[A / (A + D)] \times 100$ to give a percentage of agreement or concordance. The **concordance rate** is the degree to which the same judge (*intra*) or different (*inter*) judges agree in their scoring of the same patient (Newman et al., 2001). Newman et al. (2001) advised that for tests typically having few incorrect or multiple responses, the concordance rate may not be a valid reliability index and recommended use of another statistic, **kappa,** which measures the extent of agreement that would be expected by chance alone and ranges from –1 (perfect disagreement) to 1 (perfect agreement).

Assessment of test reproducibility is different for continuous data and is based on whether the design evaluates the agreement (e.g., means and distributions of differences between paired measurements) or variability (e.g., coefficient of variation—within-subject standard deviation divided by the mean) between test factors (Newman et al., 2001). Measures of test reproducibility are beyond the scope of this chapter and readers are referred to Newman et al. (2001). Another statistic, the **standard error of measurement,** assesses the variability of repeated measurement made on the same patients using the same test protocol. This measure has a tendency to be distributed around the ever-elusive "true" score of a participant. The larger the standard error of measurement, the poorer is the reliability of measurement. Beattie, Kenworthy, and Luna (2003) assessed the test-retest reliability of distortion product otoacoustic emissions (DPOAEs) at four frequencies (i.e., 550, 1000, 2000, and 4000 Hz) at three time intervals: (1) immediate (i.e., without repositioning the probe tip), (2) very short term (i.e., after a rest period not exceeding twenty minutes), and (3) short term (i.e., after five to ten days) on a group of participants with normal hearing. Test conditions were kept constant across trials. The standard error of measurement for 550 Hz (i.e., 4.6 dB) was nearly two times more than for the other three frequencies. Confidence intervals determined that an individual's true DPOAE threshold will be within 5 dB of values obtained for 1000, 2000, and 4000 Hz and within 10 dB of the value obtained at 550 Hz. Moreover, the amplitudes of two DPOAEs taken over a short time period have to have 18 dB difference at 550 Hz and 7 dB difference at 1000, 2000, and 4000 Hz to be significant at the $p < .05$ level.

Assessment of Test Accuracy

Investigations of test accuracy assess their efficiency in diagnosing patients with a particular disorder and dismissing those who are disease free. Typically, the instrument under evaluation, or **predictor variable,** is compared on the **outcome variable.** Sometimes the predictor variable is known as the **index test** and the outcome variable as the **reference test** (Bossuyt, Reitsma, Bruns, Gatonis, Glasziou, Irwig et al., 2003). Newman and colleagues (2001) stated that typically three different experimental designs assess test accuracy, which we have already discussed earlier in this chapter (i.e., cohort studies, case-control studies, and cross-sectional studies).

In communication sciences and disorders we most often use cross-sectional designs in assessing the accuracy of screening and diagnostic tools. The dependent variable can be categorical (i.e., nominal or ordinal) or continuous (i.e., interval or ratio) with several options for analysis, including sensitivity/specificity, receiver-operating characteristic curves, or likelihood ratios with confidence intervals. The screening test provides a pass or fail result. A diagnostic test indicates the presence or absence of a disease, with the resulting data being nominal. In these types of studies, participants are tested twice, once with the screening test (i.e., predictor variable) and then with a diagnostic test that is an accepted "gold standard" (i.e., outcome variable). The results of the testing are recorded in a matrix. Figure 12.3 shows a decision matrix demonstrating the results for a clinical scenario necessitating computation of sensitivity and specificity. The labels on the left designate the results on the predictor variable, fail (e.g., positive results) or pass (e.g., negative results). The horizontal label at the top designates the results on the outcome variable as either having the disorder or normal. The results for each participant are recorded into the four boxes labeled A through D, based on the results of the testing. For example, Box A (9) is for correct identification (i.e., hits), instances in which participants test positive on the test and are diagnosed with the disorder via the outcome variable. Box B (10) shows false positives, participants who tested positive on the test but ended up not having the condition on the outcome variable. Box C (1) shows false negatives, participants who receive negative results on the test but actually have the condition as confirmed by the outcome variable. Box D (90) shows correct rejections, participants who tested negative on the test and also tested negative via the outcome variable.

FIGURE 12.3

An Example of a Decision Matrix for Calculating Sensitivity and Specificity in a Hypothetical Clinical Situation

		Gold Standard (Outcome Variable)	
		Disorder Present	Disorder Absent
Screening Test (Predictor Variable)	Fail (Positive Results)	**A** Hits 9	**B** False Positive 10
	Pass (Negative Results)	**C** False Negative 1	**D** Correct Rejections 90

Sensitivity and specificity are measures of validity for the accuracy of a test. Sensitivity is the percent of participants who test positive on the predictor variable and actually have the disorder. The equation $[A / (A + C)] \times 100$ can be used for the results in the matrix to determine that the sensitivity of the test is 90 percent, that is, $[9/(9 +1)] \times 100 = 90$ percent. Alternatively, specificity is the percent of participants who test negative on the predictor variable and are actually disorder free. In other words, specificity is the percentage of people who are normal and would be dismissed based on the results of the predictor variable. The equation $[D/(B + D)] \times 100$ can be used for the results in the matrix to determine that the specificity is 90 percent, that is, $[90/(90 +10)] \times 100 = 90$ percent.

Another way of analyzing the data from studies assessing test accuracy is to construct a receiver-operator characteristic curve (ROC), a graph that plots coordinates of sensitivity on one axis and false positive or false alarm rates on another axis based on different criterion values and then connecting the coordinates with a line. Figure 12.4 shows an ROC curve. The horizontal axis at the top of the graph represents the false positive or alarm rate or $1 -$ specificity, ranging from 1.0 to 0 or 100 percent to 0 percent. The vertical axis is for sensitivity that ranges from 0 to 1.0 or 0 percent to 100 percent. The sensitivity and specificity of a test are plotted by finding the coordinate that represents both values for a criterion value. For example, a perfect value for a predictor variable would be one that results in 100 percent sensitivity and 0 percent false positive rate or 100 percent specificity. The coordinate

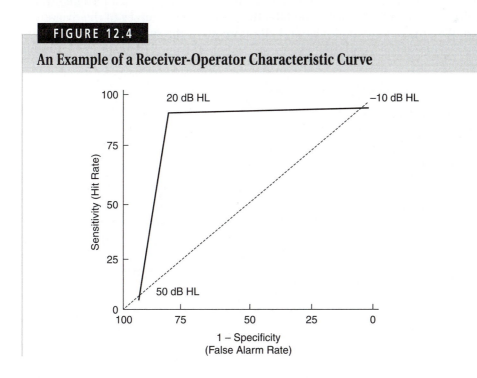

FIGURE 12.4

An Example of a Receiver-Operator Characteristic Curve

would be placed in the upper left-hand corner of the graph. Unfortunately, few if any tests are that accurate! The ROC curve plotted on the figure is from a hypothetical study whose aim was determining a criterion level (e.g., screening level) for pure-tone hearing screening that would result in the highest sensitivity and specificity. The study used three criterion levels of –10, 20, and 50 dB Hearing Threshold Level (HTL) in screening the hearing of one hundred adults with normal hearing and varying degrees of hearing loss. The results for each of the criterion levels were placed into a decision matrix so that sensitivity and specificity could be calculated and plotted on the ROC curve. Note that the 20 dB HL criterion level resulted in the highest sensitivity and specificity. The dashed line going from the lower left-hand corner to the upper right-hand corner displays an ROC of an inaccurate or worthless test.

Likelihood ratios are another way of evaluating the accuracy of a test (Newman et al., 2001). A likelihood ratio can be computed for each value or result on a test. It is the ratio of the likelihood of that result in someone with the disease to the likelihood of the result for a patient who does not have the disorder (Newman et al., 2001).

Likelihood Ratio = P(Results/With Disease)/P(Result/Without Disease), where P = probability. There are two types of ratios: **positive likelihood ratio** (LR+) and **negative likelihood ratio** (LR–). The LR+ of a diagnostic test is an index of confidence that a positive result came from a patient who has the disorder (Dollaghan, 2003). Alternatively, the LR– of a diagnostic test is an index of confidence that a negative result came from a patient who does not have the disease (Dollaghan, 2003). Therefore, the higher the LR+ and the lower the LR–, the greater the accuracy of the diagnostic tool. We can compute both LR+ and LR– if we know the sensitivity and the specificity values of the diagnostic test, 85 percent and 80 percent, respectively, in this example:

LR+ = sensitivity/(100 – specificity)

LR+ = 85/(100 – 80)

LR+ = 85/20

LR+ = 4.25

As can be seen, the LR+ is 4.25 in the example. The maximum LR+ is around 99, which is extremely rare. However, LR+'s of ten or more for a diagnostic tool indicate that persons who receive a positive test result are almost certain to have the disease or disorder. Alternatively, using the same example gives the following equation for LR–:

LR– = (100 – sensitivity)/specificity

LR– = (100 – 85)/80

LR– = 15/80

LR– = .19

The LR– for this example is .19. The smallest possible LR– for most cases is around .01, which also is quite rare. Moreover, LR–'s of less than or equal to .1 indicate that a person with a negative result on the diagnostic tool does not have the disease or disorder (Newman et al., 2001).

Some Points of Discussion about Levels of Evidence for Diagnostic Studies

Having discussed some elements of diagnostic studies, we can now explore similarities and differences among the levels of evidence for intervention. The most similarities are found at the highest and lowest levels of evidence. For example, evidence at Level I for both intervention and diagnostic studies include systematic reviews with meta-analyses fulfilling the requirement of independent confirmation of converging results (ASHA, 2004). Both rubrics also have DBPRCTs at high levels of evidence and expert opinion at the lowest levels of evidence.

Among the differences between these rubrics are the inclusion of high-quality cohort studies at the highest levels of evidence for diagnostic studies. High-quality cohort studies are those that randomly and prospectively recruit participants from populations with very specific inclusion and exclusion criteria for a double-blinded application of a well-defined index and widely accepted gold standard that are administered closely in time. Another difference between the rubrics is the inclusion of systematic reviews of homogeneous studies at Levels II and III for diagnostic studies at those specific levels of evidence, again illustrating the point that the level of evidence of a systematic review consists of the levels of the individual included studies. Lower-quality cohort studies are found at Levels II and III of evidence. At Level II are exploratory cohort studies that use statistical procedures such as regression analysis to identify significant predictor variables for adequate reference standards. Good references standards are not gold standards but are generally acceptable for use in determining presence or absence of pathological conditions, or for our purposes, communication disorders. At Level III are nonconsecutive cohort studies or those that sample from a very limited population. Nonconsecutive cohort studies do not continuously recruit participants in series but may have sporadic enrollment, possibly introducing bias into the experimental protocol (e.g., variability in project personnel and procedures). Alternatively, nonconsecutive cohort studies may be retrospective, obtaining data from chart reviews. Further, studies at Level III may sample from very limited populations or those from specific facilities, for example. Level IV of evidence involves either case-control studies or use of superseded reference standards. Case-control studies are prospective or retrospective observational investigations that compare patients' results on indices (predictor variable) versus reference standards (outcome variable) involving a smaller number of participants. Superseded reference standards use outcome variables that are no longer recognized as gold standards in a particular field. Finally, Level V of evidence is expert opinion from respected authorities.

Summary

This chapter has introduced the concept of levels of evidence used in EBM and EBP in communication sciences and disorders. Readers were shown that the rubrics for levels of evidence can vary according to the type of research study. This chapter focused on levels of evidence for intervention and diagnostic studies. Although the characteristics, advantages, and disadvantages of the types of research at each level of evidence were discussed, considerable focus was placed on studies relatively new to student and practitioners, namely systematic reviews with meta-analyses and double-blinded randomized, controlled clinical trials.

REVIEW EXERCISES

1. *Levels of Evidence for Intervention Studies:*
Please match the level of evidence to the
appropriate type of research.

A. I
B. II
C. III
D. IV
E. V
F. VI

_____ Expert opinion
_____ Nonrandomized intervention studies
_____ Systematic reviews and meta-analyses
of well-designed clinical studies
_____ Case study research
_____ Nonintervention studies (e.g., cohort
studies, case-control studies, and
cross-sectional surveys)
_____ Double-blinded, randomized, controlled
clinical trials

2. *Levels of Evidence for Diagnostic Studies:* Please
match the level of evidence to the appropriate
type of research.

A. I
B. II

C. III
D. IV
E. V

_____ Expert opinion of respected authorities
_____ Case series or superseded reference
standards
_____ Systematic reviews of Level 3 or better
diagnostic studies
_____ Systematic reviews and meta-analyses
of prospective, double-blinded, randomized, controlled clinical trials of diagnostic
studies
_____ High-quality cohort studies
_____ Exploratory cohort studies using statistical procedures (e.g., regression analysis)
to determine "significant" factors with
use of adequate reference standards
_____ Nonconsecutive cohort study or sampling
from a very limited population
_____ Systematic reviews of Level 2 or better
diagnostic studies

ANSWERS TO THE REVIEW EXERCISES

1. F, C, A, E, D, B
2. E, D, C, A, A, B, C, B

CHAPTER 13

Framing the Clinical Question and Searching for the Evidence

The important thing is to not stop questioning.

—Albert Einstein (1879–1955)

I'm searching through all that has been hoped, in praise of what can never be known.

—Real Live Preacher

Each success only buys an admission ticket to a more difficult problem.

—Henry Kissinger

A library is an arsenal of liberty.

—Unknown

I have always imagined that Paradise will be a kind of library.

—Jorge Luis Borges (1899–1986)

In earlier chapters of this book, we discussed how to develop focused research questions. One of the important points was to focus on a specific, answerable research question developed from hypotheses. Generally, students and practitioners approach the research process with very broad interests that must be honed into a feasible project that contributes to the knowledge base of the professions. Similarly, crafting a focused clinical question for evidence-based practice (EBP) saves time on the front end of the process. After all, students and practitioners are busy people and have limited amounts of time. Students in communication sciences and disorders take classes and have clinical practicum in addition to the demands of an assistantship or part-time job to help finance their educations. Similarly, practitioners have large caseloads, paperwork, and other professional commitments that limit the amount of time available for EBP. Besides saving time, a focused question can serve to clarify clinicians' understanding of clinical scenarios through careful consideration of patients, families, and their values; knowledge of viable treatments; and realistic expectations for clinical outcomes. Second, the clinical question drives the search for and retrieval of scientific evidence, an often arduous process if not carefully planned. Students and practitioners can waste hours of time searching for evidence unless they know how and where to look. This chapter discusses how to carefully frame a clinical question and strategically search for relevant evidence.

LEARNING OBJECTIVES

The chapter will enable readers to:

- List common types of questions in EBP.

- Frame a clinical question using a well-accepted rubric.

- Define information literacy and how it contributes to EBP.
- Utilize the sources of evidence in communication sciences and disorders.

- Conduct effective searches for EBP.
- Document search activities.
- Discuss the importance of a multilayered selection process.

A Rubric for Framing Clinical Questions

How do we frame a clinical research question for EBP? What elements must every question have for EBP? Because EBP is about clinical decision making, every question must relate to a patient either directly or indirectly. Although each patient is a unique individual, he or she represents a member of a particular population. Therefore, questions for EBP must contain information about a population. Additionally, clinical decision making almost always involves consideration of available options, whether they are diagnostic tests or treatments. Thus, some sort of intervention under consideration is compared to an alternative option or treatment on some clinical outcome.

One tool for framing clinical questions is the PICO framework in which each letter in the acronym stands for a key component:

- P = Population
- I = Intervention
- C = Comparative or Alternative Treatment
- O = Outcome

The PICO framework has been used in evidence-based medicine (EBM) and has been adopted for use in EBP in communication sciences and disorders (Cox, 2005; ASHA, 2008). The PICO framework is equipped with spaces for students and practitioners to write critical components (i.e., population, intervention, comparative treatment, and outcome) leading to a clinical question, as shown in Table 13.1. Before we use the PICO framework in EBP for specific clinical scenarios, we will introduce different

TABLE 13.1

The PICO Rubric

Parameter	Descriptors
Population	
Intervention	
Comparison (Intervention)	
Outcome	

types of clinical questions and then factors for defining populations, interventions, alternative treatments, and outcomes in communication sciences and disorders.

Types of Clinical Questions

Several different types of clinical questions are posed in EBP. Although broadly similar to physicians' questions for EBM, there are sufficient differences to those crafted by audiologists and speech-language pathologists for EBP that a distinct approach is required. In this chapter, we will discuss several common questions used in EBP for communication sciences and disorders. Our professions are most familiar with diagnostic and intervention questions. However, students and practitioners may come across several different types of questions as shown by the following:

- *Intervention questions* focus on the relative efficacy, effectiveness, or efficiency of two treatments for a specific patient or population.
- *Diagnostic questions* inquire about the relative efficacy, effectiveness, or efficiency of two diagnostic tools used for a specific patients or populations.
- *Etiologic questions* investigate the relative risk of certain exposures (e.g., noise) for developing a certain disease or disorder (e.g., noise-induced hearing loss).
- *Patient safety questions* evaluate the relative risks versus the benefits of clinical procedures for specific patients or populations.
- *Cost-effectiveness questions* compare the relative cost versus benefits of clinical procedures.

Questions for EBP may vary based on who is asking a question. Clinicians ask questions that focus on a specific patient for clinical decision making. Investigators ask questions in the early stages of the development of a research project. Regardless of the type of question or the reason for asking it, the PICO framework is useful in clarifying relevant issues for the decision making process. The next section describes considerations for using this framework to define the population, intervention, alternative treatment, and outcome.

Defining the Population, Intervention, Alternative Treatment, and Outcomes

Defining the population for EBP requires knowing who the patient and their family are. Most of this information is gleaned from the case history and includes such items as demographic factors (e.g., birth date, gender, ethnic background, marital status, address, phone number, and so on), medical history (e.g., general health, listing of prescription medications, record of illnesses or surgeries, allergies, and so on), and disease-specific information (e.g., type, degree, and severity of communication disorder, date of diagnosis, last evaluation, and so on). Clinicians have a plethora of information available from patients, but the key for EBP is to be able to discriminate relevant from irrelevant information in framing a question. Relevant factors are those that may directly relate to or affect clinical outcomes. What factors may or may not contribute to the relative effectiveness of two stuttering treatments in increasing fluency for a particular patient? Does the age, gender, or type of disfluency matter? Or, does a patient's prior experience with hearing aids or method of payment affect the type of hearing instruments they will consider? In some cases, clinicians must rely on their own experiences in addition to asking colleagues for their impressions of critical factors relevant for defining the population. Because the clinical question drives the search for evidence, it is important that defining characteristics for the population are neither too broad nor too narrow. For instance, being too broad may result in a recovery of a mountain of evidence that may or may not be relevant for clinical decision making. Alternatively, being too specific for defining criteria may recover little or no evidence for consideration.

Defining the population may also depend on the type of question asked. In the preceding paragraph, we discussed some considerations for defining populations for intervention questions. For diagnostic questions, defining the population may be more global and involve factors beyond patient characteristics. For example, directors of newborn hearing screening programs may be interested in the relative effectiveness of two types of screening tests for use in neonates born in hospitals similar to their own facility (e.g., same number of births per year). Defining the population for etiologic questions may involve considering patients' exposures to certain factors. For instance, history of occupational noise exposure may be a confounding factor for determining the relative risk of iPod listening behaviors in the development of sensorineural hearing loss in young-to-middle-aged adults. Therefore, defining the patient population requires only considering those adults who are not exposed to potentially excessive noise levels in the workplace. For patient safety questions, the population may focus on those individuals most likely to receive new but yet untested medical tests or treatments.

Defining the interventions for EBP involves taking into consideration available treatments, in addition to the preferences of patients and their families. Most often, the clinician, the patient, and the family consider two or more scientifically acceptable treatment options. However, sometimes patients and their families may prefer to try new or untested, experimental interventions (i.e., treatment) as opposed to a scientifically accepted standard of care (i.e., comparative treatment). For example, in many double-blinded randomized, controlled clinical trials involving cutting-edge treatments for life-threatening diseases (e.g., cancer), the comparative treatment, for ethical reasons, is usually the standard treatment protocol (e.g., recommended chemotherapy). In other words, patients with life-threatening diseases who volunteer to participate in a clinical trial should not be placed "at risk" if randomly assigned to the control group that usually receives the treatment that is the recommended standard of care rather than the experimental group that receives the cutting-edge protocol. Conversely, the alternative treatment may be no treatment at all. For example, patients diagnosed with sensorineural hearing loss must decide whether to pursue amplification (i.e., intervention) or continue on without it (i.e., comparative treatment). In summary, clinical questions may focus on comparing two scientifically acceptable interventions, unproven treatments to standard protocols, or treatment versus no treatment options.

Determining the intervention and the comparative treatment also depends on the type of question asked. For example, for diagnostic questions, the intervention may be a new type of technology for use in screening and the alternative tool may be the current tool for identifying persons with a particular communicative disorder. For etiologic questions, the intervention is the exposures or characteristics that may put patients at risk for developing a communicative disorder, whereas the comparative treatment is absence of the risk factor. For questions about patient safety, the intervention may be a new procedure that presents some risk to patients, whereas the comparative treatment may be the current procedure that poses little or no danger to participants. For cost-effectiveness studies, the intervention may be a procedure that has the potential to cut costs and conserve resources, and the alternative treatment may be the currently used protocol.

Defining the outcome in EBP deals with what is to be accomplished and determines how interventions will be compared. More often than not, the outcomes in scientific experiments are the dependent variables. Because outcomes are tied intimately to the concerns or goals of patients and their families, selection of clinical outcomes in EBP requires knowledge of the patients' and family members' values, preferences, and levels of functioning. At the level of the patient, information from diagnostic evaluations is critical for determining possible clinical outcomes. For example, outcomes for language-delayed children may focus on increasing mean length of utterance and expanding receptive and expressive vocabularies. For patients with sensorineural hearing loss, clinical outcomes may be to improve their audibility or speech recognition thresholds through the use of amplification. Most often, the outcomes are well-recognized measures in the clinical milieu that are all related to the patient's degree of impairment resulting from the communication disorder. Audiologists and speech-language pathologists are comfortable with these types of outcomes because they are familiar, well defined, and well understood. However, measures made in the clinical setting may have limited external validity and are not always related to patients' long-term functioning and quality of life.

There are several recognized outcome measures in audiology and speech-language pathology that measure the impact of communication disorders on patients' abilities to execute activities of daily living and their involvement in life situations. In Chapter 15, we will describe the World Health Organization *International Classification of Functioning, Disability, and Health* (WHO, 2001), a conceptual framework for defining, measuring, and formulating policies for health and disability. The model is also useful for defining appropriate outcomes for individual patients that reflect traditional clinical measures for impairment in addition to the impact of communication disorders on activity limitations and involvement in life situations. For example, the model incorporates the following domains:

- **Impairments** are problems in body function or structure such as a significant deviation or loss.
- **Activity limitations** are difficulties an individual may have in executing activities.
- **Participation restrictions** are problems an individual may experience in involvement in life situations. (WHO, 2001; p. 10)

Our professions have realized the importance of classifying outcome measures using these domains for EBP. Assessment of activity limitations and participation restrictions are often accomplished through self-assessment questionnaires that are specific to communication disorders. For example, activity limitations due to hearing loss are measured using tools such as the *Client Oriented Scale of Improvement* (Dillon, James, & Ginis, 1997). Similarly, participation restrictions from hearing loss are measured using the *Hearing Handicap Inventory for the Elderly* (Ventry & Weinstein, 1982). Alternatively, participation restrictions from voice disorders are measured via the *Voice Handicap Index* (Jacobson, Johnson, Grywalski, Silbergleit, Jacobson et al., 1997). In addition, some outcome measures assess multiple domains such as the *Overall Assessment of the Speaker's Experience of Stuttering* (Yaruss & Quesal, 2006). Defining patient outcomes using self-assessment questionnaires requires knowing the characteristics of viable outcome measures.

What makes a good outcome measure? Hyde (2000) stated that there are six characteristics of a good self-assessment questionnaire. First, an instrument should have a clear purpose so that it may be used appropriately by clinicians and researchers. Second, the instructions should specify the population for whom the instrument is intended and how it is to be administered. For instance, the target population should be well defined through demographic (e.g., age, sex, and socioeconomic status) and disease-specific information (e.g., type, degree, and manifestation of the communication disorder). Additionally, it should specify if the tool is to be administered via a paper-and-pencil survey, an interview, or by computer. Third, the tool should tap into a specific conceptual framework or measure (e.g., WHO, 2001) or a construct related to positive patient outcomes (e.g., satisfaction with products or health-related quality of life). Fourth, the development of the outcome measure should have had adequate pilot testing (e.g., 50 participants or less) in addition to validation and norming processes involving larger samples of participants (e.g., as many as 250 participants).

Fifth, a good outcome measure has been evaluated and determined to have adequate **reliability, validity, responsiveness,** and **feasibility** (Hyde, 2000). Recall that reliability is the degree of measurement; validity is the truth in measurement. For self-assessment questionnaires, reliability requires determination of **internal consistency** or the consistency with which its items measure the same things (e.g., domains like participation restrictions). The degree of internal consistency is determined using the following measures (Hyde, 2000):

- **Item total correlation** is the degree with which each item on the instrument correlates with the total score.
- **Split-half reliability** is the degree to which scores on a randomly selected half of the instrument correlate with those on the remaining half.
- **Cronbach's alpha** is the variance of the total score to that of the individual items.

Acceptable correlation coefficients for measures of internal consistency should range between 0.7 and 0.9 (Boyle, 1991; Hyde, 2000; Streiner & Norman, 1995). Reliability is also assessed via **test-retest reliability,** which is the degree that scores correlate with the scores obtained on a second administration of the instrument to the same participants. Correlation coefficients for test-retest reliability should be 0.85 or higher for the instrument to be of sufficient quality (Hyde, 2000).

Validity, or the accuracy of measurement in self-assessment questionnaires, has three different facets: **construct, content,** and **criterion validity.** Construct validity is the degree to which an instrument rationally and empirically measures a theoretical construct (Maxwell & Satake, 2005; Schiavetti & Metz, 2006). Construct validity is often assessed by applying special statistical procedures (e.g., factor analysis) to data to verify that patterns of responding on the questionnaire represent the intended psychological or behavioral constructs. On the other hand, content validity is the degree to which items on the instrument focus on different aspects of a behavior or domain (e.g., emotional aspects or participation restrictions resulting from hearing loss). Content validity is also known as **face validity** and is verified most often through expert opinion. For instance, often a focus group subjectively assesses content validity by determining the degree to which the instrument's items sample aspects of particular behaviors or domains. Last but not least, criterion validity is the degree to which scores on an instrument correlate with those of a recognized "gold standard" of measurement.

Feasibility and responsiveness are also characteristics of good outcome measures. Feasibility is the utility of an instrument in the real world. In developing a self-assessment questionnaire, sometimes sheer length is used to maximize reliability and validity. For instance, the *Communication Profile for the Hearing Impaired* (CPHI) (Demorest & Erdman, 1987) is a reliable and valid outcome measure that samples aspects of both the activity limitation and participation restriction domains. However, the CPHI is a 145-item instrument that has poor feasibility. In other words, most clinicians do not have the time to administer a 145-item questionnaire, particularly in a busy clinical setting. Therefore, optimal outcome measures should be feasible enough for widespread use by clinicians on a day-to-day basis. In addition, outcome measures should have a high degree of responsiveness, meaning that they are sensitive enough to measure changes in patients from pre- to postintervention.

A sixth characteristic of a good outcome measure is that norms are readily available with a clear explanation of how they were obtained (Hyde, 2000). Cox, Alexander, and Beyer (2003) provided norms for the *International Outcome Inventory for Hearing Aids* (IOI-HA) (Cox, Hyde, Gatehouse, Noble, et al., 2000), a seven-item instrument that measures several important domains for hearing aid utilization: daily use, benefit, residual activity limitations, satisfaction, residual participation restrictions, impact on others, and quality of life. Cox et al. (2003) described how the IOI-HA was normed for research and clinical purposes using patients with bilateral, single-channel, compression, analog hearing aids.

It is important to note that even though an outcome measure may meet all of the preceding criteria, if a self-assessment questionnaire is used incorrectly (e.g., with an inappropriate population or wrong purpose), the evidence gleaned from an otherwise well-conducted investigation may be invalid. This is why it is not only important for students and practitioners to acknowledge characteristics of good outcome measures but also equally important to evaluate whether researchers have applied these criteria in selecting outcome measures for use in their investigations.

Formulating Clinical Research Questions

Now that we have discussed the individual categories within the PICO rubric, it is time to practice formulating clinical questions. Despite the several types of clinical questions possible in EBP, we will use the following scenarios to focus on the two most common categories in communication sciences and disorder—intervention and diagnosis questions. The first scenario appears in Box 13.1.

Clearly, Mr. Smith's audiologist needs to apply EBP in counseling and assisting his patient in making the best decision. The first step is to formulate a focused clinical question using the PICO rubric. The population is an adult with a profound unilateral hearing loss. The intervention to consider is the BAHA versus the comparative treatment of a CROS hearing aid, and the outcomes are the ability to localize and understand speech in noise. Table 13.2 shows the PICO rubric for this scenario.

The clinical questions can be formulated from the PICO rubric. In considering this scenario, there are actually two clinical questions to ask, accounting for two different outcomes, localization and speech recognition in noise, as follows:

- What is the relative effectiveness of a BAHA versus a CROS hearing aid in improving the localization abilities of adults with profound unilateral sensorineural hearing losses?

BOX 13.1

Scenario for an Intervention Question in Evidence-Based Practice

Mr. Smith is a twenty-five-year-old man who presents with a congenital, unilateral profound sensorineural hearing loss that he has dealt with his entire life. In school, he just "got along" with preferential seating in the classroom. However, he always found it frustrating to tell where sound was coming from or to localize. In addition, he would like to have better speech recognition in noise, particularly when someone was talking at his poorer ear with noise at his better ear. He and his parents had been encouraged to pursue a CROS hearing aid, which stands for Contralateral Routing of the Signal. With a CROS hearing aid, Mr. Smith would wear a microphone and FM transmitter on the poorer ear that would send the signal coming to his nonfunctional ear to an FM receiver on his better ear. Mr. Smith asked his audiologist if there were any other options, because he did not want to wear hearing aids. Mr. Smith's audiologist knew that bone-anchored hearing aids (BAHA) were being used in patients having single-sided deafness, requiring surgery for placement of an abutment onto which the device would be attached. Not knowing the relative effectiveness of the BAHA hearing aid compared to the CROS hearing aid for localization and speech recognition in noise, Mr. Smith's audiologist needed to use EBP to aid in counseling Mr. Smith and for clinical decision making.

TABLE 13.2

Completed PICO Rubric for the Intervention Question

Parameter	Descriptors
Population	Adults with profound unilateral sensorineural hearing loss
Intervention	Bone-anchored hearing aid
Comparison (Intervention)	CROS hearing aid
Outcome	Localization and speech recognition in noise

- What is the relative effectiveness of a BAHA versus a CROS hearing aid in improving the speech recognition in noise of adults with profound unilateral sensorineural hearing losses?

Let's do this same process for a clinical scenario focusing on the diagnostic question found in Box 13.2.

EBP may be used in this scenario to assist speech-language pathologists in making a decision about whether to replace listening to voice samples with spectrographic analysis in differentiating patients with adductor-type spasmodic dysphonia from those with muscle tension dysphonia. The PICO rubric again can be used to focus a clinical question. The population is adults with either one of these vocal pathologies. The intervention (i.e., diagnostic procedure under consideration) is spectral analysis, and the alternative treatment (i.e., comparison diagnostic procedure) involves listening to speech samples. The outcome is the accuracy (i.e., sensitivity and specificity) of these two diagnostic methods in differentiating patients with adductor-type spasmodic dysphonia from those with muscle tension dysphonia. Table 13.3 shows the PICO rubric for this scenario.

The clinical question framed from the PICO rubric is "What is the relative accuracy (i.e., sensitivity and specificity) of inspecting spectral analyses versus listening

BOX 13.2

Scenario for a Diagnostic Question in Evidence-Based Practice

Speech-language pathologists at a leading university hospital were interested in comparing the accuracy of differentiating patients with adductor-type spasmodic dysphonia from those with muscle tension dysphonia using spectral analysis rather than their standard method of diagnosis by listening to patients' voice samples. If inspecting spectral analyses is found to be more accurate than listening to voice samples, the staff would purchase a computerized speech laboratory and change their diagnostic protocol.

TABLE 13.3

Completed PICO Rubric for the Diagnostic Question

Parameter	Descriptors
Population	Adults with either adductor spasmodic dysphonia or muscle tension dysphonia
Intervention	Spectral diagnostic method
Comparison (Intervention)	Listening diagnostic method
Outcome	Sensitivity and specificity

to voice samples in differentiating patients with adductor spasmodic from those with muscle tension dysphonia?" Framing the question sets the tone for the rest of the process, including searching, evaluating, and using scientific evidence in addition to clinical expertise and patient preferences for clinical decision making. Readers may find Appendix 13.A useful when framing clinical questions for their own pursuits in EBP. We will now discuss the next step in EBP, searching for the evidence.

Searching for Evidence in Communication Sciences and Disorders

Finding relevant evidence to answer a focused clinical research question may seem like trying to find a needle in a haystack. In a way it is. However, the good news is that with the development of information technology, the Internet, and the widespread availability of personal computers, searching for evidence can be relatively easy with the appropriate application of knowledge and skills. Most students in communication sciences and disorders enter graduate or professional training programs with little or no knowledge about the sources of evidence in our field. Moreover, few know how to start searching for evidence that may be of use in answering a focused question. To do so requires some acumen in **information literacy** or the knowledge and skills for effectively and efficiently finding relevant, high-quality evidence for the purposes of EBP. The primary purpose of this section of the chapter is to provide essential knowledge, skills, and resources for conducting efficient searches. However, before we get started, a few preliminary steps are necessary.

The first requirement is a personal computer with Internet access, which should be relatively easy for researchers, clinicians, and students in communication sciences and disorders. Although most faculty, clinical staff, and students have home computers and Internet access, their departments should also have such equipment available. Heads of training programs should strongly consider providing at least one personal computer with Internet access for EBP activities for students. Also, the local university library or city library probably has such resources available for little or no cost.

The next step is to identify a local comprehensive library system with extensive holdings in biomedical sciences, particularly related to speech, language, and hearing sciences and disorders. Students and faculty typically have unlimited access to the university library's staff and resources. Initial familiarity with the library may be obtained from their web pages regarding the number of libraries (e.g., main library versus those specializing in social sciences or other relevant fields), hours of operation, databases, journals, online tutorials, staff, and so on. Customarily, librarians specialize in certain subject areas and it is likely that one or more have been assigned to communication sciences and disorders, particularly if the university has a training program. Contact with one or more of these librarians is recommended, particularly before writing a paper, planning a research project, or undertaking a systematic review. These individuals are eager to share their expertise about the resources available for EBP.

Sources of Evidence in Communication Sciences and Disorders

In years past, when students went to the library, they would laboriously search the card catalog for a few books or go through key professional journals seeking articles on a certain topic. However, the days of looking through card catalogs are over. Most searching today uses computer technology to retrieve evidence for clinical decision making that might include systematic reviews, studies, and clinical practice guidelines. The goal is to find evidence with the most scientific rigor, highest level of evidence, and least amount of bias. A researcher familiar with this textbook will have examined the sources of bias and how to minimize it in research and will also be aware that threats to internal validity are often underestimated and ubiquitous in applied clinical research (Dollaghan, 2003). The goal is to search for the most relevant information to answer a focused research question using the most expeditious and systematic methods. The first step is to become familiar with possible resources to aid in searching for high-quality evidence in communication sciences and disorders.

Resources may be classified as **domestic,** originating in the United States, or **international,** coming from foreign countries. For example, some of the best resources for evidence-based medicine (EBM) are from the United Kingdom. Domestic sources provided by the federal government include PubMed or the Agency for Healthcare Research and Quality (AHRQ); entities in the private sector include the Communication Sciences and Disorders Dome; and professional organizations provide such resources as the Evidence-Based Compendium of the American Speech-Language-Hearing Association. Resources may also be **generic** or **discipline specific.** For example, generic resources are useful for physicians and allied health professionals (e.g., nurses, physical therapists, psychologists, and so on). It should be noted that audiologists and speech-language pathologists also find generic resources useful for their EBP purposes; however, discipline-specific resources provide the most benefit for EBP in communication sciences and disorders.

Before discussing specific search strategies, we will review some common EBP resources. The Cochrane Library (www.cochranelibrary.com) is published by Wiley on behalf of the Cochrane Collaboration, an international organization devoted to assisting users in making informed decisions via systematic reviews. The databases include the following:

- Cochrane Database of Systematic Reviews. Provides access to sources that assess the effects of interventions for prevention, treatment, and rehabilitation, providing full texts of systematic reviews of empirical methodological studies prepared by the Cochrane Collaboration (Methodology Reviews).
- Databases of Abstracts of Reviews of Effects (also known as DARE). Summarizes reviews that have been done by others (besides the Cochrane Collaboration) that have been assessed for quality.
- Cochrane Central Register of Controlled Clinical Trials (also known as CENTRAL). Includes specifics (e.g., title, publication information, and abstract) or publications about clinical trials from databases and other published sources.
- The Cochrane Methodology Register. Provides publications (e.g., journal articles, books, and conference proceedings) that summarize the methods used when conducting clinical trials.
- Health Assessment Database. Offers information on health technology assessments from around the world.
- The National Health Service Economic Evaluation Database. Assists in the decision-making process by providing economic evaluations and assessing their quality, strengths, and weaknesses.

To get the most out of the Cochrane Library, users should review either the online manual or view, download, or print their Quick Reference Guide.

Another source of systematic reviews is the Campbell Collaboration (www.camp bellcollaboration.org), an independent and international nonprofit organization that provides evidence-based information for making decisions regarding social, behavioral, and educational sciences. Named after Donald T. Campbell, a leader in these areas, the Campbell Collaboration (C2) works on such key principles of collaboration as building on enthusiasm of individuals, avoiding unnecessary duplication of efforts, minimizing bias, keeping current, striving for relevance, promoting access, and ensuring quality and continuity (Campbell Collaboration, 2007). The C2 reviews are frequently updated and are available electronically for any interested parties. Additional sources of EBP include their peer-review system, Register of Interventions and Policy (C2-RIPE), and a network of scholars and practitioners. The C2 works closely with the Cochrane Collaboration.

PubMed is a free and accessible online database of biomedical journal citations and abstracts provided by the United States National Library of Medicine (NLM), which indexes about 5,000 journals from around the world (NLM, 2006; 2007a). The indexing is done using NLM's controlled vocabulary or Medical Subject Headings (MeSH®) (NLM, 2007a). The MeSH consists of sets of terms or descriptors that are hierarchically arranged to enable the conduct of searches ranging from the general to the specific or vice versa (NLM, 2007b). The Medical Literature Analysis and Retrieval System Online (MEDLINE) is the largest component of PubMed containing over sixteen million references to journal articles in the life sciences with a focus on biomedical research (NLM, 2006). Relevant characteristics of MEDLINE include coverage of articles from 1950 to the present from over 5,000 journals, with 2,000 to 4,000 references added each day (NLM, 2006).

The Cumulative Index of Nursing and Allied Health Literature (CINAHL) is a database of references primarily found in professional journals published since 1982. Although most of the citations are journal articles, CINAHL also indexes books, conference proceedings, and dissertations. The database contains over one million references obtained from over 1,200 international journals. Although access to full-text articles is not provided, citations provide the title, author(s), name of the journal, along with volume, issue, page number, and abstract.

The website of the American Speech-Language-Hearing Association (ASHA) at www.asha.org can be an excellent source of evidence, particularly for members of either ASHA or the National Student Speech-Language-Hearing Association (NSSLHA) who have full access to all their journals: *American Journal of Audiology, American Journal of Speech-Language Pathology, Contemporary Issues in Communication Sciences and Disorders,* and the *Journal of Speech, Language, and Hearing Research.* Members also access to ASHA practice policy documents including practice guidelines, position statements, preferred practice patterns, and technical reports. The website also links to abstracts of convention presentations when conducting handsearches of conference proceedings. Different search options allow for specification of content including finding items from the ASHA website, American Speech-Language-Hearing Foundation (ASHFoundation) website, convention abstracts, evidence-based practice compendium, ASHA journals, NSSLHA website, and ASHA practice policies.

The Evidence-Based Compendium (EBC) can only be accessed by members of ASHA or NSSLHA at www.asha.org/members/ebp/compendium. It contains guidelines and systematic reviews that are accessible by links organized by topic headings. The EBC was created during the summer of 2005 by ASHA's Center for Evidence-Based Practice in Communication Disorders (N-CEP) because many of the clinical practice guidelines in our field have a high degree of bias. NCEP staff used the *Appraisal of Guidelines for Research and Evaluation* (AGREE), which is available online at www.agreecollaboration.org/instruments, to determine which guidelines were suitable for inclusion. The tool consists of twenty-three items in six domains (i.e., scope of agreement, stakeholder involvement, rigor of development, clarity of presentation, applicability, and editorial independence) that renders overall grades of highly recommended, recommended with provisos, and not recommended. The NCEP staff only included clinical practice guidelines rated highly recommended and recommended with provisos. The AGREE Collaboration is discussed in greater depth in Chapter 15.

The Communication Sciences and Disorders Dome (ComDisDome) has been a popular information source for audiologists, speech-language pathologists, and students. The original ComDisDome tapped into PubMed, select non-PubMed journals from *Linguistics and Language Behavior Abstracts, Seminars in Hearing,* select awarded grants from the National Institutes of Health and the National Science Foundation, dissertations from ProQuest, books from multiple select publishers, profiles of scholars, and related websites. A popular ComDisDome feature was a dictionary that provided definitions for important key words. The ComDisDome was developed, maintained, and owned by ContentScan until 2007, when it was purchased by CSA Illumina, which specializes in providing access to over 100 bibliographic and full-text databases in the natural sciences, social sciences, arts/humanities, and technologies. CSA Illumina's version of the ComDisDome has eliminated the dictionary, websites, and other features. However, subscribers to this new version will find a host of other databases to use for searches.

Macro and Micro Search Strategies

In Chapter 12, we discussed systematic reviews and the importance of their search and retrieval processes, which must be highly organized, documented, and efficient techniques. One way to characterize searches is in terms of macro and micro strategies. Macro strategies specify the order that resources (e.g., electronic databases) are searched. Micro strategies use specific features to search for evidence within an electronic database. Both the search strategies have the same goal of efficiently and effectively recovering the highest quality and most relevant evidence to answer a research or clinical question. Therefore, macro search strategies for EBP should first retrieve systematic reviews of randomized, controlled clinical trials with meta-analyses; followed by individual randomized, controlled clinical trials; then nonrandomized intervention studies and nonintervention studies (i.e., cohort studies, case-control studies, and cross-sectional surveys), and conclude with expert opinion from respected authorities. For example, Figure 13.1 shows a macro search strategy that begins with a search for systematic reviews with meta-analyses in the Cochrane Databases for Systematic Reviews (Cochrane Reviews), the Databases of Abstracts of Reviews of Effects (DARE) within the Cochrane Library, and the Campbell Collaboration and continues down the hierarchy using such resources as ClinicalTrials.Gov (www.clinicaltrials .gov), and PubMed for micro search strategies.

Some micro search strategies are particularly helpful when accessing PubMed (www.pubmed.gov), as shown by Figure 13.2, which gives a screenshot of PubMed's homepage. Note the window at the top to type in terms for searching. Above the search bar are grouped items that can be clicked to provide links. Clicking on the "MeSH Database" under PubMed permits searching for terms related to topics specific to an EBP question or systematic review. Figure 13.3 shows the MeSH data for the term *Audiology,* including a definition, year the term was introduced, subheadings (i.e., those terms that have been paired at least once with the term in MEDLINE), and previous indexing.

Sometimes it is difficult to find MeSH terms that directly relate to key concepts. In that case, the EXPLODE MeSH terms feature should be used to obtain more specific words to choose from. Sometimes even the most specific MeSH terms do not recover relevant studies for answering clinical questions. Therefore, common words found in the text of these articles should be considered for use followed by appropriate

---

FIGURE 13.1

Macro Search Strategy for Evidence in Communication Sciences and Disorders

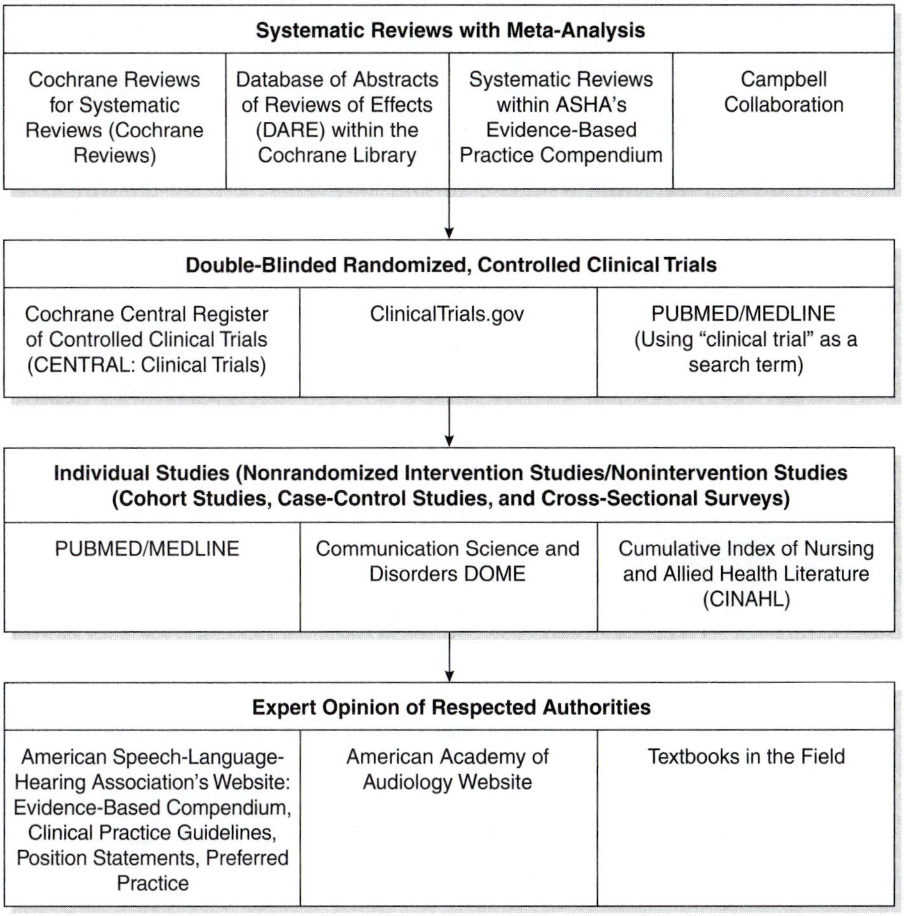

Systematic Reviews with Meta-Analysis			
Cochrane Reviews for Systematic Reviews (Cochrane Reviews)	Database of Abstracts of Reviews of Effects (DARE) within the Cochrane Library	Systematic Reviews within ASHA's Evidence-Based Practice Compendium	Campbell Collaboration

Double-Blinded Randomized, Controlled Clinical Trials		
Cochrane Central Register of Controlled Clinical Trials (CENTRAL: Clinical Trials)	ClinicalTrials.gov	PUBMED/MEDLINE (Using "clinical trial" as a search term)

Individual Studies (Nonrandomized Intervention Studies/Nonintervention Studies (Cohort Studies, Case-Control Studies, and Cross-Sectional Surveys)		
PUBMED/MEDLINE	Communication Science and Disorders DOME	Cumulative Index of Nursing and Allied Health Literature (CINAHL)

Expert Opinion of Respected Authorities		
American Speech-Language-Hearing Association's Website: Evidence-Based Compendium, Clinical Practice Guidelines, Position Statements, Preferred Practice	American Academy of Audiology Website	Textbooks in the Field

subheadings. Use of the word OR adjoining related terms will expand the search to include citations that include either term. Similarly, other strategies to broaden searches are to remove all limits, consider all publication types, choose all subject headings, and use broader terminology, or use the "See Related Articles" feature in PubMed, which is discussed a bit later in this chapter. Alternatively, the use of the word AND adjoining related terms will narrow the search to restrict citations to those that include both terms. Another micro search strategy is to click on the link "Clinical Queries" that provides opportunities to (1) search by clinical study category, or (2) find

FIGURE 13.2

Homepage for PubMed

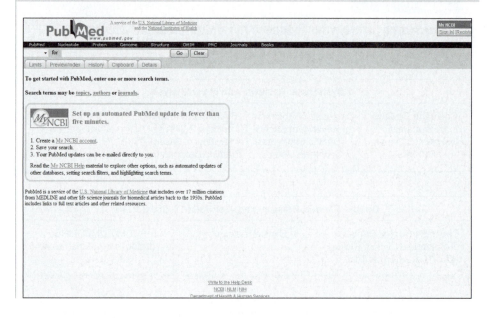

FIGURE 13.3

MeSH Results for the Term *Audiology*

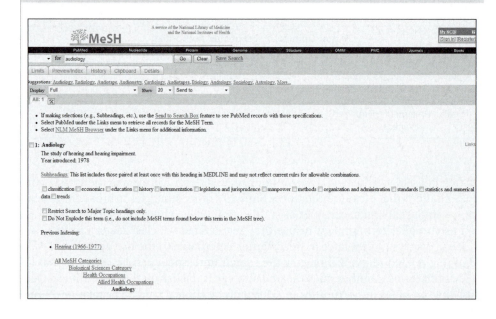

FIGURE 13.4

"Clinical Queries" Page from PubMed

PubMed Clinical Queries

| PubMed | Nucleotide | Protein | Genome | Structure | OMIM | PMC | Journals | Books |

This page provides the following specialized PubMed searches for clinicians:

- Search by Clinical Study Category
- Find Systematic Reviews
- Medical Genetics Searches

After running one of these searches, you may further refine your results using PubMed's Limits feature.

Results of searches on these pages are limited to specific clinical research areas. For comprehensive searches, use PubMed directly.

Search by Clinical Study Category   ↑

This search finds citations that correspond to a specific clinical study category. The search may be either broad and sensitive or narrow and specific. The search filters are based on the work of Haynes RB et al. See the filter table for details.

Search [   ] [Go]

Category	Scope
○ etiology	◉ narrow, specific search
○ diagnosis	○ broad, sensitive search
◉ therapy	
○ prognosis	
○ clinical prediction guides	

Find Systematic Reviews   ↑

For your topic(s) of interest, this search finds citations for systematic reviews, meta-analyses, reviews of clinical trials, evidence-based medicine, consensus development conferences, and guidelines.

For more information, see Help. See also related sources for systematic review searching.

Search [   ] [Go]

---

systematic reviews. Another option is to search on the topic of medical genetics. Figure 13.4 shows that searches may focus on one or more types of studies: etiology, diagnosis, therapy, prognosis, and clinical prediction guide. Further, the search may be broadened (increased sensitivity) or narrowed (increased specificity). The Clinical Queries page also permits a search for systematic reviews only.

Documenting the Search Strategy

Whether searching for evidence on EBP for a single patient or participating on a team conducting a systematic review, documentation of the search strategy is necessary so that replication may be possible either by a colleague or by other investigators (Appendix 13.B). The Cochrane Collaboration's *Reviewers Handbook* has suggestions for adequate documentation that varies by resource. For electronic databases, the following information should be reported (Higgins & Green, 2008):

- Title of the database
- Date of search
- Years covered by the search
- Complete strategy of the search
- Short summary of search strategy
- The absence of any language restrictions

It is imperative to report the name of the electronic database in addition to the date of the search. New articles are available every day, and the currency of the search indicates the need for, type, and scope of any updates. For example, a team updating a systematic review may restrict their efforts to the period of time elapsed since the last search. In addition, some databases may limit their inclusion of different types of information. Therefore, if coverage of key scientific journals has been chronologically limited within an electronic database, then other methods must be used to search the excluded issues. Moreover, clinicians may restrict the dates of their searches based on the availability of technology. For example, investigators conducting a search for evidence focused on assessing the relative effectiveness of transient evoked otoacoustic emissions versus distortion product otoacoustic emissions in newborn hearing screening may restrict their search to the 1990s and beyond, after the widespread implementation of OAEs. Documentation of the complete search strategy includes a list of all search terms, the number of hits, duplicates, and articles retrieved for abstract review. This information can be documented in tabular form (Appendix 13.C). The summary of the search strategy may include a short statement regarding which search terms were used for different aspects of the clinical question. Documentation of handsearching journals and conference proceedings require documenting the journal or conference name, followed by the dates of publication and or meeting, respectively. The following are examples of adequate documentation for these purposes:

- Journal: *The Hearing Journal,* January 1995 to December 2008
- Conference Proceedings: *Audiology NOW!,* 2008, April 2–5, Charlotte, North Carolina

Finally, documentation should describe the search of any miscellaneous sources, such as reference lists from bibliographies, from other books, articles, or websites, in addition to any language restrictions (e.g., English only). In the next section we discuss selection strategies for sifting the data you obtain from searches.

A Multilayered Selection Strategy

Search strategies are only the beginning of the process. The next step is screening the output obtained from electronic databases and other resources. The best approach involves a systematic step-by-step review of the evidence at multiple levels. Figure 13.5 shows a five-step process for reviewing studies to include for EBP or for

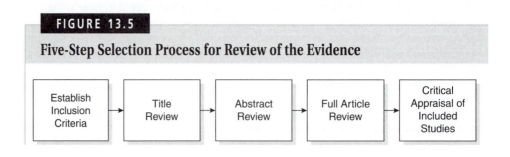

FIGURE 13.5

Five-Step Selection Process for Review of the Evidence

Establish Inclusion Criteria → Title Review → Abstract Review → Full Article Review → Critical Appraisal of Included Studies

a systematic review. Sifting through the output of electronic databases is similar to peeling an onion; one layer must be removed at a time. A multilayered approach precludes having to retrieve full-text articles of irrelevant studies. The process begins with establishing criteria that must be satisfied for a study to be used for EBP or included in a systematic review. The PICO framework discussed earlier in this chapter is useful in determining criteria for participants, independent variables, outcome measures, and level of evidence. Once inclusion criteria have been established, the review begins with a title review.

Most of the initial output from electronic databases consists of lists of titles of systematic reviews of randomized, controlled clinical trials and articles from scientific journals. We will illustrate the selection process using PubMed, although the same procedure is recommended with most electronic databases. Figure 13.6 shows typical output from an initial search conducted on PubMed using the search string "cochlear implants and health-related quality of life" for a systematic review of the health-related quality of life benefits of cochlear implants for adults with prelingual deafness.

The first step is to differentiate items for further review from those to eliminate on the basis of the relevance of the titles through ratings of (1) inclusion, (2) exclusion, or (3) for discussion. For example, titles indicating the inclusion of only pediatric patients should be excluded from the systematic review. Therefore, although not visible, the first titles listed for the PubMed output in Figure 13.6 should be eliminated.

FIGURE 13.6

PubMed Output for Search String "Cochlear Implants and Health-Related Quality of Life"

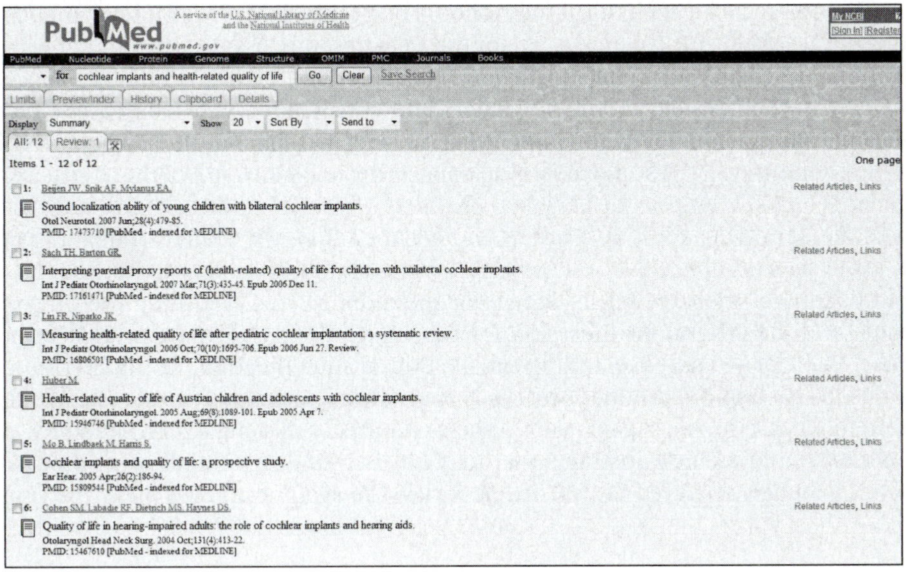

Similarly, any title not showing clear applicability to the systematic review should be labeled "for discussion" because it is not clear if it includes HRQoL results for adult patients. However, these titles should be included in the abstract review to minimize the chances of eliminating a relevant study. To avoid selection bias, two independent judges should conduct separate searches and document their results on the chart shown in Appendix 13C by recording the name of the person conducting the search, the date, the database, search strings used, the number of hits, excluded studies, and duplicates. The number of hits minus excluded studies and duplicates equals the number of included studies per search string. Using the search string "cochlear implants and health-related quality of life" on PubMed yielded twelve hits. The five excluded titles (i.e., pediatric emphasis) and no duplicates left seven titles to proceed to abstract review—that is, 12 hits – (5 excluded titles + 0 duplicates) = 7 titles to proceed to abstract review. This process should be completed for each search string.

Generally, it is best to start with the search string eliciting the greatest number of hits and then proceed in a descending fashion for each search string. At the bottom of the sheet are columns for summing the number of titles recovered, those excluded, and so on, for each database. These values are particularly useful in summarizing the study flow in a systematic review. **Study flow** describes each stage of the selection process that ultimately results in a set of included studies for use in a systematic or evidence-based review.

Point-by-point interjudge reliability for certain aspects of title review can be used to legitimize the thoroughness of search strategies for the classification of titles for inclusion or exclusion, in addition to tracking of duplicate references. Disagreements between judges should be settled through discussion or a third party. All members of search teams should maintain hard copies of their search output to include completed worksheets appended with the output from electronic databases. Several of the electronic databases permit saving electronic copies of search results.

The abstracts for each title (study) should be printed and placed into a notebook for easy access during the next stage of the selection process. Figure 13.7 shows an abstract from PubMed. Note that the abstract is structured to provide headings of objective, study design, methods, results, and conclusion. As discussed in Chapter 12, structured abstracts save time for clinicians and investigators, who can efficiently determine if the study meets inclusion criteria. To the right of the abstract are "Related Links," that provide access to abstracts of similar studies. This feature may assist in identifying additional articles not gleaned from the search strategy. Again, to avoid selection bias, two independent judges should conduct separate searches and document their results as shown in Appendix 13D by recording the person's name and the criteria for inclusion for full article review. Reviewers circle either "Yes," "No," or "Unsure" regarding satisfaction, disqualification, or undetermined status for each of the criteria. Any study that fails to satisfy all criteria is excluded from full article review. Again, to minimize chances of missing a relevant study, reviewers should include abstracts that may have an undetermined status on a few criteria. Studies retrieved for full article review are again evaluated using the same

FIGURE 13.7

A PubMed Abstract

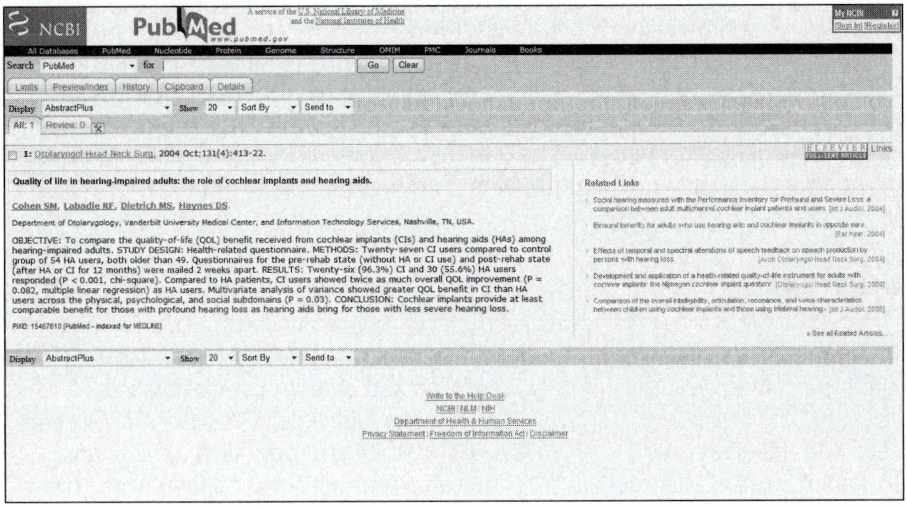

tool and are included in the critical appraisal stage of EBP, which is the topic of the next chapter. Again, point-by-point reliability can be used to calculate the percent of interjudge reliability regarding the satisfaction of inclusion criteria for each abstract. Abstracts meeting inclusion criteria proceed to full article review.

Obtaining articles for full article review may be easier for some readers than others. All articles should be rescreened for satisfaction of inclusion criteria. As mentioned earlier, memberships in AAA, ASHA, and NSSLHA provide access to their professional journals. However, much of the literature in communication sciences and disorders is found in other journals. Students and practitioners at major universities simply have to consult their libraries for access to these journals. It is advisable to search your library online before physically retrieving hard copies of journals and spending money to duplicate articles. Most libraries have purchased electronic access to journals and their articles may be obtained online with a click of the mouse. Moreover, some libraries have interlibrary loan that e-mails articles from journals available at other universities to patrons. For individuals who have no affiliation with a university, access to journal articles is limited. Some journals offer "free access" to articles, but most pertaining to communication sciences and disorders do not. Purchasing a single article can cost as much as $30. Therefore, a multilayered selection process partially precludes unnecessary expenditures by screening evidence by title and abstract before full article retrieval.

Summary

This chapter has focused on framing clinical questions and summarizing specific resources for searching, documenting, and selecting evidence in communication sciences and disorders. Specifically, the PICO rubric was discussed and illustrated for use in clarifying clinical questions. In addition, strategies and tools were provided for efficiently and effectively obtaining the highest-quality evidence for use in EBP. Particular attention was placed on documenting the search process, which provides the necessary reliability and validity for that critical step of EBP. It is hoped that readers use the knowledge and skills provided in this chapter as a starting point in exploring the resources available on the Internet and at their university libraries.

LEARNING ACTIVITIES

1. Use the PICO rubric in formulating clinical questions for actual cases involving a clinical decision.

2. Make an appointment with the reference librarian assigned to communication sciences and disorders to inquire about the resources available to students and faculty for EBP.

3. Explore and take the tutorials available on PubMed and other electronic databases to develop your skills in searching for evidence.

4. Use the strategies suggested in this chapter to search for evidence for a term paper, thesis prospectus, or other assignment.

REVIEW EXERCISES

1. *Reliability and Validity in Outcome Measure:* Please match the following terms with their correct definitions below.
   A. Validity
   B. Test-retest reliability
   C. Reliability
   D. Construct validity
   E. Face validity
   F. Internal consistency
   G. Content validity
   H. Criterion validity
   I. Feasibility
   J. Responsiveness

   _____ The degree to which an instrument rationally and empirically measures a theoretical construct (Maxwell & Satake, 2005; Schiavetti & Metz, 2006)

   _____ The degree to which items on the instrument focus on different aspects of a behavior or domain (e.g., emotional aspects or participation restrictions resulting from hearing loss)

   _____ The degree to which scores on instrument correlate with those of a recognized "gold standard" of measurement

   _____ Another name for content validity

   _____ The utility of an instrument in the real world

   _____ The sensitivity of an instrument in measuring participants' states from pre- to postintervention

   _____ The stability of a measurement over time

   _____ The truth in measurement

_____ The consistency of measurement
_____ The consistency with which the items on a questionnaire measure the same things (e.g., domains such as participation restrictions).

2. *Major Concepts in Searching for Evidence:* Please insert T for "true" or F for "false" in the blanks for the statements below.
_____ The search for evidence should begin at the highest level of evidence.

_____ It is not important to document the search process.
_____ A multilayered approach to selecting relevant evidence saves time, energy, and money.
_____ The first step in the search for evidence is to establish criteria for article inclusion.
_____ It is advisable to take advantage of pertinent tutorials available on electronic databases.

ANSWERS TO THE REVIEW EXERCISES

1. D, G, H, E, I, J, B, A, C, F
2. T, F, T, T, T

APPENDIX 13A

PICO Worksheet for Evidence-Based Practice

Clinician: _____

Patient: _____

Date: _____

PARAMETER	DESCRIPTORS
Population	
Intervention	
Comparison (Intervention)	
Outcome	

Clinical Question: _____

_____

_____

APPENDIX 13B

Documentation of an Electronic Database Search

Name of reviewer: _____

Title of database: _____

Date of search: _____

Years covered by search: _____

Complete strategy of search: _____

Short summary of search strategy: _____

_____

_____

_____

_____

List any language restrictions: _____

APPENDIX 13C

Report of Title Review

Name: _____

Date of search: _____

Electronic database: _____

Search String	Hits	Excluded Titles	Duplicates	Titles for Abstract Review (Hits – (Excluded Titles + Duplicates) =
Total: _____	Total: _____	Total: _____	Total: _____	Total: _____

APPENDIX 13D

Report of Abstract or Article Review

Name: _____

Article (Author[s] and Date) Specify:	1. POPULATION CRITERIA Specify:	2. INTERVENTION CRITERIA Specify:	3. OUTCOME CRITERIA Specify:	4. LEVEL OF EVIDENCE Specify:	5. INCLUDE?
	Yes No Unsure	Yes No Unsure	Yes No Unsure	Yes No Unsure	Yes No Unsure
	Yes No Unsure	Yes No Unsure	Yes No Unsure	Yes No Unsure	Yes No Unsure
	Yes No Unsure	Yes No Unsure	Yes No Unsure	Yes No Unsure	Yes No Unsure
	Yes No Unsure	Yes No Unsure	Yes No Unsure	Yes No Unsure	Yes No Unsure
	Yes No Unsure	Yes No Unsure	Yes No Unsure	Yes No Unsure	Yes No Unsure
	Yes No Unsure	Yes No Unsure	Yes No Unsure	Yes No Unsure	Yes No Unsure
	Yes No Unsure	Yes No Unsure	Yes No Unsure	Yes No Unsure	Yes No Unsure
	Yes No Unsure	Yes No Unsure	Yes No Unsure	Yes No Unsure	Yes No Unsure

CHAPTER 14

Evaluating the Evidence

Not a shred of evidence exists in favor of the idea that life is serious.

—Brendan Gill

The most savage controversies are those about matters as to which there is no good evidence either way.

—Bertrand Russell (1872–1970)

I'll be more enthusiastic about encouraging thinking outside the box when there's evidence of any thinking going on inside it.

—Terry Pratchett

In the previous chapters, we discussed framing the clinical research question and searching, retrieving, and managing evidence garnered for making clinical decisions. The third step in evidence-based practice (EBP) is to evaluate the quality and rigor of the evidence and provide a grade for its use in clinical practice. The level of rigor is indirectly proportional to the level of bias inherent in the study. In earlier chapters, the sources of and methods to control for bias have been thoroughly discussed with numerous examples. To review, sources of evidence may be ranked in levels by their degree of rigor and indirectly related to their degree of bias.

The purposes of this chapter are to first discuss some weaknesses in communication sciences and disorders research that may introduce bias into studies. We will then introduce checklists for evaluating sources retrieved for use in EBP. Specifically, checklists are provided for evaluating systematic reviews; randomized, controlled clinical trials; cohort studies; case-control studies; and diagnostic studies. We will conclude with a discussion of the rating of overall bias in evidence and grading of its use in clinical practice.

LEARNING OBJECTIVES

This chapter will enable readers to:

- Discuss common limitations in communication sciences and disorders research.
- Critically appraise common types of studies.

- Assign an appropriate grade to clinical recommendations provided by scientific evidence.

Common Weaknesses in Communication Sciences and Disorders Research

Throughout the chapter on EBP, controlled randomized clinical trials have been touted as the "gold standard" in biomedical research. Communication sciences and disorders researchers typically have utilized quasi-experimental designs in which groups that differ on some criteria are compared in some way. These studies do not randomly assign participants to treatment and control groups, but may use, for the sake of convenience, **intact groups** (e.g., children in two different classrooms) that may introduce a high risk of sampling bias. In addition, some investigators have felt it unethical to deny possible benefits of innovative treatments to patients who happen to be assigned to control groups. Fortunately, innovative experimental designs are available that overcome ethical issues such as assigning patients to treatment and de-layed treatment groups to serve as controls (e.g., Abrams, Chisolm, & McArdle, 2002). Common weaknesses in hearing aid research include inadequate sampling, subject self-selection bias, use of too few or too many participants, lack of blinding, failure to account for dropouts, and use of surrogate endpoints (Cox, 2005). These limitations are also inherent in most research in communication sciences and disorders. There-fore, we will discuss each of these areas below.

Inadequate sampling occurs when participants do not represent the population to which the results of the study are to be generalized. Many studies fail to recruit par-ticipants who proportionately represent the diversity of the population. Careful plan-ning and reporting of all methods of recruitment and strict adherence to inclusion and exclusion criteria assist in determining the existence of sampling bias. Whenever possible, researchers should recruit participants with the same demographics of the city or town from which the sample is drawn, especially members of minority groups. Subject self-selection, another source of sampling bias, is the tendency for partici-pants who volunteer to differ from those members of the representative population who would not opt to participate in all or part of an investigation. Participants who self-select to volunteer may be more motivated or eager to try new treatments than their nonparticipatory peers, ultimately inflating the effectiveness of an intervention for a population. For example, Kuehn, Imrey, Tomes, Jones, O'Gara, and colleagues (2002) investigated whether the hypernasality of patients with cleft palate could be reduced by eight weeks of graded velopharyngeal resistance training against continu-ous positive airway pressure. The main outcome measure was reduction of blinded expert ratings of pretreatment to immediate posttreatment hypernasality compared against a reference standard. Many patients showed an immediate reduction of hy-pernasality; some did not. Participants who showed improvement were invited for a follow-up evaluation an average of thirteen months later. Those who opted to return demonstrated long-term maintenance of their immediate posttreatment gains. How-ever, investigators admitted that the positive outcomes from the follow-up segment may have been inflated by self-selection bias.

Another weakness in communication sciences and disorders research is the re-cruitment of too few participants to detect clinically significant effects between or among groups, treatments, or other comparisons. Even experienced investigators have mistakenly believed that twelve or twenty participants were adequate sample sizes. In the other extreme, some researchers have believed that the more participants included in a study, the better. In other chapters, we have discussed the importance of and procedures for conducting analyses to determine appropriate sample sizes for adequate statistical power. Adequate sample size is a bit like Goldilocks and the Three Bears; the sample size should neither be too small nor too large, but just right. For example, Lenth (2001) stated that an undersized study is a waste of resources because it is too underpowered to yield meaningful results. Alternatively, studies that are too large also waste precious resources by being inefficient.

Another potential weakness in our research is the failure to double-blind participants and investigators to the allocation process for assignment to treatment and control groups. Failure to blind increases the likelihood of subject bias, or any conscious or subconscious influences on study outcomes due to participants' knowledge of treatment allocation (Schiavetti & Metz, 2006). Also the Hawthorne effect may influence participants to act differently when they know that they are being observed in a research study. For example, if participants know that they are receiving an innovative treatment for their communication disorder rather than no treatment, a standard treatment, or sham treatment, they may try harder or may exaggerate reductions in self-perceived activity limitations or participation restrictions. Additionally, experimenter bias, either conscious or subconscious, may influence results if investigators are not blinded to participants' treatment allocation (Schiavetti & Metz, 2006). For example, investigators may influence outcomes by being more encouraging or somehow treating participants receiving the experimental intervention differently than those in the control group. Traditionally, double-blinding has been not been done in our research due to logistical reasons (e.g., limitation of resources) and the difficulty of concealment in some treatment-no treatment comparisons (e.g., hearing aid versus no hearing aid or cochlear implants versus hearing aid).

Failure to account for and have procedures for dealing with participants who start but do not complete the study is another weakness in our research. Using only the results from participants who completed an experiment generalizes to only a subset of the original population from which the sample was drawn because the dropouts may differ in some clinically significant ways that affect outcomes. For example, participants who complete the study may have more financial resources, be more motivated, and other significant differences from those who drop out, which can result in overestimating the clinical effectiveness of the treatment based on only a segment of the population. Therefore, well-conducted studies should report and have statistical procedures to deal with dropouts. **Intention-to-treat analyses** compare the results of patients in the groups to which they were originally assigned, regardless of whether they completed the study, requiring appropriate follow-up and collection of their outcome data (Hollis & Campbell, 1999). The intention-to-treat analysis is customarily followed by and compared to an **as-treated analysis,** involving the data from participants who completed the study, in order to determine the impact of dropouts on study outcomes (Friedman, Furberg, & DeMets, 1998). For example, Roy, Weinrich,

Gray, Tanner, Stemple, and Sapienza (2003) conducted a randomized clinical trial evaluating the relative effectiveness of three voice treatment programs: (1) voice amplification using the ChatterVox portable amplifier (VA), (2) resonance therapy (RT), and (3) and respiratory muscle training (RMT). They conducted an intention-to-treat analysis and obtained pre- and postoutcome measures on a surprisingly high number of dropouts (four in the RMT group and nine in the RT group). Subsequently, using only the data collected from those participants who completed the study, an as-treated analysis was conducted that resulted in the same results as on the intent-to-treat analysis. Namely, only the VA and RT groups reported significant reductions in mean scores on the *Voice Handicap Index* (Jacobson, Johnson, Grywalski, Silbergliet, Jacobson, Benninger, et al., 1997) and voice severity scales. Moreover, the VA group reported more overall voice improvement, greater vocal clarity, and greater ease of speaking and singing than either the RT or RMT group. Due to the small number of participants who actually completed the clinical trial and identical results on both analyses, the authors chose to use the as-treated analysis when discussing the results of their study.

The final weakness we discuss in communication sciences and disorders research is the use of surrogate endpoints or dependent variables that do not actually represent the long-term status of patients or the "happily-ever-after" outcomes. For example, Cox (2005) stated that many studies investigating the effectiveness of amplification have focused on dependent variables such as insertion gain or word recognition scores that may have little or no impact on patients' long-term status as seen in health-related quality of life (HRQoL measures). Fortunately, researchers have recognized the importance of using self-report assessments focusing on HRQoL, such as in audiologic rehabilitation (Abrams, Chisolm, & McArdle, 2005). In addition, few investigators conduct longitudinal studies that show critical outcomes spanning several years. For example, Uziel, Sillon, Vieu, Artieres, Piron, Daures, and colleagues (2007) conducted a ten-year follow-up of eighty-two prelingually deafened children who received Cochlear Nucleus CI22 implants. The children were assessed on a variety of clinical measures, indices of academic achievement, and occupational status. Results of longitudinal studies like these can show that young children implanted with a cochlear implant can develop viable speech perception and production skills and achieve academic benchmarks during adolescence and young adulthood.

This section has described some common weaknesses in communication sciences and disorders research that can add sources of bias. In the next section, we will introduce and describe how to use checklists for evaluating systematic reviews, controlled randomized clinical trials, cohort studies, case-control studies, and diagnostic studies for use in EBP.

Critiquing Studies for Evidence-Based Practice

Appendices 14A through E contain checklists for evaluating most types of studies encountered in EBP in communication sciences and disorders. Each checklist was developed through synthesis of a variety of sources.

Systematic Reviews

Systematic reviews were defined and covered extensively in Chapter 12. A checklist for evaluating the quality of a systematic review is shown in Appendix 14A; it has been adapted for use from the systematic review critical appraisal sheet from the Centre for Evidence-Based Medicine (CEBM, 2006) and a similar form from the *SIGN Guideline Developers' Handbook* (SIGN-50, 2004). Generally, the introduction to the systematic review should provide the rationale for the study and a summary of previous evidence necessary to formulate focused research questions. For example, Chisolm, Johnson, Danhauer, Portz, Abrams, Lesner, McCarthy, and Newman (2007) provided an in-depth introduction explaining the effects of untreated hearing loss on the health-related quality of life of adults with sensorineural hearing loss (SNHL) that built the rationale for formulating their experimental question. What is the evidence for the health-related quality of life benefits of amplification for adults with SNHL?

The description of the methodology should be well-documented and thorough, beginning with the justification for the methodology used and the specific criteria that studies must meet for inclusion in the systematic review (e.g., the level of evidence, patient characteristics, interventions, alternative treatments, outcome measures, and so on). For example, Chisolm and colleagues (2007) mandated that in order for studies to be included in the systematic review they had to be at least at Level III of evidence (e.g., at minimum case-control or cohort studies with a high risk of confounding, bias, or chance and a significant risk that any relationships are not causal). Participants had to be eighteen years of age with normal cognitive function whose SNHL ranged from mild to profound, living in independent or assistive living conditions. The type of intervention was air-conduction hearing aids worn either monaural or binaurally without regard to the type of circuitry (e.g., analog or digital). In addition, studies had to employ either normed generic or disease-specific HRQoL outcome measures before and after hearing aid fitting. Chisolm and colleagues (2007) justified the rather lenient criteria for the level of evidence by noting the paucity of randomized, controlled clinical trials in the audiology literature. Type of circuitry was not restricted to the latest technology in hopes of retrieving all possible evidence regarding the HRQoL benefits from amplification.

The search strategy must be thorough enough to retrieve all relevant evidence pertaining to the research question. The description of the search strategy should be transparent enough to permit exact duplication and should identify who conducted the search, their training, teaming, databases and resource used, degree of reliability or validity of included results, and procedures for reaching consensus. For example, Chisolm and colleagues (2007) divided six of eight team members into three two-person teams with one team member to serve as mediator for differences among team members. One team searched the Communication Sciences and Disorders Dome (ComDisDome); another team searched the Cumulative Index to Nursing and Allied Health Literature (CINAHL), Evidence-Based Medicine Reviews (EBMR), and the Cochrane Database of Systematic Reviews (Cochrane Reviews). Each team member independently used all search strings in the same databases as their partner and made decisions regarding elimination of potential studies based first on title, then abstract, and then full article review. Study-by-study reliability agreement between team members was calculated to be over 90 percent for all phases of the search and retrieval process using the following equation: [Agreements / (Agreements + Disagreements)] × 100 = ____. Thoroughness of the search strategy is confirmed by using more than one database that taps into the same resources. Because the lag time for publications is as long as two years and not all high-quality information is found in peer-reviewed journals, systematic reviews also examine papers presented at professional meetings and in non-peer-reviewed journals. For example, Chisolm and colleagues (2007) had a third team search recent conference proceedings and non-peer-reviewed journals (e.g., *Hearing Review* and *The Hearing Journal*).

The results of the systematic review should include a graphic representation and explanation of the study flow or the summary of the search and retrieval process. For example, Figure 14.1 shows the flowchart for the search and retrieval process for Chisolm and colleagues' (2007) systematic review. The text should explain and the flowchart should depict the number of studies considered and eliminated at each stage of the process. The articles excluded after full article review should be listed in a bibliography and on a table showing their status for each of the inclusion criteria. Similarly, the characteristics for included studies should be explained in the text and depicted in tabular form (e.g., authors, year of publication, level of evidence, experimental design, and participant characteristics). For example, Chisolm and colleagues (2007) included a table of included studies presenting authors, years of publication, participant characteristics (i.e., groupings, history of hearing aid use, gender, pure-tone averages), outcome measures, and results, in addition to any pertinent notes and while thoroughly discussing the details in the text. In addition, systematic reviews should include an evaluation of the quality of included studies on level of evidence, use of control groups, power analyses, inclusion and exclusion criteria for participants, random assignment of participants to treatment and control groups, equivalence of those groups at baseline, intention-to-treat analyses, double-blinding, accounting of and provision for dropouts, and calculation of effect sizes and confidence intervals. Chisolm and colleagues (2007) assessed each of their included studies on several of these criteria with listing and discussion of the evaluation in a table and in the text, respectively.

Systematic reviews may be qualitative or quantitative. Qualitative systematic reviews generally discuss the overall trend in results of included studies and general conclusions. On the other hand, quantitative systematic reviews involve meta-analyses (see Chapter 12), which are statistical procedures that allow the aggregation of the results from several independent studies for calculation of treatment effects and confidence intervals. The combining of results should be from similar studies that share certain commonalities such as experimental designs or similar outcome measures. For example, Chisolm and colleagues (2007) had both qualitative and quantitative aspects to their systematic review. Their meta-analysis was based on combining the results of studies that utilized between versus within subject experimental designs and whether outcome measures were generic versus disease-specific. Chisolm and colleagues (2007) organized the results of the systematic review through use of

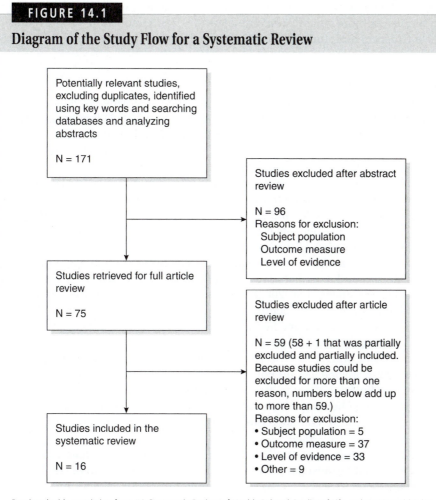

FIGURE 14.1

Diagram of the Study Flow for a Systematic Review

Potentially relevant studies, excluding duplicates, identified using key words and searching databases and analyzing abstracts

N = 171

Studies excluded after abstract review

N = 96
Reasons for exclusion:
  Subject population
  Outcome measure
  Level of evidence

Studies retrieved for full article review

N = 75

Studies excluded after article review

N = 59 (58 + 1 that was partially excluded and partially included. Because studies could be excluded for more than one reason, numbers below add up to more than 59.)
Reasons for exclusion:
• Subject population = 5
• Outcome measure = 37
• Level of evidence = 33
• Other = 9

Studies included in the systematic review

N = 16

Reprinted with permission from "A Systematic Review of Health-Related Quality of Life and Hearing Aids" by T. H. Chisolm, C. E. Johnson, J. L. Danhauer, L. J. Portz, H. B. Abrams, et al. *Journal of the American Academy of Audiology, 18,* p. 157.

tables and graphs showing the treatment effects and confidence intervals that were thoroughly discussed in the text.

Systematic reviews should conclude with an overall recommendation and a grade reflecting the strength of the evidence. For example, Chisolm and colleagues (2007) suggested a recommended grade of B as appropriate for the use of hearing aids to improve the HRQoL of adults with SNHL when considering the level of evidence and the quality of the studies included in their systematic review. Grading is discussed in more detail at the end of this chapter. Finally, systematic reviews should provide conclusions regarding clinical practice and future research. Chisolm and colleagues (2007) concluded that clinicians and researchers explore the development and use of more generic outcome measures and circumvent bias introduced by quasi-experimental studies by exploring the use of randomized, controlled clinical trials.

Randomized, Controlled Clinical Trials

Appendix 14B has a checklist for evaluating the evidence provided by a randomized, controlled clinical trial that has been adapted from the CONSORT Statement (Moher, Shulz, Altman, & CONSORT Group, 2001), a critical appraisal sheet from the Centre for Evidence-Based Medicine (CEBM, 2006), and a form available from the *SIGN Guideline Developers' Handbook* (Scottish Intercollegiate Network, 2008). As with all studies, the clinical trial should have a strong scientific foundation leading to clearly stated hypotheses and focused research questions. To accomplish these objectives, large clinical trials require considerable scientific evaluation and logistical planning. For example, clinicians and scientists from the National Institute of Deafness and Other Communication Disorders of the National Institutes of Health and the Department of Veteran Affairs collaborated in the planning of a large and extended multisite clinical trial that was conducted between 1996 and 1998 (Larson, Williams, Henderson, Luethke, Beck, Noffsinger, et al., 2002). The study began planning in 1993 after strong consideration of the available scientific evidence as reviewed by an advisory committee with the charge of facilitating hearing aid research and establishing priorities for clinical trials (Bratt, 2007). The recommendations of that advisory committee were revised, important outcomes for assessment were identified, and a grant proposal was developed by invited VA and non-VA clinicians and scientists (Bratt, 2007). The purpose of the clinical trial was to assess the relative effectiveness of three commonly used single-channel hearing aid circuits (i.e., peak-clippers, compression-limiting, and wide dynamic range compression) using a three-period, three-treatment crossover design (Larson et al., 2000).

Because randomized, controlled clinical trials are the "gold standard" in biomedical research, they must have a high degree of internal validity in the recruitment of participants (e.g., power analysis to determine sample size, inclusion/exclusion criteria and beginning and end dates for recruitment, and location of data collection); randomization, blinding, and concealment; primary outcome measures; and an accounting of and procedures (e.g., intention-to-treat analysis) for dropouts. Large multicenter studies should report how the clinical trial was conducted in addition to the safeguards ensuring uniformity of protocol administration across investigators and centers. In fact, sometimes an entire issue of a journal is needed to report the results of a large multicenter clinical trial. For example, Henderson, Larson, Williams, and Luethke (2002) wrote an entire article just to explain the organization and administration of the NIDCD-VA clinical trial. They explained that patients were recruited based on a power analysis using strict inclusion/exclusion criteria (e.g., fluent speakers of English having a sensorineural hearing loss with no evidence of outer ear, inner ear, or retrocochlear pathology) from May 1996 to June 1997 with follow-up testing completed by February 1998 (Henderson et al., 2002). The design of the study was a three-period, three-treatment crossover design in which participants were randomly assigned to use one of three hearing aid circuits during one of three ninety-day trial periods.

Procedures for random assignment, blinding, and treatment concealment must be clearly described in adequate detail. It is not sufficient to only state that participants were randomly assigned to treatment and control groups, but the description should include who generated the allocation sequence, enrolled participants, and so on. For instance, the NIDCD-VA hearing aid clinical trial had strong central coordination from an external site that randomly assigned patients enrolled at eight participating VA medical centers to experience one of six possible sequences of circuits (i.e., peak clipper, compression limiting, and wide dynamic range compression) that were counterbalanced across each block of six consecutively enrolled participants. Double-blinding was used in that neither the participant nor the investigator knew which circuit was being used, and each of the circuits was concealed in the same hearing-aid case.

Clinical trials should also clearly state primary and secondary outcome measures to include information on reliability, validity, and data collection. For instance, the primary outcome measures for the NIDCD-VA hearing aid clinical trial were tests of speech recognition, sound quality, and subjective hearing aid benefit, which were consistently administered at baseline and then after each three-month intervention period with each of the three circuits. Data collection involved identical equipment and procedures by trained personnel across VA medical centers.

One weakness of the clinical trial was that intention-to-treat analyses were not used to account for participants who did not complete testing or if the observer was unable to complete the protocol. However, the VA hearing aid clinical trial had all of the positive characteristics of a multicenter study by ensuring that the protocol was uniformly applied and results were similar across studies.

Cohort Studies

Appendix 14C is a checklist for the evaluation of cohort studies regarding background information, internal validity (i.e., selection of participants, assessment of outcomes, and accounting for confounding variables), and overall assessment of its value in EBP. It has been adapted for use from Cummings, Newman, and Hulley (2001), Newman, Browner, and Hulley (2001), and a form from the *SIGN Guideline Developers' Handbook* (Scottish Intercollegiate Network, 2008). The background information of the study should have a well-developed rationale for utilizing a cohort design. For example, Wu, Lee, Chen, and Hsu (2008) built a strong rationale for assessing genetic screening and high-resolution computed tomography of the inner ear as predictors for speech perception outcomes in children with cochlear implants. They explained that strong associations between these predictor and outcome variables warranted inclusion of genetic testing and imaging studies in the battery of preoperative evaluations. Regarding participant selection, the treatment and control groups of cohort studies should be selected from the same source populations that differ only by the presence of the predictor variable(s) under consideration. For example, the children assessed in the Wu and colleagues study (2008) were all from the same population of children having at least three years of cochlear implant experience. The study should specify the number of participants who continued on with the study in addition to those who dropped out. The number of overall dropouts, in addition to those in each subgroup, should be reported and accounted for in the statistical analyses.

Outcomes must be clearly defined and hopefully blinded to the predictor variables. In other words, persons measuring outcomes should not know the status of the predictor variables for the participants. For example, Damrose, Goldman, Groessl, and Orloff (2004) assessed long-term botulinum toxic injections on symptom severity in patients with spasmodic dysphonia. At the time, they reported being one of the first cohort studies to use blind raters to assess symptom severity from voice recordings made at several points during treatment. However, for studies in which blinding is not possible, some explanation should be provided regarding how knowledge of participants' status for predictor variables could have influenced the assessment of the outcome. Outcomes measurement must be a reliable and valid process supported by some type of external evidence. Lastly, the main potential confounding variables should have been identified and taken into account in the design and analysis of the data.

Case-Control Studies

Appendix 14D is a checklist for the evaluation of case-control studies on background information, internal validity, and overall assessment of its value in EBP (Newman, Browner, Cummings, & Hulley, 2001; Newman et al., 2001; Scottish Intercollegiate Network, 2008). First, a sound rationale should be given for using a case-control design. The experimental question should focus on assessing associative factors or possible causes for particular conditions that are somewhat rare (Newman, Browner, Cummings, et al., 2001; Scottish Intercollegiate Network, 2008). The basic logic of this design mandates that participants with the condition (i.e., cases) and those without (i.e., controls) are sampled from similar populations, because groups should only differ with regard to presence of the predictor variable. Therefore, it follows that both case and control groups should use similar exclusion criteria. Moreover, in earlier chapters, we discussed the importance of reporting and comparing both participants who completed and those who dropped out of the study. For example, intention-to-treat and as-treated analyses of the data may determine if reasons for nonparticipation may have ultimately introduced a source of bias into the results. The bottom line is that the cases are clearly defined and differentiated from controls via a process that is blinded to the status of the predictor variable for participants. Furthermore, measurement bias can be reduced through the use of more than one control group (Browner, Cummings, et al., 2001). For example, Haley, Hom, Roland, Bryan, Van Ness, and colleagues (1997) conducted a blinded case-control study to determine whether Gulf War–related illnesses are associated with peripheral nervous system dysfunction. In order to control for deployment to the Middle East, a group of twenty-three veterans with Gulf War–related illnesses was compared to ten veterans deployed to the Gulf War without the illnesses and ten healthy veterans not deployed to the Gulf War. Investigators blinded to participants' groupings administered a variety of tests that revealed a tendency for veterans with Gulf War–related illnesses to have greater interaural asymmetry in wave I to III interpeak latencies, significantly more interocular asymmetry of nystagmic velocity on rotational testing, as well as other test results indicating peripheral neurologic dysfunction.

The presence of the predictor variable in participants must be reliably and validly determined, which can be difficult from retrospective chart reviews of data that are not available for most participants. Inability to document the degree or severity of the predictor variable seriously compromises the value of case-control studies. The best confirmation is provided by reliable and valid test results that are available for all or most participants. In addition, measurement bias may be reduced by using data available prior to the development of the outcome (Newman, Browner, Cummings, et al., 2001). For example, Rubens, Vohr, Tucker, O'Neil, and Chung (2008) used a case-control design to evaluate newborns' transient evoked otoacoustic emissions results (TEOAEs) as a predictor variable for sudden infant death syndrome (SIDS). The TEOAE screening results of thirty-one babies who died from SIDS were compared to thirty-one healthy infants who were matched on critical variables of gender, term versus preterm age, and neonatal intensive care unit and well-baby nursery placements. TEOAEs are very commonly used in universal newborn hearing screening programs (Joint Committee on Infant Hearing, 2007). They found that of the babies who died from SIDS the TEOAE results for the right ear had a lower signal-to-noise ratio at 2,000 and 4,000 Hz compared to the results of the healthy infants in the control group. The authors hope that the results of this study provide a rationale for the use of TEOAE results to identify infants at risk for SIDS.

In summary, influence of confounding factors must be minimized in the design and in the analysis of the results (Scottish Intercollegiate Network, 2008). In addition, the results should contain confidence intervals if odd ratios are calculated for participants developing the disease or condition. Decisions on using a case-control study for EBP should hinge on whether the risks of bias from confounding variables inherent in sampling and measurement have been minimized and the effects, if any, were due to the predictor variable and could be generalized to the intended populations. Case-control studies can be useful in assessing the accuracy of screening and diagnostic tests.

Diagnostic Tests

Appendix 14E presents a checklist for evaluating studies of diagnostic tests, which has been adapted for use from the STARD Statement (Bossuyt, Reitsma, Bruns, Gatsonis et al., 2003), the diagnostic critical appraisal sheet (CEBM, 2006), and a form available from the SIGN Guideline Developers' Handbook (Scottish Intercollegiate Network, 2008). The first consideration is whether the introduction contains a strong rationale justifying assessment of the diagnostic accuracy of a test or index against a gold standard. In most cases, the new test has some advantages over the standard assessment tools, such as cost, feasibility, noninvasiveness, and so on.

Regarding the population, the inclusion/exclusion criteria should be adequately described in addition to the location of the data collection. Ideally, the sample should be prospectively recruited and closely resemble the population that would typically be given the index, with broad representation among those free of the disorder as well as those presenting with mild, moderate, and severe forms of the disorder in addition to those with comorbidities (Dollaghan, 2003). For example, studies evaluating the validity of a new screening test for auditory processing disorders (APD) should include children in the targeted age ranges for the instrument who are normal, in addition to children with varying degrees of severity of APD with different profiles (e.g., figure-ground problems, tolerance-memory fading) and comorbidities such as attention-deficit disorder. The study should note whether participants were selected based on presenting symptoms (prospectively) or after receipt of the index or gold standard (retrospectively).

The testing methodology should include comparing the index with a widely accepted gold standard in a field. In addition to face validity, the gold standard should be well-defined with a description of its units and categories for classification of results (e.g., −10 to 20 dBHL is normal hearing). If no gold standard is available, a validated reference standard should be justified, well-defined, and well-described, including its units and categories for classification of results. If possible, the participants should be recruited prospectively and consecutively in series or randomly from well-defined populations. Both the index and the gold standard should be administered blindly and as close in time to each other as possible.

The results should be reported for all participants and the results on the index obtained prior to confirmation with the gold standard. Moreover, the justification for the statistical procedures for assessing the validity and reliability of the index should be well-developed and include methods for determining uncertainty (e.g., confidence intervals). The results should report the participants' demographic information (e.g., age, gender, presenting characteristics, comorbidities, and so on). A flowchart and corresponding text should present the participants' progress through the study. Accounting of and procedures for participants who do not complete the study should be documented to minimize sampling bias. In addition, the time elapsed between administration of the index versus the gold standard must be reported in addition to any adverse effects. The longer the time elapsed between administration of the index and the gold standard, the greater is the likelihood of introducing confounding variables, such as those from history or maturation. Finally, the diagnostic accuracy, subject variability, and measures of statistical uncertainty must be described and interpreted appropriately. For example, the results of the specific method of assessing diagnostic accuracy (e.g., sensitivity/specificity, receiver-operator characteristic curve, likelihood ratios, and so on) must be explained in addition to standard deviations for participant subgroups and confidence intervals.

Rating of the Evidence for Bias and Grading Its Use in Clinical Practice

At the end of Appendixes 14A through E are items relating specifically to the minimization of bias and how it might have possibly contributed to the results given.

Generally, if most issues regarding internal validity are adequately addressed, then an overall rating of "++" may be made. Alternatively, if some threats to validity that were not adequately addressed were unlikely to affect the outcomes of the study, an overall rating of "+" may be made. Studies that fail to address significant threats to internal validity that are very likely to affect overall outcomes have a high risk of bias and deserve a "−" rating. These ratings are based on a rubric advocated by Cox (2005) that is shown in Figure 14.2.

The next step is to rank the level of evidence for the investigations. In Chapter 12, we discussed the levels of evidence typically used in evidence-based medicine for intervention and diagnostic studies and how these were modified for use in communication sciences and disorders. The levels of evidence for intervention and diagnostic studies were presented in Chapter 12 and are not reproduced here. Do not forget that when ranking the level of evidence for systematic reviews to consider the levels of the majority of included studies.

The studies need to be grouped according to their relevance, which is determined by how closely the populations, interventions, comparison treatments, and outcome measures correspond to those of the clinical or research question. These groupings are important for providing a grade for the overall clinical recommendations based on the evidence proposed by Cox (2005), as shown in Figure 14.3.

The results for both intervention and diagnostic studies can be put into tabular form to assist with this process. Evidence-based practice requires students and clinicians to consider the overall trends in the studies. For interventional evidence that is both relevant and consistent at Levels I and II, a grade of A may be given to the overall recommendation. A grade of B is assigned for consistent Level III or IV studies that are relevant and consistent or for studies at Levels I or II that are not directly related to the clinical or experimental question (e.g., findings for older children when the target population is preschool children). A grade of C is given to Level V evidence or extrapolated findings from Level III or IV studies. And a grade of D is given for either inconsistent results from any level of evidence or from findings of studies with a high

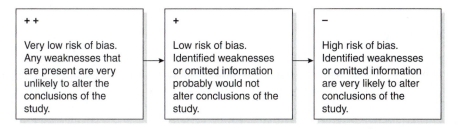

FIGURE 14.2

Ratings and Interpretations for Overall Bias in Studies

++	+	−
Very low risk of bias. Any weaknesses that are present are very unlikely to alter the conclusions of the study.	Low risk of bias. Identified weaknesses or omitted information probably would not alter conclusions of the study.	High risk of bias. Identified weaknesses or omitted information are very likely to alter conclusions of the study.

Adapted from Cox, 2005.

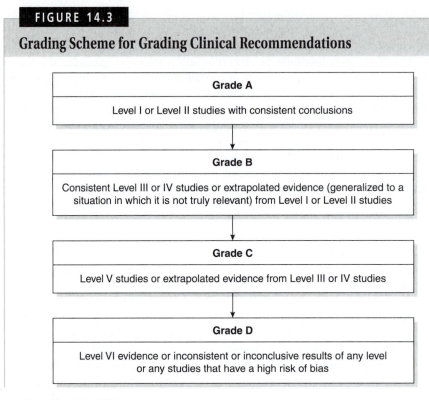

FIGURE 14.3

Grading Scheme for Grading Clinical Recommendations

Grade A
Level I or Level II studies with consistent conclusions

Grade B
Consistent Level III or IV studies or extrapolated evidence (generalized to a situation in which it is not truly relevant) from Level I or Level II studies

Grade C
Level V studies or extrapolated evidence from Level III or IV studies

Grade D
Level VI evidence or inconsistent or inconclusive results of any level or any studies that have a high risk of bias

Adapted from Cox, 2005.

degree of bias. For evidence from diagnostic studies, results that are both relevant and consistent at Level I may be given a grade of A to the overall recommendation. A grade of B is assigned for Level II or III studies that are relevant and consistent or for studies at Level I that are not directly related to the clinical or experimental question. A grade of C is given to Level IV evidence or extrapolated findings from Level II or III studies. And a grade of D, similar to interventional studies, is for either Level IV (expert opinion) evidence, inconsistent or inconclusive results from any level of evidence, or from findings of studies with a high degree of bias.

Summary

This chapter discussed some of the common weaknesses in communication sciences and disorders research that may lead to significant bias or misinterpretation of results of studies. Five checklists were provided and explained for use in critiquing systematic reviews, controlled randomized clinical trials, case-control studies, cohort studies, and diagnostic studies for EBP. In addition to determining level of evidence, these checklists can be used to determine the amount of bias in the studies so that a grade may be assigned to clinical recommendations for use in EBP. In the next chapter, a clinical scenario will help put all that we have learned into practice for doing EBP.

LEARNING ACTIVITIES

1. Use the checklists provided in the appendices to critique each of the following types of evidence: systematic reviews, controlled randomized clinical trials, cohort studies, case-control studies, and diagnostic studies.

2. Using a real clinical situation and your new knowledge and skills, complete the EBP process to arrive at a grade for the clinical recommendations provided by the evidence.

REVIEW EXERCISES

1. *Rating Bias and Clinical Recommendations from Evidence:* Place the graded evaluations with their appropriate descriptions.

A. +
B. A
C. –
D. B
E. + +
F. D
G. C

_____ Consistent Level III or IV studies or extrapolated evidence (generalized to a situation in which it is not truly relevant) from Level I or II studies

_____ Level IV evidence or inconsistent or inconclusive results of any level of evidence or from findings of studies with a high degree of bias

_____ Low risk of bias such that identified weaknesses or omitted information probably would not alter the conclusions of the study

_____ High risk of bias such that identified weaknesses or omitted information are very unlikely to alter conclusions of the study

_____ Level I or Level II studies with consistent conclusions

_____ Level V studies or extrapolated evidence from Level III or IV studies

_____ Very low risk of bias such that any weaknesses that are present are very unlikely to alter the conclusions of the study

ANSWERS TO THE REVIEW EXERCISES

1. D, F, A, C, B, G, E

APPENDIX 14A

Evaluation of Systematic Reviews

Instructions: The following items describe characteristics of well-executed systematic reviews. Please read and evaluate each statement and circle whether the issue was well-addressed, adequately addressed, not addressed, or not applicable (i.e., N/A).

Bibliographical Citation

_____

_____

_____

Background Information

The rationale for conducting a systematic review is strong based on an appropriate and clearly focused research question(s).

Well-Addressed   Adequately Addressed   Not Addressed   N/A

Notes: _____

_____

_____

Internal Validity
Description of General Methodology

• Well-documented

Well-Addressed   Adequately Addressed   Not Addressed   N/A

• Thorough

Well-Addressed   Adequately Addressed   Not Addressed   N/A

Notes: _____

_____

_____

Search Strategy

• Included criteria and rationale for article inclusion

Well-Addressed   Adequately Addressed   Not Addressed   N/A

- Conducted by adequately trained members

    Well-Addressed   Adequately Addressed   Not Addressed   N/A

- Rigorous and thorough enough to recover the necessary evidence to answer the question

    Well-Addressed   Adequately Addressed   Not Addressed   N/A

- Procedures enabling independent decisions of team members to reach consensus regarding the inclusion of studies

    Well-Addressed   Adequately Addressed   Not Addressed   N/A

- Impartial methods for settling disagreements among team members

    Well-Addressed   Adequately Addressed   Not Addressed   N/A

- Assessed reliability and accuracy of the search

    Well-Addressed   Adequately Addressed   Not Addressed   N/A

- Included handsearching of unpublished works

    Well-Addressed   Adequately Addressed   Not Addressed   N/A

Notes: _____

_____

_____

Results

Description of the study flow

- Copiously documented

    Well-Addressed   Adequately Addressed   Not Addressed   N/A

- Depicted in a flowchart

    Well-Addressed   Adequately Addressed   Not Addressed   N/A

Documentation of excluded studies after full article retrieval

- Complete bibliographical reference list

    Well-Addressed   Adequately Addressed   Not Addressed   N/A

- Table providing status on each criteria for inclusion/exclusion

    Well-Addressed   Adequately Addressed   Not Addressed   N/A

Characteristics of included studies (e.g., authors, participants' demographic data, outcome measures, etc.)

- Well-documented in tabular form

  Well-Addressed   Adequately Addressed   Not Addressed   N/A

- Thoroughly discussed in text

  Well-Addressed   Adequately Addressed   Not Addressed   N/A

Study quality assessed with careful attention to a variety of factors

- Level of evidence

  Well-Addressed   Adequately Addressed   Not Addressed   N/A

- Use of a control group

  Well-Addressed   Adequately Addressed   Not Addressed   N/A

- Power analysis

  Well-Addressed   Adequately Addressed   Not Addressed   N/A

- Inclusion and exclusion criteria of participants

  Well-Addressed   Adequately Addressed   Not Addressed   N/A

- Random assignment (e.g., treatment and control groups)

  Well-Addressed   Adequately Addressed   Not Addressed   N/A

- Equivalence of treatment and control groups at baseline

  Well-Addressed   Adequately Addressed   Not Addressed   N/A

- Intention-to-treat analysis

  Well-Addressed   Adequately Addressed   Not Addressed   N/A

- Double-blinding

  Well-Addressed   Adequately Addressed   Not Addressed   N/A

- Accounting of and provision for dropouts

  Well-Addressed   Adequately Addressed   Not Addressed   N/A

Meta-analytic procedures completed

- Results of reasonably similar studies were combined

  Well-Addressed   Adequately Addressed   Not Addressed   N/A

- Effect sizes and confidence intervals provided and discussed in table/graphical form and in the test, respectively

  Well-Addressed   Adequately Addressed   Not Addressed   N/A

Notes: _____

_____

_____

Types of Studies Included (Check all that apply)

_____ Randomized, controlled clinical trials
_____ Quasi-experimental studies
_____ Cohort studies
_____ Case-control studies
_____ Single-subject designs
_____ Case studies

Conclusions

Overall conclusion of the systematic review

- Appropriate provided the strength of treatment effects

  Well-Addressed   Adequately Addressed   Not Addressed   N/A

- Accompanied by a graded recommendation

  Well-Addressed   Adequately Addressed   Not Addressed   N/A

- Able to provide suggestions for clinical practice and future research

  Well-Addressed   Adequately Addressed   Not Addressed   N/A

Notes: _____

_____

_____

Overall Assessment of the Study

- The methodology has minimized the risks of bias from confounding studies.

  + +   +   −

- Considering clinical considerations, the study methodology, and the statistical power of the study, the effect observed was due to the intervention or treatment in the included studies.

  + +   +   −

- The results of the study are applicable to the population from whom subjects were selected.

  + +   +   −

Notes: _____

_____

_____

Adapted from CEBM, 2006; and Scottish Intercollegiate Network, 2008.

APPENDIX 14B
Evaluation of Randomized, Controlled Clinical Trials

Instructions: The following items describe characteristics of well-executed random-ized, controlled clinical trials. Please read and evaluate each statement and circle whether the issue was well-addressed, adequately addressed, not addressed, or not applicable (i.e., N/A).

Bibliographical Citation

_____

_____

_____

Background Information

The rationale for using a randomized, controlled clinical trial is based on a strong scientific foundation.

Well-Addressed   Adequately Addressed   Not Addressed   N/A

The hypotheses and objectives were specific and clear.

Well-Addressed   Adequately Addressed   Not Addressed   N/A

The research question(s) was/were clearly focused.

Well-Addressed   Adequately Addressed   Not Addressed   N/A

Notes: _____

_____

_____

Internal Validity
Recruitment of Participants
• Power analyses were used to determine sample size.

Well-Addressed   Adequately Addressed   Not Addressed   N/A

- The inclusion/exclusion criteria and sources for recruitment are clearly explained.

  Well-Addressed   Adequately Addressed   Not Addressed   N/A

- The beginning and ending dates for participant recruitment are clearly stated.

  Well-Addressed   Adequately Addressed   Not Addressed   N/A

- The locations of data collection were clearly specified.

  Well-Addressed   Adequately Addressed   Not Addressed   N/A

- Participants were randomly assigned to treatment and control groups.

  Well-Addressed   Adequately Addressed   Not Addressed   N/A

Notes: _____

_____

_____

Random Assignment, Blinding, and Concealment

- Methods for generation of random allocation procedures were well-described (e.g., who generated the allocation sequence, enrolled participants, and assigned them to their groups, etc.).

  Well-Addressed   Adequately Addressed   Not Addressed   N/A

- Participants were blinded to treatment allocation.

  Well-Addressed   Adequately Addressed   Not Addressed   N/A

- Research assistants or those administering tests were blinded to treatment allocation.

  Well-Addressed   Adequately Addressed   Not Addressed   N/A

- Methods for determining the success of blinding was described.

  Well-Addressed   Adequately Addressed   Not Addressed   N/A

- The only difference between treatment and control groups was treatment allocation.

  Well-Addressed   Adequately Addressed   Not Addressed   N/A

- The treatment and control groups were equivalent at baseline.

  Well-Addressed   Adequately Addressed   Not Addressed   N/A

Outcome Measures

- Primary and secondary outcome measures were adequately specified.

  Well-Addressed   Adequately Addressed   Not Addressed   N/A

- All outcome measures were reliable, valid, and normed for appropriate use with participants.

  Well-Addressed   Adequately Addressed   Not Addressed   N/A

- Methods (e.g., training of observers, multiple observations, and so on) were used to enhance data collection on outcome measures.

  Well-Addressed   Adequately Addressed   Not Addressed   N/A

- All outcome measures are administered in a standard, reliable, and valid way.

  Well-Addressed   Adequately Addressed   Not Addressed   N/A

Accounting and Procedures for Dropouts

- What percentage of participants in each treatment arm failed to complete or dropped out before completion of the study? _____

- An intention-to-treat analysis (all subjects were analyzed in the groups to which they were assigned) was used.

  Well-Addressed   Adequately Addressed   Not Addressed   N/A

- Details of the administration of the intervention were clear.

  Well-Addressed   Adequately Addressed   Not Addressed   N/A

- Any adverse events were reported.

  Well-Addressed   Adequately Addressed   Not Addressed   N/A

Multicenter Sites

- The experimental protocol was applied uniformly across all sites.

  Well-Addressed   Adequately Addressed   Not Addressed   N/A

- The results obtained were similar across sites.

  Well-Addressed   Adequately Addressed   Not Addressed   N/A

- Statistical procedures for analysis were appropriate and clear.

  Well-Addressed   Adequately Addressed   Not Addressed   N/A

- The flow of participants through the stages of the study was clear.

  Well-Addressed   Adequately Addressed   Not Addressed   N/A

Notes: _____

_____

_____

Overall Assessment of the Study

- The methodology has minimized the risks of bias from confounding variables.

    + +   +   −

- Considering clinical considerations, the study methodology, and the statistical power of the study, the effect observed was due to the predictor variable.

    + +   +   −

- The results of the study are applicable to the population from whom subjects were selected.

    + +   +   −

Notes: _____

_____

_____

Adapted from Moher, Shulz, Altman, and CONSORT Group, 2001; CEBM, 2006; and Scottish Intercollegiate Network, 2008.

APPENDIX 14C

Evaluation of Cohort Studies

Instructions: The following items describe characteristics of well-executed cohort studies. Please read and evaluate each statement and circle whether the issue was well-addressed, adequately addressed, not addressed, or not applicable (i.e., N/A).

Bibliographical Citation

_____

_____

_____

Background Information

The rationale for using a cohort control study has a strong basis in an appropriate and clearly focused research question.

    Well-Addressed   Adequately Addressed   Not Addressed   N/A

Notes: _____

_____

_____

Internal Validity

Selection of Participants

- The two groups of participants being evaluated are selected from source populations that are compatible in all respects other than the predictor variables under investigation.

  Well-Addressed   Adequately Addressed   Not Addressed   N/A

- The study states how many participants chose to continue on in the study from the total number recruited.

  Well-Addressed   Adequately Addressed   Not Addressed   N/A

- The possibility that some participants at the time of enrollment already had the disorder was mentioned and accounted for in the statistical analyses.

  Well-Addressed   Adequately Addressed   Not Addressed   N/A

- The percentages of individuals or clusters of individuals who were recruited into each group but dropped out of the study before completion was reported.

  Well-Addressed   Adequately Addressed   Not Addressed   N/A

- Comparison is made between full participants and those lost to follow-up, by exposure status.

  Well-Addressed   Adequately Addressed   Not Addressed   N/A

Notes: _____

_____

_____

Assessment

- The outcomes are clearly defined.

  Well-Addressed   Adequately Addressed   Not Addressed   N/A

- The assessment of the outcome is blinded to the predictor variables.

  Well-Addressed   Adequately Addressed   Not Addressed   N/A

- If blinding was not possible, the possible influence that knowledge of participants' status for predictor variables could have on assessment of the outcome is acknowledged.

  Well-Addressed   Adequately Addressed   Not Addressed   N/A

- The measure for the assessment of the outcome is reliable and valid.

  Well-Addressed   Adequately Addressed   Not Addressed   N/A

- Evidence from other sources is used to show that assessment of outcomes is reliable and valid.

  Well-Addressed   Adequately Addressed   Not Addressed   N/A

- Predictor variables or prognostic factors are assessed more than once.

  Well-Addressed   Adequately Addressed   Not Addressed   N/A

Notes: _____

_____

_____

Accounting for Confounding Factors

- The main potential confounding variables have been identified and taken into account in the design and analysis of the data.

  Well-Addressed   Adequately Addressed   Not Addressed   N/A

Notes: _____

_____

_____

Overall Assessment of the Study

- The methodology has minimized the risks of bias from confounding variables.

  + +   +   −

- Considering clinical considerations, the study methodology, and the statistical power of the study, the effect observed was due to the predictor variable.

  + +   +   −

- The results of the study are applicable to the population from whom subjects were selected.

  + +   +   −

Notes: _____

_____

_____

Adapted from Cummings et al., 2001; Newman et al., 2001; and Scottish Intercollegiate Network, 2008.

APPENDIX 14D
Evaluation of Case-Control Studies

Instructions: The following items describe characteristics of well-executed case-control studies. Please read and evaluate each statement and circle whether the issue was well-addressed, adequately addressed, not addressed, or not applicable (i.e., N/A).

Bibliographical Citation

_____

_____

_____

Background Information

The rationale for using a case-control study has a strong basis in an appropriate and clearly focused research question.

Well-Addressed   Adequately Addressed   Not Addressed   N/A

Notes: _____

_____

_____

Internal Validity

Selection of Participants

• The participants with the condition ("cases") and those without the condition ("controls") are recruited from similar populations.

Well-Addressed   Adequately Addressed   Not Addressed   N/A

• The case and control groups used the same exclusion criteria.

Well-Addressed   Adequately Addressed   Not Addressed   N/A

• The percentage of actual participants versus those who dropped out of the study was reported.

Well-Addressed   Adequately Addressed   Not Addressed   N/A

• Participants and dropouts are compared to determine possible differences between the groups that may indicate a possible source of bias in sampling procedures.

Well-Addressed   Adequately Addressed   Not Addressed   N/A

- Cases are clearly defined and differentiated from controls.

Well-Addressed   Adequately Addressed   Not Addressed   N/A

Notes: _____

_____

_____

Assessment

- Assessment procedures and personnel are blinded to the status of the predictor variable for each participant.

Well-Addressed   Adequately Addressed   Not Addressed   N/A

- Presence of the predictor variable in participants is validly and reliably determined.

Well-Addressed   Adequately Addressed   Not Addressed   N/A

Notes: _____

_____

_____

Control of Confounding Factors

- The influence of confounding factors has been well-controlled for in the design of the study and in the analysis of the results.

Well-Addressed   Adequately Addressed   Not Addressed   N/A

Notes: _____

_____

_____

Statistical Analysis

- Confidence intervals are provided.

Well-Addressed   Adequately Addressed   Not Addressed   N/A

Notes: _____

_____

_____

Overall Assessment of the Study

- The methodology has minimized the risks of bias from confounding variables.

  + +   +   −

- Considering clinical considerations, the study methodology, and the statistical power of the study, the effect observed was due to the predictor variable.

    + +   +   −

- The results of the study are applicable to the population from whom subjects were selected.

    + +   +   −

Notes: _____

_____

_____

Adapted from Newman et al., 2001; and Scottish Intercollegiate Network, 2008.

APPENDIX 14E

Evaluation of Diagnostic Studies

Instructions: The following items describe characteristics of well-executed diagnostic studies. Please read and evaluate each statement and circle whether the issue was well-addressed, adequately addressed, not addressed, or not applicable (i.e., N/A). The diagnostic tool under consideration is known as the "index."

Bibliographical Citation

_____

_____

_____

Background Information

The rationale for estimating the diagnostic accuracy of a tool (index) against a reference standard, preferably gold standard, or comparing accuracy between two tests or across participant groups is provided.

Well-Addressed   Adequately Addressed   Not Addressed   N/A

Notes: _____

_____

_____

Internal Validity of Methods

Participants

The study population is adequately described.

- Inclusion criteria

Well-Addressed   Adequately Addressed   Not Addressed   N/A

- Exclusion criteria

Well-Addressed   Adequately Addressed   Not Addressed   N/A

- Location of data collection

Well-Addressed   Adequately Addressed   Not Addressed   N/A

Basis for participant recruitment

- Presenting symptoms

Well-Addressed   Adequately Addressed   Not Addressed   N/A

- Variety of the degree of presenting disorder or condition

Well-Addressed   Adequately Addressed   Not Addressed   N/A

- Receipt of the index or reference standard

Well-Addressed   Adequately Addressed   Not Addressed   N/A

Notes: _____

_____

_____

Test Methods

- The nature of the index is clearly specified including the definition of units and categories for classification of results.

Well-Addressed   Adequately Addressed   Not Addressed   N/A

- The index is compared with an appropriate gold standard.

Yes   No

- The gold standard is well-described, including the definition of units and categories for classification of results.

Well-Addressed   Adequately Addressed   Not Addressed   N/A

- If no gold standard is available, a validated reference standard is used for comparison.

Well-Addressed   Adequately Addressed   Not Addressed   N/A

- The reference standard is well described, including the definition of units and categories for classification of results.

  Well-Addressed   Adequately Addressed   Not Addressed   N/A

- Patients for testing are selected consecutively as a series or randomly from a well-defined population.

  Well-Addressed   Adequately Addressed   Not Addressed   N/A

- The index and the gold standard are administered blindly or independently of each other.

  Well-Addressed   Adequately Addressed   Not Addressed   N/A

- The index and the gold standard are administered in as close a time period as possible with the dates provided.

  Well-Addressed   Adequately Addressed   Not Addressed   N/A

- Results are reported for all participants enrolled in the study.

  Well-Addressed   Adequately Addressed   Not Addressed   N/A

- A diagnosis is made, based on the results of the index prior to administration of the gold standard.

  Well-Addressed   Adequately Addressed   Not Addressed   N/A

Notes: _____

_____

_____

Statistical Methods

- The rationale and statistical methods for comparing the index and the gold standard were completely described and appropriate.

  Well-Addressed   Adequately Addressed   Not Addressed   N/A

- The statistical methods for describing uncertainty were provided (e.g., 95% confidence intervals).

  Well-Addressed   Adequately Addressed   Not Addressed   N/A

- The statistical methods for calculating test reproducibility were accurate.

  Well-Addressed   Adequately Addressed   Not Addressed   N/A

Notes: _____

_____

_____

Results

Participants

- The demographic information of the participants was adequately described (e.g., age, sex, spectrum of severity of disorder, presenting characteristics, comorbidity, etc.).

  Well-Addressed   Adequately Addressed   Not Addressed   N/A

- A flowchart shows and the text explains the flow of participants through the study.

  Well-Addressed   Adequately Addressed   Not Addressed   N/A

- The number of participants who failed to complete the study (i.e., dropouts) were reported.

  Well-Addressed   Adequately Addressed   Not Addressed   N/A

Notes: _____

_____

_____

Test Results

- The time elapsed between administration of the index and the gold standard was reported.

  Well-Addressed   Adequately Addressed   Not Addressed   N/A

- The distribution of patients' results according to severity of disease is provided.

  Well-Addressed   Adequately Addressed   Not Addressed   N/A

- The adverse effects of the index or the gold standard were reported.

  Well-Addressed   Adequately Addressed   Not Addressed   N/A

Notes: _____

_____

_____

Estimates

- The estimates of diagnostic accuracy and measures of statistical uncertainty were provided.

  Well-Addressed   Adequately Addressed   Not Addressed   N/A

- The procedures for accounting for indeterminate or missing data points were accounted for and provided.

  Well-Addressed   Adequately Addressed   Not Addressed   N/A

- The variability between or among subgroups of participants, tests, and so on are accounted for and provided.

Well-Addressed   Adequately Addressed   Not Addressed   N/A

Notes: _____

_____

_____

Overall Assessment of the Study

- How reliable and valid are the conclusions of this study?

++   +   −

- Was the spectrum of patients enrolled in the study comparable with the population for whom the index is intended? In other words, is the sample representative to the population regarding the proportion of those having the condition and an appropriate range of severity of cases?

++   +   −

Notes: _____

_____

_____

Adapted from Bossuyt et al., 2003; CEBM, 2006; and Scottish Intercollegiate Network, 2008.

CHAPTER 15

Evidence-Based Practice: Blending Patient Values/Preferences, Scientific Evidence, and Clinical Expertise

Where does the violet tint end and the orange tint begin? Distinctly we see the difference of the colors, but where exactly does the one first blending enter into the other. So with sanity and insanity.

—Herman Melville (1819–1891)

Formerly, when religion was strong and science weak, men mistook magic for medicine; now, when science is strong and religion weak, men mistake medicine for magic.

—Thomas Szasz, *The Second Sin* (1973)

To study the phenomenon of disease without books is to sail an uncharted sea, while to study books without patients is not to go to sea at all.

—Sir William Osler (1849–1919)

In previous chapters, we have discussed levels of evidence, skills for evidence-based practice (EBP), and how to evaluate research. You will recall that EBP is often depicted as the proverbial "three-legged stool" held up by patient values/preferences, scientific evidence, and clinical expertise. However, how do you blend the three components of patient values/preferences, clinician expertise, and evidence into clinical decision making? It depends not only on the area of professional practice but on the individual patient. For example, EBP decisions regarding the adequacy of prevention efforts, screening tests, and diagnostic batteries are more focused on clinical expertise and scientific evidence, rather than individual patient characteristics. In this chapter, we will discuss the interaction of the three components of EBP in the treatment milieu to show that these areas are not necessarily mutually exclusive in nature.

LEARNING OBJECTIVES

This chapter will enable readers to:

- Blend patient values/preferences, scientific evidence, and clinical expertise in EBP.

Patient Preferences

EBP must begin with considering patient and family needs, abilities, values, and preferences in order to integrate those factors with clinical expertise and the best current research evidence in making clinical decisions (ASHA, 2005). How do clinicians accomplish this? How do clinicians measure the preferences of patients and their families? How can their needs be matched to appropriate treatment options? How can attainment of goals be normalized to commonly used outcome measures for benchmarking? Communication sciences and disorders professionals can achieve these objectives using a model that transcends healthcare disciplines, geographical boundaries, and cultural barriers.

The World Health Organization (WHO) is the United Nations specialized agency for health. It was founded in April 1948 in order to achieve the highest possible level of health for all people in the world. **Health** is defined in WHO's constitution as a state of complete physical, mental and social well-being and not merely the absence of disease or infirmity. In other words, optimal functioning is not just being well, but having a high quality of life. WHO has established a classification system and model, the *International Classification of Functioning, Disability, and Health* (ICF) (WHO, 2001), providing a standard language and framework for describing health and health-related states. The ICF can be used for many purposes in different health-care disciplines that describe multiple health-related domains:

- Changes in body function and structure
- What a person can do in a standard environment (level of capacity)
- What a person can do in the day-to-day environment (level of performance)

These domains are classified from body, individual, and societal perspectives through the use of two lists: (1) body functions and structures and (2) domains of activity and participation. First we must define some key terms. **Functioning** refers to all body functions, activities, and participation. **Disability** is an umbrella term for impairments, activity limitations, and participation restriction. The ICF includes environmental factors that interact with all components of the model.

The other important terms noted above help in understanding the application of the ICF and the use of its model for management of communication disorders. **Body functions** are physiological functions of body systems (including psychological functions). Throughout this chapter, we will focus on the EBP as it pertains to an audiologist's treatment of a seventy-two-year-old man named Mr. Williams, who has a high-frequency sensorineural hearing loss but, despite having difficulty hearing, is not convinced he needs hearing aids. The patient's condition can be applied to the model in that hearing is a bodily function in which the auditory system takes acoustic energy, and through a series of processes, produces the function of audition. **Body structures** are anatomical parts of the body such as organs, limbs, and their components. For example, the pinna, the external auditory canal, the tympanic membrane, and the basilar membrane are only a few of the body structures involved in the function of audition.

As important as the body domain in understanding health is the general domain that includes activity and participation. **Environmental factors** are the physical, social, and attitudinal conditions that surround people as they live and conduct their lives. **Activity** is the execution of a task or action by an individual and has to do with what the patient can do. In our example, Mr. Williams could talk relatively well in face-to-face conversation with no distractions and background noise. **Participation** is involvement in life situations. Mr. Williams's involvement in life situations may include calling friends on the phone to catch up on the latest gossip, shopping at the grocery store, inviting friends over for dinner, and organizing a neighborhood watch program.

The interaction of these domains may show deficits. **Impairments** are problems in body function or structure such as a significant deviation or loss. Mr. Williams has a hearing impairment due to destruction (i.e., problems) in sensory hair cells (i.e., bodily structures) resulting in a permanent sensorineural hearing loss. **Activity limitations** are difficulties that an individual may have in executing tasks of daily living. Clinicians ask, "What can't the patient do because of their hearing loss?" In our example, Mr. Williams has difficulties with common activities of daily living, including conversing with others, whether on the telephone or with the grocery clerk, friends, or neighbors, especially in noisy situations. **Participation restrictions** are problems an individual may experience that limit involvement in life situations and interactions with other people. Audiologists ask, "How is the patient's involvement with others affected by his or her hearing loss?" Because of his hearing loss, Mr. Williams has limited interaction with people over the telephone, avoids going out to dinner with other couples, and does not participate in social events in noisy environments.

The WHO's ICF model is a biophysical social model, as shown in Figure 15.1. In this model, disability and functioning are outcomes of the interactions between health conditions (i.e., disorder or disease) and contextual factors (i.e., environmental factors and personal factors). Environmental factors include the following:

- Social attitudes
- Architectural characteristics
- Legal and social structures
- Climate
- Terrain

Personal factors also includes several characteristics:

- Gender
- Age
- Coping styles
- Social background
- Education
- Profession
- Past and current experiences
- Behavioral patterns
- Character

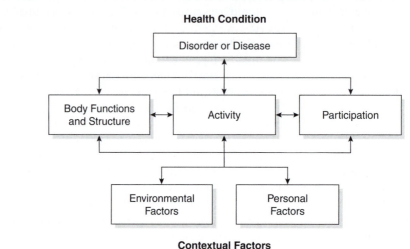

FIGURE 15.1

The World Health Organization—International Classification of Functioning

Health Condition

Disorder or Disease

Body Functions and Structure — Activity — Participation

Environmental Factors

Personal Factors

Contextual Factors

www.who.int/classifications/icf/site/beginners/by.pdf, p. 9. Reproduced by permission of WHO.

The model has three levels of human functioning classified by the ICF: (1) functioning at the level of the body or body part, (2) the entire person (i.e., activity limitation), or (3) participation (i.e., participation restriction). Therefore, disability involves dysfunction at one or more of these levels. For example, an elderly person may have a high-frequency sensorineural hearing loss that affects their activity or ability to execute a task (e.g., hearing a speaker in a large room) and their participation or involvement in life situations (e.g., taking part in bingo games). However, the effects of the hearing loss cannot be determined without considering environmental factors and personal factors. For example, the effect of hearing loss on the person's ability to play bingo will depend on the acoustics of the bingo hall, whether the sponsoring organization has an accommodating attitude toward patrons with hearing loss, and so on. Similarly, the personal actions of the bingo player can help determine the effect of hearing loss on his or her experience. For instance, will the person self-advocate by either asking the caller to speak clearly or requesting the management to install video monitors for showing the called numbers? In conclusion, the effects of communication disorders involve a multidimensional model of factors that are highly variable from person to person and across different communication contexts.

Audiologists and speech-language pathologists need to assess impairment, activity limitations, and participation restrictions not only during diagnostic evaluations for baseline measures, but also in selecting the best treatment programs via EBP. For audiologists, this means obtaining audiograms, tympanograms, acoustic reflex thresholds, speech recognition thresholds, and so on. Speech-language pathologists measure mean length of utterance, phonological processes, diadokinectic rates, and other parameters of speech and language. However, measures of activity limitations, participation restrictions, and health-related quality of life may not be as familiar to either students or practicing clinicians.

Continuing with our example, the audiologic evaluation determined Mr. Williams' type, degree, and configuration of hearing loss, speech recognition abilities, and middle ear function. His degree of activity limitation and participation restriction was assessed via self-assessment questionnaires. For example, his activity limitation was assessed via the *Client Oriented Scale of Improvement* (Dillon, James & Ginis, 1997), in which the audiologist and patient nominate and prioritize difficult listening situations involving activities of daily living. Mr. Williams targeted the following situations to improve in treatment: (1) hearing his wife and friends in a noisy restaurant, (2) talking to his grandchildren on the phone, and (3) understanding the caller in the bingo hall. Similarly, his participation restrictions were evaluated using the *Hearing Handicap Inventory for the Elderly* (HHIE) (Ventry & Weinstein, 1982), which focuses on the social and emotional impact of hearing loss. The audiologist was surprised at the profound impact that Mr. Williams's hearing loss had on his social and emotional well-being. In summary, a complete evaluation includes assessment of hearing impairment, activity limitations, and participation restrictions when using EBP in selecting treatment options for Mr. Williams.

Scientific Evidence

Recall that practicing clinicians go through a five-step process for evidence-based medicine (EBM) and EBP

- Developing a research question
- Searching for the evidence
- Critically appraising the evidence
- Integrating scientific evidence, clinical expertise, and patient factors into decision making
- Evaluating the process (Sackett, Straus, Richardson, Rosenberg, & Haynes, 2000; ASHA, 2006)

Note that the first three steps in EBP have to do with developing a research question, searching for scientific evidence, and then evaluating the evidence.

Developing a Clinical Research Question

The audiologist in our example must first construct a clinical research question in determining the best treatment option for his elderly patient. As we discussed in Chapter 13, a helpful procedure for framing clinical research questions is to use the PICO rubric, an acronym for Population, Intervention, Comparison (Treatment) and Outcome (ASHA, 2008). The population is defined by the patients under consideration, or, as in our ongoing example, patient, whom we described as an elderly man with a high-frequency sensorineural hearing loss. Mr. Williams, who is in denial about his hearing loss, is very reluctant to purchase hearing aids, but his audiogram and speech recognition thresholds as well as speech recognition scores in quiet and noise indicate that amplification may help. In addition, his hearing loss has definitely hampered his communication with family and friends. Despite his denial, the patient nominated and prioritized several difficult communication situations involving activities of daily living. Most troubling, though, was his score on the HHIE, demonstrating a significant impact of hearing loss on the patient's social and emotional well-being. Not only were the patient's activity limitations considerable with the high-frequency sensorineural hearing loss, the impact on his participation restrictions (e.g., social and emotional well-being) was profound. The audiologist felt compelled to search for evidence regarding the use of amplification on improving the social and emotional well-being of adults with sensorineural hearing loss. Therefore, the audiologist used the PICO rubric to frame the clinical research question in a relatively simple and straightforward manner, as illustrated in Table 15.1.

It may seem odd to readers that the comparison intervention for our example is to not get hearings aids, but the only treatment for most forms of sensorineural hearing loss is the use of amplification. Our patient is considering purchasing hearing aids versus doing without one rather than comparing one treatment to another as clinicians often do. With the PICO table complete, it is now possible to frame the clinical research question, streamlining the search for the evidence (Cox, 2005). A suitable clinical research question for this scenario is "What are the social and emotional benefits or improvement in quality of life for adults with sensorineural hearing loss resulting from hearing aid use in comparison to not using amplification?" The question will now be instrumental in narrowing the search for the evidence.

Searching for the Evidence

Specific strategies for searching the evidence are found in Chapter 13 and should be organized to retrieve the highest-quality evidence pertaining to the clinical question. The search strategy should always be defined to identify the highest quality evidence directly related to the clinical question. Recall that macro search strategies determine the order. As discussed earlier, the audiologist in our example used the clinical research question to develop **search strings** for use in databases such as Medline, the

TABLE 15.1

The PICO Rubric for the Clinical Example

Parameter	Descriptors
Population	Adults with sensorineural hearing loss
Intervention	Hearing aids
Comparison (Intervention)	No hearing aids
Outcome	Social and emotional well-being
	Quality of life

Cumulative Index to Nursing and Allied Health Literature (CINAHL), and so on. Search strings are words, used either singularly or in combination, that serve as input to a database in order to retrieve scientific evidence relevant to a research question. Table 15.2 shows the types of information that may be useful in EBP and search sources.

Each database is different so the audiologist in our scenario should complete any relevant tutorials on how to conduct successful searches. The PICO framework is also an excellent source for phrases to use in search strings. The audiologist in our example combined such phrases as "adults," "hearing aids," "amplification," "social and emotional," "well-being," "quality of life," and so on. As discussed in Chapter 12, there are varying levels of thoroughness of searches for EBP. However, clinicians should seek studies representing the highest level of evidence. In our scenario, the audiologist was fortunate to come across a recent systematic review with meta-analysis of the health-related quality of life benefits of amplification for adults with sensorineural hearing loss (Chisolm, Johnson, Danhauer, Portz, Abrams, Lesner, McCarthy, & Newman, 2007). Although the systematic review was relatively current and directly related to the clinical research question, the audiologist still had to appraise its quality.

Critical Appraisal of the Evidence

The third step involves formal evaluation or critical appraisal of the evidence. For example, the audiologist in our scenario needed to perform three tasks: (1) determine the systematic review's level of evidence, (2) rate the risk of bias in the individual

TABLE 15.2

Useful Information Sources for Evidence-Based Practice

Type of Information	Database
Systematic reviews	• Cochrane Collaboration. www.cochrane.org • Campbell Collaboration. www.campbellcollaboration.org • What Works Clearinghouse (U.S. Department of Education). http://ies.ed.gov/ncee/wwc • Psychological Database for Brain Impairment Treatment Efficacy. www.psycbite.com • National Electronic Library for Health (Specialist Library—ENT and Audiology). www.library.nhs.uk/ent
Research articles	• Communication Sciences and Disorders Dome. www.comdisdome.com or www.csa.com/factsheets/cdd-set-c.php • Cumulative Index to Nursing and Allied Health Literature. www.ebscohost.com/cinahl • LexisNexis. www.lexisnexis.com/us/lnacademic/home/home.do?rand=0.17859434669400087 • Medline. www.nlm.nih.gov • Pub Med. www.pubmedcentral.nih.gov
Dissertations, federally funded grants, and websites	• Communication Sciences and Disorders Dome. www.comdisdome.com or www.csa.com/factsheets/cdd-set-c.php

studies, and (3) grade the clinical recommendation under consideration. The level of evidence can be determined by using the hierarchy adapted from Cox (2005) that was covered in Chapter 12. Although systematic reviews like this are of the highest level of evidence, the individual studies contributing to the meta-analysis ultimately determine the level of rigor. Most of the studies included in the Chisolm and colleagues (2007) systematic review were of Levels II and III of evidence.

Recall that the purpose of a systematic review with meta-analysis is to weigh the evidence in support of a particular treatment for a particular population having a desired outcome. The audiologist can find the quality assessment and grading of the evidence in the conclusion of the systematic review. Members of the systematic review team typically use criteria for assessing scientific evidence similar to those found on the checklists in Appendixes 14A through E for the evaluation of different types of studies. Recall that these checklists conclude with an item that rates the quality of individual studies, similar to the paradigm Chisolm et al. (2007) adapted from Cox (2005, p. 431) that appears in Chapter 14. A rating of "+ +" characterizes studies that have a very low risk of bias and whose present weaknesses are very unlikely to alter the conclusions of the study. A rating of "+" characterizes studies that have a low risk of bias and whose identified weaknesses or omitted information probably would not alter the conclusions of the study. Alternatively, a rating of "–" is for studies that have a very high risk of bias or have omitted crucial information that probably alters the conclusions of the study.

The investigations varied in their level of bias, but their findings were deemed acceptable for combining the results of studies to compute effect sizes with corresponding **confidence intervals.** Effect sizes and confidence intervals were discussed in Chapters 6 and 12. Cox (2005, p. 432) defined effect size as a "metric that expresses the magnitude of a result, such as the differences in mean scores for two different hearing aids, within the context of the individual variation in scores." In addition, 95% confidence intervals for effect sizes are provided representing a range of where the effect size may fall ninety-five times out of every hundred the study was replicated (Cox, 2005). Effect sizes are defined such that 0.2 is a small effect size, 0.5 is a medium effect size, and 0.8 and greater is a large effect size (Cohen, 1983). It is important for deriving meaning from findings that confidence intervals should not cross the zero line. Zero for an effect size means that a treatment does not have any significant effect. If a 95% confidence interval does cross the zero line, then clinicians cannot be 95 percent sure ($p < .05$) that a treatment does have an effect.

Specifics on the computation of these values are beyond the scope of this chapter and readers are referred to other chapters in this book for additional explanations. However, readers should know that effect sizes provide some indication of the "real world" effects or impact of statistically significant differences between or among groups of participants receiving different interventions. Effect sizes from individual studies may be combined in a meta-analysis to determine the overall clinical significance of a particular intervention. Due to the quality of the individual studies included in the Chisolm et al. (2007) systematic review, overall effect sizes and confidence intervals were computed based on the type of study and outcome measures. Some of the included studies had experimental and control groups, permitting between group comparisons. The other studies used within group comparisons only. In addition, the outcome measures for health-related quality of life included both **generic** and **disease-specific measures.** Generic measures are those that are used across healthcare disciplines such as the *Medical Outcomes Survey-Short Form 36* (Ware & Sherbourne, 1992). Alternatively, disease-specific measures are those used by a particular area of healthcare such as the HHIE. Chisolm and colleagues (2007) meta-analysis found that the between subject studies supported at least a small effect for generic measures, and when measured by disease-specific instruments, hearing aids had medium-to-large effects on adults' health-related quality of life. They concluded that hearing aid use improves adults' health-related quality of life by reducing psychological, social, and emotional effects of sensorineural hearing loss. Effect sizes and confidence intervals are also good for grading clinical recommendations based on scientific evidence.

The third and final task of the appraisal process is to grade the clinical recommendation provided by the evidence. Cox (2005) developed a grading paradigm useful for this purpose that is shown in Chapter 14. A grade of "A" requires consistent evidence at Level I (i.e., systematic reviews with meta-analysis of well-designed clinical studies) and II (i.e., double-blinded randomized, controlled clinical trials that directly relate to the clinical question). A grade of "B" requires consistent evidence at Level III (i.e., nonrandomized intervention or quasi-experimental studies) or IV (i.e., nonintervention studies, cohort studies, case-control studies, or cross-sectional surveys) that directly relate to the clinical question. In addition, Level I or II evidence that may be generalized from studies that do not exactly pertain to the clinical research question also may receive a grade of "B." For example, these types of studies may have slightly different types of participants than those stated in the clinical question. A grade of "C" requires evidence at Level V (i.e., case studies) or from Levels III or IV for studies that do not directly pertain to the clinical question. Lastly, a grade of "D" is assigned for Level VI (i.e., expert opinion) or for any level of evidence that is inconsistent or has a high risk of bias.

Chisolm and colleagues (2007) used the paradigm and assigned the evidence a grade of "B" for the recommendation of adults to use amplification to reduce the social and emotional impact of sensorineural hearing loss and to improve their health-related quality of life. The audiologist in our scenario may want to search for more recent evidence because the systematic review only included studies up to 2004. However, the audiologist was fairly convinced of the appropriateness of amplification as a choice of treatment for this patient. The audiologist will use this information in counseling Mr. Williams and his family members. Once a decision to pursue amplification is made, the audiologist now needs to integrate clinical expertise with patient preference and the scientific evidence.

Clinical Expertise

Another leg of the EBP stool is clinical expertise or experience. In making clinical decisions clinicians draw on their own experiences, consult with colleagues, and attend continuing education activities. The audiologist in our scenario personally felt confident in selecting, evaluating, and fitting hearing aids but will consult the latest recommended standards of care found in clinical practice guidelines (CPGs). Field and Lohr (1990) defined CPGs as "systematically developed statements to assist practitioner and patient decisions about appropriate health care for specific circumstances." CPGs are serious business in medicine; they are considered best practice for patient care. This is also true for audiology and speech-language pathology, once again showing how relevant research guides clinical practice. We will first discuss CPGs in general and then as they are specifically dealt with in communication sciences and disorders.

The Agency for Healthcare Research and Quality (AHRQ) is the health services research arm of the U.S. Department of Health and Human Services (AHRQ, 2007). Its mission is to support research to improve the quality, safety, efficiency, and effectiveness of healthcare (AHRQ, 2007). Complementary agencies include the National Institutes of Health, the Centers for Disease Control and Prevention, the Food and Drug Administration, the Health Care Financing Administration, and the Health Resources and Services Administration (AHRQ, 2007). The AHRQ developed a partnership with the American Medical Association in developing the National Guideline Clearinghouse (NGC), whose website houses evidenced-based CPGs that must fulfill high standards for EBP to be included. The NGC has resources and links that are helpful in understanding the characteristics of rigorous CPGs. Two important groups that have established benchmarks for quality CPGs are the Conference on Guideline Standards (COGS) and the AGREE Collaboration.

Conference on Guideline Standardization

The Conference on Guideline Standardization (COGS) was an invitational meeting attracting twenty-three experts who convened in New Haven, Connecticut, on April 26, 2002, to discuss problems and propose solutions to the implementation of CPGs (COGS, 2007). One product of the conference was the COGS Statement, which provides the standard of reporting for CPGs, thereby improving their quality and streamlining the implementation process (COGS, 2007). The development of the COGS involved compiling a list of potentially desirable characteristics for CPGs gleaned from reputable sources (e.g., Institute of Medicine Professional Instrument for Assessing Clinical Guidelines, the NGC, the Guidelines Elements Model, and so on). In a two-step process, the panel of experts first rated list items on whether each was "a necessary component of a clinical practice guideline," using a nine-point scale. Subsequently, each panelist individually rated components necessary for CPG validity and practical application (Shiffman, Shekelle, Overhage, Slutsky, Grimshaw, & Deshipande, 2003). The process resulted in an eighteen-item instrument called the *COGS Statement* that is shown in Table 15.3.

The COGS Statement has eighteen desirable characteristics and corresponding descriptions that should be included in a CPG. For example, CPGs should have overview material as one desirable characteristic as well as a description of such critical components as a structured abstract, release date, status (i.e., original, revised, or updated), or print and electronic resources. Several items on the COGS Statement deal

TABLE 15.3

The COGS Statement

Topic	Description
1. Overview material	Provide a structured abstract that includes the guideline's release date, status (original, revised, updated), and print and electronic sources.
2. Focus	Describe the primary disease/condition and intervention/service/technology that the guideline addresses. Indicate any alternative preventive, diagnostic, or therapeutic interventions that were considered during development.
3. Goal	Describe the goal that following the guideline is expected to achieve, including the rationale for development of a guideline on this topic.
4. Users/setting	Describe the intended users of the guideline (e.g., provider types, patients) and the settings in which the guideline is intended to be used.
5. Target population	Describe the patient population eligible for guideline recommendations and list any exclusion criteria.
6. Developer	Identify the organization(s) responsible for guideline development and the names/credentials/potential conflicts of interest of individuals involved in the guideline's development.
7. Funding source/ sponsor	Identify the funding source/sponsor and describe its role in developing and/or reporting the guideline. Disclose potential conflict of interest.
8. Evidence collection	Describe the methods used to search the scientific literature, including the range of dates and databases searched, and criteria applied to filter the retrieved evidence.
9. Recommendation grading criteria	Describe the criteria used to rate the quality of evidence that supports the recommendations and the system for describing the strength of the recommendations. Recommendation strength communicates the importance of adherence to a recommendation and is based on both the quality of the evidence and the magnitude of anticipated benefits or harms.
10. Method for synthesizing evidence	Describe how evidence was used to create recommendations, e.g., evidence tables, meta-analysis, decision analysis.
11. Prerelease review	Describe how the guideline developer reviewed and/or tested the guidelines prior to release.
12. Update plan	State whether or not there is a plan to update the guideline and, if applicable, an expiration date for this version of the guideline.
13. Definitions	Define unfamiliar terms and those critical to correct application of the guideline that might be subject to misinterpretation.
14. Recommendations and rationale	State the recommended action precisely and the specific circumstances under which to perform it. Justify each recommendation by describing the linkage between the recommendation and its supporting evidence. Indicate the quality of evidence and the recommendation strength, based on the criteria described in 9.

(Continued)

TABLE 15.3	
(Continued)	
Topic	**Description**
15. Potential benefits and harms	Describe anticipated benefits and potential risks associated with implementation of guideline recommendations.
16. Patient preferences	Describe the role of patient preferences when a recommendation involves a substantial element of personal choice or values.
17. Algorithm	Provide (when appropriate) a graphical description of the stages and decisions in clinical care described by the guideline.
18. Implementation considerations	Describe anticipated barriers to application of the recommendations. Provide reference to any auxiliary documents for providers or patients that are intended to facilitate implementation. Suggest review criteria for measuring changes in care when the guideline is implemented.

Reprinted with permission from "Standardized Reporting of Clinical Practice Guidelines: A Proposal from the Conference on Guideline Standardization" by R. N. Shiffman et al. *Annals of Internal Medicine, 139,* 493–498.

directly with collecting, evaluating, and synthesizing scientific evidence. For instance, the methods for collecting evidence must be explicitly stated, including the search engines and the range of dates accessed. Moreover, CPGs should state the grading criteria used to rate the quality of the evidence and the system supporting the strength of recommendations. This information is similar to the rubrics used for assessing the evidence gleaned from individual studies discussed earlier in this and other chapters of this book. Because the amount of information obtained may be considerable, the methods for synthesizing relevant evidence into a cohesive CPG must be described. For instance, did reviewers construct an evidence table? Did they conduct a systematic review with meta-analysis? Did they use decision analysis? These criteria are consistent with other assessment tools such as the one discussed next.

Appraisal of Guidelines for Research and Evaluation Collaboration

An international collaboration of healthcare experts developed the *Appraisal of Guidelines for Research and Evaluation* (AGREE) *Instrument* (2001), which provides a rubric for assessing new or existing CPGs and appears in Appendix 15A. The AGREE Instrument is applicable to any type of CPG on a variety of topics such as diagnostic tools, health promotion statements, and interventions. In 1998, the AGREE Collaboration developed out of a research project under the auspices of the Biomedicine and Health Research (BIOMED 2) Programme funded by the European Union (AGREE Collaboration, 2007). The AGREE Instrument consists of twenty-three items classified into six domains:

- Scope and purpose (items 1–3) is concerned with the overall aim of the guideline, the specific overall clinical questions, and the target patient population.
- Stakeholder involvement (items 4–7) focuses on the extent to which the guidelines represent the views of its intended users.

- Rigorous development (items 8–14) relates to the process used to gather and synthesize the evidence and the methods to formulate the recommendations and then update them.
- Clarity and presentation (items 15–18) are concerned with the language used to format the guideline.
- Applicability (items 19–21) pertains to the organizational, behavioral, and cost implications of applying the guidelines.
- Editorial independence (items 22–23) is concerned with the independence of the recommendations and acknowledgements of possible conflict of interest from the guideline development group (p. 4)

The instructions advise reviewers to learn as much as possible about the development process of a CPG prior to their assessment because much of the background information should be evaluated for possible conflicts of interest, for example. Items on the AGREE Instrument consist of statements that are rated on a four-point scale from 4 (Strongly Agree) to 1 (Strongly Disagree). Each item has a user's guide that assists in the evaluation of specific criteria in relation to the CPG. For example, in item 8 in the rigor of development domain, evaluators must rate their agreement with the following statement: "Systematic methods were used to search for the evidence." Evaluators can refer to the following criteria in making their rating: "Details of the strategy used to search for evidence should be provided including search terms used, sources consulted and dates of the literature covered. Sources may include electronic databases (e.g., MEDLINE, EMBASE, CINAHL), databases of systematic reviews (e.g., the Cochrane Library, DARE), handsearching journals, reviewing conference proceedings and other guidelines (e.g., the U.S. National Guideline Clearinghouse, the German Guidelines Clearinghouse)" (p. 11).

To score the AGREE Instrument, the ratings of all reviewers should be organized on a table so that the mean score of each domain can be calculated. For example, mean evaluators' ratings of each item should be summed to obtain an overall score for the domain. A percent score is obtained by dividing the overall score by the total number of points available for that domain. These scores can be used to make recommendation for patient care, to compare CPGs on similar topics, and to guide the development of future versions. However, no definitive values are given for discriminating "good" from "bad" CPGs. The AGREE Instrument concludes with a section where reviewers rate the overall utility of the CPG by either strongly recommending, recommending (with provisos or alterations), not recommending, or registering uncertainty, along with sections for recording team comments.

Once developed, CPGs should be kept up to date through revision. How do audiologists and speech-language pathologists know when a CPG should be updated? Shekelle, Eccles, Grimshaw, and Woolf (2001) developed an evidence-based model for assessing the currency of CPGs and mentioned six possible factors that may necessitate an update: (1) evidence on the existing benefits and harms of interventions, (2) changes in outcomes considered important, (3) development of new or changes in available interventions, (4) evidence that current practices are not optimal, (5) changes in values placed on outcomes, and (6) changes in resources available for healthcare. Their model is shown in Figure 15.2.

The model shows two ways for assessing the currency of CPGs. The first method involves a literature search to identify new evidence that may suggest revision of

FIGURE 15.2

Model for Assessing the Currency of Clinical Practice Guidelines

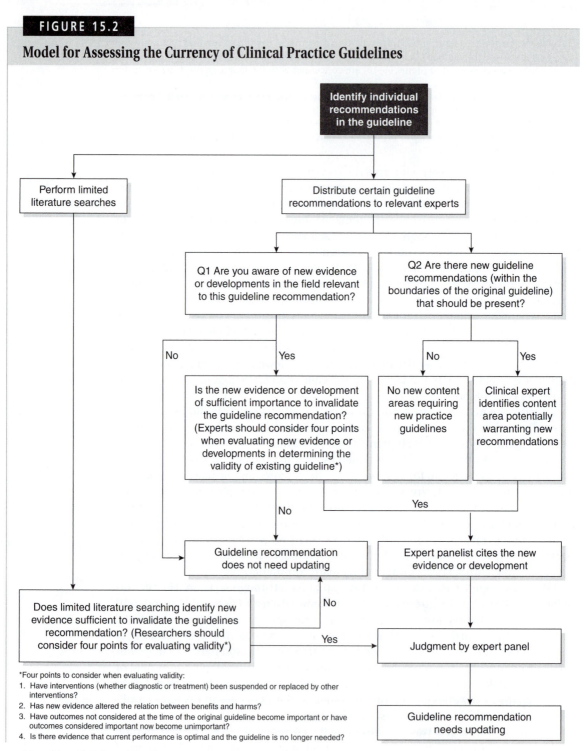

Identify individual recommendations in the guideline

Perform limited literature searches

Distribute certain guideline recommendations to relevant experts

Q1 Are you aware of new evidence or developments in the field relevant to this guideline recommendation?

Q2 Are there new guideline recommendations (within the boundaries of the original guideline) that should be present?

No   Yes   No   Yes

Is the new evidence or development of sufficient importance to invalidate the guideline recommendation? (Experts should consider four points when evaluating new evidence or developments in determining the validity of existing guideline*)

No new content areas requiring new practice guidelines

Clinical expert identifies content area potentially warranting new recommendations

No   Yes

Guideline recommendation does not need updating

Expert panelist cites the new evidence or development

Does limited literature searching identify new evidence sufficient to invalidate the guidelines recommendation? (Researchers should consider four points for evaluating validity*)

No

Yes

Judgment by expert panel

Guideline recommendation needs updating

*Four points to consider when evaluating validity:
1. Have interventions (whether diagnostic or treatment) been suspended or replaced by other interventions?
2. Has new evidence altered the relation between benefits and harms?
3. Have outcomes not considered at the time of the original guideline become important or have outcomes considered important now become unimportant?
4. Is there evidence that current performance is optimal and the guideline is no longer needed?

Adapted from Shekelle et al. (2000).

current recommendations. Search strings to use in engines and databases may be derived from specific words and phrases used in the recommendation. Shakelle and colleagues (2001) suggested using the following criteria in reviewing new evidence:

- Have interventions (whether diagnostic or treatment) been replaced by newer ones?
- Has new evidence altered the relationship between benefits and possible risks?
- Has there been a shift in the prioritization of outcomes such that once important outcomes have lessened in importance and once less important outcomes are now more important?
- Is there evidence suggesting that current CPGs are optimal and no new ones are needed?

If the answers to one or more of these questions are "yes," the evidence should be considered by a panel of experts to determine whether new CPGs are warranted.

Another method of checking the currency of existing CPGs is to assemble a panel of experts and ask the following questions:

- Are you aware of any new evidence relevant to existing CPGs?
- Are there new CPG recommendations that overlap existing CPGs that suggest revision?

If the majority of the panel answers "no" to the first question, then no new CPG is needed. However, if the answer is "yes," then the four criteria mentioned above should be applied to the evidence. If the majority of the panel replies "no" to the four questions, then no new CPG is warranted. If the majority answers "yes" to any the four questions, then that evidence is reviewed for possible CPG updating. Regarding the questions about new CPG recommendations with potential overlap, if the majority of the panel answers "no," no update is needed. However, if the majority answers "yes," the recommendations from the overlapping CPGs should be considered for inclusion.

Clinical Practice Guidelines in Communication Sciences and Disorders

The COGS Statement and the AGREE Instrument are two examples of gold standards by which to develop and evaluate CPGs. No CPG is expected to satisfy all criteria, even those for medicine. CPGs in communication sciences and disorders are less rigorous than those in medicine and understandably so. As discussed earlier in the chapter, instead of following a purely medical model, the identification, diagnosis, and treatment of communication disorders fits a more biopsychocosial model. However, our CPGs should strive to achieve at least some of these benchmarks, particularly those pertaining to EBP. However, readers first require some background information regarding CPGs and strategic documents in communication sciences and disorders.

The American Speech-Language-Hearing Association and the American Academy of Audiology have developed strategic documents related to clinical practice in our professions. ASHA has developed a series of policy statements within a conceptual hierarchy descending in scope from broad to narrow. The type of documents and their definitions appear in the following list:

- *Scope of Practice Statement:* A list of professional activities that define the range of services offered within the profession of audiology.
- *Preferred Practice Patterns:* Statements that define generally applicable characteristics of activities directed toward individual patients and that address structural requisites of the practice, processes to be carried out, and expected outcomes.
- *Position Statements:* Statements that specify ASHA's policy and stance on a matter that is important not only to the membership but also to consumers or to outside agencies or organizations.
- *Practice Guidelines:* A recommended set of procedures for a specific area of practice, based on research findings and current practice. These procedures detail the knowledge, skills, and/ or competencies needed to perform the procedures effectively. (ASHA, 2006)

The documents pertaining to standards of care most often involve preferred practice patterns (PPPs) and CPGs. The PPPs for the practice of audiology and speech-language pathology are representative of the consensus of the membership after consideration of the available scientific evidence, existing policies, current practice patterns, expert opinions, and collective input from practitioners in the field (ASHA, 2006). An example of an audiology PPP on prevention is shown in Figure 15.3.

FIGURE 15.3

Preferred Practice Pattern for the Profession of Audiology: 1.0: Prevention

---

1.0 Prevention

Procedures and programs to prevent initial or additional damage to hearing, balance, and related systems.

Prevention is conducted according to the Guiding Principles section of this document.

Expected Outcome(s)

Preventative actions avoid, eliminate, inhibit, or delay the onset and development of a hearing, balance, or related disorder.

Preventative actions may include minimizing susceptibility to hearing loss and associated auditory disorders or reducing exposure to potentially damaging events for susceptible persons.

Preventative actions are aimed at preventing hearing loss either on an individual or a group/community level.

Clinical Indications

Prevention services are indicated for the general population (e.g., community awareness or health fairs).

Prevention services are indicated for all patients and their family members/caregivers as an integral part of audiologic services.

(Continued)

FIGURE 15.3

(Continued)

Monitoring services are provided for individuals with hearing loss at risk for additional hearing loss due to toxic substances or continued exposure to occupational, environmental, or recreational noise.

Clinical Process

Prevention programs for patients with noise-induced hearing loss must be appropriate (it makes sense), adequate (it makes a difference), acceptable (one can live with it), and affordable (to the individual and/or the community).

Design, implementation, coordination, and supervision of prevention programs may include an interdisciplinary team (e.g., industrial hygienists, occupational physicians, nurses, acoustical engineers, and educators).

Prevention services may include one or more of the following:

- identifying a need for services
- establishing relationships with professionals and community groups
- selecting consultation and educational strategies
- providing general information about auditory and balance processes and related disorders and their prevention and treatment
- facilitating changes in the acoustic environment and developing programs or instrumentation for the prevention of hearing loss and associated auditory disorders
- referring to appropriate resources

Others Who May Perform the Procedure(s)

Support personnel may conduct selected procedures under the supervision of a certified audiologist but may not interpret the clinical results or provide referrals.

Setting/Equipment Specifications

Prevention services are offered in home, health care, education, business, industrial, and military settings and government agencies for individuals, families, groups, and organizations.

Safety and Health Precautions

All procedures ensure the safety of the patient and clinician and adhere to standard health precautions (e.g., prevention of bodily injury and transmission of infectious disease).

Decontamination, cleaning, disinfection, and sterilization of multiple-use equipment before reuse are carried out according to facility-specific infection control policies and procedures and according to manufacturer's instructions.

Documentation

Documentation should include prevention plans, pertinent information, educational materials, and recommendations for prevention strategies.

(Continued)

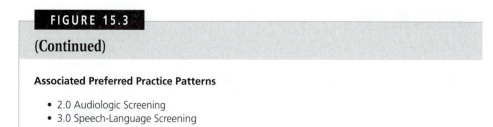

FIGURE 15.3

(Continued)

Associated Preferred Practice Patterns

- 2.0 Audiologic Screening
- 3.0 Speech-Language Screening
- 24.0 Ototoxicity
- 26.0 Occupational Hearing Loss Prevention and Conservation

All PPPs have the same format shown in Figure 15.3, with the following sections: (1) Expected Outcomes, (2) Clinical Indications, (3) Clinical Process, (4) Others Who May Perform the Procedures, (5) Setting/Equipment Specifications, (6) Safety and Health Precautions, (7) Documentation, (8) Associated Preferred Practice Patterns, and (9) ASHA Policy Documents and Related References. By using consistent formatting to facilitate their implementation, PPPs are intended to be quick reference guides for clinicians to consult that direct them to more in-depth CPGs. For example, audiologists wishing to prevent isolation caused from hearing loss in the elderly are directed to Guidelines for Audiology Service-Delivery in Nursing Homes (ASHA, 1997). PPPs are evaluated by numerous stakeholders at multiple levels of development and provide mention procedures for periodic updating. Some weaknesses in ASHA PPPs and CPGs are a failure to provide specifics on search strategies, quality assessments, and grading of the evidence that supports recommendations. Recently, however, both AAA and ASHA have recognized the importance of EBP and have focused initiatives to infuse these principles throughout all of their documents.

Toward this effort, AAA developed a strategic document, *The Clinical Practice Guidelines Development Process* (AAA, 2006a), to provide a framework for developing evidence-based CPGs, as shown in Appendix 15B. The process for development includes a consensus approach involving academy members at multiple levels. Customarily, the president of AAA, on recommendation of the board of directors, contacts a recognized expert in the particular area of practice who is also a member of the Academy and offers the opportunity to serve as chair of a task force charged with developing a CPG. The chair of the Strategic Documents Committee (SDC) contacts the chair of the new task force to discuss the purpose and the timeline for development of the CPG. The chair selects and recommends members of the academy to serve on the task force that begins preparation of the document.

Members of the task force must consider the following questions in development of the CPG (AAA, 2006a):

- What is the purpose of the CPG?
- What is the CPG's targeted procedure or intervention?

- What are the important clinical objectives related to the CPG topic?
- Who is the target population?
- Are there potential benefits or risks for individual patients associated with the procedure or treatment?
- Who are the CPG's intended users or stakeholders?
- What is the epidemiology of the topic?
- Will the new CPG be related in any manner to existing CPGs established by the academy?

The task force then develops the CPG using a special format that has six sections: (1) Title Page, (2) Introduction, (3) Methodology, (4) Discussion—Results—Recommendations, (5) Conclusion—Summary, and (6) References. Appendix 15B shows the recommended CPG format that has a log for recording the names of the members of the task force and timetable for logging the completion of critical steps of the process. A major advantage of this process is the detail required for describing the search for and use of scientific evidence in CPG development. For example, the systematic methods for searching for the evidence must be specified, including the range of dates, the databases accessed, and so on. Furthermore, the level of evidence hierarchy and the system for quality rating of individual studies is stipulated for consistent use across development of all CPGs for audiologic practice. Indeed, the AAA (2006a) document on the development of CPGs implements many of the evidence-related criteria from the COGs Statement and the AGREE Instrument, in addition to requirements for stakeholder review.

The review process begins with the submission of the initial document via the chair of the Strategic Document Committee (SDC) to the academy's board of directors, who approves it for peer review. The chair of the task force recommends to the chair of the SDC a minimum of three members who provide an expert review and make suggestions for improvement. The suggested revisions are sent to the task force for revision of the candidate CPG. The revised document is then sent to the chair of the SDC who sends it to the academy's director of communication, who, in turn, sends it to the editor of *Audiology Today* and the webmaster of its Internet site for widespread dissemination and peer review for at least one month. In addition, an e-mail is sent to the membership alerting them to the availability of the CPG for peer review. Moreover, the contact information for the director of communication and the chair of the SDC is provided so that any suggestions may be sent for forwarding to the task force for consideration in their final revision of the CPG. The chair of the task force forwards the final version of the CPG to the chair of the SDC, who, in turn, sends it to the board of directors for approval by vote. If the document receives a favorable review, the final version is posted on the academy's website and published in one of the organization's journals. If the document does not receive a favorable vote, it is sent back to the task force for subsequent revision and further review by the board of directors.

So far we have discussed tools for evaluating CPGs and the AAA's relatively new CPG development process, which brings up the question of how many current CPGs in communication sciences and disorders would meet the stringent criteria discussed above? The answer is few, but this will gradually change. *The Guidelines for*

FIGURE 15.4

Grading of the Evidence for Recommendation 2.2 of the Guidelines for the Management of Adult Hearing Loss

Recommendations

1. Each patient should receive formal self-assessment instrument(s), inventory(s) prior to fitting to establish communication needs, function, and goals.
2. Goals should be patient specific and composed of both cognitive and affective characteristics.
3. Post-fitting administration of these instrument(s) is necessary to validate benefits/ satisfaction from amplification.

Summary of Evidence for Needs Assessment

Recommen-dations	Evidence	Source	Level	Grade	EF/EV
1	A formal self-assessment inventory/instrument test battery determines patient-specific communication needs/function and detailed hearing aid features (e.g., directional microphones).	1–4	3	B	EV
1	Test battery addresses user expectations of hearing aid use.	1–4	3	B	EV
1, 2	Both cognitive and affective patient needs/goals can be assessed with the test battery.	1–4	3	B	EV
3	Test battery is proven useful in validating the patient's goals and expectations following the use of amplification.	1–4	3	B	EV

References

[1]Dillon H. James A. & Ginis J. (1997). The client oriented scale of improvement (COSI) and its relationship to several other measures of benefit and satisfaction provided by hearing aids. *J Am Acad Audiol* 8:27–43.

[2]Cox R. Alexander G. (1995). The abbreviated profile of hearing aid benefit. *Ear Hear* 16:176–186.

[3]Ventry I. Weinstein B. (1982). The hearing handicap inventory for the elderly: a new tool. *Ear Hear* 3:128–134.

[4]Cox RM. Alexander GC. (2000). Expectations about hearing aids and their relationship to fitting outcome. *J Am Acad Audiol* 11:368–382.

Reprinted by permission from the American Academy of Audiology.

the Management of Adult Hearing Impairment, created by an AAA Task Force and chaired by Michael Valente, Ph.D., exemplifies the incorporation of EBP by describing how members searched for, evaluated, and graded the evidence for specific recommendations that were labeled as "effective" (i.e., EV = measured in the real world) or "efficacious" (i.e., EF = measured in laboratory or ideal conditions) (AAA, 2006b). Figure 15.4 shows an example from the recommendation section from the CPG for part of the following objective:

2.2 Self-Perception of Communication Needs, Performance, and Selection of Goals for Treatment

Objective   The objective of this portion of the selection process is to establish patient-specific communication needs and realistic expectations from treatment. An additional objective of this component in the hearing aid selection process is to create patient-specific fitting goals. These are developed following the assessment of the patient's communication status. Goals are critical to quantify the benefits of amplification. This is the initial stage in the "validation" process, where treatment outcomes are established and measured. Specific measurement of treatment outcomes is a necessity to provide a basis for evidence-based clinical practice guidelines.

The notation used in the CPG makes it easy for clinicians to practice EBP by showing the recommendation, sources of the evidence, level of evidence, grading of the supporting evidence, and labeling of the effectiveness or efficaciousness of the recommendation. For example, clinicians who are curious about the recommendation of formal self-assessment inventory or instrument test batteries for determining patient-specific communication needs and functions can be confident of a grade of "B" when justifying the time spent during the diagnostic evaluation. In fitting Mr. Williams with hearing aids, the audiologist in our scenario frequently consulted this CPG, which provides recommendations throughout the entire treatment continuum for the management of adult hearing loss through amplification. Hopefully, this section of the chapter has provided necessary background information in considering the role of clinician expertise in EBP.

Putting It All Together for Evidence-Based Practice

So far, we have discussed patient preferences, scientific evidence, and clinician expertise, but how do you put these all together for clinical decision making? Well, there are no easy cookbook answers. Even the so-called "experts in the field" do not agree on all aspects of the identification, diagnosis, and treatment of communication disorders. However, most clinicians would agree that the best place to start is with the patient. Who are they (e.g., age, gender, ethnicity, and so on)? What is their communication disorder? Recall that we started the chapter considering patient preferences first in EBP. We proposed using the WHO-ICF (2001) model as a paradigm for assessing the patient's impairment, activity limitations, and participation restrictions. Therefore, part of the assessment process should include not only clinical measures of impairment (e.g., number of disfluencies per minute in conversational speech), but self-assessments of activity limitations, participation restrictions, and health-related quality of life. Clinicians should interview patients regarding their feelings about and personal goals (i.e., outcomes) for management in order to determine acceptable treatment options. In our scenario, the audiologist discovered that not only had sensorineural hearing loss interfered with Mr. Williams' activities in daily living, but it had also profoundly impacted his social and emotional well-being.

Only after the clinician has gone through this process can EBP be used in deciding the best treatment plan *with* the patient and his or her family. Recall that Mr. Williams was not convinced that he was ready for hearing aids. The audiologist knew how difficult it is for reticent patients to accept and benefit from amplification and therefore wanted to know the strength of the evidence for the possible benefits of amplification in improving patients' quality of life. From his weighing of the scientific evidence, the audiologist was convinced that it was worth the effort and counseled the patient and his family about the benefits of using amplification. So once the course of treatment has been selected, the audiologist wants to use the best clinical expertise in providing the best care possible. Therefore, the audiologist must consider his past experiences with similar types of patients, consult with colleagues, and examine CPGs on the topic.

Clinicians can access CPGs on AAA's and ASHA's website that pertain to most areas of practice. For example, the clinician may select a PPP in a particular area of practice and use its listed resources for additional references or even use the search option on the ASHA website. Once CPGs and related documents have been found, the currency of the information must be assessed, possibly necessitating a search for information on PubMed. Use of the PICO rubric discussed earlier may assist the clinician in framing the research question and constructing relevant search strings to use in various databases. Unfortunately, because most CPGs in communication sciences and disorders do not yet have evidence in the form necessary for EBP, clinicians may even have to assess the evidence for specific recommendations in current documents.

Once the evidence for various treatment options has been reviewed, the clinician should bring the information full circle in consulting with patients and their families. Skills in EBP practice include melding the three areas of patient preferences, clinical expertise, and scientific evidence into a clear, unbiased explanation of the advantages and disadvantages of appropriate treatment options at the patient's and family's level of understanding. Mr. Williams and his family elected to pursue amplification. Three months later, the EBP process was completed during a follow-up appointment in which the audiologist evaluated Mr. Williams's progress with hearing aids and found a significant improvement in key communication situations and a reduction in the social and emotional impact of hearing loss. For students, EBP may seem like an unachievable goal; for clinicians, it may seem like an extra chore to do. However, in communication sciences and disorders, EBP is a work in progress. Each individual is different, and clinicians vary as do our CPGs in various areas of practice, while scientific evidence changes daily. Therefore, students and clinicians may prepare themselves by being sensitive to the needs of their patients; by honing their knowledge, skills, and intuition; and keeping up with the scientific literature.

Summary

EBP was defined as the integration of patient preferences, scientific evidence, and clinical expertise in clinical decision making. On the surface, these components seem to be equally important, and thus, we would assume that our efforts to apply and integrate the best from each area will achieve positive patient outcomes. Unfortunately, clinicians rarely reach the ideal combination of the three components. Sometimes patients may have extenuating circumstances that affect the appropriateness of a particular treatment. Sometimes, the highest quality of evidence in our research is not there. Sometimes, our clinical expertise with a particular approach is lacking, or there are no CPGs defining best practices with certain types of patients with rare disorders. Other times we may not spend enough time asking the right questions to gain insight into the patient's situation, or we may fail to perceive a patient's concerns on many levels. We try to make certain that the patient mirrors the particular clinical profile (e.g. specific type of disorder, severity, age, etc.) used in the assessment and treatment procedure that represents the highest level of evidence. We also must always take into account the needs (effects of the disability), preferences (cultural, personal), resources (finances, time) that the patient brings to the table. There is sometimes an inexact fit. The ideal use of the EBP model is having the highest level of research evidence, clinical expertise in all of these high-level approaches, and a keen sensitivity to the patient's goodness of fit for a particular treatment or assessment. As mentioned, there will always be mismatches among the three levels of the EBP model and therein lies the "art" of EBP, the realization that scientific approach cannot operate in the real world without a clinician having to take stock of inadequacies in the various components and provide the best care for the patient, despite less than ideal conditions. Our goal in these chapters is to make you aware of the ideal conduct of EBP, especially in gathering of high-quality research evidence. Your abilities in perfecting your clinical expertise and developing effective interpersonal relationships with patients will allow you to make the EBP model work in the clinical setting. Unfortunately, no textbook can help you with such attributes; only clinical experience will allow you to steadily develop those skills.

LEARNING ACTIVITIES

1. Use your skills in EBP to aid in the clinical decision making for an actual patient.

2. Interview an audiologist and speech-language pathologist in how they use EBP for clinical decision making.

REVIEW EXERCISES

1. *The WHO-ICF Model:* Please match the parts of the model with the correct components.

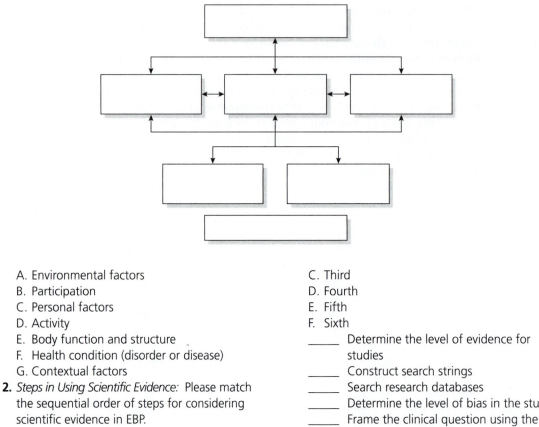

A. Environmental factors
B. Participation
C. Personal factors
D. Activity
E. Body function and structure
F. Health condition (disorder or disease)
G. Contextual factors

2. *Steps in Using Scientific Evidence:* Please match the sequential order of steps for considering scientific evidence in EBP.
A. First
B. Second

C. Third
D. Fourth
E. Fifth
F. Sixth

_____ Determine the level of evidence for studies
_____ Construct search strings
_____ Search research databases
_____ Determine the level of bias in the studies
_____ Frame the clinical question using the PICO rubric
_____ Grade the clinical recommendation

ANSWERS TO THE REVIEW EXERCISES

1. See Figure 15.1
2. D, B, C, E, A, F

APPENDIX 15A

The Clinical Practice Guidelines Format

Clinical Practice Guidelines Format

I. Title Page
   A. Full title for condition, procedure, or treatment intervention
   B. Full names of authors (members of the task force)
   C. Describe how the writing group was selected (include a description of the credentials for each group member)
   D. Date of completion (release date)
   E. Print and electronic sources
II. Introduction
   A. Purpose/Focus of the guideline—the condition, disease, treatment, procedure, technology, etc. addressed in the guideline
   B. Goal—what is the guideline expected to achieve; describe need for the guideline
   C. Describe intended users and settings in which guideline will be used
   D. Describe intended target patient population
III. Methodology
   A. Describe the systematic methods used to search for evidence; include range of dates and databases searched (e.g., MEDLINE/PubMed; Cochrane Library, etc.); include the criteria for article inclusion
   B. Provide the criteria used to rate the quality and strength of evidence to support conclusions and recommendations.

Level of Evidence Hierarchy for High-Quality Studies

Level	Type of Evidence
1	Systematic reviews and meta-analyses of randomized controlled trials
2	Randomized controlled trials
3	Nonrandomized intervention studies
4	Nonintervention studies: cohort studies, case-control studies, cross-sectional surveys
5	Case reports
6	Expert opinion

System for Quality Rating of Individual Studies

Rating	Interpretation of Rating
++	Very low risk of bias. Any weaknesses that are present are very unlikely to alter the conclusions of the study.

| + | Low risk of bias. Identified weaknesses or omitted information probably would not alter the conclusions of the study. |
| — | High risk of bias. Identified weaknesses or omitted information are likely or very likely to alter the conclusions of the study. |

Source: Adapted from Cox, 2005.

IV. Discussion/Results/Recommendations
   A. Provide and discuss the evidence that lead to the conclusions.
   B. Make recommendations that are specific and unambiguous.
      1. All recommendations will be written in complete sentences.
      2. Separate recommendations that apply to specific clinical objectives.
      3. Include information regarding areas of uncertainty or controversy in the recommendation as necessary.
      4. To the extent possible, quantify benefits, harms, and/or timeframes.
      5. Include flexibility in applying recommendations (e.g., special populations), where appropriate.
   C. Assign classification level to individual recommendations.

Classification of Recommendations

Class

1	Conditions for which there is evidence and/or general agreement that a given procedure or treatment is useful and effective.
2	Conditions for which there is conflicting evidence and/or divergence of opinion about usefulness/efficacy of a specific procedure or treatment.
3	Conditions for which there is evidence and/or general agreement that the procedure/treatment is not useful and/or effective.

Source: Adapted from American Heart Association.

   V. Conclusion/Summary
   A. Provide an overview of presented data.
   B. Highlight gaps in existing literature.
   C. Describe areas that need further study.
   D. Provide recommendations that will encourage research related to guideline topic area.
   E. Provide suggested timeline for review of guideline.
VI. References (provide a comprehensive list of references and related readings)

Reprinted by permission from the American Academy of Audiology.

Appendix A

Clinical Practice Guidelines Format and Process

Title of document: _____

Task Force:

(Chair) _____   _____

_____   _____

_____   _____

_____   _____

_____   _____

Actions/Steps	Date Due	Date Completed
1. President contacts Academy member (as recommended by the BOD) to chair the task force.		
2. Academy member accepts position as chair of task force.		
3. Chair of the Strategic Documents Committee contacts task force chair to review purpose of document. An estimated timetable for completion is discussed.		
4. Chair of task force selects committee members and provides names of members to chair of the Strategic Documents Committee.		
5. Completion of initial document by task force. This document is submitted to the Chair of Strategic Documents and distributed to the BOD. After review by the BOD, permission is granted to begin the review process.		
6. Chair of the task force recommends a minimum of three peer reviewers to the chair of the Strategic Documents Committee. The chair of the Strategic Documents Committee forwards document to peer reviewers for comments. Reviewers' comments are incorporated into the document by the task force prior to widespread review.		
7. Revised document is emailed to the chair of the Strategic Documents Committee, who forwards the document to the Academy Director of Communications.		
8. Director of Communications contacts the Editor of Audiology Today (AT) so that an announcement can be printed in AT indicating that there is a document available for widespread review.		
9. Director of Communications posts the document on the Academy Web site and alerts the membership via email that there is a document available for review.		

Actions/Steps	Date Due	Date Completed
10. The document posts for at least one month on the Web site under the appropriate content category. The Director of Communication's phone number is made available so members can request hard copies. The e-mail address of the Strategic Documents Committee chair is also made available so that comments can be directed to him or her.		
11. After one month of widespread review, all comments received from the membership are forwarded to the chair of the task force for consideration in the preparation/editing of the final document.		
12. The revised version of the document is emailed to the Publications Manager for stylistic editing. The resultant version is emailed to the Strategic Documents Committee chair and then forwarded to the chair of the task force for final editing.		
13. The final document is emailed by the chair of the task force to the chair of the Strategic Documents Committee, who e-mails copies to the entire BOD for review. The BOD takes a vote to either accept or decline the final document.		
14. A negative vote would result in returning the document to the chair of the task force with the comments from the BOD for review/editing. The revised version would then be returned to the BOD for re-review and another vote.		
15. A positive vote results in the document being posted on the Academy Web site as a document of the Academy and being published in AT or in another Academy publication (e.g., Journal of the American Academy of Audiology)		

References

American Heart Association. AHA Statement and Guideline Development. http://americanheart.org/presenter.jhtml?identifier=3023366 (accessed April 15, 2006).

Cox, R. M. (2005). Evidence-based practice in provision of amplification. *Journal of the American Academy of Audiology, 16*(7), 414–438.

CHAPTER 16

Producing Research as a Student or Practitioner

Writing a book is an adventure. To begin with, it is a toy and an amusement. Then it becomes a mistress, then it becomes a master, then it becomes a tyrant. The last phase is that just as you are about to be reconciled to your servitude, you kill the monster, and fling him to the public.

—Sir Winston Churchill (1874–1965)

Writing is easy. All you do is stare at a blank sheet of paper until drops of blood form on your forehead.

—Gene Fowler (1890–1960)

We have a habit in writing articles published in scientific journals to make the work as finished as possible, to cover up all the tracks, to not worry about the blind alleys or describe how you had the wrong idea at first, and so on. So there isn't any place to publish, in a dignified manner, what you actually did in order to get to do the work.

—Richard Feynman (1918–1988)

A new idea is delicate. It can be killed by a sneer or a yawn; it can be stabbed to death by a joke or worried to death by a frown on the right person's brow.

—Charles Brower

It may be difficult for you to conceive of yourself conducting research and writing an article for a professional journal. We are here to testify, however, that every day throughout the world both students and practitioners are submitting articles describing scientific investigations. These articles may be based on a thesis, dissertation, capstone project, or research conducted in a public school or medical setting by interested practitioners. Moreover, many of these articles are accepted for publication. As we stated in Chapter 1, conducting research and publishing the results carries with it many positive effects for both the scientist and the workplace. This chapter describes the process by which students or practitioners can carry out and write the results of their research for submission to professional venues such as conventions or journals. We encourage you not to underestimate yourself and make a contribution to our professional literature.

LEARNING OBJECTIVES

This chapter will enable readers to:

- Understand the basic process a student will go through to produce a capstone project, thesis, or dissertation.

- Understand the basic process a practitioner might go through to collaborate on a research project.

Theses, Capstone Projects, and Dissertations

The Beginning

Students can find themselves involved in a research project through various means. Some training programs offer an opportunity to design and carry out an undergraduate honors thesis under the direction of a faculty advisor. On the master's level, many programs give students the option to produce research in the form of a **thesis** under the direction of a faculty member who serves as director. Many professional doctorate programs in audiology and speech-language pathology require some sort of research project prior to graduation. These projects go by various names, such as *doctoral research project,* **capstone project,** *optional research experience, doctoral project, research lab experience, Au.D. research,* and so on, but all require the student to engage in some form of research or project in evidence-based practice under the direction of a faculty member. In Ph.D. programs students are also required to produce a **dissertation,** which is a larger and more in-depth research project than usually seen in a master's thesis. Another way that students can become involved in research without producing a project of their own is through graduate assistantships. Graduate assistants are assigned to assist faculty members with their conduct of ongoing research. Although assistants may get to participate in gathering and analyzing research data as directed by a faculty member, they are usually not involved in planning the research or in the reporting of an investigation for a convention presentation or journal article. Hence, graduate research assistants are not required to produce their own "product" such as a capstone project, thesis, or dissertation. However, despite the limitations of some forms of involvement, there is no shortage of research involvement on some level available for students in training. One commonality of thesis, capstone, or dissertation experiences is that these products are typically not due until the final stages of a student's program, leaving time for the student to come up with research ideas from early coursework and to take a course in research methods to aid in planning a project.

No matter what type of research project a student is preparing to undertake, he or she almost always feels overwhelmed at the outset. First comes the haunting feeling of stepping into the unknown. Most have never done research before and have no clue where to begin. Second comes the sheer size of the choice. In a field like communication sciences and disorders there are many possible areas of interest to focus on in research. Combine the possible study subjects in speech-language pathology and audiology with the functions of development, assessment, and treatment. When you join these with other interdisciplinary factors that can interact with communication disorders from anatomy, physiology, education, psychology, acoustics, cognition, multicultural issues, and so on, the permutations of study possibilities are mind-boggling. It is a daunting task just to choose a single topic to study in a research project. Even a student who has selected a general area of study is likely to be overwhelmed when besieged by the sheer volume of the literature in virtually every area of inquiry. There are hundreds of articles, books, and convention presentations on even the narrowest aspect of our field. It is no wonder that most students interested in research stare glassy-eyed at journals as they wander with no direction through the literature. Some make the mistake of using a search engine and typing in a search string such as "language." We can assure you that by the time you scroll through the results of *that* search, your clothes will be out of style.

Defining a General Area of Research Interest

One pathway out of the overwhelming array of choices is trying to focus at least on a *general* area of interest so that you can recruit some help in the form of a faculty member who will direct your efforts. It is not difficult to choose a general area based on your interest and on the coursework you have taken. For example, in speech-language pathology, a very basic choice is among voice, phonology, language, and fluency. Whether you are interested in development, assessment, or treatment, you must first find a general area of interest. Students who enter a training program with a preexisting interest in a general area can schedule a meeting with the faculty member specializing in teaching or researching that topic to discuss more specific research questions. Students having difficulty even choosing a general area might consider chatting with faculty members in *each* of the general areas to determine which topics are "hot" in the current research literature. After meeting with a variety of faculty members you should have a good idea about the breadth and scope of research in all of the general research areas, and you can narrow your choice to one or two. A similar process can be applied to audiology, among such fields as pediatric audiology, hearing instruments, assessment, industrial audiology, balance, aural rehabilitation, and so on. You must narrow these categories down to one or two for consideration as your research topic. Committing to a general area is the first step in narrowing your focus of research, and it also moves you toward selecting a thesis director who specializes in your interest area.

The Director

Your research director, who is the mentor who will guide you through your thesis, capstone project, or dissertation, must have the obvious attributes of expertise in your area of interest and additional expertise in research. Clearly, a history of publishing and presenting research in the general area you want to study is an important qualification. Another variable to consider is whether the person has had experience in successfully directing student research. The more student research the person has been involved with, the better. If other students further advanced in the program are completing research projects with your prospective director, that is also a good sign. You should ask these students about their experiences. For example, you might want to ask if they are graduating on time. You might want to ask if the faculty member provided assistance when needed in finding literature, analyzing data, and helping with other aspects of the project. Obviously, no research director is expected to do the project for a student, but they should be expected to guide students through the process and assist them if they begin to flounder. A thesis project is a long-term commitment that takes over a year of close collaboration with a faculty member. You might ask other students if they got along well interpersonally with the research director. A thesis is difficult enough, but it can be a real trial if there are major personality conflicts between a director and the student. In most cases, faculty are delighted to participate in student research. It is an opportunity to do one-on-one teaching, to study a topic of interest, and to be involved in a presentation or publication at the end of the process. Once you choose your research director, you are ready to narrow the focus of your project.

As mentioned earlier, a person who chooses a general area such as language has only narrowed the focus to the point where a research director can be selected. In discussions with the faculty member it will become clear that you can study preschool language, school-age language, adolescent language, or adult language. In each of those segments, you could study development, assessment, or treatment. Within these permutations are all the various subfields of language, such as phonology, syntax, semantics, morphology and pragmatics, as well as other ancillary but critical aspects such as cognitive development, literacy, social development, caretaker–child interaction, and many others. In a series of discussions with your research director you should be able to determine, for example, that you are interested in school-age language. Your director indicates that assessment of narratives in school-age children is a topic that has received increased research attention. So you start reviewing literature on narrative assessment in school-age children, and you find studies that have elicited narratives in many different ways. Notice at this point that although you have narrowed your focus somewhat and at least can begin to search the literature more specifically, you have not yet arrived at your specific research question.

The Specific Research Idea

In our experience, students who are new to the research process have difficulty narrowing their idea down to the point of posing answerable questions. (You will recall from Chapter 3 that only certain types of questions are answerable using the scientific method.) There are several useful processes to achieve this narrowing. First, it is important to meet frequently with the research director to discuss your general area of interest and the ways to focus on researchable problems. A good strategy is to set a weekly meeting time during which you talk about the progress made in the past week and any questions or problems encountered. A second process critical to narrowing your focus is to voraciously read the pertinent literature. As soon as you define a more specific area within your general area, you should be searching the literature for studies that have explored that issue. Figure 16.1 shows some selected processes you can use to arrive at a more focused research idea. Your research director will no doubt have more, but these are a beginning. A major point to make at the outset, however, is that you are not trying to design a research project that *no one* has ever done before. Certainly, we want students to do original research, but "original" does not have to be totally unique. You might recall that the way science builds is by taking into account the results of prior studies and taking the next step. All you have to do is change one aspect of a previous investigation and you have a new study. Thus, one of the branches in Figure 16.1 involves looking at prior studies and consider changing some aspect, such as the task. If the previous study used imitation in a language task, you could use delayed imitation or spontaneous productions. If one study used story retelling

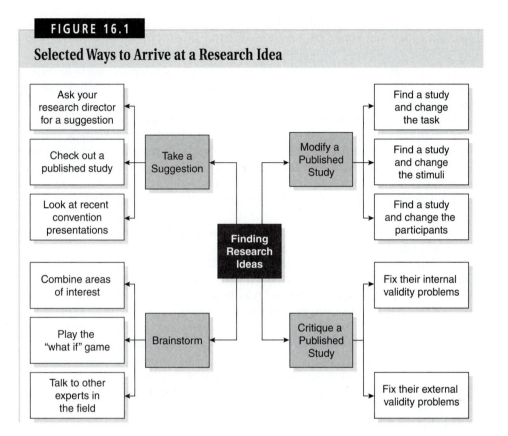

FIGURE 16.1

Selected Ways to Arrive at a Research Idea

of narratives, you could use personal narratives about vacations. Another variable to manipulate might be stimuli. If a prior study used objects, you could use pictures or video. A final variable is the participants. If a previous investigation used white children, you could use children from another culture. If the study used first graders, you could use preschoolers or eight year olds. Such thinking about tasks, stimuli, and participants gets your focus on variables to be manipulated in research, which will be good when it comes time to choose independent and dependent variables.

Another branch in Figure 16.1 has to do with taking suggestions. An obvious source of ideas is your research director. Many times, a faculty member has an abiding interest in a particular research area, sometimes having just completed a study and knowing of a research avenue just begging to be traveled as a follow-up. Clearly, this will be of interest to the research director, and it gives you an opportunity to focus your efforts on a topic if you are interested in it as well. Other research directors are not shy about suggesting research ideas to students, and again, if you are interested in those ideas it is a great way to narrow your focus. Almost every research article in print ends with a section in which the authors suggest pathways for future research, either in a separate section with a title like Suggestions for Future Research or other times embedded in the final few paragraphs of the article. Do not underestimate the value of such suggestions. Usually they have to do with the author's intentions to follow up the results of the current study. A good strategy for students trying to find ideas is to look at pertinent journals from the last year or two and specifically examine the suggestions for future research. There is nothing wrong with capitalizing on these suggestions because the authors may never pursue them, and even if they did, you are not doing anything wrong by studying a particular interest area. Actually, you can even use their suggestion as part of your rationale for studying the particular topic. A similar process is to consider ideas presented at professional conventions. If you attend the convention, you can talk with the researcher and ask about future research directions. Every researcher likes to be asked about plans to follow up the study being presented.

Another source of research ideas comes from critically examining existing studies. From Chapter 4 you learned that there are many threats to internal and external validity. Any time you read a scientific investigation, you should be thinking about such threats that, if not controlled for, can compromise integrity of an investigation. So if you find a study that did not counterbalance the order of conditions in a repeated-measures design, you certainly have the right to say that their conclusions are equivocal. You also have the right to design a study that corrects any uncontrolled threats and make it your own. If you haven't thought of it yet, there is an advantage to "spinning off" an existing study, which is the possibility of using similar procedures, controls, and statistical analyses in your study so that you can compare your results to prior research. Thus, instead of having to design a study from scratch, you might make certain decisions about the conduct of your study based on similarities to existing research. That is just good procedure.

The final branch of Figure 16.1 concerns brainstorming. One way to brainstorm is to look at general areas that relate to one another and design a study to combine both aspects. For example, language overlaps with many areas in communication disorders. There are linguistic influences on fluency and phonology. There are uses of voice measurements and instruments with fluency as well as voice disorders. Cognition and memory are important to child language, adult language, and auditory processing disorders. Think about your area of interest and the other factors that influence it; there may be a study in there somewhere. Play a "what if" game by asking yourself that question as you put two seemingly unrelated areas together as shown in the following possibilities: "What if we used electrical stimulation to increase swallowing ability?" "What if we did therapy via the Internet or videophone?" "What if children's narratives have very low test-retest reliability?" You can go on for a long time asking "what if" questions. Sometimes the research has already been done. Sometimes even if the question is too harebrained to even be investigated ("What if we did fluency therapy in geodesic domes?"), it gets your mind working and thinking about research, and that is what matters. A final source of brainstorming is to chat with faculty members other than your director as well as other students who have engaged in research. You may even want to talk with experts from other departments (e.g., psychology, education, child development, aging, etc.) about your area of interest and see if there is research in other fields that bears on your topic. You would be surprised to learn how many other fields deal with communication and areas related to it.

One more very practical point should be made here. Students who elect to do thesis, capstone, or dissertation research are on a fixed timeline. Most master's programs last about two years. Most professional doctorate programs last four years. Most Ph.D. programs last from three to five years. One of the most important constraints on any student research project is time. The student has not been hired as a full-time researcher and is taking classes and doing practicum at the same time as the thesis, capstone, or dissertation work is progressing. Also, many Au.D. and master's programs include an internship at the end of the curriculum, often taking students to geographically distant locations, far from their research populations. Since Ph.D. programs usually do not necessarily require internships, they afford the most time for research. However, in any format student research is conducted simultaneously with coursework and practicum and is a constant juggling act of balancing all of these activities. Another important fact is that students, no matter what type of program they are in, want to graduate on time. They should not be in the business of languishing in a training program for an indefinite period just to complete a research project. Although there are some instances in which a project may experience difficulty and the student's graduation may be delayed by a semester, there is no reason for this to happen. In directing over thirty master's theses, I have never had a student fail to graduate on time. It is all in the planning and selection of the study. Obviously, a student with a limited time frame should not select a longitudinal investigation that would last a year. It is clearly better to select a project with available participants rather than having to travel around the region looking for people to take part in your study. The notion of "doability" is very important to consider in arriving at your research idea.

Hopefully, you have been able to narrow the focus of your research project by following some of these suggestions. Remember, narrowing the focus does not necessarily mean that you have crafted an answerable research question. It just means that you now know what types of literature you need to gather to review the existing research. With every study you read, you should be thinking how your final methodology will be affected by decisions the researchers made.

The Committee

In formal student research enterprises such as theses, dissertations, and capstone projects, a faculty committee is formed to oversee the investigation. We have already talked about the research director, but typically there are one or two other faculty members involved. Choosing the members of your committee can be very important for several reasons. First of all, the other committee members have the potential to be sources of additional guidance for you as the project unfolds. Thus, selecting members who have expertise in your area of interest is very useful. Most faculty members "specialize" in certain areas of communication disorders; an expert in voice and speech science would have limited knowledge about child language. Such an expert might not provide much help for your project regarding language and might even refuse to be on your committee in the first place because of lack of expertise and interest. Therefore, it is useful to choose faculty members who have some connection to your area of interest. A second consideration might be to take the advice of your research director when selecting a committee. Do not underestimate the importance of forming a committee that has a history of working well together with the goal of getting the project completed and the student through graduation. Nothing is worse than choosing a committee that does not agree on issues theoretically or scientifically and is constantly at odds. Each member tells the student something different, and meetings can lead to frustration and stress. Guess who gets caught in the middle of a dysfunctional committee: That's right, the student. So, the lesson is to make sure that your committee knows about your topic of interest before you sign them up and to ask your director for suggestions on faculty members who have a history of working together and being helpful.

Format and Submission Requirements

Any student engaged in research that will produce a "product" such as a thesis, dissertation, or capstone project is faced with format issues, by which we refer to established requirements for issues such as margins, fonts, titles, subtitles, table of contents, required sections, and references, among many other factors. Most schools even have guidelines for the weight of the paper on which your thesis will be printed. Submission requirements refer to the timeline for turning in various drafts to your committee and other administrative offices such as the graduate school. Submission requirements also include the wide variety of forms that must accompany phases of your project from its inception to its completion.

It takes a certain type of person to keep track of these kinds of requirements, who, in the case of one of the authors, was an administrator in the graduate school named Orvis G. Tyree. Orvis had only a thumb and little finger on his right hand since the other three fingers were cut off in an unfortunate mishap with a table saw. At any rate, he scrutinized every thesis as if it were part of a crucial national security project. When it came time to turn a page, he would put his thumb and remaining finger in his mouth to moisten them and rub them together, rather like a fly cleaning its wings, and then the page was turned. He also used a ruler to measure the four margins of every page and the number of spaces that each beginning paragraph was indented. As I sat there watching this spectacle and the growing list of red circles and arrows on *every page* of my thesis, I could not believe it was actually happening. But it did, and massive changes had to be made before I was allowed to graduate. The reason I bring this up is that I know many students cannot possibly imagine such requirements are actually required or enforced. But let me assure you that you will have your own counterpart of Orvis G. Tyree up in some office at your university taking the job every bit as seriously.

Fortunately, your research director will no doubt tell you early on in the project that the graduate school or department has a booklet or web page elucidating the formatting requirements for your research. Most often you are asked to select a format such as APA (American Psychological Association), which has a manual all its own that goes into even more detail than the graduate school guidelines. It is probably a good idea to start writing your project in the correct format even in the early stages of developing your literature review and methodology, so that when you finish you will not have many last minute surprises from your committee or the graduate school.

Submission requirements have to do with due dates for various project-related events, such as scheduling a prospectus meeting, submission of a protocol to the institutional review board for protection of human subjects (IRB), and scheduling the oral defense of the thesis before graduation. Additionally, most universities require that early drafts of theses are submitted to the graduate school for a format check early in the semester a student plans to graduate. Final drafts of theses, with all corrections made, are typically due in the graduate school several weeks prior to graduation. Some of these events are scheduled for you by the university calendar that may stipulate final dates for submission of thesis drafts for a format check, oral defenses, and final drafts. Other aspects such as the prospectus meeting and IRB are decided based on your progress with the research. For example, you cannot write an IRB protocol until you have developed your methodology stating what you will do with your participants.

The Literature Review

After you have focused your area of interest to a manageable scope, you will begin to search for scientific literature on the topic. Remember, manageable means that our hypothetical student is not searching in broad strokes for something general such as "language." From discussion with the research director, he or she will have already decided to pursue a narrowed interest in the assessment of narratives produced by children with language impairment between the ages of four and six. A literature review, however, must provide evidence that the student is familiar with the major concepts that underlie the potential research question. These aspects help to organize the literature review into logical sections, and not unimportantly, provide an opportunity to divide the work into doable portions. The student writing a literature review may start with a section on the definition of narratives and their components. The focus is only on certain types of articles that define narratives and different ways of explaining what they include. When this section is finished, the student can then focus on another topic in the review. The student, continuing to do one section at a time, pretty soon will realize that the review is nothing more than chaining these sections together and making transitions between them. The task of writing an entire review of the literature is not as daunting when completed one section at a time. For example, a preliminary organization of a literature review for our example of assessing narratives in children with language disorders might look like this:

• *Definition of a narrative and its components.* If we are doing a research project on narratives, we need to demonstrate that we know what they are and what a good narrative is composed of.

• *Research on development of narratives in children with normal language development.* If we are going to do a study on assessment of narratives in children with language disorders, we had better be familiar with the literature on normal development. Assessment, after all, is locating a child in developmental space.

• *Research on methods used in narrative assessment.* Again, if we are studying assessment of narratives, we should demonstrate that we know the most common techniques used in such evaluations.

• *Research on narrative production in children with language impairment.* It naturally follows that a study of assessing narratives in children with language impairment should include common symptoms and deficits in narrative production in this population.

These four sections are clearly related to the research problem being investigated and are presented in a logical order. Note that the sections do not include areas that are too broad or tangential to our research topic. For instance, a general section on language development would be far too broad and go into details on syntax, vocabulary, and morphology that are not directly related to narrative production. We also would not want a general section on the assessment of child language; it is clearly too broad. There are several guidelines to bear in mind when choosing sections for the literature review. First, most of the review should stick closely to the specific problem you hope to address. The sections most directly related to your problem should be the densest in terms of number and coverage of research articles. The student can be quite general in "the definition of narratives" section without coming up with a definition from every major authority who ever lived. On the other hand, when assessing narratives, the student should spend more time reviewing articles that use different stimuli and tasks in this process and should spend considerable time on the literature dealing with the types of errors children with language problems exhibit in their narratives. It is all a matter of focus and depth of coverage; the more the section is specifically related to your research problem, the deeper and more detailed that section should be. A second point to remember when choosing sections for your literature review is that you will be referring back to this review in later sections of your research project, such as the discussion of your findings. You do not want to review the literature in your discussion section of the thesis but rather refer back to your review of the literature. Thus, choose sections for your review that make logical sense in terms of explaining your results. A classical goal of the discussion section in a research project involves putting the results into the context of prior research. How are your results similar to and different from previous studies? You can only discuss these important factors if you have spent time in your review providing the details of the studies that are similar to your own.

The Justification

Either in a separate section of your thesis or at the end of the literature review some sort of justification for conducting the research is expected. The justification typically flows from the review of the literature and is a logical extension of the studies that were examined. In the justification the researcher states why the exploration of a particular subject is reasonable. There are many ways that researchers can justify their investigations, but we will only provide three general examples. First, the investigator may demonstrate in the review of the literature that there is a gap in extant research that could be filled by a new study. This can only be shown by a thorough review of existing research, which, if done in the correct way, can be clearly demonstrated. As stated earlier, gaps can be found in a lack of scientific study of particular types of participants (e.g., culture, age) or of certain types of stimuli and tasks. In other words, the justification for doing your study is to provide data in an area that has not been directly investigated by others. A second way to justify your investigation is to point out conflicts in the existing literature that form at least two points of view. For example, you might find one group of investigations showing that males and females process information differently and another cluster of studies that shows no difference between genders. In reviewing the literature you might note that the two sides in this issue used different types of tasks when evaluating information processing. This finding leaves an opening for you to investigate the gender issue with two types of tasks in your own study to determine whether a gender or a task difference is operating. A final example of justification involves controlling for internal validity. Let's say that during the review of the literature you find a study that reports very interesting findings. On reading it closely, however, you determine that the investigators did not control for certain threats to internal or external validity. As a result, the findings are not easily interpreted in terms of the independent variable accounting for the results. If you can make this case in your review, then you are justified in exploring the same issue, but in your study you will control for the previously uncontrolled threats. Whatever you decide to study, there must be some sort of compelling reason to go forward with the investigation. One purpose of the review of the literature is to set the stage for you to justify conducting your research.

Crafting Answerable Questions

After justifying your study, you will be expected to delineate the specific questions that your study is setting out to answer. You might be wondering why we are just now getting to developing answerable questions. After all, haven't we already said that our hypothetical student is studying the assessment of narratives in children with language impairment? Hasn't he or she already done the literature review? It may seem like the student is putting the proverbial cart before the horse by reviewing the literature prior to developing research questions. There are, however, a few reasons for doing this. First of all, the student did have a fairly specific guide in reviewing the literature based on an interest in methods of assessing narratives in children with language impairment. Thus, the student knows that this is the area of interest and he or she probably is not wasting time reviewing literature on the sections outlined earlier. A second reason not to lock in on the *exact* question posed for research until after reviewing the literature is that the review might provide insights that affect question development. For instance, let's say that the literature review demonstrated that there are two most common methods used for assessing narratives. One method involves story retelling with picture support, in which a child listens to an adult tell a story and then retells it while looking at pictures. The second method involves the child telling a story while looking at the pictures in a book with no model from the adult.

The student researcher might decide after reviewing the literature that no one has specifically compared these two elicitation methods in the same study. Some studies used one method, and other studies used the other. Thus, the student may form a research question such as: *What differences in story grammar elements and structural measures (MLU, number of different words, syntactic complexity) exist between the two narrative elicitation methods of story telling with picture support and story retelling with picture support in children with specific language impairment and those with normal language?* Notice that the question is far more specific than earlier generalities about narrative assessment methods in children with language impairment. From the review of the literature the student can determine which dependent variables (e.g., MLU, number of different words, story grammar elements) had been studied in past research. The review also helps the student define the independent variables (the two elicitation methods and SLI versus normal groups) in the study. These specifics could not have been decided prior to a thorough review of the literature.

Designing the Method

One of the first steps in designing a methodology is to take stock of independent and dependent variables. In the suggested study, we have two independent variables. One is group with two levels (SLI/normal). The other independent variable is elicitation method (story retelling/story telling). Our dependent variables are MLU, number of different words (NDW), and number of story grammar elements. Going back to Chapter 8, you might recognize this as a possible 2×2 factorial design. Another decision is whether investigation should be between subjects, within subjects, or mixed. Obviously, the group factor must be between subjects because a child cannot both be normal and language impaired at the same time. For illustrative purposes, let's make the other factor within subjects or repeated measures resulting in a mixed design, as shown in Figure 16.2. Classically, the methodology section has several important components.

Participants. Once the basic design has been decided, the next major task is to decide the selection criteria for participants. This means that the researcher needs to decide who will be included in the study and who will be excluded. The participants are important because they make up one of our independent variables. Any

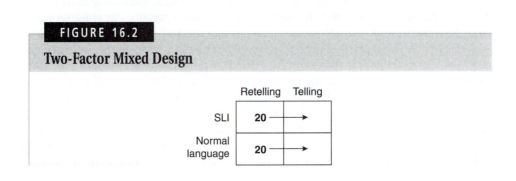

FIGURE 16.2

Two-Factor Mixed Design

differences found between children with SLI and those with normal language need to be interpreted on the basis of their language abilities and not on other confounding factors. In Chapter 4, we discussed threats to internal and external validity. You might remember that differences between groups such as gender, age, SES, intelligence, MLU, hearing acuity, ethnicity, and many others represent threats to internal validity by giving alternative explanations for the independent variable. Thus, the participants section of the methodology must address as many of these issues as possible. Also, it needs to be determined whether participants can be randomly selected from a larger group or a sample of convenience that will just be matched on relevant variables (e.g., hearing, SES, etc.) prior to the study. Finally, the measurement of language ability is a critical variable. We want the group with SLI to be clearly defined by standardized and nonstandardized testing (e.g., language sample). The group with normal language should also be documented using the same procedures. A complete description of both groups and their demographic and test information should be provided in a table.

Instrumentation. Any instrumentation being used in the study should be detailed in this section. To some degree, any study uses instrumentation, even if it is merely a tape recorder or human judges. The calibration of instruments should also be discussed in this section, whether they are human judges or pieces of research equipment. In a study of narrative assessment we have several "instruments" that must be described in detail. For instance, the books used to elicit narratives should be described and a rationale for their use provided (e.g., they have been used in prior research). This description should include the reference for the book, its length and physical properties (e.g., dimensions, color/black and white, worded, wordless, etc.). The environment where the samples are taken is also part of the instrumentation (e.g., a quiet room in the school building, university clinic, etc.) Any electronic instrument such as a tape recorder and microphone should be described by model number and its positioning in relation to the participants explained.

Procedure. The procedure section describes all of the events that occur while conducting the study. It should be described in enough detail so that the reader can get a sense of what the participants experienced during the conduct of the study. In our example, the first thing experienced by the participants is testing to determine whether they had normal or impaired language. The procedure should indicate when the testing was done in relation to the actual experiment. Perhaps the tests were administered during a first session and the rest of the tasks were saved for subsequent sessions. Remember, we are testing the language of these participants to determine if they qualify for membership in a particular group. It is not a good idea to mix up testing for participant classification with the actual experiment. In a second session three to five days later we might schedule the first of the experimental conditions. Since the independent variable of task (telling/retelling) is a repeated-measures factor, it would be a good idea to counterbalance the two levels in order to control for order effects, learning, and fatigue. Thus, we should present a table showing the order in which each participant experienced the two conditions of telling and retelling. In a third session three to five days later, each participant would experience the condition not used in session two. There are many other details that should be explained in the procedure section, such as the specific instructions given to the participants as they engaged in each task or which books were used for stimuli in the telling and retelling conditions. It would be a good idea to counterbalance the books between story telling and retelling conditions so that any results could not be attributed to a particular book, but to the tasks themselves.

Data Analysis.   The analysis of data typically involves several levels. First, the raw data must be obtained from the participants. In the case of our example, the participants generate narratives from pictures during a story telling and retelling task. The narratives are captured on tape or by digital recorder. These recordings must be transcribed by someone involved in the project so that more specific analyses of the story grammar elements and structural measurements can be taken. One issue then is who will transcribe the information from the recorder. To avoid experimenter bias it would be wise to have a transcriber who does not have a vested interest in the outcome of the experiment, such as an assistant. It would also be prudent to not identify the participant as being a member of the normal language or language-impaired group. Although it may be difficult to blind the transcriber to whether the generated narrative was in the telling or retelling task, it would be an excellent idea to do so. Thus, we should end up with similarly transcribed narratives for each participant in the telling and retelling conditions. The next level of analysis is for someone to make the determinations about the story grammar elements produced in each narrative. Some sort of established system from prior research should be used to assign portions of utterances story grammar element status. For the structural measurements (MLU, number of different words, syntactic complexity), procedures used in prior research should be selected to reflect these variables. The researcher might use Brown's calculation guidelines for MLU and Miller's guidelines for NDW and compute the DSS for complexity. Once the specific measurements have been decided, we need to know who will calculate them. The same guidelines mentioned previously apply here. Whoever calculates the structural measures and story grammar elements should be blind to the group membership of the speaker and elicitation condition from which the narrative was generated. Note that the data extracted from these procedures represent the raw data from the study prior to any statistical analysis. We must have the raw data in some usable form before we can plan the statistical analysis.

Reliability.   In Chapter 3 we mentioned the importance of reliability computations in all types of research. Just because someone has transcribed the recordings, identified story grammar elements, and computed structural measurements does not mean that we are ready to get into statistical analysis. A scientist cannot rely on the judgment and perception of one person to count and interpret reality. Thus, we need to check the reliability of the transcriber to see if another person would come up with the same utterances. We need to determine if the computation of structural measurements and story grammar elements are similar between two independent judges. Our reliability measurements and procedures must be described in detail.

The Prospectus

Any thesis or dissertation proposal requires the student to write a **prospectus** outlining the proposed research. Sometimes capstone projects also require some form of research plan or prospectus, depending on the university and departmental policies. The prospectus is essentially the front end of the thesis or dissertation and includes a title page, a general introduction, a review of the literature, a justification, and a methodology section. Thus, it encompasses everything but the results and discussion portions of the project. The good news is that when you are done writing the prospectus, you have essentially completed the bulk of the thesis or dissertation project since results and discussion sections are often shorter than the review of the literature and methodology. In some cases, however, the project has many figures and tables explaining the statistical analysis and this can add enough pages to the project that some results and discussion sections can be longer than the front portions of the work. Typically, the student and major professor work closely as a team to develop the prospectus, which will be distributed to the thesis committee several weeks prior to a prospectus meeting. Wise professors and students maintain good communication with committee members during the development of the prospectus, especially regarding major or controversial decisions on how to approach the research project. It is well worth asking your committee for their input on such issues before you spend time writing the prospectus and getting blindsided in your prospectus meeting. It is better to know the feelings of your committee along the way so there are few surprises at the meeting. Once the prospectus has been developed, it can be distributed to committee members. The committee typically takes several weeks to critically read the prospectus and will share their suggestions and concerns at the prospectus meeting.

The Prospectus Meeting

The prospectus meeting is often a source of angst for students and professors alike. Remember that the prospectus represents many months of thinking, planning, reading, and writing not only for the student but for the thesis director. It is easy to see that if the student and thesis director have maintained good communication with committee members and the committee has worked together on other thesis projects, the likelihood of a surprise at the meeting is minimized. If, on the other hand, the committee has not worked together before and little communication has occurred while developing the prospectus, the possibility of some difficulty is increased.

It is important to remember that the prospectus meeting represents an opportunity for the student to present his or her proposal and for the committee to make suggestions that will help to make the project a success. Most prospectus meetings are not designed to play "gotcha" with the student and impede his or her research. The committee should be interested in helping the student design a project that will be successful and make a legitimate contribution to the research literature. From all you have read about research thus far, it is easy to see how certain aspects of an experiment can be overlooked during the planning and writing process. Sometimes the student and thesis director are too close to the project to see more objective points of view. Often, committee members come up with very important suggestions that can control for sources of error or make the conduct of the study easier or more effective. It is always healthier to go into a prospectus meeting with the thought that everyone is working together to make the project the best that it can possibly be and not view it as an adversarial situation. It has been my experience that most of these meetings have resulted in a research project that was better than the ideas proposed in the original prospectus.

The prospectus meeting usually opens with the student delivering an oral presentation of the proposed study, which takes thirty to forty-five minutes, depending on the particular practices followed by the university. The presentation provides an opportunity for the student to explain his or her proposal to the committee, each of whom has just spent a couple of weeks reading the written version of the prospectus in painful detail. The goal of the presentation is not, therefore, communication, but rather a chance for the student to gather together a lot of theoretical and technical information and coherently organize it into an oral format. This is good practice for other venues where the student might be asked to discuss his or her research, such as convention presentations or the oral defense of the thesis or dissertation project. We usually recommend that the student not simply read or paraphrase the prospectus but encapsulate important issues in a PowerPoint presentation that summarizes the project. In this way the material is less redundant for the committee while giving the student practice synthesizing the material into understandable chunks. Obviously, in a thirty-minute presentation at a prospectus meeting, most of the time should be devoted to the justification and methodology and the review of the literature should only be summarized in general terms unless some particular studies are critical to the research project. Although this presentation is a valuable experience for the student, it is not quite as meaningful for the committee, whose members often are thumbing through the prospectus and writing marginal notes during the entirety of the student's presentation. This should not be construed by the student as rudeness or disinterest. After all, the committee has already read the prospectus and they are thinking about the next step in the meeting, which involves their asking questions about the project. Sometimes their questions have not been finalized before the meeting and sometimes the student will say something in the oral presentation that may provoke a question in a committee member. Students should remember that committee members will not feel as if they have done their job effectively unless they have some questions. It should also be remembered that these committee members are being asked to make a significant contribution to the project in front of their peers, and they do not want to be in the position of giving no relevant input. Thus, there is some pressure on committee members to ask scintillating questions and show their own research expertise in front of the student and other faculty. No matter how "perfect" the prospectus, there will *always* be questions and concerns brought up by the committee. It is the nature of committees, and there is no way around it. Some members come in with notes in the margins, others will have a fringe of Post-It notes sticking out from the side of the prospectus, and some will come to the meeting with a separate sheet of questions and concerns. In most cases these questions are constructive and a legitimate attempt to make the research project a more tightly controlled, practical, and meaningful exercise.

When the student presentation concludes, the thesis director usually opens the meeting to questions from the committee. Sometimes one member at a time is allowed to exhaust his or her questions before going on to another member, but other times all members may contribute questions on a particular issue. For example, if one member questions whether it is appropriate to control for socioeconomic level in the participants, other members may chime in and say that they shared that concern. The questions may range from theoretical issues and experimental design concerns to grammatical errors. Many committee members mark grammatical errors in their copy of the prospectus and simply give the marked copy to the student at the end of the meeting. There is usually discussion surrounding the questions from the committee in an effort to problem-solve any issue that has been raised so that the proposed study will be improved. Sometimes several options will be suggested and the student and thesis director will have to decide what to do after further reading and discussion.

One good thing about the prospectus meeting is that it is rather like a contract between the student and the committee. After all the issues have been resolved, the committee is basically saying, "If you do the study as put forth in the prospectus with the modifications we have suggested at this meeting, your project is approved to go forward." Thus, the student is somewhat protected from a situation in which some member of the committee suggests a procedural change halfway through the study. Similarly, when the study is completed as planned, the committee should not be able to disapprove the project on methodological grounds, because they have given their blessing to the experiment during the prospectus meeting.

Appendix 16A includes a number of questions that a student or practitioner might ask when writing up a research proposal (e.g., thesis prospectus, capstone project) or when writing an article based on the study after it is completed. For a research proposal the portions on the title, review of the literature, justification, and methodology are the basic components. The other sections on the results and discussion are for projects that have been completed. The list of questions is not all inclusive, but it does serve to jog your memory about most of the important elements that should be included in a proposal or article. Obviously, if you are new to research you will not be able to anticipate every possible query from your committee or peer reviewers, but these questions address the most critical aspects of a research proposal.

The Midpoint

The IRB

In Chapter 2 we discussed the importance of the institutional review board (IRB) approving any research involving human participants. Most studies in communication sciences and disorders involve human participants. At the earliest possible time after the prospectus is finalized and approved by the thesis committee, the project should be submitted for IRB approval because the data cannot be gathered until the study is approved. Institutional review boards have many similarities across universities, but there are also some local procedural differences that you should be aware of. The IRB will typically have unique procedures and formats for submitting research protocols, and these are usually available on the university website. Although there is considerable variation in the time needed to obtain approval, it is not unreasonable to expect that the IRB may take several weeks to a month to make a judgment about your project. Most IRBs have specific deadlines for submission of protocols each month and if you miss the deadline, you may be moved into the following month's group of protocols. It is unusual for the IRB to approve a research protocol without questions and concerns. Most of the time you can expect ten to twenty specific concerns that you will have to address before you obtain final IRB approval. Most of these are usually fairly trivial and easily corrected. The IRB research protocol tends to focus mainly on the methodology to be used in the proposed study. Certainly, there is a brief section for mentioning pertinent literature and a section for justification, but this is typically not more than a page or two. Fortunately, with the approved prospectus in hand, the student is in the position of electronically "cutting and pasting" the information from the prospectus into the IRB protocol format. This most often involves reducing the amount of information in the prospectus rather than expanding it. Since IRB protocols may vary by institution, we will not provide examples here, but we encourage you to go to your university's website and download the specific protocol format used by your institution.

Finding Participants

Hopefully, you will have thought about your research population prior to designing your study and submitting the prospectus for approval. One of the basic premises of a student research project is that it is "doable." Thus, a most practical matter is that a study should be designed with a certain population of participants in mind that you will have access to in order to conduct your research. Many facilities may be available in your geographical area, including public schools, private schools, daycares, hospitals, rehabilitation centers, university lab schools, nursing facilities, private clinics, community clinics, headstart programs, industry, and many variations. In some of these settings, there may be yet another IRB panel that you must satisfy in order to gain approval to conduct the research. In most cases your IRB protocol will contain all the information these other panels might require, and it just needs to be reconfigured to adhere to any unique format. In some cases, however, the IRB approval from the university will suffice.

Informed Consent

One hallmark of the IRB process is the notion that participants have the choice about whether or not to participate in a research project. Therefore, attracting participants may begin with a simple announcement of the study so that participants may consider participating. For example, the researcher may leave flyers announcing the project at local daycare facilities. A flyer might be sent home with children from school for their parents to consider. When dealing with participants who have disorders, it is important that they do not feel coerced to take part in the study just because they are receiving services from a clinic or other facility. This is an important part of the informed consent procedure. In many cases, the student may not find all the participants needed in a single setting, and some travel to different facilities is necessary to obtain the number of subjects required for the study.

The first time you meet a potential participant, the initial step is to complete the informed consent procedures. This involves letting the participant, or parents of participants in the case of young children, read the informed consent form and providing an opportunity to ask questions about the study. In cases of school-age children who may not be able to fully read and understand the informed consent, it is sometimes necessary to explain the study verbally to them (sometimes called an "assent" procedure) and have them initial a simple form that says they have heard the explanation of the project and want to participate. The form also says that they can quit at any time if they so desire. Thus, the informed consent is a prerequisite part of a participant's folder that must be dealt with prior to any testing or experimental procedures.

Gathering Data

Even though you may think that your research project is the most important thing in the world, we can assure you that the people working in the facilities where your participants are found do not share this view. In fact, your project is an interruption to the normal operation of whatever setting you enter to gather data. Thus, it is always important to remember that you represent an intrusion on the normal routine in any setting and an interruption to the usual activities of your participants. When designing your study, it is a good idea to make sure that the tasks you use are not too intrusive and the amount of time your participants will be needed is kept to a minimum. You are a guest in these facilities and should act as such during every visit. You represent not only yourself, but the university and department you come from. You certainly do not want to compromise a research site for future students who want to conduct a similar project.

As mentioned earlier, there may be several stages to data gathering, all of which take time. First, you may have to administer tests to people in order to "qualify" them for inclusion in the study. For instance, you may need to confirm that they have language disorders or hearing impairments. Once you have done any preliminary testing to group your participants, the second stage involves administering the experimental tasks that are part of your particular research project. This may involve one or more sessions, depending on the length and difficulty of the tasks and design of the study. A third time-consuming task may involve arranging the experimental environment for your research, such as setting up equipment, moving furniture, and arranging stimulus items, instructions, and data forms to be used in the study. Finally, there is more time spent transporting participants from classrooms or hospital rooms to the experimental setting. Remember that every minute that you are spending with a participant is time that he or she is not able to be in the classroom, some form of therapy, or recreational activities.

The ultimate goal of gathering data is to get your data "in the can," as some researchers are prone to saying. This means that you get your participant's voice on audiotape, video, or on a data sheet while performing your experimental tasks. These data, then, are captured in a format that can later be analyzed. Without capturing the data in such a way as to preserve it and transport it back to your laboratory, you will have nothing to analyze. Ideally, the data you have gathered were obtained under the specific conditions outlined in your prospectus.

Organization in Gathering and Safeguarding Data

In Chapter 1 we indicated that organizational ability was a major characteristic of a competent researcher. In all of the previous sections you can easily see that organization permeates the designing of the study, writing the prospectus, and developing the IRB protocol. If you are not organized in any of these activities, the research project will be far more difficult than it should be. As the study progresses from its idealized form in the prospectus to the real world of participants and data gathering, organization becomes even more important. Just the process of finding participants takes a lot of scheduling and organization. Gathering data from participants means that you have organized the environment and your materials and adhered to your experimental procedures. In some studies you will not even know what to do with a participant without consulting a table of random numbers or counterbalancing sheet. If you miss a condition or fail to give instructions appropriately, you have effectively lost a participant. This means that the person is unusable due to your inability to follow procedure. Thus, organization is critical in running participants in your study. Once you have your data "in the can," organization becomes even more important. The way that you organize data you have obtained is critical for later retrieval and analysis. You cannot simply throw all of the tapes and paperwork into your backpack and move on to the next participant. What if you have not numbered audiotapes with a code so that you know which group a participant is from? What if you have not filled out the identifying information on test forms and then do not know who took the test? What if the data sheet you marked during the task had no participant code on it so it is not identifiable later on? Researchers must become compulsive and meticulous about keeping track of the data they obtain during an experiment because there is always the possibility of error and confusion. The more data that have been collected, the more paranoid researchers become and the more organized they need to be. There is an old story about doctoral students who keep their data in plastic bags in their refrigerators as the study progresses. This is presumably to safeguard the data in case their house burns down. Just imagine, worrying about your data when all of your other belongings have been incinerated in a house fire! But, as you will see, you have so much invested in the project that you do not want to lose those data, especially as you are approaching the end of the study.

Another aspect of safeguarding your data comes from one of the important components of the IRB protocol: maintaining the confidentiality of participants throughout the study. Thus, the IRB will want you to specify how you are safeguarding data as the study progresses. Typically, they want limited access to the data by the researcher and trusted research assistants. The data should be locked in a file cabinet or safe in a controlled environment such as an office so that others cannot access the materials.

Data Analysis

As mentioned in an earlier section, the analysis of the data takes place in several steps. First, the raw data such as scores on tests, language samples, video recordings, performance on experimental tasks, and so on must be reduced down to a manageable form so that quantitative analysis can take place. This means that in our example, the narratives must be scored for their macrostructure (story grammar elements) and their grammatical complexity (MLU, NDW, etc.). This scoring may involve the experimenter and research assistants and should include some estimates of reliability in scoring.

The second step in data analysis involves statistics. For students doing a thesis, dissertation, or capstone project we assume that they will have taken one or more courses in statistics and research design. Obviously, Ph.D. students will take more research courses than any other group because they are working on a research degree. Thesis and capstone students may have only taken one course in research, such as the one that the present textbook is designed for. As we have said throughout the text, we have taken a conceptual approach to statistical methods rather than exclusively focusing on how to perform the quantitative methods. Thus, thesis and capstone students must rely on their major professor for some guidance in statistical analysis. Every thesis director has different levels of expertise with quantitative methods and computer programs that perform statistical analyses. Some major professors are familiar with one major statistical analysis program, and others may have expertise in several different programs.

Table 16.1 shows some common statistical analysis programs that can be used to analyze your data. The programs have some similarities and some differences in terms of the statistics computed, methods of data input, and types of output (e.g., graphs, tables, etc.). Some of the programs are extensive and quite expensive. Other programs are more limited and may even be free to download from the Internet. The bottom line is that you need to find a program that will do the statistical analysis appropriate for your study. If all you are doing is an independent *t*-test, you can probably get by

TABLE 16.1

Selected Statistical Analysis Software Programs

ASP (a statistical package)	DMC Software 6169 Pebbleshire Dr. Grand Blanc, MI 48439	www.dmcsoftware.com
MODSTAT	Dr. Robert C. Knodt 1414 37th Street Bellingham, WA 98279	www.members.aol.com/rcknodt/pubpage.htm
NCSS	328 N. 1000 East Kaysville, UT 84037	www.ncss.com
SPSS	233 S. Wacker Drive 11th Floor Chicago, IL 60606	www.spss.com/spss
Statistica	2300 E. 14th Street Tulsa, OK 74104	www.statsoft.com
Online statistical freeware programs		www.statpages.org

with a freeware program. If you are doing a multiple regression or MANOVA you will require a program that offers more options and is more powerful. Your best bet where statistical analysis is concerned is to stick with your major professor, who will already have access to a statistical program through the university and will know how to help you input scores to analyze the data from your study. Most thesis directors are happy to lend their expertise in data analysis for thesis and capstone students, whereas dissertation students are expected to be more independent in data analysis since they have taken multiple courses on the subject. If you are a practitioner doing research, it is fine to perform your own statistical analysis if you have the expertise, but if you do not, you always have the option of hiring a consultant from a nearby university. Although there is no shortage of statistical consultation companies advertised on the Internet, it is usually better to have a resource that you can meet with, explain your study to, and even go back to for help in interpreting the analyses.

When entering data into any program for statistical analysis it is important to check the reliability of data input to make certain that you have not mistyped numbers into the program. Statistical software will always give you an answer, even if you have typed in the wrong numbers. Whichever program you use, remember that the first step in data analysis is to examine summary statistics to determine the means and standard deviations of your data. This is an important factor in establishing whether or not you meet the assumptions of parametric statistics such as homogeneity of variance.

The End Game

Writing the Results

The results section of a thesis, dissertation, or capstone project is usually much more detailed than the results section of a research article. Because these types of projects are meant to be learning experiences for students, we usually require them to put in all of the painful details of statistical analyses. This includes entire ANOVA summary tables with sums of squares, mean squares, degrees of freedom, sources of variation, and F-ratios. This makes for a very repetitive results section since many of the tables look similar and go through the same process over and over for each independent and dependent variable. You will recall from prior chapters that in a research article, all of these data are not presented, just degrees of freedom, F-ratios, and probabilities, and these can even be placed in parentheses within a sentence.

The results section is typically organized to some degree in terms of the independent and dependent variables included in the study. Usually, each section begins with some depiction of summary statistics, including means and standard deviations. The summary statistics are usually depicted in tabular form and can combine several dependent variables within the same table for the sake of economy. This is sometimes done in a separate section, but it can also be included in parts of the results section dealing with hypothesis testing. In our example of narrative production, the results section could be divided by independent variables. Recall that one IV was elicitation mode (telling/retelling) and language status (normally developing/language disordered). Thus, the results section could begin by comparing the two types of elicitation on the various dependent variables (story grammar, MLU, NDW, etc.) for the participants regardless of their group. Another section could then deal with the IV of the group and describe differences between language ability groups on the dependent variables. A third section might deal with the interaction effects of the two IVs to determine if the elicitation methods differed in terms of group performance. This, of course, is only one way to organize the results section. Another tactic might be to organize the results in terms of dependent variables. In this variation we might talk about story grammar elements in terms of elicitation method, group performance, and interactions between the two. Then we move on to the next dependent variable such as MLU and present results for elicitation method, group performance, and interaction effects. Whatever way results are presented, they must be orderly and clear with some sort of logic to the section. It is not possible to really illustrate a "typical" results section, mainly because the results will differ markedly depending on the type of statistic and experimental design that was used in the analysis. The results section showing the analysis of variance will look quite different from a section showing the results of a multiple regression or factor analysis. The point here is that the section must be orderly and logical so that readers can understand the findings of the study. Often, researchers will add figures in the form of graphs to clarify the results of a study.

Writing the Discussion

The discussion section of a thesis, dissertation, or capstone project is where the researcher puts the findings of the study into the context of prior research. We mentioned earlier that the review of the literature was important because it needed to be detailed enough that the researcher can refer back to the information during the discussion. One way to place research into context is to discuss how the current results agree or disagree with prior studies. In cases of disagreement, it is incumbent on the researcher to suggest why the findings were different. The usual suspects to examine for disagreement among studies revolve around methodological differences. The studies disagreed because the participants were different in some critical way such as age or ethnicity. The studies could have disagreed because the dependent variables used were different or the tasks were dissimilar in the two studies. Whatever the reason, the researcher tries to account for differences in the extant research and play up similarities between the current results and prior studies.

Another goal of the discussion section is to suggest clinical or practical implications of the results for practitioners. It could be that the results suggest important assessment or treatment implications. It is important, however, that the researcher not go beyond his or her data and make recommendations not warranted by the results of the study. One common way that researchers go beyond their data is to make assessment and treatment recommendations for disordered clients when their study only involved normally developing participants. Despite some possible connection between such results and clinical practice, the researcher should remember that people with communication disorders may react quite differently from people with normal communication. In our example of narratives, we studied both people with normal language and those with disordered language. A finding that all participants produced simpler narratives during story telling as compared to retelling could suggest that the elicitation methods presented differing degrees of difficulty to both normal and disordered participants.

Limitations of the Study and Suggestions for Future Research

Although we would all like to believe that our study was perfect and every possible variable was controlled optimally, such is rarely the case. You will recall from Chapter 4 that there are almost always some compromises in the conduct of research. You wanted pristine groups in your study that were balanced on every pertinent variable. In reality, however, you had to accept some participants who were older than wanted or had some degree of hearing impairment. Initially you had set out to gather data on thirty participants, but you could only muster eighteen for your study. You wanted all middle-SES children, but you had to take some from lower socioeconomic levels. Ideally, you wanted to use the most expensive equipment, but you had to settle for what was available in the laboratory at the time of your study. You might have liked to do a longitudinal study that lasted a year, but you only had the time to do a study that lasted four months if you were to graduate on time. Thus, in every thesis, dissertation, and capstone project there is some mention of limitations related to the study. They may be limitations in how the study was conducted, in the participants, or in how the results can be applied clinically. Sometimes there is a separate section in the thesis for limitations, and other times these issues are folded into the discussion section of the thesis. The limitations are put there so that everyone knows that the researcher is aware of potential problems with how the results might be interpreted. You should not think of this section as a negative one, because it actually allows you to show your acquaintance with the research process and it lets you guard against a potential over-interpretation of your results by others.

Another issue that the researcher should address is suggestions for future research. These can take several forms. First, a research avenue might be to improve on the study that you have just completed. Maybe you found that some parts of the project did not go well and you have suggestions for improvement. A second research implication might be that your findings were important and you feel that further investigation needs to be conducted with other types of participants, tasks, or stimuli. A third example might be to discuss the next logical step in the research progression. Thus, in our example which found story telling to be more difficult than retelling, a logical extension might be to expand into different narrative genres such as personal narratives. Another logical extension might be to study story telling/retelling with and without pictorial cues. Whatever the advice, it is helpful to nascent researchers, like you were before your project, to have some suggestions about further research avenues. And so, you can see, we have come full circle.

The Defense

We know what you are thinking. If they call it a **defense,** that implies an attack. Let's spend some time softening that notion a bit. First of all, you have been working with your committee from the beginning in designing your study. They have helped you to design a study that was empirically sound and they are invested in it to some degree. Second, at the prospectus meeting the committee approved your project and essentially indicated that if you completed it as planned, you have fulfilled your obligations in doing your project. Third, your major professor has been through this before and would not let you go into your defense unprepared. In order to remove some of the mystery from the thesis defense, we will outline what happens in this meeting.

The first step in preparing for your defense is to add sections to the prospectus that you developed before you started your research project. Even before you add the new sections, however, it is a good idea to make *certain* that you have incorporated the feedback received from your committee at the prospectus meeting. Remember, your committee spent considerable time putting those notes in the margins of your prospectus and placing sticky notes on the pages, and they expect that their input has been incorporated into the prospectus. After cleaning up the review of the literature, justification, and methodology, you are ready to add new sections. The results and discussion sections, along with the limitations and recommendations for future research, will all have to be added to the prospectus to assemble the final product. You and your thesis director will spend some time and effort in crafting these new sections so that your results will be explained and interpreted in an appropriate fashion. Also, remember our old friend Orvis G. Tyree? The prospectus was only an editorial appetizer; the completed thesis project is the main course. This is format crunch time in terms of making sure you have all the title pages, acknowledgments, dedication, table of contents, lists of tables and figures, bibliography, and appendixes in line with university policy.

The completed research project is again submitted to the committee with at least two weeks allowed for review and a room reserved for the defense. In many universities the thesis defense is a public meeting announced by disseminating flyers to interested parties. In this way, students and other faculty can become familiar with departmental research, and students who are beginning the program can see how impressive a more advanced student can be. In most cases, however, attendance is meager and the only other attendees are other thesis, dissertation, or capstone students who want to be there for moral support and to see what a defense is like. Many thesis directors will hold a mock defense in which the student has the opportunity to make his or her presentation and practice answering questions. In the defense, the student will again have thirty to forty-five minutes to make a presentation to the committee and any other attendees. This presentation, unlike the prospectus meeting, will focus on the results and discussion. There will be a small portion of time devoted to the review, a small portion focusing on the method, and a large emphasis on the results and discussion. Again, the committee will have made marginal notes on the thesis in preparation for their questions, which will be asked after the student completes the presentation. The only questions about methodology will be related to any deviations from the original approved procedures discussed in the prospectus meeting. Predictably, most questions will revolve around how the statistics are presented and how well the discussion stuck to the actual findings of the study. Sometimes the committee will ask some theoretical questions related to the project or some sort of question involving "what if" scenarios. Most questioning is not done in a threatening manner but is directed at making sure that the student presents data clearly and fairly but does not go beyond the legitimate implications of the study. At the end of the defense the committee members will give the student their copies of the project so that any comments or concerns can be incorporated into the thesis before it is submitted to the graduate school. Often, there are forms to be signed by committee members and the thesis director that will be submitted with the thesis, indicating that the project is approved. In some cases the committee members want to see final copies prior to submission to the graduate school and in other instances this work is left up to the student and thesis director to ensure all concerns have been taken into account.

Writing Up a Presentation or Journal Article

You may be thinking, "Why would a student want to write an article right after completing a thesis project?" Well, we are not talking about immediately starting on an article or presentation without taking a break. We are really just advocating that you develop a *plan* with your thesis director for transforming your thesis, dissertation, or capstone project into a presentation or article. Some people feel that it is best to stay in the writing mode while they are in the mood. Others would prefer to make a plan to develop a draft of an article within a matter of months postgraduation. The worst thing to do is to make no plan. Think about what happens after you turn in your thesis. First of all, you heave this immense sigh of relief that you have accomplished everything you set out to do. Second, you will graduate and move away to begin your first job or go on for more graduate school. You will enjoy the luxury of not having to study every night and take tests. You will actually have time to read novels, resume hobbies, watch television, and have a social life! The last thing on your mind will be to come up with a draft of an article based on your research, unless, that is, you have planned to do so. Remember that in an earlier section of this book we said that science should be shared with others. We also said that articles and presentations are good vehicles for improving your resume. The process of developing an article is not as onerous as one might think.

In most cases the process of editing is easier than generating written work when faced with a blank page. Luckily, you have produced a thesis, dissertation, or capstone project and it contains far more detail than is ever going to be published in an article. It sits on your parents' coffee table as a monument to your research acumen. It may be a few hundred pages long. An article submission, on the other hand, is usually no more than forty pages double spaced. Editors want articles to be economical in order to reduce publication costs and to fit as many different articles as possible into an issue of a journal. Thus, you are faced with cutting your hundreds of pages of text, figures, and tables into a lean, mean article. As we said above, this is far easier than writing the project in the first place. It is beyond the scope of the present chapter to tell you everything you need to know to write a competitive article for a professional journal. We will only provide a few general guidelines. Most of the time, the largest cuts come in the review of the literature. Articles do not have the luxury of spending many pages reviewing previous research. If you look at articles in journals, the review may be only one to three pages of the article. (Here we are talking "printed" pages in the journal itself, not the double-spaced pages on which you submitted the article.) The methods section may be another three to five printed pages. The results and discussion may encompass six to seven pages. A good procedure is for the student to develop a draft of the article and send it to the thesis director for comments, additions, or deletions. This can easily be done electronically via e-mail. After several exchanges, a reasonable draft of the article based on your research project should take shape.

Depending on the journal you intend to submit your article to, there are particular format requirements that must be met. Most of the time, these can be found on the journal website under "Instructions for Authors" or inside the front or back cover of the actual journal if you have a copy. Some journals allow and encourage electronic submission, and others want you to submit five copies of the paper so they can disseminate the manuscript to reviewers. At any rate, it is good to submit your article soon after graduation so that your results are not old news to the scientific community and before you forget the details of the project with time.

If you are submitting your work for a presentation, the editorial task is even more daunting. In the previous example, we condensed several hundred pages of a thesis project down into under forty pages of double-spaced manuscript. Most presentation submission formats for organizations such as ASHA or AAA require *less than* 1500 words describing the project and its results for consideration as a convention paper. You can see how this is really an editorial challenge, and why it is impossible to include all of the relevant information for peer review, which is why, as stated in an earlier chapter, many convention papers are not subject to the same strict peer review as journal articles, simply because it is impossible to present enough information for a thorough critique in 1500 words. Most word-processing programs have "word counters" that will tell you how many words you have placed in a particular document. The best advice is to keep cutting information until you reach the limit set for the presentation submission. Obviously, you will find that some information is superfluous and can be easily cut. You will also find that scientific writing is often cumbersome and you can say things in a much more economical way. In presentation submissions the most cutting usually comes in the review of the literature and the discussion. This leaves your justification, method, and results. You will soon discover that describing all the frequencies you tested in a hearing screening, which were so critical in your thesis, are expendable in a 1500-word convention submission.

Whether you submit your student research as an article, convention presentation, or both, it is a great reward for you, your thesis director, and the university you graduated from to have increased visibility due to your efforts.

Another Perspective on Ethics for Students and Practitioners

You will recall that in Chapter 2 we spent some time talking about ethics in the conduct of research. In that chapter we emphasized protection of human participants and outlined the components of informed consent. We also discussed the ethical violations seen in scientific misconduct in which unscrupulous researchers may have fabricated their data or intentionally misinterpreted the findings of an investigation.

The present section has to do with ethical considerations that revolve around the process of publishing research. The American Speech-Language-Hearing Association has published a guidelines document prepared by the ASHA committee for research integrity and publication practices (ASHA, 2007). In the guidelines, the focus is on the process of publication rather than on protection of human participants. Some of the ASHA view is based on the work of the American Association for the Advancement of Science guidelines. We elaborate on some of the important points in the following sections.

Ethical Considerations in Planning the Study and Specifying Roles.   When a study is planned, there should be some thought put into determining who will be making contributions to the investigation, because this bears on who will receive authorship on any published version of the project. Obviously, this consideration applies more to practitioners who collaborate on research than it applies to thesis/dissertation/ capstone students. Even students, however, will be faced with issues of authorship to some degree. For example, even though the student will take the primary responsibility for a research project such as a thesis, the major professor will doubtless spend considerable time in helping to plan the study and perhaps in the data analysis, depending on the student's familiarity with statistical methods. The major professor will also contribute to the editing process as the thesis goes through the various stages of development. A thesis director may also play a major role in helping to cut down the thesis project into a reasonable draft of an article for submission to a journal. Thus, depending on the input contributed by the involved parties, the student should consider at the outset of the thesis project that he or she and the major professor might have to decide on authorship of an article. Typically, the student is first author on his or her thesis project, with the major professor as the second author, just based on the workload during the project. It is always a good idea at the outset of a thesis project to mention the future publication of the results and discuss how authorship will be handled. It is especially important when practitioners collaborate in research to define roles and contributions and determine who will get authorship and in what order the authors will appear on the manuscript to reflect their contributions. The ASHA guidelines mentioned indicate that we should guard against "ghost authorships" or "honorary authorships" of published articles. This means that we should not simply tack someone's name onto an article if they did not make a substantive contribution. An example might be to give authorship to thesis committee members who did not make substantial contributions to the project other than reading the prospectus and making a few suggestions, which is part of their normally expected role as a committee member. An example from practitioner research might be to give authorship to a professional such as a school principal who allowed access to participants in his or her school system but had nothing to do with actually conducting the research. Of course, anyone who helped in an ancillary way with the project can be noted in an acknowledgement at the end of the article to give credit for limited participation.

Another ethical consideration in conducting a research project is the attitude of the investigators and their professional behavior throughout the study. It is expected that all members of the research team will have respect for the scientific process, coinvestigators, procedures, and participants. Furthermore, it is expected that all research data will be safeguarded to protect confidentiality both during the experiment and after the study has concluded, as mentioned in an earlier section.

Ethics in Writing the Research Article.   Resnik (2001) discusses several practices that have definite ethical implications. First, he says that an article should report the complete results of the study. A researcher should not eliminate data that do not go along with his or her hypotheses by eliminating extreme scores. Resnik calls this "trimming" the data. Second, Resnik says we should not engage in "fudging" of data that involves making a finding appear more important than it actually is. One example might be to construct a graph showing a large difference between data points because of the scale used, when the difference was actually small. Third, a researcher should avoid "cooking the data" by selecting a statistical procedure that shows a significant result when other, more accepted methods may show no significant difference. Fourth, Resnik decries the practice of "salami science," in which a researcher takes a single study and turns it into several articles in order to earn more publications. If the study was done as a whole, it should not be "sliced and diced" into multiple studies unless the project was so large that it is not possible to present it in a single article.

Even after a study is submitted and accepted for publication in a journal, it is incumbent on the researcher to retain some degree of control over the data so that other scientists can ask questions about the investigation or actually see the data to verify specific conclusions. If a researcher finds that an error was made in analyzing data or writing up the results, even after the study is published, it is important to report this error to the journal so that appropriate errata can be printed in some future issue alerting consumers of the problem.

Submission of the Manuscript for Publication.   When the article is being prepared for submission, several ethical considerations are important. A rather obvious ethical issue is to avoid plagiarism. Although on the surface this can seem fairly simple, let's take a closer look. Over the course of reviewing the literature, an investigator will take copious notes about a host of different investigations. Sometimes it is easy to jot down phrases from an article because at the time they seem to crystallize the essence of a procedure or finding. After amassing notes on scores of different articles, it is easy to overlook the fact that you may have written some statements verbatim. It all gets mixed in with your own unique notes, and you may not remember that some statements were actually taken from an article. This is why it is important to always put verbatim statements in your notes in quotation marks and note the page you took them from. Then there will be no mistake. Paraphrasing of results or procedures is fine, but do not make the mistake of forgetting which lines are your own and which came from an article. Plagiarism is a serious ethical problem, so try to err on the side of caution. Interestingly, it is even an ethical problem to plagiarize *from your own writings* (i.e., "self-plagiarism") if they are copyrighted in a journal.

Most journals will ask authors submitting manuscripts to indicate whether they have any conflicts of interest in the research outcome. For example, if a researcher was acting as a consultant for a company that manufactured a new device for the treatment of swallowing disorders, which was the subject of the research, it should be indicated that the researcher was receiving such support. If there is any way that the researcher could have a vested interest in the outcome of the study, it should be admitted at the outset to the journal editor.

Another ethical issue involved in submitting an article is that you will only submit a particular manuscript to one journal at a time. Duplicate submissions are not allowed, so you cannot send out multiple copies of a manuscript and simply wait until one is accepted by some journal. When you do submit an article, make sure that the manuscript is prepared in accordance with the guidelines of the journal to which you are submitting the work. Most journals will ask authors to sign a cover letter indicating that they are not submitting their work to multiple journals simultaneously, that they actually did the work, and that they have no conflict of interest in the outcome of the project.

Interestingly, even the editorial process engaged in by journals is under ethical guidelines. For example, reviewers and editors must indicate whether they have a bias or conflict of interest related to a study that will be the subject of their review. If a reviewer is acting as a consultant for a company that makes a new device to reduce stuttering and the study to be reviewed has found that the device does not work very well, this could constitute a conflict of interest in the review process. Similarly, if the reviewer simply has a well-known bias against a particular theory and the study to be reviewed is attempting to validate that theory, the reviewer should consider abstaining from the process.

Collaborative Research by Practitioners

Early in the present text we suggested that collaboration between professionals working in the field either with other colleagues in their setting or with university faculty is an excellent way to engage in applied clinical research. Some issues that are pertinent to such collaborations will be discussed next. This section will be shorter than the student research portion presented previously because some of the issues are similar to those already discussed.

Finding a Collaborator

The work setting of which you are a part may offer many opportunities for joint research efforts. Whether you work in a medical or school setting, there are typically other specialists in communication disorders who may be interested in developing and implementing a research project. This is especially true if there are issues that a research project can help to resolve, such as development of new screening procedures, determining the efficacy of an existing treatment program, or instituting a new one. Also, within the work setting, professionals from other disciplines such as physical therapy, occupational therapy, education, special education, psychology, medicine, and social work all have issues that could be illuminated by interdisciplinary research.

Outside the work setting, we have already indicated that nearby colleges or universities have faculty members who are interested in conducting research and would most likely jump at the chance to collaborate with workers in "real-world" settings. If nothing else, such faculty might be willing to serve as a consultant in your research even if they do not participate as collaborators. Also, collaboration with other settings similar to your own school system or medical facility may be productive avenues to explore.

The first step in developing a research collaboration is to make it known that you are interested in conducting a scientific investigation. Collaboration will not happen until at least one person projects an interest in research and talks about the possibilities with other people. Thus, your willingness to "talk it up" is important, and it is also crucial that you reinforce other professionals when they mention an idea for a research project. In some work settings professionals set aside time each month to discuss current research trends in meetings such as journal clubs to facilitate continuing education. Sometimes professionals are asked to provide a recap of a conference they attended, and this is also a good platform to suggest research ideas to colleagues. If there is a university in your area, pay a visit to the faculty members you might collaborate with and let them know of your interest. The point here is that a research project will never happen without an ongoing effort to discuss research and brainstorm ideas. It is a good idea to invite professionals from other disciplines as well as university faculty to some of these meetings so that a broader perspective can be considered in potential research projects. You might be surprised at how receptive these other professionals will be to the prospect of engaging in a joint research project.

The Idea and Research Questions

The notion of collaboration implies a two-way street in terms of developing ideas and research questions. It is ideal if the research idea can encompass perspectives from all of the people involved. There is often much common ground to be discovered when people start talking about their jobs, their interests, and their past experiences. The group members will also have many questions that have occurred to them over the years and avenues of research that have been stimulated by articles, books, and conferences. It is good to have this general discussion at the beginning of a potential research collaboration and jot down areas of common interest that could be studied using resources available within the community. Once you have a list of general areas, it is only a matter of deciding to follow through on the design and implementation of a research project.

Designing the Study and Defining Roles

Once you have committed to doing a project with someone, it is important to outline the experimental design and the roles and responsibilities of everyone involved. As we discussed in the thesis/dissertation/capstone section, there are many details that need to be attended to in a research project. Luckily, in research done by practitioners, you do not have to worry about writing a prospectus that contains a lengthy literature review and detailed methodology. This, however, does not absolve you of the responsibility to review the literature to determine what has been done in your area of research interest. You don't have to write it up in the form of a prospectus, but you certainly should take notes on the articles you find that relate to your project. These notes will be used later when you write up the results of the project for an article or presentation. The research question, including independent and dependent variables, should be clearly stated just as it is done in a thesis or dissertation. As we will mention later in this section, the methodology should be written up with enough detail to serve as an IRB protocol. Also, any materials and equipment to be used in the study must be developed and assembled.

Sometimes the roles of collaborators will be defined by their work setting, their interest area, or their access to resources. A good idea is to divide up the responsibilities at the outset of the project. Each task can be done by a single person or in collaboration with another researcher, but the work should be divided equally so that no one feels as if they are doing a disproportionate amount of the work. The following major tasks have to be accomplished:

- *Review of the literature.* This does not have to be a lengthy paper that is written up formally, but notes should be taken about resources for later reference.
- *IRB protocol.* Once the study is designed, the researchers will have to obtain approval of the IRB either at the university, public school system, or hospital. As mentioned in the section on writing student research projects, the IRB protocol largely consists of the methods to be used in the study and development of an informed consent document. This is roughly equivalent to the methodology section of a thesis, with about a one-page review and justification for the study.
- *Obtaining equipment/instrumentation.* In some cases, equipment will already be available in the university setting, school system, or hospital. If not available, arrangements must be made to get any equipment necessary to conduct the study. In some cases a small grant can be written to obtain funds. Other necessities such as data sheets, stimuli, instruction sheets, counterbalancing schedules, and so on should be developed prior to the conduct of the study.
- *Finding participants.* In many cases, one of the collaborators may already have access to a population that could be used in the research. Collaborators who work in a school system or medical environment may find some potential participants already available. In other cases, a person who works in a school system or medical setting may have connections with other professionals who work in similar environments and can use these personal contacts to obtain permission to gather data in those settings.
- *Gathering data.* The gathering of data from participants can be done by a variety of people. If a university faculty member is involved, perhaps research assistants will be available for such duties. If not, collaborators can divide the time for gathering data in a way that is fair to all concerned.
- *Analyzing data.* If data analysis such as coding of audio or video tapes or disks is involved, any trained person can participate in this phase of the study. Statistical

analyses may best be left to the person on the team with access to computer programs and expertise in quantitative methods.

Writing up a Presentation and Journal Article

Writing a presentation or journal article is essentially similar to the general guidelines provided in the section on thesis/dissertation/capstone research. The major difference in writing an article with a colleague is that you will not have a large thesis or dissertation to work from. You will recall that turning a thesis into an article involves mainly cutting information from the detailed version presented to the graduate school. If you are writing an article with a colleague, the only part that is already written is probably the methodology section that you turned in to the IRB for approval. Thus, sections such as the review of the literature, the results, and the discussion are not yet written and must be produced for purposes of an article. The writing must be economical because you do not have an infinite number of pages as in a dissertation when crafting an article. You must think of the finished product as an article, not as a thesis or dissertation. As such, the review of the literature will probably be less than ten typed pages, double spaced. The method will probably be another five to ten pages. Finally the results and discussion should total another ten pages, depending on the extent of the analyses performed. Thus, the double-spaced, typed manuscript will probably be less than forty to fifty pages. Many articles can be substantially less than that if the study was more limited in scope. The guideline for presentations is similar to our earlier section in which the product is even more abbreviated.

Summary

As mentioned in Chapter 1, the production of research and its publication is an important scientific contribution. But beyond the science, such publications bring the attention of colleagues to the people who perform the research and the institutions with which they are affiliated. There is excitement at every step in the research process, from coming up with the idea, to gathering the data, to analyzing the data, to writing up the results and seeing the finished product appear in a journal or convention program. Both students and practitioners can participate in this exciting process for both personal and professional gratification.

LEARNING ACTIVITIES

1. Examine three finished theses/dissertations/capstone projects from your department in your area of interest.

2. Interview a student who is currently engaged in graduate-level research.

3. Download your university's guidelines for thesis or dissertation projects.

APPENDIX 16A

Selected Questions to Address in Writing Research Proposals or Articles Based on Student/Practitioner Research

Title

- Did you include enough appropriate descriptors so that search engines can identify your research?
- Did you mention the types of participants and the independent and dependent variables?

Introduction

- Did you provide a general statement of the problem area to be studied?
- Did the introduction set the stage for a more detailed review of the literature?

Review of Literature

- Did you include the most current research related to the research area?
- Did you include enough older research to provide a historical perspective and evidence of a thorough review of the literature?
- Did you include peer-reviewed research from journals, textbooks, and convention presentations showing an exhaustive examination of the area?
- Did you include operational definitions of the variables you are interested in studying?
- Did you include any theoretical perspectives that might be important to understanding the research area?

Justification

- Did you present a logical argument from the review of the literature that leads to the research questions?
- Are your research questions answerable with the scientific method?
- Do your research questions specify some relationship or difference between two or more variables?
- Do the questions allow for the specification of the independent and dependent variables?

Methodology

Participants

- Did you specify the number of participants?
- Did you determine the statistical power of the study when selecting number of participants?

- Did you use random selection of participants?
- Did you use random assignment of participants to conditions?
- Was your sample selected based only on convenience?
- Did you have specific exclusion and inclusion criteria for participants?
- If participants were normally developing, how was this determined?
- If participants were disordered, how was this determined?
- What were the participant demographics in terms of culture, gender, SES, age, intelligence, bilingualism, geography, or other relevant variables?
- Did the participants sign an informed consent form and was the project approved by the IRB?
- Did you include a table summarizing relevant characteristics of the participants?
- Did you control for other relevant factors in the participants such as background history, time post-onset of problem, medications, habits (e.g., smoking), medical problems, psychological problems, history of treatment, noise exposure, and any other specific behaviors related to your study?
- Did you control for any threats to internal and external validity that could be a product of participant selection, exclusion, inclusion, or grouping?

Instrumentation

- Did you describe all instrumentation used in the study in terms of brand and model number, including every piece of equipment (microphones, speakers, filters, amplifiers, etc.)?
- If human judges were used, did you describe how they were selected, trained, and used in the study?
- Did you provide evidence of validity for the measurements you took, whether they were electronic instruments, standardized tests, human judges, or mechanical devices?
- If you developed a new measurement for the study, did you describe how it was constructed, piloted, and validated?
- Did you describe the calibration of equipment and how often calibration was checked during the study?
- Did you describe the experimental environment in detail, including location of the study, room size, ambient noise, room arrangement, reverberation, specifications of sound-treated booths, and the physical locations of participants, experimenters, and equipment?
- Did you describe in detail all types of stimuli used in the study such as sounds, tones, reading material, pictures, masking noise, and so on?
- Did you provide some measure of inter- or intrajudge reliability of measurements taken in the study?
- Did you provide some measure of test-retest reliability of measurements taken in the study?
- Did you implement single, double, or triple blinding when appropriate in the study?
- Did you control for instrumentation threats to internal and external validity?

Procedures

- Is your description of the methodology specific enough for the reader to understand the actual procedures a participant went through in the study?
- Is the order of procedures clearly explained?
- Were any counterbalancing or randomization procedures clearly explained?
- Did you explain instructions given to participants for each condition in the study and provide verbatim transcripts of such instructions?
- Did you adequately describe any interfacing of equipment with the participants, such as placement of electrodes, distance from speakers, distance from microphones, and so on?
- Did you adequately describe any breaks between conditions or time elapsed between multiple experimental sessions?
- Did you control threats to internal and external validity related to procedures such as order effects, experimenter bias, maturation, history, or regression effects?

Data Reduction

- Were the specific procedures for reducing participant performance down into quantifiable data adequately explained (including scoring of tests, obtaining electronic readouts of performance from instruments, collating judge's ratings, examining video or audio tapes for specific behaviors of interest, transcribing language samples, or live coding of events under study)?
- Who translated participant behaviors into quantifiable data for statistical analysis?
- Was blinding implemented when appropriate to control for experimenter bias?
- Was interjudge reliability computed to ensure that behaviors were reliably observed and counted?

Selection of Statistical Analyses

- Did you indicate which statistical analyses would be used to evaluate the data and why these were selected?
- Did you specify the alpha level used to determine significant differences or relationships?
- Were the selected statistics appropriate for the experimental design and the level of measurement represented by the data?
- Were appropriate summary statistics (central tendency, variation) selected to provide a general description of the groups under study?
- Were appropriate tests of homogeneity of variance considered in the case of diverse group variations?
- Were appropriate follow-up statistics considered such as post hoc tests following the analysis of variance?
- Were measures of effect size and variance accounted for considered to determine practical significance?

Results

- Were statistical analyses reported in tabular form and did they include all relevant data (e.g., degrees of freedom, *F*-ratio, etc.) necessary to interpret the results?
- Were measures of central tendency and variability reported?
- Were follow-up tests for homogeneity of variance used when groups were obviously different on summary statistics?
- Were measures of effect size reported?
- Were figures included when appropriate to illustrate results of study?

Discussion

- Did the discussion focus on the specific findings of the study and not go beyond the data?
- Did the discussion place the research findings into the context of prior research on the topic in terms of comparing and contrasting results to previous studies?
- Did the discussion make attempts to account for reasons why the results either agree or disagree with prior research (e.g., methods, measurements, etc.)?
- Did the discussion raise clinical implications of the results?
- Did the discussion deal with limitations of the study?
- Did the discussion suggest future research avenues?

CHAPTER 17

Grantsmanship: Funding Research Endeavors

Nothing in the world can take the place of Persistence. Talent will not; nothing is more common than unsuccessful men with talent. Genius will not; unrewarded genius is almost a proverb. Education will not; the world is full of educated derelicts. Persistence and determination alone are omnipotent. The slogan 'Press On' has solved and always will solve the problems of the human race.

—Calvin Coolidge (1872–1933)

If I had to select one quality, one personal characteristic that I regard as being most highly correlated with success, whatever the field, I would pick the trait of persistence. Determination. The will to endure to the end, to get knocked down seventy times and get up off the floor saying, "Here comes number seventy-one!"

—Richard M. DeVos

Persistence is the twin sister of excellence. One is a matter of quality; the other, a matter of time.

—Marabel Morgan, *The Electric Woman*

Does the thought of writing grants make your palms sweat? The process of designing a study, writing a proposal, preparing a budget, and then submitting the grant to a nameless, faceless panel of reviewers who may shoot holes in it is an intimidating prospect! Sound like fun? Well, it can be, and it may provide the necessary resources for completion of a project that is near and dear to your heart. Funding for research is available for investigators at all experience levels, from undergraduate students to seasoned research investigators.

LEARNING OBJECTIVES

The chapter will enable readers to:

- List some funding sources in communication sciences and disorders according to the experience level of the investigator.

- Prepare a grant application within the parameters of a specific competition.
- Discuss the grant review process.

Funding Sources in Communication Sciences and Disorders

Sources of funding in communication sciences and disorders depend on the background and experience level of the grant writer. Specific grant competitions or mechanisms vary based on an investigator's experience, profession, and area of expertise. Sources of funding are available for all levels of research, from beginners to independent researchers. Table 17.1 shows sources of funding and various grant mechanisms that are identified for various levels of investigative experience.

Four Types of Funding

There are four broad sources of funding for research in communication sciences and disorders: (1) intramural, (2) private industry, (3) the federal government, and (4) private foundations and professional organizations and societies. Intramural funding resources include support that come from within one's own college, university, or place of employment. For example, assistant professors may compete for internal grants aimed at collecting preliminary data for studies that will set the stages for future external grant proposals.

Private industry also funds research projects, particularly those aimed at conducting clinical trials of new products or devices. For example, the Janus Corporation of Greenville, North Carolina, recently funded several investigators to conduct clinical trials on their SpeechEasy, a device that fits in the ear much like an in-the-ear

---

TABLE 17.1

Some Funding Sources and Granting Mechanisms Based on the Experience Level of the Investigator

Source	Undergraduate	M.A./Ph.D./Au.D. Student	Post-Doc/New Investigator	Independent Investigator
Intramural	Research grant		Seed grant	
Private Foundations				
American Academy of Audiology		Student research grant	New investigator grant	
American Speech-Language-Hearing Foundation		Student research grant in audiology	New investigator grant	
		Student research grant in early childhood language	Speech science grant New Century Scholars Research grant	New Century Scholars Research grant
Deafness Research Foundation				
National Hearing Conservation Association	Research grant	Research grant		
National Organization for Hearing Research			Research grant	Research grant
Federal		F-31 T-32, T-35	Small grant (R-03) K-08, K-23, F-32	R-01

The "Level" spanning header covers the Undergraduate, M.A./Ph.D./Au.D. Student, Post-Doc/New Investigator, and Independent Investigator columns.

hearing aid and provides altered auditory feedback (AAF) to persons who stutter. One advantage of private funding sources is a reduction in the amount of time from grant submission to receipt of funding seen in government grant competitions. Private funding sources also may not require adherence to high standards of rigor typically required for approval from government offices such as the Food and Drug Administration (Cummings, Holly, & Hulley, 2001). Some of the disadvantages of private funding are adherence to company research protocols and a tendency to discount negative results.

The federal government supports research in communication sciences and disorders through agencies such as the National Institutes of Health (NIH). The National Institute on Deafness and Other Communication Disorders (NIDCD) is one of twenty-four different components of the National Institutes of Health (NIH). The NIDCD supports biomedical and behavioral research on both normal and disordered processes of balance, hearing, language, smell, speech, taste, and voice (NIDCD, 2007). The research can be conducted intramurally (i.e., within the NIH) or extramurally (i.e., by nonfederal scientists). It should be noted that some speech, language, and hearing scientists are funded through other institutes than the NIDCD, such as through the National Institute on Aging (NIA/NIH) or the National Institute of Neurological Disorders and Stroke (NINDS/NIH).

Private foundations frequently provide funding for research, particularly on topics in their designated areas of focus. For example, the Deafness Research Foundation (DRF) funds research projects on the following topics:

- Hearing and balance restoration
- Cochlear reenergization
- Genetic hearing loss
- Acoustic trauma (noise-induced hearing loss)
- Tinnitus (ringing in the ears) and hyperacusis (decreased tolerance of sound)
- Vestibular and balance disorders (dizziness and vertigo)
- Temporal bone research

Some foundations are focused on audiology/hearing science, some on speech-language pathology. The American Academy of Audiology Foundation (AAAF) has a mission of supporting promising programs in education, research, and public awareness in audiology and hearing science. Alternatively, the Voice Foundation, more pertinent to speech-language pathology, has a mission of promoting "the gift of vocal communication" on many fronts, including the support of research through grants. In addition, the American Speech-Language-Hearing Foundation (ASHF) has a mission to "advance knowledge about the causes and treatment of hearing, speech, and language problems" in several areas, including funding the research of investigators at various stages of training or career. We will discuss some of these foundations' grant problems later in the chapter.

Studies that do not directly pertain to these areas of focus may be of lower priority for funding.

Levels of Investigative Experience

Funding mechanisms are frequently defined by the level of experience of the investigator. Figure 17.1 shows the continuum of investigative experience for students and clinicians as well as the inverse relationship between the need for supervision and the level of independence. For example, most undergraduates need direct one-on-one supervision during their first experiences as a research assistant for a faculty member or in the completion of a senior honors thesis. Graduate students in speech-language pathology typically need less supervision in completing a master's thesis, maybe only requiring weekly meetings with their major professor. Likewise, students may need similar amounts of supervision in undertaking a capstone project in partial fulfillment of requirements for their doctor of audiology (Au.D.) degree.

As mentioned in other chapters of this textbook, the doctor of philosophy (Ph.D.) is for students interested in a career in research and university teaching. The culmination of these programs is the defense of the doctoral dissertation, an original research project completed under the direction of the student's major professor with the advisement of a committee. In addition to completing their dissertation, new Ph.D.s may be coauthors on a few articles but are just beginning to develop their own research programs.

Sometimes, attainment of a Ph.D. is followed by two or three years of postdoctoral training in a productive research laboratory headed by a senior scientist who has a track record of external funding. Alternatively, some new Ph.D.s may forgo

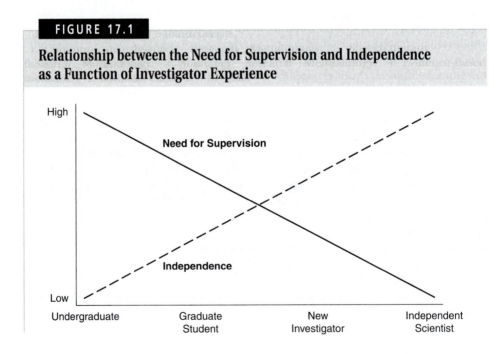

FIGURE 17.1

Relationship between the Need for Supervision and Independence as a Function of Investigator Experience

postdoctoral training and accept assistant professorships at colleges or universities. Both postdoctoral trainees and assistant professors are considered new investigators for at least five but usually no more than seven years beyond receipt of their terminal degrees. Moreover, this period of time is equivalent to most probationary periods for junior faculty, culminating with a tenure and promotion decision. Hopefully, at this point, individuals have developed a focused and independent research program as a senior faculty member. Students and clinicians interested in developing their research skills either through executing a single project or planning a research career should be aware of the availability of various sources of funding.

Specific Granting Mechanisms Appropriate for Various Levels of Investigative Experience

Undergraduate Students

Funding for undergraduate students is frequently available through intramural campus sources and from private foundations. For example, many universities have competitive undergraduate research fellowship programs that fund projects lasting from one to two years. Students in university honors programs frequently use these funding mechanisms to support their senior honors theses. Customarily, these programs have some minimum criteria for participation such as advanced class standing and a 3.0 grade point average. Students require a mentor to assist with proposal preparation and supervision of the research effort. Finding a mentor may seem intimidating to undergraduate students. However, most faculty members are aware of these programs and enjoy mentoring young scholars, particularly if the topic of investigations is related to their area of expertise. Faculty sponsors are usually required to attend an orientation session on effective mentoring and must agree to supervise the fellow in the execution of the research. The selection committee is often composed of faculty from a broad range of disciplines, thus accommodating a breadth of topic areas and research.

An example of a private foundation or society providing funding for undergraduate research includes the National Hearing Conservation Association (NHCA). For example, the National Hearing Conservation Association Scholarship Foundation annually awards two $1500 scholarships to undergraduate or graduate students focusing on applied or practical studies in hearing-loss prevention or hearing conservation at regionally accredited U.S. institutions. The funds are designed to assist with student research studies such as special projects, theses, or dissertations relating to hearing-loss prevention and hearing conservation.

Graduate Students

Funding for graduate students can be internal to the university or external through private foundations or federal programs. Faculty members are excellent resources in directing students to potential funding sources, such as the American Speech-Language-Hearing Foundation grant programs for graduate students (e.g., the Student Research Grant in Audiology and the Student Research Grant in Early Childhood Language for speech-language pathology students). Both grant programs require a mentor to supervise the research project. Customarily, mentors must write a letter of support to append to the student's grant proposal. Typically, the mentor is the chair of the student's master's thesis or doctoral dissertation committee. However, students wishing to do a research project for an independent study may also apply (see www .ashfoundation.org). Audiology students enrolled in Ph.D. or Au.D. programs may also compete in the Annual Student Research Competition sponsored by the American Academy of Audiology Foundation (see www.audiologyfoundation.org). These are all excellent programs for funding of graduate or professional student research.

So far, we have discussed funding mechanisms through private foundations. The federal government also has funding sources for students completing a Ph.D. program. The NIDCD-NIH may seem like a cold, uncaring governmental agency that could not possibly be sensitive to the needs of graduate students seeking funding. However, nothing could be farther from the truth! In fact, initial contact with appropriate program officers is but one e-mail or phone call away. **Program officers** are staff members at the NIDCD who assist applicants by serving as a contact person, preapplication advocate, postreview guide, and postaward activity manager (Sklare, 2007). These individuals can assess the appropriateness of a proposal's scientific focus to the funding agency. For doctoral students, the NIDCD has research training and development awards for pre- and postdoctoral training known as the Ruth L. Kirschstein National Research Service Awards. Awards can be individual fellowships (e.g., F-31) or traineeships on institutional training grants (e.g., T-32 or T-35). In particular, the Ruth L. Kirschstein National Research Awards for Individual Predoctoral Fellows, F-31, provide two to three years of support during the dissertation stage (see www.nidcd.nih.gov). Alternatively, students may find research funding through their departmental training grants. For example, the Institutional National Research Service Awards Training Grants (T32) are awarded to nonprofit or public institutions or to predoctoral and/or postdoctoral trainees. Similarly, the Ruth L. Kirschstein National Service Award Short-Term Training Grants (T35) are awarded to the same types of entities as the T32 awards and provide short-term, intensive training for students in the health professions (e.g., Au.D. students).

New Investigators

The next level involves new investigators or those having less than about five years of experience past obtaining their doctoral degrees. The NIDCD-NIH's Ruth L. Kirschstein National Service Awards for Postdoctoral Fellows (F-32) offer a stipend, tuition and fees, and an institutional allowance for additional research training. Postdoctoral fellows should consult their program directors about sources of funding. New faculty members are advised to plan a visit to their university's office of sponsored programs, which has staff who actively seek sources of funding for investigators. It is important that these staff personnel are aware of investigators' areas of expertise so that they may relay information about potential funding sources. Investigators should also consider subscribing to services that provide information about public and private sources of funding, such as the Community of Science (COS), The Foundation Center, and Sponsored Projects Information Network (SPIN). Appendix 17A has web addresses for these resources.

New investigator research programs typically offer smaller of amounts of money for one to two years of support of projects whose purpose is collecting pilot data for larger grant applications. For example, the American Speech-Language-Hearing Foundation (ASHF) has two such grant competitions. The New Investigator Grant Competition is open to audiologists and speech-language pathologists who have graduated within the last five years. In addition, the Research Grant in Speech Science is for speech scientists who have also graduated within the past five years. Similarly, the American Academy of Audiology Foundation also has a New Investigator Research Grant program for audiologists who received their doctoral degrees within the same time frame.

The NIDCD-NIH has programs aimed at developing new investigators into senior scientists. The NIDCD's Mentored Clinician-Investigator Career Development Programs (i.e., K-08—Mentored Clinical Scientist Development Award and K-23—Mentored Patient-Oriented Research Career Development Award) are awarded to applicants who have significant prior research experience and have the highest potential to develop into an independent clinician-investigator (Sklare, 2007). Applicants must have a primary sponsor (i.e., mentor) within the same institution or within a reasonable distance. The Small Grant Program (R-03) through the NIDCD-NIH is for new investigators who are no more than seven years beyond receipt of their terminal degrees. R-03 grants require relatively short proposals (ten pages or less) and can prepare new investigators for writing future full-scale grants (Firszt, 2007). This grant program provides resources (e.g., $100,000 annually for up to three years) for research projects of limited scope that may result in preliminary data for a competitive R-01 grant, the funding program for independent researchers.

Independent Investigators

Experienced investigators may also compete for grants from nearly all of these sources of funding. However, they are often held to higher standards than new investigators. For example, university competitive grant-in-aid programs tend to give priority to new faculty in awarding seed money, but senior faculty are also considered if they are embarking on a new line of research. In addition, seasoned investigators may compete for the New Century Scholars Research Grant Competition sponsored by the ASHF, but the proposed project should not be for any established or funded research efforts. Similarly, the Deafness Research Foundation accepts new and innovative projects developed by established scientists, but they may only apply for one year of support. The NIDCD expects experienced investigators to compete for funding through the R-01 funding mechanism.

Preparing a Grant Application

The old adage, "A failure to plan is a plan to fail" especially applies to preparing a grant application. Besides perseverance, other important qualities for successful grant applications are time management and the ability to follow directions. We will use the New Century Scholars Research Grant Competition (NCSRG) announcement for an example of how to prepare a grant application. It is important to note, however, that many of the basic procedures and components of this type of grant application, and indeed, the process of applying, can be representative of any funding competition. So those of you who will seek grant support working in schools or medical settings will have similar issues to deal with. We chose the NCSRG to use as our example because it involves procedures found in more rigorous grant applications. Some intramural or other private funding sources may not require such rigor, but we would rather that readers see a more comprehensive process as an example. In addition, it is advised that readers interested in this specific grant program should contact the American-Speech-Language-Hearing Foundation.

Let's pretend that the investigator is an associate professor in communication sciences and disorders at a major university who is considering establishing a focused line of funded research. The proposed project is for the purpose of collecting pilot data for submitting a large federal grant application. The investigator was alerted to this competition by a colleague, has downloaded the grant announcement, and is in the preproposal stage. We will examine the document closely to demonstrate how to prepare a grant application. Figure 17.2 presents the grant announcement and a discussion of the nature of the competition.

FIGURE 17.2

Example Grant Application: Nature of the Competition

The American Speech-Language-Hearing Foundation (ASHF) invites investigators to submit proposals in competition for five $10,000 research grants. This grant initiative is designed to advance the knowledge base in communication sciences and disorders. The competition does not restrict proposal type or content area, but will give priority to studies that are innovative, groundbreaking, or that can meet research needs not yet addressed. The intent of this grant is to initiate new research in the field and funding can be applied to a one- or two-year investigation.

The ASHFoundation is able to offer this special competition as a result of its *Dreams and Possibilities Campaign* initiative. This campaign raised over $1.9 million to support doctoral education and research in the field of communication sciences and disorders. The intention of this research program is to support investigations by individuals who are committed to teacher-investigator careers in the university/college academic environment or in external research institutes or laboratories.

The research grants are not intended to provide additional or extended support for an established and funded research effort. They are intended to support new research ideas and directions for investigators who are not currently funded in the proposed area of investigation, including new investigators. Proposals for work that can be accomplished in 1–2 years with the $10,000 grant and/or for pilot work in a demonstrably new area by experienced investigators are also welcomed.

Deadline for receipt of applications and proposals is **April 9, 2007.** Selection of recipients will be completed and funding will be disbursed in November of 2007. Potential applicants should read the section on eligibility carefully and, upon determining that all criteria are met, follow application procedures on page 2.

Reprinted by permission of American Speech-Language-Hearing Foundation. www.ashfoundation.org.

The description of the nature of the competition helps investigators determine if the grant mechanism suits the needs of their project. For example, the NCSRG program invites investigators to compete for five $10,000 grants for projects lasting from one to two years. The general spirit of the program is to expand the knowledge base in communication sciences and disorders and is particularly suited for applicants committed to teacher-investigator careers in university or college academic environments or external research institutes. Therefore, the program is not intended for clinician-scientists working in hospital settings, for example. The program is aimed at supporting new research ideas for investigators who are not currently funded in the particular area of investigation. Therefore, the grant program is not designed to provide funding for established lines of research for seasoned investigators, although they may submit proposals for work outside their current line of inquiry. In summary, investigators should use information about the nature of the competition to determine if their circumstances meet the spirit of the grant program. For our hypothetical example, in general, the NCSRG seems well-suited for the purpose of our investigator who must consider other eligibility criteria presented in Figure 17.3.

The investigator in our example, now serious about preparing a proposal for this competition, inspects the eligibility requirements. It is important to note that

FIGURE 17.3

Example Grant Application: Eligibility

In order to be eligible to receive the 2007 Research Grant, individuals must meet the following criteria:

1. The applicant must have received a PhD or equivalent research doctorate within the discipline of communication sciences and disorders.

   Note: Due to availability of student research grant and scholarship competitions through the ASH-Foundation, students enrolled in a degree program or working on dissertation research are **not** eligible for this award.

2. The applicant must demonstrate the potential for and commitment to conducting independent research.

3. The research must have significance and direct application to communication sciences and disorders.

4. The setting where the research will be pursued must be an environment conducive to completing the investigation.

5. Experienced investigators should provide an explanation of why the proposed work represents new effort that is not fundable from existing research support nor an extension of funding that is currently supporting the work. With regard to funding, experienced investigators are those whose current or recent professional history indicates "principal investigator" or "co-investigator" status on research funding with direct costs exceeding $50,000 from agencies other than the investigator's host institution.

6. Preference for funding consideration will be given to ASHA members.

Reprinted by permission of American Speech-Language-Hearing Foundation. www.ashfoundation.org.

criteria are either **objective** (e.g., concrete requirements of the competition such as deadlines) or are more **subjective** (e.g., those influencing reviewers' impressions), mandating greater effort on the part of the applicant for qualification within the proposal. For example, items 1, 5, and 6 are objective criteria that are easily verifiable, such as earning a Ph.D., experience of the investigator, and ASHA membership, respectively. However, applicants must ensure that their proposals *convince* reviewers regarding the more subjective criteria of their potential to conduct independent research and their commitment to the process (item 2), the significance and direct application of the proposal to communication sciences and disorders (item 3), and the suitability of the proposed environment for conducting the experiment (item 4) in appropriate sections of the application.

Next, the investigator reviews the application and submission procedures, which are shown in Figure 17.4. Investigators need to follow these instructions very carefully,

---

FIGURE 17.4

Example Grant Application: Application and Submission Procedures

Providing that all eligibility requirements are met, applicants should prepare a research proposal following the attached *Guidelines for Preparation of Proposals.*

The applicant should provide a letter of application addressed to "Grant Review Committee." Indicate briefly why you are pursuing the proposed study, the aims of the proposed research, and how the project fits into your career development plan. Include, as appropriate, information relative to your research interests and activities to date. Specifically indicate how your institution will support your research efforts.

Submit the original application form with all accompanying documents and six additional complete sets of the original packet to the address shown below. Please attach each individual packet with paperclips, *do not* use staples. The ASHFoundation must receive these seven assembled packets no later than April 9, 2007.

American Speech-Language-Hearing Foundation
New Century Scholars Program
2007 Research Grant Competition
10801 Rockville Pike
Rockville, MD 20852
Attn: Emily Diaz

In addition to hard copy submissions, applicants should transmit an electronic version of the entire proposal (Guideline Sections 1–9) to newcenturygrants@ashfoundation.org. A PDF file is preferred but a Word or Rich Text File is also acceptable. Please place the title "NCSRG proposal" in the subject box. This process will enable expert grant reviewers using an NIH study section process to access investigator submissions.

No extensions will be granted beyond the April 9 deadline and FAX copies will not be accepted. Confirmation that your application has been received will be sent by e-mail if you include an e-mail contact address.

Reprinted by permission of American Speech-Language-Hearing Foundation. www.ashfoundation.org.

because no matter how innovative and meritorious a proposal may be, failure to comply with rules of submission may preclude review of the grant application. For example, principal investigators must submit the original and six paper-clipped, not stapled, copies of the proposal, which must be received by April 9 at the ASHF. Investigators must carefully check their calendars to ensure that a quality proposal can be prepared in time. Often, it is better to forgo the opportunity rather than submit a poorly prepared grant application. Principal investigators should send their packets to the address *exactly* as specified in the instructions so that it arrives on time in the hands of the appropriate official. In addition, an electronic copy (i.e., PDF file is preferred, but a Word or Rich Text file is also acceptable) should be sent to newcentury grants@ashfoundation.org with the title "NCSRG" in the subject window. Failure to follow directions may disqualify an otherwise competitive grant application.

Each proposal must contain a letter addressed to the grant review committee. The cover letter is an opportunity to explain why the project is being done, its specific aims, how it fits into the investigator's overall career development plan, and how the institution will support the research effort. The letter is an excellent way to convince reviewers of the fulfillment of the subjective eligibility criteria mentioned earlier. For example, applicants should convey with enthusiasm their suitability to conduct the investigation, the significance and application of the project to the profession, and how the institution will support their efforts.

Next, the investigator should carefully examine the evaluation criteria used by the reviewers in assessing grant proposals. Figure 17.5 shows the evaluation criteria

---

FIGURE 17.5

Example Grant Application: Evaluation Criteria

An evaluation of proposals by an expert review panel will follow these weighted criteria.

CRITERIA	VALUE
a. Evidence of the applicant's potential for and commitment to conducting research activities.	20
b. Clearly stated project objectives and significance of the research, including its impact on communication sciences and disorders.	20
c. Scientific and technical merit of the research question, design, and methodology for addressing the research need, completing the project within the identified time period, and evaluating the project results.	30
d. Indication of the facilities, resources, subjects, and/or professional affiliation to which the applicant would have access in order to carry out the activities described in the proposal.	10
e. Management plan that clearly outlines the proposed project activities and related timeliness. The plan must be accompanied by a budget detailing the allocation of the $10,000 grant to specific project expense items.	20
Maximum Points Possible	100

Reprinted by permission of American Speech-Language-Hearing Foundation. www.ashfoundation.org.

that are based on a point system, with weighted values assigned to different criteria. Applicants are advised to keep the evaluation criteria at hand when preparing the actual grant application.

The next step involves carefully preparing the proposal in accordance with the guidelines that appear in Figure 17.6. Note that the proposal has nine sections: (1) Investigator Application Form, (2) Abstract, (3) Investigator's Research Experience, (4) Research Plan, (5) Management Plan, (6) Budget, (7) Human Subjects, (8) Bibliography and Appendices, as appropriate, and (9) Letters of Support. For this competition, proposals must be typed and double spaced using a 12-point noncompressed font and margins of at least one inch. Notice that each section has page limitations (e.g., Research Plan must be six pages or less). Investigators must resist any temptation to violate formatting requirements in order to meet page limitations. The administrative staff checks for formatting violations and will disqualify proposals from the competition if they occur. Revising a proposal into a clearer and more concise document is always a better plan.

The first component of the proposal is the Investigator Application Form, shown in Appendix 17B. Applicants may find it difficult to come up with a title that best reflects their project. Developing a title may be easier at the end of the grant-writing process when investigators have a clearer vision of their project. Section IV on Research Feasibility asks for a description of the investigator's time distribution among research, teaching, and service responsibilities. Typically, in academic settings time allotment is designated by full-time equivalent (FTE) units in which 1.0 represents full-time employment, working 40 hours per week. For example, academic faculty may have 0.6 FTE (60%) for teaching, 0.3 FTE (30%) for research, and 0.1 FTE (10%) for service. Department or unit heads should be consulted to determine the amount of time to allot to the project. For those employed in other settings, investigators should specify how much time may be devoted to the project.

The Abstract section should concisely describe the project's focus, specific aims, methodology, and long-term objectives, specifying its impact on the field of communication sciences and disorders. The clearer the investigator's vision of the project, the easier the abstract is to write. Applicants may find use of a structured format helpful in organizing pieces of information into different sections of an abstract. Briefly, recall that a structured abstract is a format in which headings (e.g., Purpose, Methods, Results, and Conclusions) are used in summarizing a study. Investigators might consider using the following headings for their abstract: Project Focus, Specific Aims, Methodology, Long-Term Objectives, and Impact on the Profession. Similar to devising a title for the proposal, some may find it easier to write the abstract last.

The Investigator's Research Experience section should be limited to one page and address interests, past training, and productivity in the specific area of pursuit. Recall that the evaluation criteria allotted twenty out of the hundred maximum points possible for reviewers' assessment of the applicant's potential for and commitment to conducting research activities. Again, this part of the proposal is another opportunity to convince reviewers of the investigator's enthusiasm and preparedness to complete the proposed project. Investigators should mention any special training

FIGURE 17.6

Example Grant Application: Guidelines for Preparation of Proposals

Proposals should be typed, double spaced, and should include the following information in the order indicated. Font size should be set at 12 point, noncompressed font with margins of at least 1 inch. Please include section headings in your proposal and number pages. Carefully follow page limits for each section. Any page(s) exceeding the limitation will be removed before circulation to the review panelists.

1. **Investigator Application Form** (2 pages, form attached) Complete all sections on the investigator application form.

2. **Abstract** (limit to 1 page)
   Concisely describe the project's focus, specific aims, methodology, and long-term objectives. Address the clinical application(s) of the study's outcome. Describe the impact of the project and its activities on the field of communication sciences and disorders.

3. **Investigator's Research Experience** (limit to 1 page)
   Address your interests, experiences, and productivity in the area of clinical research. Append a current copy of your professional *curriculum vitae* and include a listing of scientific or professional presentations and publications.

4. **Research Plan** (limit to 6 pages)
   a. Objectives and Significance
   Present the problem or issue to be addressed and the specific objectives for addressing it within the proposed investigation. This section should also outline the significance of the clinical need which exists and the importance of the proposed project in understanding, diagnosing, remediating or compensating for the problem. Address the potential impact of the project's activities on the field of communication sciences and disorders.

   b. Design and Methodology
   Provide a description and justification for the project design. Include subjects, measurement techniques (including reliability and control measures), instrumentation, data analysis, and evaluation procedures. This section should provide sufficient detail to enable reviewers to make informed judgments about the soundness of the proposed research procedures.

   c. Facilities and Resources
   Describe the facilities, resources, and subjects available to the applicant for carrying out the proposed project. Note evidence of collaborative relationships that will promote the completion of the research study.

5. **Management Plan** (limit to 2 pages)
   Describe project activities, timelines, and dissemination plans for research results. Please be specific about travel required for research activity and indicate why it is essential to the investigation. Incorporate ASHFoundation report deadlines into the management timeline.

6. **Budget** (limit to 1 page)
   State the importance of the requested funds to the project objectives and indicate how funds will be allocated to specific expense items. The grant will not cover indirect costs. There are not other restrictions, but the case must be clear on how the funds are essential to conduct the research.

7. **Human Subjects** (limit to 3 pages)
   If the project will utilize human subjects, include consent form and copy of Institutional Review Board (IRB) approval.

(Continued)

FIGURE 17.6

(Continued)

If the IRB approval is not available at time of grant submission, the investigator should explain the status of the IRB approval process and ensure that approval documents are mailed to the ASHFoundation as soon as IRB approval is granted, but not later than the conclusion of the grant review.

If there is no IRB process and the project will utilize human subjects, the applicant should provide the following information.

a. Describe the characteristics of the subject population, including the anticipated number, age ranges, gender, ethnic background, and health status;

b. Identify sources of research materials in the form of specimens, records, and/or data;

c. Describe plans for the recruitment of subjects and the consent procedures to be followed (include copy of consent form to be used);

d. Describe the potential risks to subjects (e.g., physical, psychological, social, legal, or other);

e. Describe the procedures for protecting against or minimizing potential risks to subjects, including risks to confidentiality; and

f. Discuss why risks to subjects are reasonable in relation to the anticipated benefits and to the importance of the knowledge that may result.

8. **Bibliography and/or Appendices, as appropriate** (limit to 6 pages)

9. **Letters of Support**
Submit a letter to the Grant Review Committee from the administrator of your current employment setting indicating that the proposed project is endorsed and will not present a conflict of interest with your current responsibilities and commitment. If a research project involving a colleague or mentor is proposed, include a letter and credentials from the individual(s) indicating commitment to participate in the research study.

Reprinted by permission of American Speech-Language-Hearing Foundation. www.ashfoundation.org.

and presentations or publications and explain how the project fits into developing a focused line of research. As with most grant applications, the investigator is instructed to append **curriculum vitae** (CV) to the proposal. A CV is a type of resume in academic and research settings and includes education, professional positions, publications, and so on. Granting agencies and programs have different formats for CVs. For example, NIH requires the use of biosketches that are two-page resumes containing academic degrees, current and previous employment, honors, and federal committee service in addition to references to related publications and presentations (Cummings et al., 2001).

The Research Plan is the most critical part of the proposal, consisting of three sections: (1) Objectives and Significance, (2) Design and Methodology, and (3) Facilities and Resources. Applicants are instructed to state how the specific aims or objectives of the project will contribute to the understanding, diagnosis, remediation, or compensation for a problem in communication sciences and disorders. **Specific aims** are "statements of the research question using a format that specifies in concrete terms the desired outcome" (Cummings et al., 2001, p. 289). Successful projects are hypothesis driven, meaning that their specific aims are designed to test theories that are based on sound scientific research (National Institute of Allergy and Infectious Diseases, 2007). There should be no more than two specific aims for a grant of this size and each should be highly related and tightly focused (Firszt, 2007). Each specific aim should be no more than two sentences and presented in some logical sequence based either on (1) importance, (2) chronological order of events, or (3) type (e.g., descriptive followed by analytical) (Cummings et al., 2001). The Significance section includes a critical review of previous research and sets the context for the proposed work. Obviously, with a limit of six pages, only the most recent studies directly relating to the proposed investigation should be included to show that the hypotheses to be tested are appropriate and evidence based. Investigators that have some **preliminary data** from pilot work supporting the research plan should include it in this section.

The Design and Methodology section should provide both a description and justification for the project design, including a discussion of the participants, measurement techniques (reliability and control measures), instrumentation, data analysis, and evaluation procedures. Sufficient detail should be provided so that reviewers are able to judge the fitness of the study. Many of the earlier chapters in this textbook presented critical information for designing a study and selecting methods for data analysis. This section of the grant is often the most scrutinized by reviewers (Cummings et al., 2001). For example, thirty out of the hundred maximum points possible are for reviewers' evaluations of the scientific and technical merit of the experimental question, design, and methodology for addressing the research need; probability of completing the project on time; and methods for evaluating the project results. Investigators should also discuss any anticipated problems with the project and corresponding contingency plans. Reviewers are impressed by investigators with realistic expectations who are able to foresee problems and potential solutions in the completion of a project. The Design and Methodology section should be reviewed by several colleagues, preferably by someone well-versed in grantsmanship, prior to submission.

The Facilities and Resources section should describe the laboratory (e.g., space and equipment), resources, and participants in addition to the existence of collaborative relationships available to complete the proposed investigation. Ten of the hundred maximum points has been allocated to this area of the grant. Grant reviewers must be convinced that the investigator has everything needed to be successful in the execution of the project. For example, a proposal investigating the speech and language development of children with cochlear implants requires access to such participants. Moreover, the letters of support (discussed later in the chapter) from the applicant's administrator and collaborators should confirm the existence of necessary resources.

The Management Plan is a timetable that lists all the steps of a project and graphically represents the starting and ending date. Figure 17.7 shows a management plan for a hypothetical grant. Notice how some steps are relatively short (e.g., Step 1: Training of the Research Assistant) and may last only one month, whereas some steps last several months (e.g., Step 4: Recruiting of Participants). A good management plan

FIGURE 17.7

A Management Plan for a Hypothetical Study

The proposed project on the topic of the effects of noise and reverberation on speech perception will last two years. The major steps for project completion and an accompanying graphic timeline are presented below.

A. Steps for Completion

- *Step 1:* Training of research assistants will occur during month 1

- *Step 2:* Preparation of the lab and materials will occur during month 1

- *Step 3:* Preparation of speech stimuli and pilot testing with young adults with normal hearing to set equivalency for degree of reverberation time and signal-to-noise ratio for the noise for consonant identification will occur during month 2

- *Step 4:* Recruitment of participants will occur from month 3 of year 1 to month 4 of year 2

- *Step 5:* By December 31, 2008, a progress report will be sent to ASHF

- *Step 6:* Execution of the experimental protocol will occur from month 4 of year 1 to month 5 of year 2

- *Step 7:* Listeners' errors will be converted to confusion matrices for later submission to sequential information analysis program (SINFA) month 4 of year 1 to month 5 of year 2

- *Step 8:* Data analysis and interpretation will occur during months 6 to 8 of year 2

- *Step 9:* Preparation of a journal article to the *Journal of Speech, Language, and Hearing Research* will occur from months 9 to 12 of year 2

- *Step 10:* Preparation and submission of a final report to the ASHF will occur during months 11 and 12 of year 2.

B. Graphic Timeline:

```
Year 1:  1 2 3 4 5 6 7 8 9 10 11 12       Year 2:  1 2 3 4 5 6 7 8 9 10 11 12

Step 1:**
Step 2:**
Step 3:    **
Step 4:     ********************        ********
Step 5:                       **
Step 6:     ******************          **********
Step 7:     ******************          **********
Step 8:                                           ******
Step 9:                                             **********
Step 10:                                               ****
```

accomplishes two things. It helps the investigator plan the execution of the project and it shows the reviewers that the research plan is plausible. It is important for investigators to mention important deadlines for the fulfillment of responsibilities in the management timeline. For example, Steps 5 and 10 involve submissions of progress and final reports to the ASHF, respectively.

The Budget section specifies and justifies how the funds are to be spent. Note that funds will not be provided for **indirect costs,** which are expenses (or overhead) that are incurred by all research projects but are not directly attributable to any one project (e.g., utilities such as electricity in buildings where research is conducted). Typically, academic institutions require retrieval of indirect costs from funding agencies as a function of a fixed percentage of the direct costs of the grant. **Direct costs** are those that are directly related to a specific grant. The word *direct* should remind investigators that budget items should be directly related to that which is necessary to complete the project. Customarily, funds for high-end pieces of equipment are strongly discouraged and may cast doubts on the adequacy of the investigator's existing facilities and resources. More appropriate expenditures include funding for research assistants, compensation of participants, expendable supplies, and so on. An appropriate motto is, "If you can't justify, modify."

The Human Subjects section is for approvals obtained for participants. Academic institutions, hospitals, and research institutes often require submission of a protocol to their institutional review boards (IRBs) for any research involving the use of human subjects (see Chapter 2 regarding protection of human subjects). In this section of the proposal, investigators should include approval letters and informed consent forms. If no IRB exists, investigators must discuss items a through f. Although investigators have until completion of the review process to secure IRB documentation, reviewers may be impressed by investigators who have secured necessary approvals prior to grant submission.

The Bibliography and Appendices section may not exceed six pages. The bibliography should include citations of all references mentioned in the grant application to indicate the currency of the investigator's knowledge of the topic (Cummings et al., 2001). Care should be taken to ensure accuracy of the citations. Appendices can include technical and other supporting material such as charts, block diagrams, and so on (Cummings et al., 2001). Investigators should be aware that any pages over the limit will be discarded prior to grant review.

Supporting letters from the administrator of the principal investigator's place of employment as well as any collaborators should be addressed to the grant review committee and appended to the proposal. The administrator's letter should enthusiastically endorse the proposal and mention how it enhances the applicant's career development, as well as corroborate what has been described in the Facilities and Resources section. For example, administrators may openly state the project does not present any conflict with the applicant's job responsibilities or commitments. Administrators should also mention release time, laboratory space and equipment, and other support allocated to the project. Junior faculty should be well advised that keeping their administrator "in the loop" during the grant preparation process increases the likelihood of garnering a letter conveying strong support of the research endeavor. Letters from collaborators, particularly if they are mentors, should also demonstrate enthusiasm for the project in addition to a description of how they will participate in the project. Investigators should append a brief biosketch of each collaborator.

The last step is for investigators to submit the proposal to the agency and wait for a response. If the investigator supplied an e-mail address, the agency often will send confirmation of receipt of the proposal. From time to time, administrative staff may contact the applicant in case there are any questions or if additional documentation is needed. For example, an agency will remind investigators of the deadline for when verification of IRB approval must be received. Investigators are advised to keep a log and hard copies (e.g., e-mail) of any communication from the granting agency during the grant submission and review process.

Grant Review Process

The grant review process takes place behind the scenes and varies based on the source of funding. For example, the process for the NIH is different from those of private foundations, as shown in Figure 17.8.

When a grant proposal is received at the NIH, the Center for Scientific Review (CSR) logs it, assigns it an identification number, and sends it to an institute and appropriate review committee or **study section.** A study section is a group of scientists

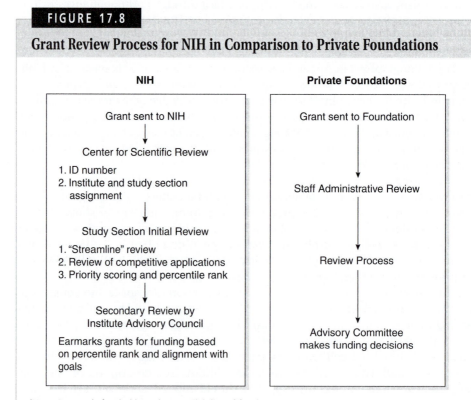

FIGURE 17.8

Grant Review Process for NIH in Comparison to Private Foundations

NIH

Grant sent to NIH

Center for Scientific Review

1. ID number
2. Institute and study section assignment

Study Section Initial Review

1. "Streamline" review
2. Review of competitive applications
3. Priority scoring and percentile rank

Secondary Review by Institute Advisory Council

Earmarks grants for funding based on percentile rank and alignment with goals

Private Foundations

Grant sent to Foundation

Staff Administrative Review

Review Process

Advisory Committee makes funding decisions

Note: Proposals funded based on availability of funds.

Adapted from Cummings et al., 2001; and NIAID, 2007.

(i.e., experts in a particular area of investigation) who have volunteered to serve as grant reviewers. The CSR mails all proposals to members (i.e., reviewers) in the study section for initial **streamlining,** a review process that separates competitive applications (i.e., those considered to be in the top half of the group in terms of merit) from the noncompetitive applications. Assigned primary and secondary reviewers have the job of carefully scrutinizing and presenting all competitive applications to the study section for discussion and scoring. Each member scores competitive applications with a numerical rating of 1 (best) to 3 (worst). A mean priority score is calculated and used to determine a percentile rank. This information is then sent back to the institute for a secondary review by members of the advisory council, who ultimately determine funding decisions.

Applications are funded until the money is depleted. Investigators can track the review of their proposal online and may inspect priority scores, percentile ranks, and **summary statements,** which are feedback from the study section presenting the strengths and weaknesses of an application. If possible, new investigators should review the summary statement with an experienced investigator who may be able to "read between the lines" regarding whether a resubmission is advisable. Investigators should realize that most applications are not funded on the first submission and that reviewers' comments can assist in preparing a tighter revision. The comments on the summary sheet are an opportunity for professional and scientific growth.

The grant review process for private foundations also uses peer review in evaluating proposals. Customarily, submitted grants undergo an administrative review to determine whether investigators meet eligibility requirements and the proposals are complete. Then experts evaluate the proposals using standard evaluation criteria. A review committee may meet to discuss, evaluate, and prioritize the proposals for funding. However, the advisory committee of the foundation ultimately makes the funding decisions.

Summary

This chapter has discussed funding sources, how to prepare a proposal, and the grant review process. Although many audiologists and speech-language pathologists have had very productive research careers without ever even applying for a grant, hopefully, the general outline of grant application procedures provided in this chapter has shown students and practitioners that applying for funding is another achievable way to support their research efforts.

LEARNING ACTIVITIES

1. Explore the websites listed in Appendix 17A for possible grant programs to fund your research efforts.

2. Interview a professor or colleague who has been successful in attracting research funding and ask, "What are the five most important pieces of advice for someone preparing a grant application?"

REVIEW EXERCISES

1. *True or False:* Please insert T or F appropriately in the blanks next to each statement below.

_____ Most grant competitions are for investigators at specific levels of research experience.

_____ Most granting agencies will not notice if an 11-point font is used instead of the required 12-point font.

_____ Page limitations are most often suggestions rather than requirements for proposals.

_____ "Failure to plan is a plan to fail!"

_____ Streamlining separates competitive applications (i.e., those considered to be in the top half of the group in terms of merit) from the noncompetitive applications.

_____ If an investigator becomes aware of a grant competition close to the deadline, it is better to submit an inferior proposal than none at all.

_____ It is imperative for an experienced colleague to read and provide feedback prior to submission of a grant proposal.

_____ The management plan specifies how the grant money will be spent.

_____ If items on the budget cannot be justified, then modification is necessary.

_____ Program officers at the NIDCD-NIH are committed to assisting young researchers prepare successful grant applications.

ANSWERS TO THE REVIEW EXERCISES

1. T, F, F, T, T, F, T, F, T, T

APPENDIX 17A
Useful Internet Sites

American Academy of Audiology Foundation: www.audiologyfoundation.org
American Speech-Language-Hearing Foundation: www.ashfoundation.org
National Hearing Conservation Association: www.hearingconservation.org
National Institute of Health (Sklare, 2007)
- National Institute on Deafness and Other Communication Disorders: www.nidcd.nih.gov
- All About Grants Tutorial (NIAID): www.niaid.nih.gov/ncn/grants

National Organization for Hearing Research: www.nohrfoundation.org
Subscription Services:
- Community of Science: www.cos.com
- The Foundation Center: www.foundationcenter.org
- Sponsored Programs Information Network: www1.infoed.org

APPENDIX 17B
Application Form for a Hypothetical Grant Application

American Speech-Language-Hearing Foundation
New Century Scholars Program

Investigator Application Form

Form is available electronically at www.ashfoundation.org/foundation/grants. Scroll down to the New Century Scholars Program section and click on New Century Scholars Research Grant.

Section I: **Proposal Title**

Effects of Auditory Maturation and Minimal Hearing Loss on Qualitative and Quantitative Aspects of Children's Phoneme Identification in Reverberation and Noise

Section II: **Investigator Information**

Carole E. Johnson _____   Ph.D., Au.D. _____
Name   Degree

Professor _____
Title

Auburn University _____
Institution

Department of Communication Disorders; 1199 Haley Center _____
Preferred Mailing Address

Auburn University, AL 36830 _____
City, State Zip Code

(334)663-6947 _____   johns19@auburn.edu _____
Daytime Area Code and Telephone Number   Email Address

Section III: **Educational History**

Degree Granted	Year	Institution	Field
Au.D.	2006	Pennsylvania College of Optometry	Audiology
Ph.D.	1989	University of Tennessee, Knoxville	Hearing Science
M.A.	1986	Same	Audiology

Title of Completed Dissertation:

Loudspeaker-to-Listener Distance and Speech Recognition in a _____

Reverberant Lecture Hall _____

Director: Anna K. Nabelek, Ph.D., and Carl W. Asp, Ph.D. _____

Section IV: **Research Feasibility**

If you are in a academic setting, describe your time allotment among teaching load, research, community service and other assigned duties.

If you are not in an academic setting, what percent of your workload time is devoted to research?

   25% Research, 65% Teaching, and 15% Service and Administration

Section V: **Research Design**
Is the proposed investigation an interdisciplinary study?

[ ] Yes    No

GLOSSARY

A priori method: Learning about the world through discussion and reasoning.

Activity: Execution of a task or action of an individual; has to do with what the patient can do (WHO, 2001).

Activity limitations: Difficulties that an individual may have in executing tasks (WHO, 2001).

Additive designs: Designs evaluating the effectiveness of a treatment protocol (e.g., B) when compared with an addition of another component (e.g., C), using the following component arrangement: B-BC-B-BC (Kearns, 1986).

Advisory Council: A review panel that actually determines which proposals get funded at the National Institutes of Health.

Agency for Healthcare Research and Quality: The AHRQ is the lead federal agency for research focusing on healthcare quality, costs, outcomes, and patient safety.

Alternative hypothesis: Hypothesis that predicts a particular outcome in a research project as contrasted to the null hypothesis.

Analysis of covariance (ANCOVA): A parametric statistical procedure related as a counterpart to ANOVA that evaluates group differences while taking into account pretest differences or statistically controlling for other characteristics (covariates).

Analysis of variance (ANOVA): A parametric statistic designed to determine differences among group means when there are more than two groups.

Animal Care Use Committee (ACUC): A panel that evaluates the ethical aspects of research on animals.

ANOVA1: One-factor analysis of variance examining group differences on multiple levels of one independent variable.

ANOVA2: Two-factor analysis of variance examining group differences on multiple levels of two independent variables.

ANOVA3: Three-factor analysis of variance examining group differences on multiple levels of three independent variables.

Associations: Relationships between variables (e.g., predictor and outcome) that may range from no relationship to cause and effect.

As-treated analysis: An analysis involving the data from participants who actually completed a study which is compared to the results of an intention-to-treat analysis to assess the effects of dropouts.

Between subjects: Use of independent groups in research in which each participant only experiences one level of an independent variable.

Biserial correlation coefficient: A nonparametric statistic used to determine relationships between two variables.

Bivariate regression: A regression analysis involving two variables in which one variable is used to predict the value of the other.

Body functions: Physiological functions of body systems (including psychological functions) (WHO, 2001).

Body structures: Anatomical parts of the body such as organs, limbs, and their components (WHO, 2001).

Bonferroni procedure: An adjustment procedure in which the alpha level is made more stringent when a statistical analysis is used multiple times on data gathered from the same participants, done to reduce Type I errors.

Calculated *t*: Calculated by a researcher using a formula or a computer program for the *t*-test, this value is compared to a critical value of *t* in order to determine statistical significance.

Canonical correlation analysis: A multivariate procedure in which several predictor (independent) variables are used to predict a number of dependent variables taken as a unit.

Capstone project: A research project used as a culminating experience in many professional doctoral programs, typically a pilot study that is not as involved as a thesis or dissertation but serves as a research requirement prior to graduation.

Case-control studies: Retrospective investigations that seek to identify factors or predictor variables associated with a particular disorder or affliction.

Case-study research: Research investigating individual participants in detail and comparing their profile to typical cases of a particular patient population.

Changing-criterion designs: Designs investigating the effectiveness of treatment with ever-increasing criterion levels of performance achieved on a gradually acquired behavior (Kearns, 1986).

Chi-square test for *K* independent samples: A nonparametric statistic used to determine differences between more than two independent groups.

Chi-square test for two independent samples: A nonparametric statistic used to determine differences between two independent groups.

Clinician-researcher: A clinician who engages in collaborative research with others or independent research on applied clinical issues.

Cochran *Q* test: A nonparametric statistic used to find differences in related samples of more than two groups.

Cochrane Collaboration: An international nonprofit and independent organization dedicated to making up-to-date, accurate information about the effects of healthcare readily available to healthcare providers and patients around the world.

Cochrane Library: A collection of high-quality evidence-based healthcare databases, providing instant access to over 2000 full-text articles reviewing the effects of healthcare interventions.

Cochrane review groups: These are groups of healthcare professionals composed of both researchers and clinicians with a common area of expertise who oversee area-specific systematic reviews.

Coefficient of determination: A value of r squared indicating the amount of variance accounted for by the relationship when evaluating Pearson product-moment correlations.

Cohen's d: A measure of effect size or practical significance.

Cohort studies: Studies that follow a group of participants over time.

Component-assessment designs: Designs evaluating the degree to which individual components of a treatment package contribute to a change in behavior (Kearns, 1986).

Concordance rate: Degree to which the same judge (i.e., intra) or different judges (i.e., inter) agree in their scoring of the same patient (Newman et al., 2001).

Confidence intervals: Measures of the precision of the summary effect estimate that should be reported.

Confidentiality: The ethical responsibility of researchers to safeguard personal information of participants in scientific investigations.

Construct validity: The degree with which an instrument rationally and empirically measures a theoretical construct (Maxwell & Satake, 2005; Schiavetti & Metz, 2006).

Content validity: The degree with which items on an instrument focus on different aspects of a behavior or domain (e.g., emotional aspects or participation restrictions resulting from hearing loss).

Continuing education: The acquisition of knowledge and skills via sanctioned events for practicing audiologists and speech-language pathologists.

Control group: A group of participants who do not receive the experimental treatment.

Correlated t-test: A t-test performed on within subject (repeated measures) designs in which participants are tested in multiple conditions.

Correlation matrix: A method of displaying multiple correlation coefficients.

Counterbalancing: A method of alternating the exposure of participants to various conditions in the experiment to control for threats to internal validity.

Covariate: The variable controlled for in the analysis of covariance (ANCOVA).

Criterion level of performance: The performance required for mastery of the particular goal, which must be achieved over the course of at least two data-collection sessions.

Criterion validity: The degree with which scores on an instrument correlate with those of a recognized "gold standard" of measurement.

Critical value: The value that must be exceeded by the calculated value when performing certain quantitative analyses to determine statistical significance.

Cronbach's alpha: A statistic reflecting the variance of the total score to that of the individual items.

Cross-sectional designs: Designs *that* entail sampling to enroll participants who may be likely to have the condition and who are administered an accepted gold standard for the condition.

Curriculum vitae: A type of resume in academic and research settings that includes education, professional positions, publications, and so on.

Curve fitting, time-series analysis, autoregressive integrated average technique, C-statistic, and nonparametric smoothing: Statistical procedures used in analyzing data gleaned from single-subject-design research.

Data extraction: Carefully excising and gathering statistical results from studies included in the review that directly pertain to the research question posed in the systematic review.

Data reduction: The procedure by which a researcher converts the behavior of participants into numerical values for statistical analysis.

Data transformation: The process of converting participant data into a different metric (e.g., square roots, logarithms) to compensate for lack of homogeneity of variance or other violations in parametric statistics.

Deductive reasoning: The process of moving from the general to the specific in research, such as using a general theory to design an investigation.

Defense: The last stage of a thesis or dissertation in which the student presents and defends the results of his or her investigation in front of a committee.

Degrees of freedom: This term is very difficult to define in a sentence or two, but the essence is that after knowing specific information about the number of variables to be studied and the numbers of participants, certain values in the data set are free to vary in the experiment.

Dependent variable: The measurement taken from participants that is expected to vary as a result of the independent variable in a scientific investigation.

Descriptive discriminant analysis: Using the multivariate technique of discriminant analysis to find a set of predictor variables that will identify a categorical group of people (e.g., stutterers/nonstutterers) whose status is known at the outset of the study.

Descriptive single-subject designs: These designs involve observing trends in patients' behavior over time without experimental manipulation.

Direct costs: Costs directly related to a specific grant.

Direct measures: Measures of the actual manifestations of the communicative disorder (e.g., the number of disfluencies per minute, percent correct production of a phoneme).

Disability: An umbrella term for impairments, activity limitations, and participation restrictions.

Discipline-specific resources: Resources for evidence-based practice that are mostly useful in communication sciences and disorders.

Discriminant function analysis: A multivariate procedure in which several predictor variables are used to predict a categorical variable such as a specific grouping of participants.

Disease-specific health-related quality of life measures: Measures such as the Hearing Handicap Inventory of the Elderly used in a particular area of healthcare.

Dissertation: A research project that is the culmination of a Ph.D. program.

Domestic resources: Resources for evidence-based practice originating in the United States.

Double blind: A procedure in which both the participant and the researcher are not aware of the specific condition (e.g., control group/experimental group) the participant represents in a scientific investigation, used as a way to control for bias in a study.

Dunn-Sidak modification: An adjustment of the alpha level to compensate for running multiple analyses of the same statistic on data gathered from the same participants, done to avoid Type I errors.

Duration measures: Measures of how long an event or behavior lasts.

Effect sizes: Statistical calculations that estimate the clinical significance of a particular intervention.

Eigenvalue: A value calculated in factor analysis used to define factors.

Empirical testing: The process of gathering data to evaluate a scientific question.

Engineering question: A question asking how to do something that is not directly answerable by use of the scientific method.

Environmental factors: The physical, social, and attitudinal factors that surround people as they live and conduct their lives (WHO, 2001).

ETA squared: A measure of practical significance used with the analysis of variance.

Evidence-based medicine: The "conscientious, explicit, and judicious use of current best evidence in making decisions about the care of individual patients" (Sackett, Rosenberg, Gray, Haynes, & Richardson, 1996, p. 71).

Evidence-based practice: An approach by which current high-quality research evidence is integrated with practitioner expertise, patient preferences, and patient values into the process of making clinical decisions (ASHA, 2005).

Exclusion criteria: Characteristics that eliminate a study from inclusion in a systematic review.

Experimental arrangement: A threat to external validity in which the conditions of participant performance in a study were so artificial in laboratory conditions that they do not relate to performance in the natural environment.

Experimental control: The efforts of the researcher to compensate for threats to internal validity.

Experimental designs: Used in single-subject designs to observe patients' behavior before, during, and then after treatment, seeking to establish causality between changes in the dependent variable and the treatment.

Experimenter bias: Anything the experimenter does having measurable influence on the dependent variable that is not attributable to the independent variable.

Expert clinical opinion: The expertise of recognized leaders in the professions who have established themselves through clinical work and/or scholarly activity.

External validity in single-subject-design research: The degree to which the study represents possible effects of treatment on behavior with specific patients in the real world.

External validity: The generalizability of research results from the laboratory to the real world.

Face validity: Another name for content validity.

Factor analysis: A multivariate analysis that determines individual factors that make up or underlie broad constructs.

Factorial design: An experiment that involves two or more independent variables with multiple levels.

Factors: Synonymous with independent variable; a two-factor design is the same as a design that has two independent variables.

Feasibility: The utility of an instrument in the real world.

Fisher Exact Probability Test: A nonparametric procedure for finding differences between two independent groups.

Frequency measures: The number of times a behavior occurs during a period of time.

Friedman Two-Way Analysis of Variance by Ranks: A nonparametric statistic for finding differences among more than two related samples.

Functioning: All body functions, activities, and participation (WHO, 2001).

Funnel plot: Special graphs whose shape denotes presence or absence of publication bias in a systematic review.

Generic health-related quality of life measures: Measures used across healthcare disciplines such as the *Medical Outcomes Survey—Short Form 36.*

Generic resources: Resources for evidence-based practice that are useful for physicians and allied health professionals (e.g., nurses, physical therapists, psychologists, and so on).

Glass's delta: A measurement of practical significance.

Handsearching: The search for articles in journals or for unpublished studies.

Hawthorne effect: A change in the behavior of participants attributed to the fact that they are being observed or studied.

Health services research: Investigation of how people get access to health care, how much care costs, and what happens to patients as a result of this care.

Health: Defined in the World Health Organization Constitution as a state of complete physical, mental and social well-being and not merely the absence of disease or infirmity.

Hedge's g: A measure of practical significance.

Hierarchial multiple regression: A type of multiple regression in which the researcher systematically enters predictor variables into the prediction equation based on a particular theory or construct.

History threat: A threat to internal validity in which participants who are sampled multiple times are affected by an external influence between samples, impacting the outcome of the study.

Homogeneity of variance: A basic assumption of parametric statistics in which variances of groups are required to be similar prior to analysis.

Homoscedasticity: Refers to the notion of homogeneity of variance in multivariate research.

Hotelling's T^2: A multivariate equivalent of the t-test.

Hypothesis: A conjectural statement that specifies the relationship between independent and dependent variables.

Hypothesis statements: The formal declaration of the null hypothesis and all alternative hypotheses in the investigation.

Impairments: Problems in body function or structure, such as a significant deviation or loss (WHO, 2001).

Incidence: The number of people who develop a particular condition during a specific period of time per the number of those at risk (e.g., the number of new cases of preschoolers diagnosed with autism this year).

Inclusion criteria: Characteristics a study must have in order to be included in a systematic review.

Independent t-test: A parametric statistical procedure that evaluates differences between the means of two independent groups.

Independent variable: The variable manipulated by the researcher that affects the dependent variable in an investigation.

Index test: The predictor variable under assessment in a diagnostic study.

Indirect costs: Expenses (or overhead) incurred by all research projects but not directly attributable to any one project (e.g., utilities such as electricity in buildings where research is conducted).

Indirect measures: Measures that are not directly observable or are physiological in nature and are measured in the laboratory setting.

Inductive reasoning: Moving from the specific to the general in designing a scientific investigation (e.g., using specific controlled observations to ultimately arrive at a theory).

Information literacy: The knowledge and skills to find relevant high-quality evidence for the purposes of EBP using effective and efficient search strategies.

Informed consent: The document signed by a participant in a research project explaining the details of the study and communicating the ethical responsibilities of the researcher and rights of the participant.

Institutional Review Board (IRB): Committee that evaluates research proposals for the ethical treatment of human participants.

Instrumentation threat: A threat to internal validity that can influence the outcome of a study due to improper or uncalibrated instrumentation whether mechanical, electronic, or human.

Intact groups: Already existing groups of participants that are used for the sake of convenience in nonrandomized intervention research (e.g., quasi-experimental research).

Item total correlation: A correlation that assesses the degree with which each item on the instrument correlates with the total score.

Intention-to-treat analyses: Statistical procedures that include all of the participants recruited for a study, precluding biased results that include only those patients who complete the protocol or those with positive outcomes.

Interaction effects: The combined effects of two or more independent variables on a dependent variable in a factorial design.

Interjudge reliability: The agreement between two or more judges on the occurrence of behaviors sampled or analyzed in a research project.

Internal consistency: The consistency with which the items on a questionnaire measure the same things (e.g., domains like participation restrictions).

Internal validity: The ability of a study to rule out competing explanations for the results other than the effect of the independent variable on the dependent variable by using experimental control to compensate for confounding or nuisance variables in a study.

International Classification of Functioning, Disability, and Health (ICF): A system for describing health and health-related states (WHO, 2001).

International resources: Resources for evidence-based practice that originate in foreign countries.

Interobserver reliability for the dependent variable: The degree of agreement (e.g., percent) between the judgments of the same target behaviors by two independent judges who evaluate the same session.

Interobserver reliability of the independent variable: The degree to which two judges agree that the treatment has been consistently applied when evaluating the same session.

Interval data: Scores representing distinct groups, with ordered levels and equal distances between values.

Interval scoring: Breaking an observation period into consecutive, equal segments and then counting occurrences of the target behavior during each portion.

Intramural funding resources: Support that comes from within one's own college, university, or place of employment.

Intraobserver reliability for the dependent variable: The degree of agreement (e.g., percent) between the judgments of the same target behaviors by the same judge at two different times.

Intraobserver reliability of the independent variable: The degree of agreement between the evaluations of the application of treatment within the same session by the same judge.

Item total correlation: An index of how each item on an instrument correlates with the total score.

Junk science: Research produced in a shoddy, superficial manner and passed off as scientific investigation.

Kappa: A statistic that assesses the extent of agreement that would be expected alone and ranges from -1 (perfect disagreement) to 1 (perfect agreement) between judgments (i.e., intra- and interjudge) and is used when there are few incorrect or multiple responses.

Kendall rank-order correlation: A nonparametric statistic to determine relationships among variables.

Kruskal-Wallis one-way analysis of variance: A nonparametric statistic used to find significant differences among three or more groups.

Kurtosis: A measurement of the shape of a distribution.

Leptokurtic: A kurtosis measurement describing a distribution that is tall and narrow with a small amount of variability.

Level of measurement: The type of data gathered in an experiment such as nominal, ordinal, interval, or ratio.

Levels: Groups or conditions associated with an independent variable; an independent variable (factor) that is comparing four groups has four levels.

Levels of evidence: Hierarchies for categorizing the scientific rigor of research studies.

Likelihood ratio: Assesses the accuracy of a test; for a specific result, it is the ratio of the likelihood of a score being obtained by someone who has the condition to the likelihood of the score being obtained by someone who does not have the condition (Newman et al., 2001).

Line of best fit: The line drawn on a scattergram that represents the midpoints between data points and shows whether the relationship is positive or negative.

Linear relationship: Variables that show a relationship in a straight line either positive or negative.

Macro search strategies: The order in which resources (e.g., electronic databases) are searched for evidence-based practice.

Main effects: Differences between groups or conditions on one independent variable that are not influenced by other independent variables (interaction effects).

Management plans: Timelines that denote when specific objectives of grant projects are initiated and completed.

Mann-Whitney *U* test: A nonparametric statistic used to find differences between two independent groups.

MANOVA1: Multivariate analysis of variance that is the counterpart of the ANOVA1; MANOVA1 analyzes multiple dependent variables whereas ANOVA1 is concerned with only one.

Marginal means: Means of the performance of groups or conditions collapsed across independent variables. For instance in a 2 × 2 factorial design with gender (M/F) and age (4/6) as independent variables, the marginal mean for males would "collapse" the two age groups and include the average performance of both four and six year olds who are male.

Matching: The process by which a researcher populates groups of participants in an investigation to make them similar on relevant variables (e.g., IQ, gender, age, etc.).

Maturation threat: A threat to internal validity in which participants who are sampled multiple times are affected by an internal influence between samples, impacting the outcome of the study (e.g., maturation, spontaneous recovery, fatigue, etc.).

McNemar's test: A nonparametric statistic used to find differences between two related groups on nominal data.

Mean: The arithmetic average of a group's performance on a dependent variable.

Measures of central tendency: The mean, median, or mode of a distribution of scores.

Measures of variability: The range, variance, or standard deviation of a distribution of scores.

Median: The middlemost score in a distribution in which 50 percent of scores lie above and below this value.

Mesokurtic: A measure of kurtosis often called a "bell curve" in which the distribution resembles the shape of a bell.

Meta-analyses: Statistical procedures that combine the results of individual studies in order to weigh the evidence regarding the efficacy of a particular procedure or intervention.

Method of authority: Reliance on authority figures or institutions to learn about the world.

Method of science: Using the scientific method to learn about the world.

Method of tenacity: Persistence in a particular view just because it is a long-standing belief.

Micro search strategies: The use of specific features within an electronic database (e.g., PubMed) for evidence-based practice.

Miniseminar: A format at national professional meetings in which information on a particular topic that may involve research and tends to be instructional in nature is presented for several hours.

Mixed design: A factorial design in which at least one independent variable is between subjects and at least one is within subjects.

Mode: The most frequently occurring score in a distribution.

Mortality: A threat to internal validity in which participants leave an investigation due to relocation, disinterest, or some other reason for discontinuing participation in the study.

Multicollinearity: The degree of intercorrelation among predictor variables in a multiple regression analysis

Multiple-baselines single-subject designs: Options in which treatment need not be removed in order for the patient to relapse as evidence of the effectiveness of an intervention.

Multiple-baselines-across-subjects designs: Assessments of the effectiveness of an intervention on changing the same behavior across a group of homogeneous subjects.

Multiple-baselines-across settings designs: Evaluations of the effectiveness of a treatment on a target behavior in the same subject(s) across treatment settings.

Multiple-baselines-across-behaviors designs: Assessments of the effectiveness of a treatment in changing two functionally independent behaviors within the same subject.

Multiple-probe techniques: Assessments that probe performance of multiple behaviors at continuous intervals.

Multiple regression analysis: A multivariate procedure in which several independent (predictor) variables are simultaneously used to predict a dependent variable.

Multivariate statistics: Statistical methods that can analyze multiple independent and dependent variables.

National Institute on Deafness and Other Communication Disorders (NIDCD): One of twenty-four different components of the National Institutes of Health (NIH) that supports biomedical and behavioral research on both normal and disordered processes of balance, hearing, language, smell, speech, taste, and voice (NIDCD, 2007).

Negative likelihood ratio: An index of confidence for a diagnostic test that a patient who tests negative is actually free of the disease or disorder (Dollaghan, 2003).

Negative relationship: A correlation in which one variable increases as another decreases such that the variables are moving in opposite directions.

Negative skew: A distribution in which the median and the mode are higher than the mean.

New investigators: Researchers that have less than about five years of experience past their doctoral degrees.

Neyman bias: Effect of variations in incidence on prevalence estimates (e.g., estimating prevalence when the sample is drawn from an increasingly at-risk population).

Nominal data: Scores that represent distinct groups or categories.

Nonparametric statistics: Quantitative methods that are distribution free and do not require a normal distribution as in parametric methods.

Normal distribution: A mesokurtic distribution or bell-shaped curve.

Null hypothesis: A hypothesis indicating that there is no difference between groups or relationships among variables that is rejected or not rejected during hypothesis testing.

Objective grant criteria: Concrete requirements in the submission process such as deadlines, page limitations, and so on.

Occam's Razor (Law of Parsimony): The rule that a theory should be able to account for phenomena with the least amount of unsupported assumptions.

Omega squared: A measure of practical significance.

One-tailed test: A statistical procedure that hypothesizes a directional approach to analysis.

Operational definition: A working definition used by researchers to operationalize their study; for example, "social skills" might be operationally defined as the score on a teacher rating scale.

Ordinal data: Scores that represent distinct groups with ordered levels.

Outcome measures: Data collected to determine the benefit of treatment.

Outlier: A participant in a study who earns a particularly high or low score in comparison to the mean; outliers can have an important effect on measures of central tendency or correlation coefficients.

Parametric statistics: Quantitative methods that assume a normal distribution and have other assumptions of normality, in contrast to nonparametric or "distribution-free" statistics.

Participant bias: Anything a participant does that has a measurable influence on the dependent variable that is not attributable to the independent variable.

Participant selection bias: A threat to internal validity in which a researcher's selection of participants results in groups that are not equated for relevant factors. These confounding variables could represent competing explanations for the results of the study.

Participation: Involvement in life situations (WHO, 2001).

Participation restrictions: Problems an individual may experience that restrict involvement in life situations (WHO, 2001).

Path analysis: A multivariate statistical procedure used to study cause-effect relations among variables.

Pearson product-moment correlation coefficient: A parametric statistic is used to determine the strength and direction of the relationship between two variables.

Personal factors: Characteristics specific to individual patients, such as gender, age, coping styles, social background, education, profession, past/current experiences, behavioral patterns, and character (WHO, 2001).

Phi coefficient: A nonparametric statistic used to determine relationships among variables.

Pillai's trace: A statistic used to determine if a multivariate F-ratio is statistically significant.

Placebo effect: A change in the behavior of research participants in a control group presumably due to their belief they have received a treatment when in reality they have not.

Platykurtic: A measure of kurtosis in which a distribution is wide and flat with a lot of variability.

Point-biserial correlation coefficient: A nonparametric statistic used to determine the relationship between variables.

Population, intervention, comparison (intervention), and outcome rubric: A format used for framing an experimental question for evidence-based practice.

Positive likelihood ratio: An index of confidence for a diagnostic test that a patient who tests positive actually has the disease or disorder (Dollaghan, 2003).

Positive relationship: A correlation in which two variables move in the same direction, whether up or down.

Positive skew: A distribution in which the mode and the median are below the mean.

Post hoc means comparison tests: When an F-ratio for a main effect including more than two groups or an interaction effect is found to be significant in the analysis of variance, post hoc tests determine which groups or cells in the design are significantly different from one another.

Poster session: A format at professional meetings in which researchers and clinicians present their work on poster boards and discuss results with attendees.

Power analysis: The process of evaluating the statistical power of a research design by taking into account the alpha level, effect size, and sensitivity of the measurement, among other things, to determine how many participants are necessary to include in the study in order to avoid a Type II error.

Practical significance: The real-world importance of study outcomes, which can be statistically significant but not meaningful beyond the study context; measures of practical or clinical significance such as effect size are an indication of how important group differences or relationships are in the real world.

Practice effect: A possible result for participants engaged in several different conditions in a repeated measures study, in which earlier conditions can have an effect on later conditions due to practice.

Predictive discriminant analysis: Using the multivariate technique of discriminant analysis to find a set of predictor variables that will identify a categorical group of people (e.g., stutterers/nonstutterers) whose status is unknown at the outset of a study.

Preliminary data: Pilot data included in a grant application to demonstrate feasibility of a proposed experimental protocol.

Prevalence: The number of persons who have a disease as a function of the number of those at risk.

Primary measurement methods: Methods by which an experimenter collects and analyzes the data.

Private foundations: Nonprofit organizations that may offer funding for research related to its scope of interest (e.g., the American Speech-Language-Hearing Foundation).

Probabalistic knowledge: A characteristic of science in which the results of most experiments are viewed in terms of probability and not absolute truth.

Probability level: Also called alpha level, level of confidence, or significance level, the probability that results of an experiment could be due to chance or sampling error.

Problem: A general statement or question relating to the topic of a research project.

Program officers: Staff members at NIDCD who assist applicants by serving as a contact person, preapplication advocate, postreview guide, and postaward activity manager (Sklare, 2007).

Prospective cohort studies: A recruited group of participants who are measured on predictor variables and potential confounders and then followed over time to measure outcome variables.

Prospective randomized clinical trial (PRCT): Studies in which patients are (1) enrolled as participants prior to conducting the experiment, (2) randomly assigned to groups receiving either the treatment or a placebo, (3) measured after some period of time, and (4) compared for any statistically significant differences attributable to the treatment or intervention.

Prospectus: A research proposal for a thesis or dissertation that includes a review of the literature, justification for the study, and the proposed methodology.

Pseudoscience: Any practice that simulates science or claims to have a scientific basis but in reality does not (e.g., astrology).

Publication bias: The tendency for journals to only publish statistically significant findings.

Publication lag: The delay between an article's submission date to a professional journal for consideration for publication and the date that the paper is actually published.

Quackery: A special category of pseudoscience usually related to the medical profession.

Qualitative analysis: An analysis of how many studies showed certain results for various outcomes in a systematic review.

Quantitative analysis: The application of statistical procedures of individual studies in a meta-analysis to determine the sum total effect of an intervention across different investigations.

Random assignment: The procedure by which each participant has a 50-50 chance of being assigned to receive a placebo or the treatment, which ensures that the experimenter does not bias certain groups with participants that may respond to the treatment in a predictable way.

Range: The spread of scores from low to high in a distribution.

Rate measures: The ratio of the number of times a target behavior occurred per specific period of time (e.g., the number of instances of secondary stuttering behaviors per minute).

Ratio data: Scores that represent distinct groups, have ordered levels, equal distances between levels, and a zero point.

Reactive testing: Exposure to a test or measurement early in a study that can affect the way participants respond in later conditions of the investigation.

Receiver-operator characteristic curve: A graph that plots coordinates of sensitivity on one axis and the false positive rate on the other to show the accuracy of a diagnostic test using various criterion levels.

Reduction designs: The assessment of the effectiveness of an entire treatment regimen (e.g., BC) against a single component (e.g., B) in an interaction design (e.g., BC-B-BC-B) (Kearns, 1986).

Reference test: An outcome variable in a diagnostic study that serves as a gold standard.

Regression equation: The mathematical formula in which a researcher can place known variables in order to predict unknown related variables.

Reliability: An index of the consistency of measurement.

Repeated measures: An experimental design, also known as a within subjects design, in which participants experience all levels of an independent variable.

Replication: A major tenet of science that says research findings become stronger and more valid if an experiment is repeated many times by different researchers on different participants using similar as well as different methods.

Research plan: The most critical part of a grant proposal, consisting of three sections such as (1) Objectives and Significance, (2) Design and Methodology, and (3) Facilities and Resources.

Research question: A statement of the relationship between independent and dependent variables in the form of a question.

Responsiveness: The sensitivity of an instrument in measuring participants' states from pre- to postintervention.

Residuals: Differences between predicted scores and actual scores in a regression analysis.

Retrospective cohort studies: Studies that recruit a group of participants and compare measured predictor variables from past data against measured outcomes occurring at a later date (Cummings et al., 2001).

Reversal designs: Used in single-subject research having baseline, treatment, and baseline phases in which, instead of removing treatment during the second baseline phase, treatment is applied to a second behavior and if performance on the first behavior returns to baseline performance, treatment is assumed to be effective.

Rev-Man 5.0 software: A tool developed by the Cochrane Collaboration for documenting a systematic review.

Rosenthal effect: Change in behavior due to the experimenter setting up certain expectations either intentionally or unintentionally in the participants.

Rotated factor matrix: A step in factor analysis in which factor loadings are adjusted in order to facilitate their interpretation.

Roy's largest root: A statistic used to determine if a multivariate F-ratio is statistically significant.

Sampling bias: The measurable influence on the dependent variable by assignment of participants to treatment or control groups that is not attributable to the independent variable.

Scattergram: A graphical plot of scores on two variables.

Scientific misconduct: Intentional fabrication of data or misrepresentation of results by a researcher.

Search strings: Words used either singularly or in combination that serve as input to a database in order to retrieve scientific evidence relevant to a research question.

Secondary measurement methods: Methods in which the experimenter uses data collected by other researchers.

Selection criteria: Criteria by which people are selected for participation in a scientific investigation, possibly including demographic variables and many other attributes.

Sensitivity: The percentage of participants who test positive on the predictor variable and the outcome variable or the proportion of patients who test positive on the index who actually have the condition as measured by the reference test.

Short course: A course of study on a specific topic presented at a professional meeting that may include a summary of existing research and clinical implications on a topic.

Shrinkage: In performing multiple regression analysis the prediction model developed with one set of participants is expected to "shrink" when the study is replicated with other groups. Shrinkage is dealt with by use of shrinkage formulas or by performing a cross-validation study using other participants to support the regression model.

Simultaneous multiple regression: A type of multiple regression in which the investigator enters all variables into the regression model at the same time as opposed to in a stepwise fashion.

Single blind: An experimental arrangement in which the participant does not know to which condition of a study he or she is assigned.

Single-subject design research: This involves measuring the same participant, serving as his or her control, over time.

Slope: The change in the dependent variable per unit of time in single-subject research that may be accelerating (i.e., increasing with time with respect to starting value), decelerating (i.e., decreasing with time), or zerocelerating (i.e., no change with time) (Maxwell & Satake, 2005).

Spearman rho: A nonparametric statistic that specifies the strength and direction of a relationship between two variables.

Specific aims: "Statements of the research question using a format that specifies in concrete terms the desired outcome" (Cummings et al., 2001, p. 289).

Specificity: The percentage of participants who test negative on the predictor variable and negative on the outcome variable or the proportion of patients who test negative on the index who actually do not have the condition as measured by the reference test.

Split-half reliability: A correlation that assesses the degree to which scores on a randomly selected half of an instrument correlate with those on the remaining half.

Stability: A variation of no more than 5 percent in the dependent variable over time when measured in single-subject design research.

Standard deviation: A measure of variability in a distribution.

Standard error of measurement: The variability of repeated measurements made on the same patients using the same test protocol.

Standard error of the estimate: The average amount of error in the predictions made by a regression formula.

Statistical power: Using the alpha level, effect size, and sensitivity of the measurement, among other things, to determine how many participants are necessary to include in the study in order to avoid a Type II error.

Statistical regression: A threat to internal validity in which participants who are selected due to extreme scores on a measurement, if tested again on this measurement, will regress toward the mean.

Stepwise multiple regression: Entering variables into a multiple regression in a systematic way to determine the prediction ability of these variables singly or in specific combinations to account for the best prediction model. Some regressions start with all variables and remove them systematically (backward stepwise) and others insert predictor variables one at a time (forward).

Streamlining: An early part of the grant review process that separates competitive from noncompetitive applications.

Stringency of alpha level: The lower the significance level, the smaller the probability that the results were due to chance or sampling error. An alpha level of .05 is less stringent than .01.

Structured abstracts: The use of separate headings to emphasize the critical elements of an investigation.

Study flow: A description of each stage of the selection process that ultimately results in a set of included studies in a systematic or evidence-based review.

Study sections: Groups of scientists (i.e., experts in a particular area of investigation) who have volunteered to serve as grant reviewers.

Subjective grant criteria: Subtle qualities of an application that influence reviewers' impressions of the merit of the principal investigator(s) and their proposed research efforts.

Successive-level analyses: Assessments of whether treatment results in the acquisition of successive steps as part of a chaining sequence of behaviors (Kearns, 1986).

Summary statements: The feedback from the study section that presents the strengths and weaknesses of an application.

Summary statistics: Statistics including some measure of central tendency (e.g., mean) and some measure of variability (e.g., standard deviation) that should be present in every study to allow consumers to determine the shape of the distribution.

Surrogate outcomes: Measures that capture the treatment effect on an important clinical endpoint but do not directly measure the main clinical benefit of the intervention.

Systematic reviews: Observational research designs that can be helpful in weighing the evidence regarding the efficacy of specific diagnostic measures or treatments for patients with or without meta-analyses.

Test-retest reliability: The stability of a measurement over time.

Theory: A systematic account of phenomena that allows prediction and explanation.

Thesis: A research project typically associated with a master's degree program.

Three-way interaction: The significant combination of three independent variables on a dependent variable in the analysis of variance.

Traditional platform presentation: A format in a professional meeting in which different researchers present their results on a specific topic in a fifteen- to twenty-minute speech.

Treatment-treatment designs: Investigations of the relative effectiveness of two or more rapidly alternating treatments that are counterbalanced in their presentation to equally distribute possible influences of different clinicians, regimen order, and time of presentation (Kearns, 1986).

Trial scoring: The proportion of number of times a target behavior occurred per the number of opportunities calculated as percent correct.

Triple blind: A situation in which the experimenter and participants are unaware of the condition in the study to which they are assigned, and those who analyze data do not know which condition or participant the data represent.

Two-tailed test: A statistical procedure that does not hypothesize directionality in data analysis.

Two-way interaction: The significant combination of two independent variables on a dependent variable in the analysis of variance.

Type I error: A decision that a result was statistically significant when in fact it was due to chance.

Type II error: A decision that a result was not statistically significant when in fact it was significant.

Uncontrolled observation: Nonscientific observation of phenomena.

Univariate statistics: Statistical methods that examine the effects of independent variables on only one dependent variable.

Validity: An index of the truth or accuracy in measurement.

Value question: A question about the nature of morality or good and evil which is not answerable by the scientific method.

Variance: A measure of variability or dispersion in which deviations from the mean of the distribution are squared, summed, and divided by $N - 1$.

Wilcoxon matched-pairs signed ranks test: A nonparametric statistic used to determine differences between two related groups.

Wilk's lambda: A statistic used to determine if a multivariate F-ratio is statistically significant.

Withdrawal designs: Used in single-subject research for using a baseline, treatment, and then withdrawal phase (e.g., A-B-A) in which treatment is removed during the second baseline phases to see if patients' behaviors return to baseline performance levels, indicating effectiveness of the treatment.

Within subjects: An experimental design in which participants experience all levels of the independent variable, also known as a repeated measures design.

REFERENCES

Abrams, H., Chisolm, T. H., & McArdle, R. (2002). A cost-utility analysis of adult group audiologic rehabilitation: Are benefits worth the cost? *Journal of Rehabilitation Research and Development, 39*, 549–558.

Abrams, H. B., Chisolm, T. H., & McArdle, R. A. (2005). Health-related quality of life and hearing aids: A tutorial. *Trends in Amplification, 9*, 99–109.

Agency for Healthcare Research and Quality (AHRQ). (2002). Retrieved January 5, 2007, from www.ahrq.gov

Agency for Healthcare Research and Quality (AHRQ). (2007). Retrieved July 6, 2007, from www.ahrq.gov

AGREE Collaboration. (2007). Retrieved July 6, 2007, from www.agreecollaboration.org

American Academy of Audiology. (2006a). *The clinical practice guidelines developmental process.* Retrieved July 12, 2007, from www.audiology.org/publications/documents/positions/guidelines.html

American Academy of Audiology. (2006b). *Guidelines for the management of adult hearing impairment.* Retrieved July 12, 2007, from www.audiology.org

American Heritage Dictionary. (1985). Boston, MA: Houghton-Mifflin.

American Speech-Language-Hearing Association (ASHA). (1995). *Preferred practice patterns for the profession of audiology.* Rockville, MD: Author.

American Speech-Language-Hearing Association. (1997). *Guidelines for audiology service delivery in nursing homes.* Retrieved July 7, 2007, from www.asha.org/policy

American Speech-Language-Hearing Association. (2004). Evidence-based practice in communication disorders: An introduction [technical report]. Retrieved January 1, 2008, from www.asha.org/members/deskref-journals/deskref/default

American Speech-Language-Hearing Association. (2005). *Evidence-Based Practice in Communication Disorders* [position statement]. Retrieved July 7, 2007, from www.asha.org/policy

American Speech-Language-Hearing Association. (2006). *Preferred Practice Patterns for the Profession of Audiology* [Preferred Practice Patterns]. Retrieved July 7, 2007, from www.asha.org/policy

American Speech-Language-Hearing Association. (2007). Guidelines for the responsible conduct of research: Ethics and the publication process. Retrieved February 9, 2008, from www.asha.org/policy

American Speech-Language-Hearing Association. (2008). *Evidence-based practice.* Retrieved June 1, 2008, from www.asha.org/members/ebp.default

Anastasi, A. (1958). *Differential psychology.* New York: Macmillan.

Anderson, T. W. (1984). *An introduction to multivariate statistical analysis* (2nd ed.). New York: Wiley.

Aydin, E., Akdogan, V., Akkuzu, B., Kirbas, I., & Ozgirgin, O. N. (2006). Six cases of Forestier syndrome, a rare cause of dysphagia. *Acta Otolaryngologica, 126*, 775–778.

Bachrach, A. (1969). *Psychological research: An introduction.* New York: Random House.

Bartholomew, D. J. (1984). The foundations of factor analysis. *Biometrika, 71*, 221–232.

Batavia, M. (2001). Clinical research for health professionals. Boston: Butterworth-Heinemann.

Beattie, R. C., Kenworthy, O. T., & Luna, C. A. (2003). Immediate and short-term reliability of distortion-product otoacoustic emissions. *International Journal of Audiology, 42*, 348–354.

Becker (2000a). Effect Size (ES). Retrieved March 12, 2008, from http://web.uccs.edu/lbecker/psy590/es.htm

Becker, L. (2000b). Effect size calculators. Retrieved March 12, 2008, from http://web.uccs.edu/becker/psy590/es-calc3.htm

Beecher, H. (1955). The powerful placebo. *Journal of the American Medical Association, 159*, 1602–1606.

Bentler, R. A., Niebuhr, D. P., Johnson, T. A., & Flamme, G. A. (2003). Impact of digital labeling on outcome measures. *Ear and Hearing, 24*, 215–224.

Blalock, H. M. (1972). *Social statistics* (2nd ed.). New York: McGraw-Hill.

Bland, J. M., & Altman, D. G. (1996). Transforming data. *British Medical Journal, 312*, 770.

Blodgett, J., & Cooper, E. (1987). *The analysis of the language of learning (ALL).* Moline, IL: Linguisystems.

Bock, R. D. (1975). *Multivariate statistical methods in behavioral research.* New York: McGraw-Hill.

Bolton, P. (2002). *Chapter 16: Scientific ethics.* Retrieved September 3, 2007, from www.sc.doe.gov/sc-5/benchmark/ch%2016%20scientific%20ethics%2006.10.02.pdf

Bordens, K., & Abbott, B. (1999). *Research design and methods: A process approach.* Mountain View, CA: Mayfield.

Bordens, K., & Abbott, B. (2002). *Research Design and Methods: A Process Approach.* Boston: McGraw-Hill.

Bossuyt, P. M., Reitsma, J. B., Bruns, D. E., Gatsonis, C. A., Glasziou, P. P., Irwig, L. M., Moher, D., Rennie, D., de Vet, H. C. W., & Lijmer, J. G. (2003). The STARD statement for reporting studies of diagnostic accuracy: Explanation and elaboration. *Clinical Chemistry, 49*, 7–18.

Box, G. E. P., Hunter, W. G., & Hunter, S. J. (1978). *Statistics for experimenters: An introduction to design, data analysis, and model building.* New York: Wiley.

Boyle, C. M. (1991). Does item homogeneity indicate internal consistency or item redundancy in psychometric scales? *Personality and Individual Differences, 12*, 291–294.

Bratt, G. W. (2007). NIDCD/VA hearing aid study. *Journal of the American Academy of Audiology, 18*, 272–273.

Brockman, J. (1995). *The third culture.* New York: Touchstone.

Brown, B. (1993). STPLAN (Version 4.0) Calculations for sample sizes and related problems. University of Texas, Department of Biomathematics.

Bruning, J., & Kintz, B. (1997). *Computational handbook of statistics.* New York: Longman.

Buchner, A., Faul, F., & Erdfelder, E. (1996). GPower: A priori, post-hoc, and compromise power analyses for MS-DOS (Version 2.1.1). Trier, Germany: University of Trier.

Campbell, D. (1957). Factors relevant to the validity of experiments in social settings. *Psychological Bulletin, 54,* 297–312.

Campbell, D., & Stanley, J. (1963*). Experimental and quasiexperimental design for research.* Chicago: Rand McNally.

Carey, S. (1994). A beginners guide to scientific method. Wadsworth: Belmont, CA.

Carrier, R. (2001). Test your scientific literacy. Retrieved January 5, 2008, from www.infidels.org/library/modern/richard_Carrier/SciLit.html

Casby, M. W. (1992). An intervention approach for naming problems in children. *American Journal of Speech Language Pathology, 1,* 35–42.

Centre for Evidence-Based Medicine (CEBM). (2006). *Critical appraisal.* Retrieved December 20, 2006, from www.cebm.net/index.aspx?0=1157

Centre for Evidence-Based Medicine. (2007). Study designs. Retrieved December 31, 2007, from www.cebm.net/index.aspx?o=1039

Centre for Evidence-Based Medicine. (2008). *Levels of evidence.* Retrieved January 5, 2008, from www.cebm.net/index.asp?0=1025

Chalmers, A. (1990). *Science and its fabrication.* Minneapolis: University of Minnesota Press.

Champlin, C. A. (2007). Launching your research career: Navigating the NIH/NIDCD. Learning module presented at Audiology NOW!, Denver, CO.

Chisolm, T. H., Johnson, C. E., Danhauer, J. L., Portz, L. J., Abrams, H. B., Lesner, S., McCarthy, P. A., & Newman, C. W. (2007). A systematic review of health-related quality of life and hearing aids: final report of the American Academy of Audiology Task Force On the Health-Related Quality of Life Benefits of Amplification in Adults. *Journal of the American Academy of Audiology, 18,* 151–183.

Cline, D., & Clark, D. (2000). A Writer's Guide to Research and Development Proposals. Retrieved December 8, 2007, from http://mutans.astate.edu/dcline/guide/problem.html

Cochrane Collaboration. (2008). Retrieved January 6, 2008, from www.cochrane.org

Cohen, J. (1965). Some statistical issues in psychological research. In B. Wolman (Ed.), *Handbook of Clinical Psychology.* New York: McGraw-Hill.

Cohen, J. (1983). *Statistical power analysis for the behavioral sciences.* (2nd ed.). Mahwah, NJ: Lawrence Erlbaum Associates.

Conference on Guideline Standardization (COGS). (2007). *COGS: The COGS statement.* Retrieved December 20, 2007, from www.med.yale.edu/cogs

Connell, P. J., & Thompson, C. K. (1986). Flexibility of single-subject experimental designs. Part III: Using flexibility to design or modify experiments. *Journal of Speech and Hearing Disorders, 51,* 214–225.

Cooley, W. W., & Lohnes, P. R. (1971). *Multivariate data analysis.* New York: Wiley.

Cox, R. M. (2004). Page 10: Waiting for evidence-based practice for your hearing aid fittings? *The Hearing Journal, 57*(8), 10, 12, 14, 16, 17.

Cox, R. M. (2005). Evidence-based practice in the provision of amplification. *Journal of the American Academy of Audiology, 16,* 419–438.

Cox, R. M., Alexander, G. C., Gray, G. M. (2005). Hearing aid patients in private practice and public health (Veterans Affairs) clinics: Are they different? *Ear and Hearing, 26,* 513–528.

Cummings, S. R., Grady, D., & Hulley, S. B. (2001). Designing an experiment: Clinical trials I. In S. B. Hulley, S. R. Cummings, W. S. Browner, D. Grady, N. Hearst, & T. B. Newman (Eds.), *Designing clinical research* (2nd ed., pp. 143–156). Philadelphia: Lippincott, Williams, and Wilkins.

Cummings, S. R., Holly, E. A., & Hulley, S. B. (2001). Writing and funding a research proposal. In S. B. Hulley, S. R. Cummings, W. S. Browner, D. Grady, N. Hearst, & T. B. Newman (Eds.), *Designing clinical research* (2nd edition, pp. 285–300). Baltimore: Lippincott, Williams, & Wilkins.

Cummings, S. R., Newman, T. B., & Hulley, S. B. (2001). Designing an observational study: Cohort studies. In S. B. Hulley, S. R. Cummings, W. S. Browner, D. Grady, N. Hearst, & T. B. Newman (Eds.), *Designing clinical research* (2nd ed., pp. 95–106). Philadelphia: Lippincott, Williams, and Wilkins.

Damrose, J. F., Goldman, S. N., Groessl, E. J., & Orloff, L. A. (2004). The impact of long-term botulinum toxin injections on symptom severity in patients with spasmodic dysphonia. *Journal of Voice, 18,* 415–422.

Demorest, M. E., & Erdman, S. A. (1987). Development of the communication profile for the hearing impaired. *Journal of Speech and Hearing Disorders, 52,* 129–143.

Demorest, M., & Erdman, S. (1989). Relationships among behavioral, environmental and affective communication variables: A canonical analysis of the CPHI. *Journal of Speech and Hearing Disorders, 54,* 180–188.

Deng, H. (2005). Does it matter if non-powerful significance tests are used in dissertation research? *Practical Assessment, Research & Evaluation* [Electronic], *10*(16).

Diamond, W. J. (1981). *Practical experimental design.* Belmont, CA: Wadsworth.

Dickoff, G. (1996). *Basic Statistics for the Social and Behavioral Sciences.* Upper Saddle River, NJ: Prentice-Hall.

Dillon, H., James, A., & Ginis, J. (1997). Client Oriented Scale of Improvement (COSI) and its relationship to several other measures of benefit and satisfaction provided by hearing aids. *Journal of the American Academy of Audiology, 8,* 27–43.

Dixon, W. J., & Massey, F. J. (1983). *Introduction to statistical analysis* (4th ed.). New York: McGraw-Hill.

Dooley, J., & Kerch, H. (2000). Evolving research misconduct policies and their significant for physical scientists. *Science and Engineering Ethics. Special Issue on Scientific Misconduct: An International Perspective, 6,* 1.

Dollaghan, C. A. (2003). *The handbook for evidence-based practice in communication disorders.* Baltimore: Paul H. Brookes.

Draper, S. (2005). *The Hawthorne, Pygmalion, placebo and other effects of expectation: Some notes.* Retrieved June 9, 2008, from www.psy.gla.ac.uk/~steve/hawth.htm

Drucker, P. (1998). *Harvard business review on knowledge management.* Boston: Harvard Business School Press.

Duarte-Silva, A., & Stam, A. (2004). Discriminant analysis. In L. Grimm and P. Yarnold, *Reading and Understanding Multivariate Statistics* (pp. 277–318). Washington, DC: American Psychological Association.

Dupont, W. D., & Plummer, W. D., Jr. (1990). Power and sample size calculations: A review and computer program. *Controlled Clinical Trials, 11,* 116–128.

Dworkin, J. P., Abkarian, G. G., & Johns, D. F. (1988). Apraxia of speech; the effectiveness of a treatment regimen. *Journal of Speech and Hearing Disorders, 53,* 280–294.

Eddy, D. M. (2005). Evidence-based medicine: A unified approach. *Health Affairs, 24,* 9–17.

Edgerton, B. A., & Danhauer, J. L. (1979). *Clinical implications of speech discrimination testing using nonsense stimuli.* Baltimore: University Park Press.

Eisenberg, L. S., Fink, N. E., & Niparko, J. K. (2006, November 28). Childhood development after cochlear implantation: Multicenter study examines language development. *ASHA Leader, 11*(16), 5, 28–29.

Ferguson, G. A. (1971). *Statistical analysis in psychology and education.* New York: McGraw-Hill.

Field, M. J., & Lohr, K. N. (1990). *Clinical practice guidelines: directions for a new program, Institute of Medicine.* Washington, DC: National Academy Press.

Firszt, J. B. (2007). Launching your research career: A clinician scientist's view. Learning module presented at AudiologyNOW!, Denver, CO.

Fisher, R. (1928). Moments and product moments of sampling distributions. *Proceedings of London Mathematical Society, 30,* 199–238.

Fisher, K. V., Ligon, J., Sobeks, J. L., & Roxe, D. M. (2001). Phonatory effects of body fluid removal. *Journal of Speech, Language, and Hearing Research, 44,* 354–367.

Flanagan, D., & Harrison, P. (2005). *Contemporary Intellectual Assessment: Theories, Tests and Issues.* New York: The Guilford Press.

Flower, R. (1983). Keynote address: Looking backwards and looking forward: Some views through a four decade window. In N. Rees and T. Snope (Eds.), *Proceedings of the 1983 national conference on undergraduate, graduate and continuing education* (Rep. No. 13, pp. 9–13). Washington, DC: American Speech-Language-Hearing Association.

Frattali, C. M. (1998). Outcomes measurement: Definitions, dimensions, and perspectives. In C. M. Frattali (Ed.), *Measuring outcomes in speech-language pathology* (pp. 1–27). New York: Thieme.

Friedman, L. M., Furberg, C. D., & DeMets, D. L. (1998). *Fundamentals of clinical trials* (3rd ed.). New York: Springer.

Gibbons, J. D. (1976). *Nonparametric methods for quantitative analysis.* New York: Holt, Rinehart, & Winston.

Gibbons, J. D. (1985). *Nonparametric statistical inference* (2nd ed.). New York: Marcel Dekker.

Gibbs, A., & Lawson, A. (1992). The nature of scientific thinking as reflected in the work of biologists and biology textbooks. *American Biology Teacher, 54*(3), 132–152.

Giolas, T. G., Owens, E., Lamb, S. H., & Schubert, E. D. (1979). Hearing Performance Inventory. *Journal of Speech and Hearing Disorders, 44,* 169–195.

Gjertsen, D. (1989). *Science and philosophy past and present.* New York: Penguin.

Glass, G. V., & Hopkins, K. D. (1996). *Statistical methods in education and psychology.* Boston: Allyn & Bacon.

Goodstein, D. (2002). Scientific misconduct. Retrieved August 3, 2002, from www.aaup.org/publications/academe/2002/02JF/02jfgoo.htm

Grady, D., Cummings, S. R., & Hulley, S. B. (2001). Designing an experiment: Clinical trials II. In S. B. Hulley, S. R. Cummings, W. S. Browner, D. Grady, N. Hearst, & T. B. Norman (Eds.), *Designing clinical research* (2nd ed., pp. 157–174). Philadelphia: Lippincott, William, & Wilkins.

Gravetter, F., & Wallnau, L. (2000). *Statistics for the behavioral sciences* (5th ed.). St. Paul, MN: West.

Grievink, E. H., Peters, S. A., van Bon, W. H., & Schilder, A. G. (1993). The effects of early bilateral otitis media with effusion on language ability: a prospective cohort study. *Journal of Speech, Language, and Hearing Research, 36,* 1004–1012.

Haley, R. W., Hom, J., Roland, P. S., Bryan, W. W., Van Ness, P. C., Bonte, F. J., Devous, M. D. Sr., Mathews, D., Fleckenstein, J. L., Wians, F. H. Jr., Wolfe, G. I., & Hurt, T. L. (1997). Evaluation of neurologic function in Gulf War veterans: A blinded case-control study. *Journal of the American Medical Association, 277,* 223–230.

Hanson, M. J. (1997). Ethnic, cultural, and language diversity in intervention settings. In E. W. Lynch and M. J. Hanson (Eds.), *Developing cross-cultural competence: A guide for working with children and their families* (2nd ed., pp. 3–22). Baltimore: Paul H. Brookes.

Harbour, R., & Miller, J. (2001). A new system for grading recommendations in evidence-based guidelines. *British Medical Journal, 323,* 334–336.

Harris, M. (1998). *Basic statistics for behavioral science research.* Durham, NC: Sage Publications.

Haynes, W., & Pindzola, R. (2008). *Diagnosis and evaluation speech pathology.* Boston: Allyn and Bacon.

Hays, W. L. (1988). *Statistics* (4th ed.). New York: CBS College Publishing.

Hearst, N., Grady, D., Barron, H. V., & Kerlikowske, K. (2001). Research using exisiting data: Secondary data analysis, ancillary studies, and systematic reviews. In S. B. Hulley, S. R. Cummings, W. S. Browner, D. Grady, N. Hearst, & T. B. Newman (Eds.), *Designing clinical research* (2nd ed., pp. 195–214). Philadelphia: Lippincott, William, & Wilkins.

Hegde, M. (2003). *Clinical research in communicative disorders: Principles and strategies.* Pro-Ed: Austin, TX.

Heiss, G., Wallace, R., Anderson, G. L., Aragaki, A., Beresford, S. A., Brzyski, R., Chlebowski, R. T., Gass, M., LaCroix, A., Manson, J. E., Prentice, R. L., Rossouw, J., Stefanick, M. L., & WHI Investigators. (2008). Health risks and benefits 3 years after stopping randomized treatment with estrogen and progestin. *Journal of the American Medical Association, 299,* 1036–1045.

Henderson, W. G., Larson, V. D., Williams, D., & Luethke, L. (2002). Organization and administration of the NIDCD/VA hearing aid clinical trial. *Ear and Hearing, 23,* 277–279.

Higgins, J. P. T., & Green, S. (2008). *Cochrane handbook for systemic reviews of interventions, version 5.0.0.* Cochrane Collaboration.

Holden, C. (1987). NIMH finds a case of "serious misconduct." *Science, 235,* 1566–1567.

Holland, A. L., Fromm, D. S., DeRuyter, F. D., & Stein, M. (1996). Treatment efficacy: Aphasia. *Journal of Speech, Language, and Hearing Research, 39,* S27–S36.

Hollis, S., & Campbell, F. (1999). What is meant by intention to treat analysis? Survey of published randomised controlled trials. *British Medical Journal, 319,* 670–674.

Hopkins, K. (1996). *Basic statistics for the behavioral sciences* (3rd ed.). Boston: Allyn & Bacon.

Horner, J., & Wheeler, M. (2005). HIPAA: Impact on research practices. *ASHA Leader, 10*(15), 8–10.

Houser, N., & Kloesel, C. (Eds.) (1992). *The essential Peirce: Volume 1.* Bloomington, IN: University of Indiana Press.

Howell, D. (1992). *Statistical methods for psychology.* Belmont, CA: Duxbury Press.

Howell, D. (1995). *Fundamental statistics for the behavioral sciences* (3rd ed.). Belmont, CA: Duxbury Press.

Hrobjartsson, A., & Gotzsche, P. (2001). Is the placebo powerless? An analysis of clinical trials comparing placebo with no treatment. *New England Journal of Medicine, 344,* 1594–1602.

Huck, S. (2004). *Reading statistics and research* (4th ed.). Boston: Allyn & Bacon.

Hyde, M. L. (2000). Reasonable psychometric standards for self-report outcome measures in audiological rehabilitation. *Ear and Hearing, 21*(Suppl. 4), 24S–36S.

Ingham, R. J., Kligo, M., Ingham, J. C., Moglia, R., Belknap, H., & Sanchez, T. (2001). Evaluation of a stuttering treatment based on reduction of short phonation intervals. *Journal of Speech, Language, and Hearing Research, 44,* 1229–1244.

Jaccard, J., & Becker, M. (1997). *Statistics for behavioral sciences.* Pacific Grove, CA: Brooks-Cole.

Jacobson, B. J., Johnson, A., Grywalski, C., Silbergleit, A., Jacobson, G., Benninger, M. S., & Newman, C. W. (1997). The voice handicap index: Development and validation. *American Journal of Speech-Language Pathology, 6,* 66–70.

Janosky, J. E. (1991). *An overview of the analysis of a single-subject design with recommendations.* Paper presented at the Annual Meeting of the American Educational Research Association, Chicago, IL.

Jerger, J., Chmiel, R., Florin, E., Pirozzolo, F., & Wilson, N. (1996). Comparison of conventional amplification and an assistive listening device in elderly persons. *Ear and Hearing, 17,* 490–504.

Johnson, C. E., & Danhauer, J. L. (2002). *Handbook of outcomes measurement in audiology.* Clifton Park, NJ: Thomson-Delmar Learning.

Joint Committee on Infant Hearing. (2007). Year 2007 position statement: Principles and guidelines for early hearing detection and intervention programs. *Pediatrics, 120,* 898–921.

Jones, M., Gebski, V., Onslow, M., & Packman, A. (2002). Statistical power in stuttering research: A tutorial. *Journal of Speech, Language and Hearing Research, 45,* 243–255.

Kachigan, S. K. (1986). *Statistical analysis: An interdisciplinary introduction to univariate & multivariate methods.* New York: Redius Press.

Kearns, K. P. (1986). Flexibility of single-subject experimental designs. Part II: Design selection and arrangement of experimental phases. *Journal of Speech and Hearing Disorders, 51,* 204–214.

Keith, R. (1999). Clinical issues in central auditory processing disorders. *Language, Speech and Hearing Services in Schools, 30,* 339–344.

Kent, R. (1983). Issue-IX. Role of research: How can we improve the role of research and educate speech-language pathologists and audiologists to be competent users of research? In N. Rees & T. Snope (Eds.), *Proceeding of the 1983 national conference on undergraduate, graduate and continuing education* (Rep. No. 13, pp. 76–86). Washington, DC: American Speech-Language-Hearing Association.

Keppel, G. (1982). *Design and analysis: A researcher's handbook* (2nd ed.). Englewood Cliffs, NJ: Prentice Hall.

Kerlinger, F. (1973). *Foundations of behavioral research.* New York: Holt, Rinehart and Winston.

Kerlinger, F., & Lee, H. (2000). *Foundations of behavioral research.* New York: Thomson Learning.

Kienle, G. S., & Kiene, H. (1997). The powerful placebo effect: Fact or fiction? *Journal of Clinical Epidemiology, 50,* 1311–1318.

Kim, J. O., & Mueller, C. W. (1978). *Introduction to factor analysis: What it is and how to do it.* Beverly Hills, CA: Sage Publications.

Kim, Y. T., & Lombardino, L. J. (1991). The efficacy of script contexts in language comprehension intervention with children who have mental retardation. *Journal of Speech, Language, and Hearing Research, 34,* 845–857.

Kirk, R. (1996). Practical significance: A concept whose time has come. *Educational and Psychological Measurement, 56,* 746–759.

Kirk, R. E. (1995). *Experimental design: Procedures for the behavioral sciences.* Pacific Grove, CA: Brooks-Cole.

Kroll, R., & Chase, L. (1975). Comunication disorders: A power analytic assessment of recent research. *Journal of Communication Disorders, 8,* 237–247.

Kuehn, D. P., Imrey, P. B., Tomes, L., Jones, D. L., O'Gara, M. M., Seaver, E. J., Smith, B. E., Van Demark, D. R., & Wachtel, J. M. (2002). Efficacy of continuous positive airway pressure for treatment of hypernasality. *Cleft Palate-Craniofacial Journal, 39,* 267–276.

Larson, V. D., Williams, D. W., Henderson, W. G., Luethke, L. E., Beck, L. B., Noffsinger, D., Bratt, G. W., Dobie, R. A., Fausti, S. A., Haskell, G. B., Rappaport, B. Z., Shanks, J. E., & Wilson, R. H. (2002). A multi-center, double blind clinical trial comparing benefit from three commonly used hearing aid circuits. *Ear and Hearing, 23,* 269–276.

Larson, V. D., Williams, D. W., Henderson, W. G., Luethke, L. E., Beck, L. B., Noffsinger, D., Wilson, R. H., Dobie, R. A., Haskell, G. B., Bratt, G. W., Shanks, J. E., Stelmachowicz, P., Studebaker, G. A., Boysen, A. E., Donahue, A., Canalis, R., Fausti, S. A., & Rappaport, B. Z. (2000). Efficacy of 3 commonly used hearing aid circuits: A crossover trial. NIDCD/VA: Hearing Aid Clinical Trial Group. *Journal of the American Medical Association, 284,* 1806–1813.

Law, J., Garrett, Z., & Nye, C. (2003). Speech and language therapy interventions for children with primary speech language delay or disorder. *Cochrane Database of Systematic Reviews (3):* CD004110.

Lenth, R. V. (2001). Some practical guidelines for effective sample size determination. *The American Statistician, 55,* 187–193.

Licht, M. (2004). Multiple regression and correlation. In Grimm, L. and Yarnold, P. (Eds.), *Reading and understanding multivariate statistics.* Washington, DC: American Psychological Association.

Liles, B. Z., Duffy, R. J., Merritt, D. D., and Purcell, S. L. (1995). Measurement of narrative discourse ability in children with language disorders. *Journal of Speech and Hearing Research, 38,* 415–425.

Lock, S., Wells, F. and Farthing, M. (2001). *Fraud and misconduct in biomedical research.* London: BMJ Books.

Lord, F. (1953). On the statistical treatment of football numbers. *American Psychologist, 8,* 750–751.

Lynch, E. W. (1997). Developing cross-cultural competence. In E. W. Lynch and M. J. Lynch (Eds.), *Developing cross-cultural competence: A guide for working with children and their families* (2nd ed., pp. 47–89). Baltimore: Paul H. Brookes.

Lyons, L. & Morris, W. (2007). The meta-analysis calculator. Retrieved October 23, 2007, from www.lyonsmorris.com/lyons/metaAnalysis/index.cfm

Marsa, L. (1992). Scientific fraud. *Omni, 14,* 38–43.

Martin, J. S., Jerger, J. F., Ulatowska, H. K., & Mehta, J. A. (2006). Complementing behavioral measures with electrophysiological measures in diagnostic evaluation: A case study in two languages. *Journal of Speech, Language, and Hearing Research, 49,* 603–615.

Matarazzo, J. (1990). Psychological assessment versus psychological testing: Validation from Binet to the school, clinic and courtroom. *American Psychologist, 45,* 999–1017.

Maxwell, D. L., & Satake, E. (2005). *Research and statistical methods in communication sciences and disorders.* Clifton Park, NY: Cenage Delmar Learning.

Mayo, E. (1933). *The human problems of an industrial civilization.* New York: Macmillan.

McKibbon, A., Easy, A., & Marks, S. (1999). *PDQ: Evidence-based principles and practice.* St. Louis, MO: B. C. Decker.

McReynolds, L. V., & Kearns, K. P. (1983). *Single-subject experimental designs in communicative disorders.* Baltimore: University Park Press.

McReynolds, L. V., & Thompson, C. K. (1986). Flexibility of single-subject experimental designs. Part I: Review of the basics of the single-subject designs. *Journal of Speech and Hearing Disorders, 51,* 194–203.

Medawar, P. (1963). *The threat and the glory.* New York: Harper-Collins.

Meline, T., & Paradiso, T. (2003). Evidence-based practice in schools: Evaluating research and reducing barriers. *Language, Speech and Hearing Services in Schools, 34,* 273–283.

Meline, T., & Wang, B. (2004). Effect-size reporting practices in AJSLP and other ASHA journals, 1999–2003. *American Journal of Speech-Language Pathology, 13,* 202–207.

Moher, D., Schulz, K. F., Altman, D. G., & CONSORT Group (Consolidated Standards of Reporting Trials). (2001).

The CONSORT Statement: Revised recommendations for improving the quality of reports of parallel-group randomized trials. *Journal of the American Medical Association, 285,* 1987–1991.

Montgomery, D. C. (1991). *Design and analysis of experiments* (3rd ed.). New York: Wiley.

Mook, D. (1983). In defense of external validity. *American Psychologist, 38,* 379–387.

Morrison, D. F. (1990). *Multivariate statistical methods.* (3rd ed.). New York: McGraw-Hill.

Muma, J. (1998). *Effective speech-language pathology: A cognitive socialization approach.* Mahwah, NJ: Lawrence Erlbaum Associates.

National Academy of Sciences (NAS), National Academy of Engineering (NAE), & Institute of Medicine (IOM). (1996). *On being a scientist: Responsible conduct in research.* Committee on science, engineering and public policy: Washington, DC: National Academy Press.

National Institute of Allergy and Infectious Diseases. (2007). All about grants tutorial (NIAID). Retrieved June 1, 2007, from www.niaid.nih.gov/ncn/grants

National Institute on Deafness and Other Communication Disorders. (2007). Retrieved June 1, 2007, from www.nidcd.nih.gov

National Library of Medicine. (2006). Fact sheet: MEDLINE. Retrieved July 15, 2007, from www.nlm.nih.gov/pubs/factsheets/medline.html

National Library of Medicine. (2007a). Fact sheet: Medical subject headings (MeSH). Retrieved July 15, 2007, from www.nlm.nih.gov/pubs/factsheets/mesh.html

National Library of Medicine. (2007b). Fact sheet: What is the difference between MEDLINE and PubMed? Retrieved July 15, 2007, from www.nlm.nih.gov/pubs/factsheets/dif_med_pub.html

New awards address doctoral shortage. (2004). *ASHA Leader, 9*(8), p. 21.

Newman, T. B., Browner, W. S., & Cummings, S. R. (2001). Designing studies of medical tests. In S. B. Hulley, S. R. Cummings, W. S. Browner, D. Grady, N. Hearst, & T. B. Newman (Eds.), *Designing clinical research* (2nd ed., pp. 175–194). Philadelphia: Lippincott, Williams, and Wilkins.

Newman, T. B., Browner, W. S., & Hulley, S. B. (2001). Enhancing causal inferences in observational studies. In S. B. Hulley, S. R. Cummings, W. S. Browner, D. Grady, N. Hearst, & T. B. Newman (Eds.), *Designing clinical research* (2nd ed., pp. 125–142). Philadelphia: Lippincott, Williams & Wilkins.

Newman, T. B., Browner, W. S., Cummings, S. R., & Hulley, S. B. (2001). Designing an observational study: Cross-sectional and case-control studies. In S. B. Hulley, S. R. Cummings, W. S. Browner, D. Grady, N. Hearst, & T. B. Newman (Eds.), *Designing clinical research* (2nd ed., pp. 107–124). Philadelphia: Lippincott, Williams & Wilkins.

Nunnally, J. (1978). *Psychometric theory.* New York: McGraw-Hill.

Oratio, A. (1976). A factor analytic study of criteria for evaluating student clinicians in speech pathology. *Journal of Communication Disorders, 9,* 199–210.

Palmer, C. V., Adams, S. W., Bourgeois, M., Durrant, J., & Rossi, M. (1999). Reduction in caregiver-identified problem behaviors in patients with Alzheimer's disease post-hearing-aid fitting. *Journal of Speech, Language, and Hearing Research, 43*, 312–328.

Park, R. (2003). The seven warning signs of bogus science. *The Chronicle of Higher Education, 49*(21), B20.

Pearson, K. (1937). *The grammar of science*. Dalton: London.

Peirce, C. S. (1877). The fixation of belief. *Popular Science Monthly, 12*, 1–15.

Peirce, C. S. (1878). How to make our ideas clear. *Popular Science Monthly, 12*, 286–302.

Pedhazur, E. J. (1982). *Multiple regression in behavioral research* (2nd ed.). New York: Holt, Rinehart, & Winston.

Pezzei, C., & Oratio, A. (1991). A multivariate analysis of the job satisfaction of public school speech-language pathologists. *Language, Speech and Hearing Services in Schools, 22*, 139–146.

Pezzullo, J. (2006). Web pages that perform statistical calculations. Retrieved June 5, 2007, from http://statpages.org

Pocock, S. (1983). *Clinical trials: A practical approach*. Chichester, UK: Wiley.

Pouryahoub, G., Mehrdad, R., & Mohammadi, S. (2007). Interaction of smoking and occupational noise-exposure on hearing loss. *BMC Public Health, 7*, 137.

Reefhuis, J., Honein, M. A., Whitney, C. G., Chamany, S., Mann, E. A., Biernath, K. R., Broder, K., Manning, S., Avashia, S., Victor, M., Costa, P., Devine, O., Graham, A., & Boyle, C. (2003). Risk of bacterial meningitis in children with children with cochlear implants. *New England Journal of Medicine, 349*, 435–445.

Resnik, D. (2001). *The ethics of science: An introduction*. New York: Routledge.

Roberts, R. (1989). *Serendipity: Accidental discoveries in science*. New York: John Wiley & Sons.

Robey, R. R. (1999). Speaking out: Single-subject versus randomized group design. *ASHA Leader, 41*(6), 14–15.

Robey, R. (2004, April 13). Levels of evidence. *ASHA Leader*, 5.

Robey, R., & Schultz, M. (1998). A model for conducting clinical outcome research: An adaptation of the standard protocol for use in aphasiology. *Aphasiology, 12*, 787–810.

Robey, R. R., & Dalebout, S. D. (1998). A tutorial on conducting meta-analysis of clinical outcome research. *Journal of Speech, Language, and Hearing Research, 41*, 1227–1241.

Roethlisberger, F., & Dickson, W. (1939). *Management of the worker*. Cambridge, MA: Harvard University Press.

Rosenthal, R., & Rosnow, R. (1975). *The volunteer subject*. New York: Wiley.

Rosnow, R., & Rosenthal, R. (1996). Computing contrasts, effect sizes and counternulls on other peoples published data: General procedures for research consumers. *Psychological Methods, 1*, 331–340.

Roy, N., Weinrich, B., Gray, S. D., Tanner, K., Stemple, J. C., & Sapienza, C. M. (2003). Three treatments for teachers with voice disorders: A randomized clinical trial. *Journal of Speech, Language, and Hearing Research, 46*, 670–688.

Rubens, D. D., Vohr, B. R., Tucker, R., O'Neil, C. A., & Chung, W. (2008). Newborn oto-acoustic emission hearing screening tests: Preliminary evidence for a marker of susceptibility to SIDS. *Early Human Development, 84*, 225–229.

Ryan, T. P. (1997). *Modern Regression Methods*. New York: Wiley.

Sackett, D. L., Rosenberg, W. M. C., Gray, J. A. M., Haynes, R. B., & Richardson, W. S. (1996). Evidence-based medicine: What it is and what it isn't. *British Medical Journal, 312*, 71–72.

Sackett, D. L., Straus, S. E., Richardson, W. S., Rosenberg, W. M., & Haynes, R. B. (2000). *Evidence-based medicine: How to practice and teach EBM, second edition*. New York: Churchill Livingstone.

Satake, E., Jargaroo, V., & Maxwell, D. L. (2008). *Handbook of statistical methods: Single-subject design*. San Diego, CA: Plural Publishing.

Schiavetti, N. and Metz, D. (2002). *Evaluating Research in Communicative Disorders* (4th ed.). Boston: Allyn & Bacon.

Schiavetti, N. and Metz, D. (2006). *Evaluating Research in Communication Disorders* (5th ed.). Boston: Allyn & Bacon.

Scottish Intercollegiate Network. (2008). SIGN-*50: A guideline developer's handbook*. Edinburgh, Scotland: Author.

Sedlmeier, P., & Gigerenzer, G. (1989). Do studies of statistical power have an effect on the power of studies? *Psychological Bulletin, 105*, 309–316.

Shekelle, P., Eccles, M. P., Grimshaw, J. M., & Woolf, S. H. (2001). When should clinical guidelines be updated? *British Medical Journal, 323*, 155–157.

Shiffman, R. N., Shekelle, P., Overhage, J. M., Slutsky, J., Grimshaw, J., & Deshipande, A. M. (2003). Standardized reporting of clinical practice guidelines: A proposal from the Conference on Guidelines Standardization. *Annals of Internal Medicine, 139*, 493–498.

Sidman, M. (1960). *Tactics of scientific research*. New York: Basic Books.

Siegel, S. (1956). *Nonparametric statistics for the behavioral sciences*. New York: McGraw-Hill.

Silverman, F. H. (1998). *Research design and evaluation in speech-language pathology and audiology* (4th ed.). Boston: Allyn & Bacon.

Skinner, B. (1972). Cumulative record: A selection of papers. New York: Appleton-Century-Crofts.

Sklare, D. A. (2007). NIDCD/NIH 101 for the new and budding audiologist-investigator: Challenges and opportunities. Learning module presented at Audiology NOW!, Denver, CO.

Snow, C. (1998). *The two cultures*. Cambridge, UK: Cambridge University Press.

Sprague, R. (1989). A case of whistleblowing in research. *Perspectives on the Professions, 8*, 1–3.

Stevens, S. (1946). On the theory of scales of measurement. *Science, 103*, 677–680.

Stevens, S. (1951). Mathematics, measurement and psychophysics. In S. S. Stevens (Ed.), *Handbook of Experimental Psychology*. New York: John Wiley & Sons.

Stevens, S. (1968). Measurement, statistics, and the schemapiric view. *Science, 161*, 849–856.

Streiner, D. L., & Norman, G. R. (1995). *Health measurement scales: A practical guide to their development and use*. New York: Oxford University Press.

Thompson, B. (2000). A suggested revision to the forthcoming 5th edition of the APA publication manual. Retrieved from www.coe.tamu.edu/~bthompson/apa effec.htm

Thompson, C. K. (2006). Single subject controlled experiments in aphasia: The science and the state of the science. *Journal of Communication Disorders, 39,* 266–291.

Thorndike, R. (1963). *Concepts of over- and underachievement.* New York: Teachers College Press.

Turner, R. (1998). The hearing aid expert: Audiologist, dealer, or otolaryngologist? *American Journal of Audiology, 7,* 1–16.

Tye-Murray, N. (2008). *Foundations of aural rehabilitation: Children, adults, and their family members* (3rd ed.). Clifton Park, NJ: Thomson.

Uziel, A. S., Sillon, M., Vieu, A., Artieres, F., Piron, J. P., Daures, J. P., & Mondain, M. (2007). Ten-year follow-up of a consecutive series of children with multi-channel cochlear implants. *Otology & Neurotology, 28,* 615–628.

Ventry, I. M., & Weinstein, B. E. (1982). The hearing handicap inventory for the elderly: A new tool. *Ear and Hearing, 3,* 128–134.

Walker, D. (2006). David Walker's effect size calculator. Retrieved June 9, 2008, from www.cedu.niu.edu/~walker/calculators/index.html

Wambaugh, J. (1999). Speaking out: Single-subject versus randomized group design. *ASHA Leader, 41*(6), 14–15.

Wambaugh, J., & Bain, B. (2002). Make research methods an integral part of your clinical practice. *ASHA Leader, 7*(21), 1.

Ware, J. E., Jr., & Scherbourne, C. D. (1992). The MOS 36-item short-form health survey (SF-36). I. Conceptual framework and item selection. *Medical Care, 30,* 473–483.

Warnes, E., & Allen, K. D. (2005). Biofeedback treatment of paradoxical vocal fold motion and respiratory distress in an adolescent girl. *Journal of Applied Behavior Analysis, 38,* 529–532.

Weinfurt, K. (1995). Multivariate analysis of variance. In Grimm, L. and Tarnold, P. (Eds.), *Reading and Understanding Multivariate Statistics.* Washington, DC: American Psychological Association.

Williams, A., & Fagelson, M. (2003). Fostering a community of scholars in a graduate program. *ASHA Leader, 8*(4), 4.

Windsor, J., Doyle, S. S., & Siegel, G. M. (1994). Language acquisition after mutism: A longitudinal case study of autism. *Journal of Speech, Language, and Hearing Research, 37,* 96–105.

Winer, B. (1971). *Statistical principles in experimental design.* New York: McGraw Hill.

Winer, B. J., Brown, D. R., & Michels, K. M. (1991). *Statistical principals in experimental design* (3rd ed.). New York: McGraw-Hill.

World Health Organization. (2001). *International classification of functioning, disability, and health.* Geneva: World Health Organization.

Wu, C. C., Lee, Y. C., Chen, P. J., & Hsu, C. J. (2008). Predominance of genetic diagnosis and imaging results as predictors in determining the speech perception performance outcome after cochlear implantation in children. *Archives of Pediatric Adolescent Medicine, 162,* 269–276.

Yaruss, J. S., & Quesal, R. (2006). *OASES: Overall assessment of the speaker's experience of stuttering.* Boston: Pearson.

NAME INDEX

Abbott, B., 76, 132–133, 144, 156, 162, 168–170, 178, 227
Abkarian, G. G., 277, 279, 281, 283
Abrams, H. B., 366, 368–372, 403–405
Abrams, J., 297
Ackoff, R. L., 221
Adams, S. W., 273, 274, 283, 289
Akdogan, V., 331
Akkuzu, B., 331
Alexander, G. C., 330, 416
Allen, K. D., 279, 282
Altman, D. G., 163, 372, 384–387
Anastasi, A., 115
Anderson, G. L., 320, 321
Anderson, T. W., 255
Aragaki, A., 320, 321
Artieres, F., 368
Avashia, S., 328
Aydin, E., 331

Bachrach, A., 78
Bain, B., 37
Barron, H. V., 316–318
Bartholomew, D. J., 255
Batavia, M., 178
Beattie, R. C., 333
Beck, L. B., 325, 372
Becker, L., 182, 183, 185
Becker, M., 199
Beecher, H., 122
Belknap, H., 273, 275, 276, 279
Benninger, M. S., 344, 368
Ben-Shlomo, Y., 311–312
Bentler, R. A., 323–324
Beresford, S. A., 320, 321
Berra, Y., 243
Biernath, K. R., 328
Bigelow, J., 267
Billings, J., 305
Bland, J. M., 163
Blodgett, J., 172
Bolton, P., 62
Bonte, F. J., 374
Bordens, K., 76, 132–133, 144, 156, 162, 168–170, 178, 227
Borges, J. L., 339
Bossuyt, P. M., 333–334, 375, 392–396

Bourgeois, M., 273, 274, 283, 289
Box, G. E. P., 190
Boyle, C. M., 328, 344
Boysen, A. E., 325, 372
Bradbury, R., 139
Bratt, G. W., 325, 372
Breuning, S., 60, 61
Breyer, S. G., 71
Brockman, J., 67
Broder, K., 328
Brower, C., 425
Brown, B., 179
Brown, D. R., 190
Brown, P., 305
Browner, W. S., 323, 324, 328–330, 332–334, 336, 373–375, 387–392
Bruning, J., 157, 225
Bruns, D. E., 333–334, 375, 392–396
Bryan, W. W., 374
Brzyski, R., 320, 321
Buchner, A., 179

Campbell, D. T., 107, 108, 114, 135, 137, 327, 350
Campbell, E., 367
Camus, A., 150
Canalis, R., 325, 372
Carey, J., 48
Carlyle, T., 189
Carrier, R., 51, 52
Carter, F. A., 221, 243
Cartmill, M., 1
Casby, M. W., 272–273
Chalmers, A., 48
Chamany, S., 328
Chase, L., 179
Chen, P. J., 373–374
Chisolm, T. H., 366, 368, 369–372, 371, 403–405
Chlebowski, R. T., 320,321
Chmiel, R., 316–317
Chung, W., 375
Churchill, W., 221, 425
Clark, D., 75–76
Clarke, C. E., 311–312
Clay, H., 165
Cline, D., 75–76
Clinton, W. J., 63
Cochrane, C., 297

Cohen, J., 179, 180, 182, 185–186
Connell, P. J., 287
Cooley, W. W., 255
Coolidge, C., 463
Cooper, E., 172
Copernicus, N., 76
Costa, P., 328
Cox, R., 416
Cox, R. M., 303–304, 306, 308, 330, 340, 366, 368, 377, 378, 402, 404–405, 416, 421–424
Cruise, T., 73, 74
Cummings, S. R., 319, 320, 323, 324, 327–330, 332–334, 336, 373–375, 387–392, 465, 476–477, 479, 480

Dalebout, S. D., 310
Damrose, J. F., 374
Dangerfield, R., 4
Danhauer, J. L., 326, 333, 369–372, 403–405
Darsee, J., 59–60
Daures, J. P., 368
Dawson, C., 59
Deane, K. H. O., 311–312
De Mets, D. L., 367
Demorest, M., 260–261, 345
Deng, H., 179
DeRuyter, F. D., 289
Deshipande, A. M., 406–408
De Vet, H. C. W., 333–334, 375, 392–396
Devine, O., 328
DeVos, R. M., 463
Devous, M. D., Sr., 374
Diamond, W. J., 100
Dickson, W., 120
Dillon, H., 344, 401, 416
Disney, W., 221
Disraeli, B., 165
Dixon, W. J., 190
Dobie, R. A., 325, 372
Dollaghan, C. A., 303, 336, 349, 376
Donahue, A., 325, 372
Dooley, J., 61
Doyle, A. C., 189
Doyle, S. S., 330
Draper, S., 120

Drucker, P., 11
Duarte-Silva, A., 262
Duffy, R. J., 262
Dupont, W. D., 179
Durrant, J., 273, 274, 283, 289
Dworkin, J. P., 277, 279, 281, 283

Easy, A., 310
Eccles, M. P., 409–411
Eddy, D. M., 297
Edgerton, B. A., 333
Einstein, A., 76, 139, 339
Elsenberg, L. S., 328
Emerson, R. W., 267
Erdfelder, E., 179
Erdman, S., 260–261, 345

Fagelson, M., 37
Farthing, M., 60
Faul, F., 179
Fausti, S. A., 325, 372
Ferguson, G. A., 163–164
Feynman, R., 425
Field, M. J., 406
Fink, N. E., 328
Firszt, J. B., 469
Fisher, K. V., 271
Fisher, R., 161
Fisher, R. A., 201
Flamme, G. A., 323–324
Flanagan, D., 129, 130
Fleckenstein, J. L., 374
Florin, E., 316–317
Flower, R., 7
Foster, J., 150
Fowler, G., 425
Frattali, C. M., 288–289, 328
Friedman, L. M., 367
Fromm, D. S., 289
Furberg, C. D., 367

Garrett, Z., 309, 315
Gass, M., 320, 321
Gatsonis, C. A., 333–334, 375, 392–396
Gebski, V., 179
Gibbons, J. D., 207
Gibbs, A., 48
Gigerenzer, G., 179
Gill, B., 365
Ginis, J., 401, 416
Giolas, T. G., 310
Gjertson, D., 48

SUBJECT INDEX

511